Integrative
Control
Functions of
the **BRAIN**
Vol. I

Integrative
Control
Functions of
the BRAIN
Vol. I

QP376
I 517
v.1
1978

1978

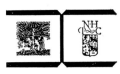

KODANSHA LTD.   **ELSEVIER/NORTH-HOLLAND BIOMEDICAL PRESS**
TOKYO   AMSTERDAM · NEW YORK · OXFORD

353526

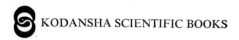 KODANSHA SCIENTIFIC BOOKS

ISBN 0444-80101-4 (series)

Library of Congress Cataloging in Publication Data

Main entry under title:

Integrative control functions of the brain.

    Includes index.
    1. Brain. 2. Biological control systems.
3. Neural circuitry. 4. Sensory-motor integration.
I. Ito, Masao, 1928-
QP376.I517   591.1'88   78-31615
ISBN 0-444-80115-4 (v. 1)

Copublished by
KODANSHA LTD.
12–21 Otowa 2-chome. Bunkyo-ku, Tokyo 112, Japan
and
ELSEVIER/NORTH-HOLLAND BIOMEDICAL PRESS
335 Jan van Galenstraat, P.O. Box 211,
Amsterdam, The Netherlands
Distributors for the United States and Canada:
ELSEVIER NORTH-HOLLAND INC.
52, Vanderbilt Avenue, New York,
N. Y. 10017, U.S.A.

PRINTED IN JAPAN

PREFACE

Due to the rapid growth of recent developments in brain research, the future outlook in this endeavor is extremely promising as well as exciting. As emphasized on many occasions, brain research is multilateral, and so it requires the close cooperation of several diverse disciplines. The decision by the Japanese Ministry of Education, Science and Culture to fund the special grant-in-aid project "Integrative Control Functions of the Brain", was a fortunate and timely one, indeed. Supporting more than a hundred neuroscientists organized into ten teams, the three-year project began in April of 1977. Three similar projects in the past, "Brain" (1964–67), "Brain Disorders" (1967–73), and "Neurosciences" (1973–76) have contributed greatly to the progress of brain research in Japan.

The current project, "Integrative Control Functions of the Brain", focuses on the elucidation of several aspects of the brain in connection with the diverse functional subsystems in the living body, such as sensation, motor control, respiratory and cardiovascular functions, digestion, intrinsic behavior, sleep-wakefulness control, neuroendocrine regulation, memory, and learning. The actual work is being carried out in three steps. The first step is to analyze the structure of the neuronal circuitry essential for each subsystem; secondly, to study the dynamic characteristics of performance of the neuronal circuitry; and finally, to reveal the plasticity of the neuronal circuitry and the adaptability of its dynamics. Thus, the project requires the combined efforts of investigators in a wide range of disciplines.

Besides the activity in the individual teams, workshops and symposia were held before and during the course of the project to organize and synthesize the aims and progress of the group as a whole. In the summer of 1977, a week-long workshop was held at Kiryu in order to discuss the various strategies in brain research, and in the summer of 1978, another workshop at Tateyama was devoted to exploration of methods of conceptualization in brain research. As a prelude to the project, a symposium was held in Tokyo in the winter of 1976 on "Neuronal Control of the Cardiovascular System" and "Central Neuronal Networks". In the winter of 1977, another symposium was held in Tokyo on the "Concept of Paraneurons", together with a number of lectures on topics ranging from phylogenetical development of the brain to recent developments in psychophysics.

The progress and results of these research activities, a part of which are presented here, will comprise a total of three volumes. In each volume, organized into eight sections, the ten teams will present their research reports and review articles. The team leaders act as the Section Editors, in addition to the overall responsibilities given to the four members of the Editorial Board.

I sincerely hope that these volumes will contribute significantly not only to national, but also international communication and cooperation so greatly needed for the accomplishment of our goals.

September, 1978

MASAO ITO
Editor-in-Chief

CONTENTS

Preface v

PART I: ELEMENTARY PROCESS OF THE NERVOUS SYSTEM

Editor's Commentary (M. Otsuka) 3
Current Review
    Properties of Na and Ca channels in the tunicate egg cell membrane (K. Takahashi)............5

Short Papers

    Three dimensional observations of neurons and glia cells by means of the high voltage
        electron microscopy (K. Hama and T. Kosaka).......................................26
    Kinetics of the inhibitory postsynaptic current in crayfish muscle (K. Onodera and A.
        Takeuchi)..30
    Dopamine release in reconstituted synapses from rat cerebrum (M. Takeda, R. Tanaka and
        K. Konno)..32
    Acetylcholine synthesis in a stretch receptor cell of crayfish *in vivo* (H. Koike and K. Tsuda) 36
    Cholinergic agents and synaptic transmissions in the striatum (M. Takagi and C. Yamamoto).....38
    Development of acetylcholine sensitivity in cultured embryonic chick atrium (K. Obata and
        M. Oide)...40
    The GABA receptor and GABA-induced anion permeability in mammalian primary afferent
        neurons (S. Nishi and H. Higashi)...42
    Calcium measurement in axons with a fluorescent probe (K. Aizawa and S. Iwasaki) 44
    A study of the mechanism of synaptogenesis in the inner ear and cerebellar cortex of chick
        embryo through chronic treatment and immunocyochemistry with β-bungarotoxin (N.
        Hirokawa and J. Nakai)..48
    Interpeduncular nucleus: multiple innervation by fibers of the fasciculus retroflexus Meynerti
        (K. Kataoka, K. Sunayashiki, C. Nakata, H. Yoshimi, S. Matsukura and Y. Imura) 51
    Fluorographic and quantitative analyses of slowly migrating axonal polypeptides in bifurcat-
        ing axons (M. Kurokawa. Y. Komiya and H. Mori)....................................53
    Scanning electron microscopic studies on developing brain of mouse and man (S. Fujita and
        S. Fushiki) 55
    A search for neurogenetic genes among behaivora' and lethal mutations in *Drosophila me-*
        lanogaster (Y. Hotta) 58

PART II: NEURAL MECHANISMS OF SENSATION AND ITS DISORDERS

Editor's Commentary (K. Tasaki) 63
Current Review
    Interneuronal connectivity in cat visual cortex: studies by cross-correlation analysis of the
        responses of two simultaneously recorded neurons (K. Toyama) 65
    Neuronal mechanisms of active and passive touch (Y. Iwamura) 73

Short Papers

    Rod and cone convergence to carp bipolar cells (A. Kaneko, M. Tachibana and E. V. Fa-
        miglietti, Jr.) 82
    Some relations between receptive-field properties and afferent conduction velocities in relay
        cells of the rat lateral geniculate nucleus (Y. Fukuda, I. Sumitomo, M. Sugitani and K.
        Iwama) 85
    Unitary responses in the nucleus centralis lateralis toelectrical stimulation of the visual path-
        ways in chloralose-anesthetized cat (T. Ogawa and T. Takimori) 87

Vestibular and visual influences on superior colliculus neurons in the cat (M. Maeda, T. Shibazaki and K. Yoshida) 90

Origin of the mossy fiber projection to the cerebellar flocculus from the optic nerves in rabbits (K. Maekawa and T. Takeda) 93

High amplitude photic driving evoked by red-flicker and flickering-pattern (T. Takahashi and T. Okuma)...96

Morphology of the eye and brain in anophthalmic rats (K. Otani, K. Kobayashi and G. Kato) 100

How are optic impulses transfered to the cerebellum? (K. Kawamura) 102

Role of the hair cell-afferent fiver synapse in the coding of afferent impulses (T. Furukawa)....104

An electron microscopic study of spinothalamic fibers which end at the centrolateral nucleus neurons sending their axons to the motor cortex in the cat and monkey: the use of horseradish peroxidase as a neuronal marker for electron microscopy (N. Mizuno, A. Konishi, K. Itoh and S. Nomura) 106

Somatotopic trigeminal projection onto the caudal medulla oblongata. Part I. Tactile representation within the pars magnocellularis of the trigeminal subnucleus caudalis (T. Yokota, N. Nishikawa and Y. Nishikawa) 109

Central monoaminergic neurons in sensory transmission—An electrophysiological study— (S. Takaori, M. Sasa, Y. Chikamori and I. Matsuoka) 112

Selective action of enkephalins on lamina V neurons of the spinal dorsal horn: a microelectrophoretic study (M. Satoh, S. Kawajiri, M. Yamamoto and H. Takagi) 114

Morphology of mitral cell dendrites in the rabbit olfactory bulb: intracellular Procion Yellow injection (K. Mori, M. Satou, and S. F. Takagi) 117

Neurons in the solitary tract—parabrachial nucleus pathway (H. Ogawa, T. Akagi, H. Ito and M. Sato) 120

Electrophysiological studies of gustation in the honeybee (*Apis mellifica* L.) (K. Aoki and M. Kuwabara)..122

The site of origin of the abortive spikes in terminals of the frog muscle spindle afferent nerve (F. Ito and Y. Komatsu) 124

Statocyst-driven interneurons in crayfish circumesophageal commissure (M. Hisada and M. Takahata) 126

Morphological study of a small nucleus in the posterolateral hypothalamus of the cat (M. Fujii, T. Kusama, N. Yoshii and T. Mizokami) 128

Brain-stem evoked potentials elicited by electrical stimulation of the vestibular and cochlear nerves: an animal experiment (N. Furuya, A. Saito, M. Ishikawa and J. Suzuki) 130

PART III: MOTOR CONTROL AND ITS DISORDERS

Editor's Commentary (H. Shimazu and M. Yoshida)..135

Current Review

Intraspinal multiple projections of single corticospinal neurons in the cat and monkey (Y. Shinoda) 137

Anatomy and physiology of the thalamic nucleus ventralis intermedius (C. Ohye) 152

Short Papers

The mode of tapering and distribution of nodes of Ranvier in group Ia fiber collaterals in the cat spinal cord (T. Hongo, N. Ishizuka, H. Mannen and S. Sasaki)........................164

Antagonist inhibition in sequential voluntary movements of ankle extension and flexion in man (R. Tanaka) 168

Changes in monosynaptic EPSPs of quadriceps motoneurons in monkeys with the spinal cord chronically hemisected at the thoracic level (M. Aoki and S. Mori) 170

Statistical analysis of 'locked' motor unit spikes in the stretch reflex (S. Homma and Y. Nakajima) 172

Neuronal activity in cortical supplementary motor area responding to motor instructions
(J. Tanji) 174
Compensatory activities of pyramidal tract neurons after sudden target position shifts in
awake monkeys (K. Matsunami, S. Funahashi and K. Kubota) 177
Corticospinal collateral actions on pontine nuclei of the cat (T. Oshima) 180
Automatic and reliable discrimination between simple and complex spikes of a cerebellar
Purkinje cell (N. Mano and K. Yamamoto) 182
Cerebrocerebellar connections through the parvocellular part of the red nucleus (H. Oka and
K. Jinnai) 184
Neuronal circuits of cerebro-cerebellar interactions (K. Sasaki, K. Jinnai and H. Gemba) 187
The distribution of cerebellar projection neurons in the spinal cord of the cat, as studied by
retrograde transport of horseradish peroxidase (M. Matsushita, Y. Hosoya and M. Ikeda)...190
Electrophysiological analysis of neuronal circuit in the cerebellar cortex of rolling mouse
Nagoya (T. Ohno and S. Sasaki)..194
Antidromic responses of thalamic VL neurons to cortical stimulation in cats (M. Uno, N.
Ozawa and K. Yamamoto) 196
Clinicophysiological studies of ocular movement in Parkinson's disease (H. Shibasaki and
S. Tsuji) 199
Cerebellar modification of involuntary movements (H. Narabayashi) 202
EMG study of human reflex blinking by air puff stimulation (M. Hiraoka and M. Shima-
mura) 205
A brain-stem mechanism responsible for cortical control of trigeminal motoneurons (Y.
Nakamura and S. Nozaki) 207
Lower brain-stem "locomotor region" in the mesencephalic cat (S. Mori, H. Nishimura, C.
Kurakami, T. Yamamura and M. Aoki) 209
Differential effects on locomotor movements of fore- and hindlimbs of the decerebrate cat
induced by partial cooling of cerebellar intermediate and vermian cortices (M. Udo and
K. Matsukawa)...212

PART IV: CENTRAL NERVOUS SYSTEM CONTROL OF CARDIOVASCULAR AND RESPIRATORY FUNCTIONS

Editor's Commentary (H. Irisawa) 217

Current Review

Regional differentiation of sympathetic efferents (M. Iriki and E. Simon)....................221

Short Papers

Effect of carotid sinus stimulation on the excitation of afferent cardiac sympathetic fibers
during myocardial ischemia (Y. Uchida) 239
Depressor and pressor responses produced by muscular thin-fiber afferents (T. Kumazawa,
K. Mizumura, E. Tadaki and K. Kim) 242
Origin of the cardio-inhibitory motoneurons in the medulla of the cat (M. Miura and T.
Kitamura) 244
Effects of cord section on blood pressure in different experimental hypertensive rats (J.
Iriuchijima and Y. Numao) 247
Inhibition of renal sympathetic discharge during trigeminal depressor response (N. Terui,
M. Kumada and D. J. Reis) 249
Role of the central monoaminergic system in the control of arterial blood pressure in the rat
(M. Ozaki, K. Sugawara Y. Fujita and N. Takami) 252
Bulbar neural mechanisms originating intrinsic respiratory rhythms in the central respira-
tory mechanisms (T. Hukuhara, S. Kageyama, Y. Kiguchi, K. Goto, Y. Nishikawa and
K. Takano) 254
Effects of picrotoxin on vagal respiratory inhibition in the rabbit (K. Shimada, Y. Kitada
and Y. Yamada)...257

A quantitative evaluation of hypoxic drive in ventilation from the peripheral chemoreceptors (Y. Honda, N. Hata, Y. Sakakibara and S. Akiyama) 260

PART V: NEURAL CONTROL OF THE DIGESTIVE SYSTEM

Editor's Commentary (Y. Matsuo) 265

Current Review

Central nervous regulation of motility of alimentary canals in the dog (T. Semba and K. Fujii) 267

Short Papers

Rhythmic fluctuations of postsynaptic potentials recorded in masseteric neurons during mastication (T. Sumi) 281
Role of the myenteric plexus in the control of defecation in the guinea pig (S. Nakayama, T. Yamasato, M. Mizutani, T. Neya and N. Takaki) 283
Reflex facilitation and inhibition of gastric motility from various skin areas in rats (H. Kamatani, A. Sato, Y. Sato and K. Ueki) 285
Interdigestive motor activity and gut polypeptides (Z. Itoh, S. Takeuchi and I. Aizawa).........288
Central noradrenergic neuron system: its relation to gastric mucosal blood flow and acid secretion in rats (Y. Osumi, Y. Nagasaka and M. Fujiwara) 290
Secretory responses to stimulation of the vagus nerve and to acetylcholine in rat pancreas perfused *in situ* (T. Kanno, A. Saito and Y. Habara) 292
Inhibition of gastric acid secretion of somatostatin, secretin and CCK-PZ (Y. Matsuo and A. Seki) 294
Effect of intraluminally administered lidocaine upon the pancreozymin—producing endocrine cells of the canine duodenum (T. Fujita, Y. Matsunari, S. Muraki, K. Sato and K. Shimoji) 296
The effects of glucose, mannose and 2-deoxyglucose on the efferent discharge rate of the hepatic nerve in the rabbit (A. Niijima) 298
Central cholinergic regulation of hepatic enzymes (T. Shimazu, M. Ozawa. K. Ishikawa and H. Matsushita) 301

PART VI: NEUROENDOCRINE CONTROL MECHANISMS

Editor's Commentary (K. Yagi) 307

Current Review

Membrane electrical properties of anterior pituitary cells and their relation to hormone secretion (S. Ozawa) 311

Short Papers

Ultrastructural changes of stellate cells in rabbit anterior pituitary gland under various endocrine conditions (T. Ban and Y. Shiotani) 325
Effect of sex steroid hormones on rat anterior pituitary LH-RH receptor (M. Taga, H. Minaguchi, T. Kigawa and S. Sakamoto) 327
Function of tanycytes in the hypothalamic median eminence (H. Kobayashi, M. Nozaki and H. Uemura) 329
Constant illumination blocks the effects of infundibulo-preoptic pathways in female rats (Y. Sawaki and K. Yagi) 331
Projection from the arcuate nucleus to the preoptic areas revealed by retrograde transport of horseradish peroxidase (Y. Ibata, H. Kinoshita, H. Kimura, K. Watanabe, Y. Nojyo and H. Fujisawa) 333
Vasopressin release from guinea-pig hypothalamo-neurohypophysial system in organ culture (S. Yoshida, S. Ishikawa and T. Saito) 336

Neural inputs from the limbric structure to preoptic area and the preovulatory release of gonadotrophin in rats (M. Kawakami and F. Kimura)....................................338
Indoleamine 2,3-dioxygenase in the brain (O. Hayaishi, M. Fujiwara, M. Shibata, Y. Watanabe, T. Nukiwa, F. Hirata and N. Mizuno) 341
Morphological studies on the circadian cycle of the pineal gland of the rat (W. Mori, K. Kurumado and A. Hasegawa)...343
Control of the circadian rhythm of serotonin N-acetyltransferase activity in the pineal gland of chicken (T. Deguchi) 345

PART VII: NEURAL MECHANISMS OF INTRINSIC BEHAVIOR; SLEEP-WAKEFULNESS CONTROL

Editor's Commentary (Y. Oomura and S. Torii) 351

Current Review

Neuroendocrine regulation and sexual differentiation of lordosis behavior in rats (Y. Arai, K. Yamanouchi and A. Matsumoto) 355

Short Papers

Effect of sequential destruction of amygdala and septum on hypothalamic rage in cats (H. Maeda and H. Nakao) 370
Functional relationship between the frontal cortex and lateral hypothalamus (Y. Oomura, T. Ono, M. Ohta, N. Shimizu, H. Kita and S. Ishibashi) 373
Lateral hypothalamus—motor cortex relations in the chronic monkey (T. Ono, Y. Oomura, H. Nishino, M. Ohta, K. Sasaki, N. Shimizu and H. Kita) 376
Semi-automatic measurements of neuronal processes by a computer controlled optical microscope (M. Nakamura, K. Taniguchi, K. Tsuchida, Y. Oomura and N. Shimizu) 379
Electrophysiological studies on the depolarization shift of hippocampal pyramidal cells *in vitro* (N. Hori and N. Katsuda)...381
The laminated organization of the cytoarchitecture of the dog brain in relation to domestication (H. Masai, K. Takatsuji and Y. Sato) 384
Sleep-related growth hormone secretion in dogs after 8-hr forced wakefulness (Y. Takahashi, S. Ebihara, Y. Nakamura and K. Takahashi)..389
Sleep-pormoting fractions obtained from the brain-stem of sleep-deprived rats (K. Uchizono, A. Higashi, M. Iriki, H. Nagasaki, M. Ishikawa, Y. Komoda, S. Inoue and K. Honda) 392
The circadian rhythm of tryptophan hydroxylase in rat pineal gland (M. Toru, S. Watanabe, H. Shibuya and Y. Shimazono) 397
Nervous and humoral factors in sleep mechanisms (J. Matsumoto, Y. Morita, A. Sano, N. Ishikawa, H. Seno and E. Uezu) 400

PART VIII: BRAIN MECHANISMS FOR LEARNING AND MEMORY

Editor's Commentary (M. Ito)..405

Current Review

Neuron activity in the dorsolateral prefrontal cortex of the monkey and initiation of behavior(K. Kubota) 407
The visual learning area in the inferotemporal cortex in monkeys(E. Iwai) 419

Short Papers

Effect of destruction of microtubules upon the memory function of mice (T. H. Murakami) ...428
Neurochemical correlates of learning disability in experimental phenylketonuric rats and postnatal undernourished rats (Y. Tsukada and S. Kohsaka) 431

A neurochemical analysis of hemispherectomized rats (Y. Komai, Y. Kobayashi, Y. Nagano, S. Araki, M. Okuda and M. Satake) 434

Reorganization of the cerebello-cerebral response following hemicerebellectomy or cerebral cortical ablation in kittens (S. Kawaguchi, T. Yamamoto and A. Samejima) 436

Control of the cerebellar reverberatory activities by local cooling of the cerebellar peduncles (N. Tsukahara, T. Bando, F. Murakami and N. Ozawa) 439

Neuronal correlates of timing behavior in the monkey (H. Niki and M. Watanabe)..........441

Change in visual responsiveness of prefrontal cortical neurons related to gazing behavior (H. Suzuki and M. Azuma) 443

A hemispheric asymmetry of performance of a visual conditional discrimination task in split-brain monkeys (K. Murofushi) 445

Analysis of memory disturbance using speech tests in human cerebral disorders (K. Ueki and K. Konno) 448

Mathematical theory of self-organizing nerve cells (S. Amari) 450

Index 453

PART I

ELEMENTARY PROCESS OF THE NERVOUS SYSTEM

MASANORI OTSUKA

*Department of Pharmacology, Faculty of Medicine, Tokyo Medical and Dental University,
Bunkyo-ku, Tokyo 113, Japan*

The papers in Part I deal with the elementary processes of nervous functions. Most of them are concerned with synapses, transmitters, and receptors, and several others deal with developmental aspects. These studies were carried out at the cellular or molecular level, and some of them might at first sight appear still remote from the ultimate understanding of the brain. Yet it is becoming more and more certain that the higher functions of the central nervous system, such as perception, will eventually be understood in cellular and molecular terms.

Neuronal membranes are diverse. Some are sensitive to certain special chemicals, and others are permeable to particular ions in specifically voltage- and/or time-dependent manners. As shown by the studies of Takahashi and his colleagues, it is remarkable that the egg membrane is already endowed with sodium and calcium channels. Furthermore, with ingenious techniques it is possible to perfuse these egg cells intracellularly. These studies showed that the functions of the ion channels are critically regulated by intracellular calcium and anions, and this may give a hint to how the excitable membrane differentiates during development to eventually display either sodium or calcium spike. An interesting merit of egg membrane is that a relatively large amount of homogeneous material can be obtained, and this might be useful for isolation and chemical characterization of ion channel molecules.

The pursuit of neurotransmitters has attracted many neuroscientists for more than seventy years. Particularly in the central nervous system an increasing number of substances are being proposed as transmitter candidates. Some ten years ago, people tended to believe that the number of existing neurotransmitters is probably less than ten. Nowadays, it is perhaps more general to suppose that the number is perhaps much larger. It may even be possible that the concept of neurotransmitters will be broadened. The study of Kataoka and his colleagues suggests that β-endorphin, a peptide of relatively large molecular weight, plays a functional role in a particular pathway of the central nervous system. When the number of transmitters increases one might feel that the discovery of a new transmitter is less exciting. What is the rationale of continuing the pursuit of new transmitters? I think, however, one may imagine that the discovery of certain transmitters in the future might suddenly give us a breakthrough for the solution of some major brain functions or diseases, such as sleep, schizophrenia, etc. One of the merits of understanding the chemical mechanisms of nervous functions rather than of clarifying the wiring of neuronal pathways is that the former approach might produce means for exogenously manipulating the brain functions.

The study of the central nervous sytem is usually much more difficult than that of the peripheral nervous system. Some major obstacles can be removed when the studies are performed *in vitro* using the slice preparation as introduced by Yamamoto and his colleagues. In the near future it may become possible to study central synapses under visualization of pre- and postsynaptic elements with electrical recordings therefrom, just as it is possible now in peripheral synapses.

In addition, further improvement of cell culture techniques of central neurons will be very important.

Whenever we see the detailed whole image of a single neuron with its long luxuriant dendritic trees together with innumerable spines, as described by Hama and Kosaka using a high-voltage electron microscope, we are led to contemplate how a neuron can efficiently integrate the full information conveyed onto these dendrites. It is probably far too inefficient if the synaptic potential occurring at the peripheral ends of dendrites is propagated to the soma by a simple electrotonic mechanism. On the other hand, the usual all-or-nothing type action potential along the dendrite may not be the best way to transmit all the finely graded inputs to the cell soma, either.

Hotta and his colleagues attempt the genetic dissection of the *Drosophila* nervous system using mosaics and lethal gene techniques. As in higher animals, the number of synapses in the *Drosophila* central nervous system is larger by several orders of magnitude than the number of genes which take care of the development of the nervous system. How these genes can program the precise formation of a vast number of neuronal connections is one of the most attractive targets in neuroscience. Studies of the nervous system in this genetically most thoroughly clarified animal may give useful information for this purpose.

Many studies described in Part I again emphasize the importance of multidisciplinary approaches in the neurosciences, using electrophysiological, chemical, histological, genetic, and other techniques focused on single targets.

Properties of Na and Ca channels in the tunicate egg cell membrane

KUNITARO TAKAHASHI

Department of Neurophysiology, Institute of Brain Research, Faculty of Medicine, University of Tokyo, Bunkyo-ku, Tokyo 113, Japan

Modern ionic theory of the excitable membrane accounts for action potentials in terms of selective permeability to the major cations, Na and K[23]. During the past fifteen years, several types of excitable membrane have been reported to be able to elicit action potentials in the presence of Ca ions without Na ions[9,12,17,27,30,34,60]. The existence of both Na and Ca components in an action potential has been demonstrated in various types of excitable cells[12,16,27,30]. These components have been identified not only by their different ionic dependences but also by the differential effects of pharmacological agents such as tetrodotoxin and transition metal ions.

It has been reported that the Na- and Ca-dependent action potential is also evoked in the tunicate egg membrane[36,37] and that two components of the transient inward current, major and minor ones, were found under voltage-clamp conditions[44]. The major component was identified as Na current and the minor one as Ca current[45]. A series of experiments on tunicate egg and embryo in our laboratory has suggested the importance of quantitative changes in the relative amounts of Na, Ca and K channels rather than qualitative alterations of the properties of these channels during embryonic development. In particular, the ion channels in the egg membrane were found to be identical with those of other differentiated excitable membranes, and Na and Ca channels in the tunicate egg membrane had discrete critical membrane potentials and different kinetic properties[44,45]. This was of great advantage in identifying the ionic currents through the respective channels. Thus, studies on the egg cell membrane provide a good opportunity to compare the properties of two types of ionic current which may enter the "Na" and "Ca" channels separately in the same cell membrane under voltage-clamp conditions.

Major and minor components of the transient inward current in the tunicate egg membrane

On the removal of Na ions in the external solution by replacement with either choline or Tris ions, most of the inward current found in standard artificial sea water disappeared in the tunicate egg membrane, as shown in Fig. 1A. In addition to abolition of the inward current a reverse transient outward current was observed above -15 mV as shown in 10 Ca choline ASW (Fig. 1A). At the $+8$ mV level, the fast and major component of the inward current was clearly reversed to an outward current (arrow), but the slow and minor component which had been seen in the falling phase of the major component in standard ASW remained unchanged in its polarity and amount even after the removal of Na ions. It can be concluded that the major component was Na current and the reversed outward transient current was probably the outward flux of Na ions in the absence of external Na ions.

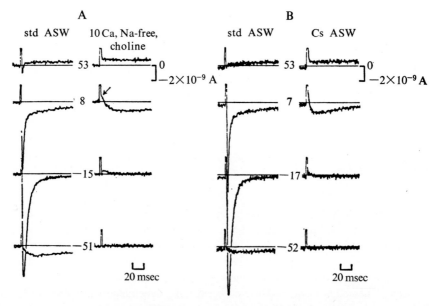

Fig. 1.   A: the effect of Na removal from the external solution upon the transient inward   currents under voltage-clamp conditions. The temperature of the egg was 12°C. The left-hand traces were obtained in standard (std) ASW while the right-hand traces were obtained in choline ASW without Na. Each set of traces was observed at the same potential level as indicated in mV in the middle of two traces in Fig. 1A and 1B. The arrow indicates the reversed major component of the transient inward currents. B: the effects of the replacement of Na in standard ASW with Cs upon the major component of the inward current. 14.5°C. The left-hand traces were obtained in standard ASW while the right-hand traces were obtained in Cs ASW. (From Okamoto, H., Takahashi, K., and Yoshii, M., *J. Physiol.*, 254 (1976) 607–638.)

The minor component of the inward current was activated at around −10 mV in standard ASW, the critical level being far more positive than the value of −55 mV of the major component or Na current. When the test pulse was preceded by a prepulse to −15 mV of 400 msec duration, the major component which would have been evoked by the test pulse alone was completely abolished, while the minor and slow component remained[44]. It was noted that the *V-I* relation at the peak of the minor component isolated with the prepulse in standard ASW was exactly the same as that obtained in Na-free choline ASW. The peak current of the minor component was about 5% of that of the major one and its level of activation was at least 40 mV more positive than that of the major one.

Effects of replacement of Na with Li or other alkaline cations and tetrodotoxin upon the major component

As shown in Fig. 2B, the replacement of external Na with Li ions did not affect the transient inward current significantly. This is in agreement with the fact that Li can be substituted for Na of the inward current in other excitable membranes[25,46]. The *V-I* relation at the peak of the major component in Li ASW was similar to that in standard or Na ASW (Fig. 2A). However, a small positive shift of the reversal potential was noted. Other alkaline cations, Cs, Rb and K, were also used to replace Na in ASW. In Cs ASW the major component was mostly reversed in polarity (Fig. 1B), as in Na-free choline ASW (Fig. 1A), though a residual inward

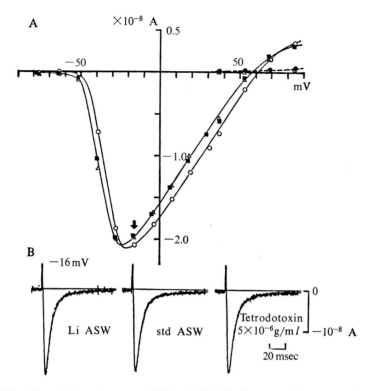

Fig. 2. The effects of the replacement of Na in ASW with the same molar concentration of Li and of the addition of tetrodotoxin (5×10^{-6} g/ml) to standard ASW upon the major component of the inward current at -16 mV (B: see arrow in A) together with the *I-V* relations at the peak of the inward current (continuous line) and at the steady state (interrupted line (A). ■, □, Standard ASW; △, standard ASW with tetrodotoxin 5×10^{-6} g/ml; ○, ●, Li ASW. Temp. 12.5°C. (From Okamoto, H., Takahashi, K., and Yoshii, M., *J. Physiol.*, (1976) 607–638.)

current was seen at about -40 mV, indicating slight permeability to Cs. In K and Rb ASW, small transient inward currents were visible around the potential range in which the major component was expected to be dominant. The permeability sequence of the egg Na channel was in the order Li>Na>K>Rb>Cs. An estimate of the permeability ratio of the egg Na channels among alkaline cations was obtained from the apparent shifts of the reversal potential of the major component in various ASWs from that in standard or Na ASW. The resulting values, 1:0.088: 0.045:0.027 for Na:K:Rb:Cs, coincided well with those for squid axons or myelinated fibers[7,11, 21,38].

The specific Na channel inhibitor tetrodotoxin[39,40] had no effect on this Na inward current of the tunicate egg even at the high concentration of 1.6×10^{-5} M. The *I-V* relations at the peak of Na current were still the same in the presence of tetrodotoxin.

Identification of the minor current as Ca current

The significant difference between the critical membrane potentials of the two components of the inward current allowed us to record the minor component isolated from the major one by means of a conditioning depolarization above -30 mV. The isolated minor component was greatly enhanced by an increase of Ca concentration in ASW, as shown in a series of current traces on the left-hand side of Fig. 3A.

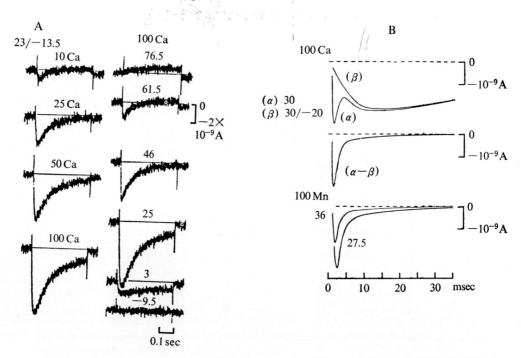

Fig. 3.   Dependency of the minor component upon the external Ca concentration and upon the membrane potential. A, left-hand side: the Ca concentration was raised from 10 to 100 mM by replacing NaCl in ASW with $CaCl_2$ isotonically; right-hand side: the minor component in 100 Ca ASW at various membrane potential levels. The conditioning depolarization was -13.5 mV for the currents in both cases. 13.5°C. This identifies the egg Ca current. B, the abolition of Ca current by the replacement of Ca with Mn^{2+} in 100 Ca ASW (PIPES buffer, pH 7.0). For the significance of (α), (β) and $(\alpha-\beta)$, see the text. 12°C. The figures on the current traces indicate the potential levels of the test voltage pulses in mV and the denominators of the fractional numbers indicate those of the conditioning depolarization. The holding potential was -90 mV in this and succeeding figures unless otherwise noted (From Okamoto, H., Takahashi, K., and Yoshii, M., *J. Physiol.*, 255 (1976) 527–561).

On replacement of 100 mM Ca with $10Mn^{2+}$, the minor component was lost, while the major component remained almost intact (Fig. 3B, 100 Mn). Although the replacement of Ca with Mg abolished the minor component as well, it induced a significant negative shift of more than 7 mV in the critical membrane potential of Na current and the Na current was frequently reduced irreversibly. On the other hand, Mn^{2+} ions maintained the critical membrane potential at almost the same level and Na current was essentially intact during and after the use of Ca-free Mn^{2+} ASW, as reported in squid axons[61]. Fig. 3B shows the value of (α) traced from the current record obtained by a voltage pulse to 30 mV in 100 Ca ASW; (α) thus include both components of inward current. (β) was similarly traced from the current record using the same test pulse but preceded by a conditioning depolarization to -20 mV. Therefore, (β) is considered to be a minor compoment isolated by inactivation of Na current. If this view were correct, the $(\alpha - \beta)$ trace obtained by subtracting (β) from (α) should represent Na current free from the minor component. As expected, the trace $(\alpha - \beta)$ was identical with the uncontaminated Na current in 100 mM Mn^{2+} ASW, in which all Ca was replaced by Mn^{2+} (Fig. 3B, 100 Mn). This gave further evidence that (β) obtained after the conditioning prepulse represented Ca current.

Effects of replacement of Ca with Sr or Ba upon the minor component

Sr and Ba can replace Ca in the production of "Ca" action potential of crustacean muscle fiber[9,14,17]. In the present egg Ca current, Sr and Ba could also replace Ca, as shown in Fig. 4C. The illustrated current traces were obtained with a test potential pulse to 25 mV preceded by conditioning depolarization of −29 mV in 100 mM Ca, 100 mM Sr and 100 mM Ba ASWs without Mg. The current intensity was increased with Sr and reduced with Ba. The apparent selectivity sequences were in the order Sr > Ca > Ba. The selectivity ratios were 1.0:1.7:1.1 for

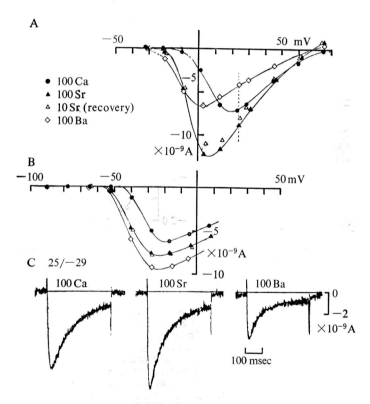

Fig. 4. Ion selectivity of the "Ca channel" among alkali earth cations, Ca, Sr, and Ba. A, *V-I* relations in 100 Ca Mg-free, 100 Sr Mg-free and 100 Ba Mg-free ASWs. Conditioning depolarization, −28 mV and 400 msec in all ASWs. B, *I-V* relations of Na current. The symbols have the same meaning as in A. C, Examples of Ca, Sr and Ba currents at the same potential level of +25 mV (the vertical interrupted line in A). A, B, and C are all from the same egg. 12.5°C. (From Okamoto, H., Takahashi, K., and Yoshii, M., *J. Physiol.*, 255 (1976) 527–561.)

Ca:Sr:Ba as determined by measuring the peak inward currents in appropriate ASWs. The replacement of Ca with foreign divalent cations altered not only the amplitude of the current, but also shifted the V-I relations. On replacing Ca with Sr and Ba in ASW, the V-I relations of "Ca" channels shifted in a negative direction by 11 and 17 mV, respectively (Fig. 4A). Similar shifts of 8 and 9 mV occurred in the V-I relations of Na currents of the same egg (Fig. 4B) upon replacement with Sr and Ba, respectively. These results suggest that there was a stabilizing effect of divalent cations independent of their role as charge carriers through "Ca" and "Na" channels. The sequence of stabilizing power was Ca > Sr > Ba.

Effects of Co^{2+}, La^{3+} and Mg^{2+} on the egg Ca current

It is well-known that the Ca spike is inhibited by polyvalent cations, Mn^{2+}, Co^{2+}, La^{3+} and to a lesser extent by Mg^{2+} [9,18,20]. The egg Ca current was also inhibited by those polyvalent cations. For example, 1 mM La^{3+} in 100 mM Ca ASW at pH 7.0 inhibited the Ca current completely and reversibly, leaving the Na current relatively intact, as shown in Fig. 5A. With conditioning depolarization to inactivate Na current, the isolated Ca current was observed and the effect of 1 mM La^{3+} was further examined; the complete abolition of Ca current was confirmed (Fig. 5A, c' and d'). The presence of 50 mM Mg^{2+} reduced the Ca current by 20% at the maximum current in comparison with the control in 100 mM Ca, Mg-free ASW.

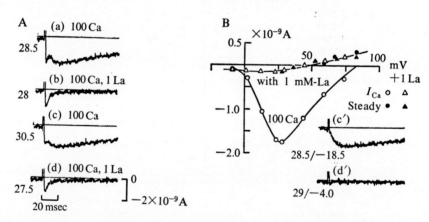

Fig. 5.   Inhibition of Ca current in 100 Ca ASW with La^{3+}. A, Demonstration of the inhibition of Ca current by 1 mM La^{3+}. Traces from (a) to (d) Na and Ca currents induced by the test pulses without the conditioning prepulses to the potential levels indicated by the figures to the left of the traces (mV). The external solutions were exchanged from 100 Ca ASW (a) to 100 Ca ASW with 1 mM La^{3+} (b), 100 Ca ASW (c) and 100 Ca ASW with 1 mM La^{3+} (d) successively. All ASWs were buffered with PIPES at pH 7.0. The (c') and (d') traces were obtained with the same external solutions as in (c) and (d), respectively, but the Ca currents of (c') and (d') were isolated from the Na currents by the conditioning depolarization indicated by the denominators (mV). B, V-I relation of Ca currents (open symbols) and the steady currents (filled symbols) in 100 Ca ASW (PIPES, pH 7.0) (circles) and in 100 Ca ASW (PIPES, pH 7.0) with 1 mM La^{3+} (triangles). (From Okamoto, H., Takahashi, K., and Yoshii, M., *J. Physiol.*, 255 (1976) 527–561).

Potential dependence and external Ca dependence of the kinetic parameters of Na and Ca currents

The time constants of both activation and inactivation processes (τ_{mCa}, τ_{hCa}, τ_{mNa}, and τ_{hNa})

of Ca and Na currents were calculated by applying the Hodgkin-Huxley type formula[24] for *mh* and m^2h in the egg membrane[44,45]. They are plotted against the membrane potential in Fig. 6. Open symbols and interrupted lines indicate the time constants obtained in 100 mM Ca ASW. Maximum τ_{mCa} at +10 mV was 15 msec and was almost 2.5 times that of Na at −40 mV. The sensitivity to the membrane potential was 18 mV for *e*-fold change of τ_{mCa} and was the same as that of τ_{mNa}, while the potential dependency of τ_{hCa} was quite different, *e*-fold change being observed for every 15 mV in the potential range below 20 mV and for every 100 mV beyond that level. The sensitivity of τ_{hCa} to membrane potential beyond 20 mV was apparently much less than that of τ_{hNa}.

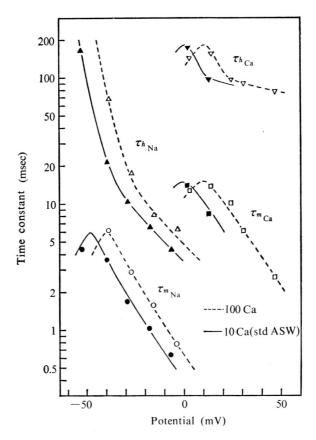

Fig. 6. The relation of the time constants for both activation and inactivation of Na and Ca currents (τ_{mNa}, τ_{mCa}, τ_{hNa}, τ_{hNa}) to the membrane potential. Ordinate: logarithmic scale in msec; Abscissa: membrane potential (mV). The continuous line and filled symbols correspond to standard ASW (Tris, pH 7.8). The interrupted line and open symbols correspond to 100 mM Ca ASW (Tris, pH 7.8). 13.5°C. (From Okamoto, H., Takahashi, K., and Yoshii, M., *J. Physiol.*, 255 (1976) 527–561.)

Comparing the values in 100 mM Ca ASW with those in 10 mM Ca (standard) ASW, the changes in the potential dependence of the parameters τ_m and τ_h of Na and Ca currents along the voltage axis are indicated by the distance between the continuous line (10 mM) and the interrupted line (100 mM). All parameters showed a parallel shift in a positive direction by 10 to 12 mV with an increase in Ca concentration from 10 to 100 mM. As described above, the stabilizing effect of Ca was roughly the same for Na and Ca currents.

Two types of Ca current in Na-free Ca ASW

Since the major component of the inward currents was Na current, one would expect that no major component would be observed in Ca ASW in which all NaCl in standard ASW was replaced isotonically with $CaCl_2$. However, a residual inward current with a relatively negative critical membrane potential of -25 mV and with a time course comparable to that of Na current was obtained in 267 mM Ca, Na-free solution, in addition to the "Ca" or minor component with the relatively positive critical potential of $+3$ mV (Fig. 7). The residual inward current was inactivated by a conditioning depolarization to -26 mV just as in the case of Na current, leaving

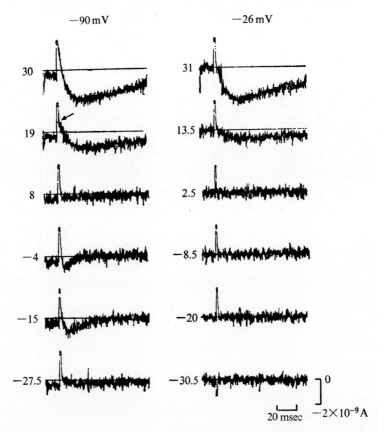

Fig. 7. Demonstration of two components of Ca current in Na-free 267 mM Ca ASW. The left-hand side; current traces obtained by the test voltage steps without the conditioning prepulse. The right-hand side, the current obtained by the test voltage steps preceded by conditioning depolarization of 400 msec to -26 mV. In the traces to the left, the component with the lower threshold and with the faster time course is clear, but it is completely inactivated in the right-hand traces. 13.3°C. Holding potential was -90 mV in both cases. (From Okamoto, H., Takahashi, K., and Yoshii, M., *J. Physiol.*, 255 (1976) 527–561.)

the "Ca" or minor component unchanged. Thus, the current seemed to be closely related to the "Na" channels. The following findings strongly suggest that the current was a Ca current flowing through the egg "Na" channels, as has been reported in the case of the squid axonal membrane.[2,35]

Firstly, the residual current reversed its polarity at about $+10$ mV in 267 mM Ca ASW and the reversal level shifted in a negative direction with decrease in Ca concentration in Na-free ASW.[45] The reversal point could be explained by the balance between Ca influx and Na efflux. Secondly, in choline Na-free ASW the transient residual current was dependent upon Ca and the amplitude increased with increase of Ca from 10 to 200 mM[45]. Thirdly, the apparent difference of the critical potentials between -25 mV for the residual current in Ca ASW and -55 mV for the Na current of the same egg in standard ASW could be explained by the fact that the critical potential is raised in isotonic Ca ASW. Fourthly, when 175 mM choline in 200 mM Ca ASW was replaced with 175 mM Na, the residual inward current increased considerably while the minor or "Ca" component remained almost unchanged (Fig. 8A and B). The increased inward current was simply the "Na" or major component, and its critical membrane potential, or the potential level at which the inward current became maximum, was the same as for the residual inward current under Na-free conditions (Fig. 8B). The time course of the inward current at the same potential level was scarcely affected by addition of Na to the external medium, as shown in Fig. 8A.

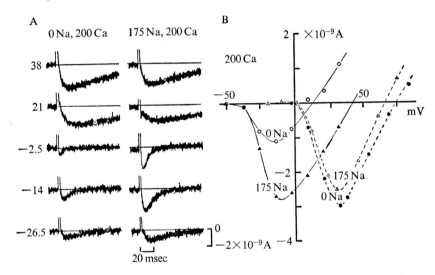

Fig. 8. Comparison of the currents through "Na channels" in 200 mM Ca ASWs without Na and with 175 mM Na. A, the left-hand side: without Na but with 175 mM choline. The right-hand side: with 175 mM Na. B, *V-I* relations of the current through "Na channels" (continuous lines) without Na (open circles) and with 175 mM Na (filled triangles), and the Ca current through "Ca channels" interrupted lines) without Na (filled circles) and with 175 mM Na (open triangles). (From Okamoto, H., Takahashi, K., and Yoshii, M., *J. Physiol.*, 255 (1976) 527–561.)

Selectivity of divalent cations through the egg "Na" channels

Fig. 9 shows the changes of both the residual inward current and the "Ca" or minor component during the replacement of Ca with Sr or Ba in Na-free media. The 200 mM Ca was successively replaced with 200 mM Sr, 200 mM Ca, 200 mM Ba and 200 mM Ca in choline Na-free

ASW. As described above, the changes in the critical potential and current intensity at the peak of the inward current of the minor component were similar to those in the case of Na ASW. The residual current may also have shown shifts in the critical potential, but it is remarkable that the residual inward current was almost abolished in Sr or Ba ASW and changed into an outwardly directed one. Upon close inspection, the *V-I* relation at the peak of the reversed residual current in Sr ASW was more inwardly shifted in any range of the membrane potential compared to that in Ba ASW (Fig. 9). It seems reasonable to postulate a higher permeability to Sr than to Ba. Thus, the permeability sequence of divalent cations through Na channels may be Ca ≫ Sr > Ba (Fig. 9, continuous lines). The sequence is different from that of divalent cations through minor or "Ca" channels: Sr > Ba > Ca (Fig. 9, interrupted lines, at the maximum currents), suggesting further

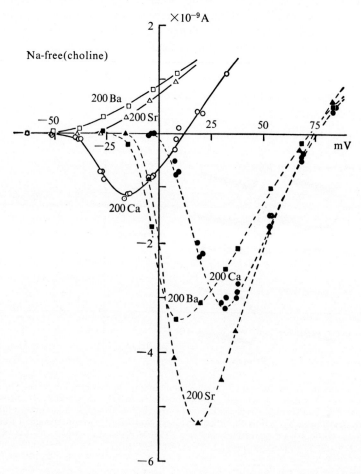

Fig. 9.   *V-I* relations of the currents through Na and Ca channels in Na-free choline ASWs with different alkaline earth cations at 200 mM (Ca, Sr, Ba). 14°C. The full lines and open symbols show the current through "Na channels". The interrupted lines and filled symbols show the current through "Ca channels". Triangles, Sr; circle, Ca; squares, Ba. *V-I* curves for 200 mM Ca include the data from three series of experiments in 200 Ca Na-free ASW. (From Okamoto, H., Takahashi, K., and Yoshii, M., *J. Physiol.*, 255 (1976) 527–561.)

that the Ca current through "Na" channels was qualitatively different from that through "Ca" channels.

Effects of internal Cl⁻ and F⁻ ions upon the Na and Ca channels

In our previous study[51] the egg cell of the tunicate was successfully perfused intracellularly by a method similar in principle to that described by Kostyuk *et al.*[32] and Lee *et al.*[33] In our experiments, however, the cleaned surface of the egg was brought into contact with a smooth Pyrex glass wall inside a small funnel, instead of using a hole in the polyethylene sheet or a suction pipette. Close contact was facilitated by coating a positively charged protein, protamine, on the glass wall. The intact membrane free from this contact was estimated to amount to half of the total surface of the intact egg and was used for the internal perfusion experiments. After contact, the lower membrane at the lower orifice of the funnel was ruptured by slight negative pressure of 2–3 mm H_2O and the inside of the egg was perfused with the internal solution, in which free Ca ions were regulated by means of Ca-chelating agents, such as GEDTA or DPTA-OH. The remaining free membrane appeared to behave in just the same way as in the intact egg, despite the fact that the membrane on the opposite side had a hole amounting to almost a quarter of the egg diameter. The degree of exchange of the intracellular solution was monitored in terms of the shift in the reversal potential for Na current and was found to be 80 – 90 % complete within 30 min.

Fig. 10 shows that significant differences exist in the behaviour of various membrane currents in the presence of Cl⁻ ions and F⁻ ions in the internal perfusates. The lower trace in Fig. 10A indicates the membrane potential, and the upper one the holding current. Immediately after rupture, the membrane potential was voltage-clamped and held at −90 mV. The initial perfusate was Cl⁻ solution and this was later replaced by F⁻ perfusate. During the initial 10 min, the holding current was as low as 0.3 nA even in the Cl⁻ perfusate, but thereafter it increased gradually and, at around 20 to 30 min, it increased abruptly. However, when the internal Cl⁻ perfusate was changed to F⁻ perfusate just before the destruction of the membrane, the holding current, which had first increased, decreased again and finally became stable at a low level of less than 0.2 nA. During the phase of the relatively stable and low holding current in Cl⁻ perfusate step changes in the potential revealed both Na and Ca current with Na and Ca ASW as an external solution. Essentially the same results were obtained when Ca was replaced by Sr in the external solution. Actually in Fig. 10A, left-hand insets, the Sr current through "Ca" channels is illustrated by isolating with a conditioning prepulse. After changing the perfusate to F⁻ solution, the Sr current was completely abolished, as shown in the right-hand insets. The current-voltage relations at the peaks of Na and Sr currents are presented for internal F⁻ (filled circles) and Cl⁻ (open circles) perfusates in Fig. 10B (Na Current) and Fig. 10C (Sr current) for the same experiment as in Fig. 10A. The maximum inward Na current in F⁻ perfusate was usually 1.5 to 2 times that in Cl⁻ perfusate. The reversal potential of Na current in Cl⁻ perfusate was shifted in the negative direction when the perfusate contained 400 mM Na and the time after rupture was more than 10 min. The reversal potential in F⁻ perfusate was +6 mV and was slightly more negative than the value of +9 mV in Cl⁻ perfusate. This is simply due to the longer perfusion time for the recordings in F⁻ perfusate.

As shown in Fig. 10B, the $V_{1/2}$ and the $V_{p\text{-max}}$ values of the Na current in F⁻ perfusate were clearly shifted in the negative direction by 5 to 10 mV in comparison with those in Cl⁻ perfusate. The values in Cl⁻ perfusate were similar to those found in the intact egg (Fig. 4B). The $V_{1/2}$ and

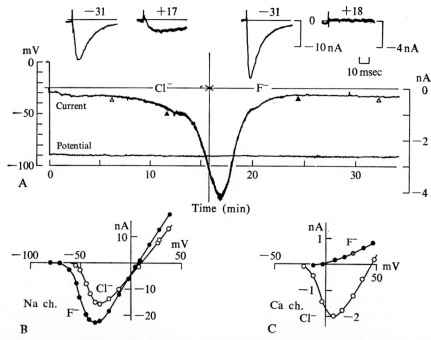

Fig. 10.   Comparison of the holding current, Na current and Sr current for internal Cl⁻ and F⁻ per-fusions. A illustrates the holding current at −90 mV and the membrane potential on a multi-channel DC recorder in an egg cell perfused initially with Cl⁻ solution and later with F⁻ solution. Insets are sample records of Na current at −31 mV and Sr current at +17 mV isolated from Na current by a conditioning depolarizing pulse of 400 msec to −34 mV in the Cl (left) and F (right) perfusates. The times at which the samples were obtained are indicated by triangles on the DC current records. △, Na currents; ▲, Sr currents. B and C illlustrate *I-V* relations of the Na and Sr currents, respectively, with internal Cl (open circles) and F (filled circles) perfusates. Sr currents were also isolated by condition-ing depolarization to −34 mV. (From Takahashi, K., and Yoshii, M., *J. Physiol.*, 279 (1978) 519–549)

the $V_{\text{p-max}}$ values of the Ca or Sr current in Cl perfusate were also similar to those in the intact egg. In F⁻ perfusate the "Ca" channel current was completely abolished and only the outward current was observed.

Fig. 11 shows typical examples of the changes occurring in Na and Sr currents during the initial phases of F⁻ and Cl⁻ perfusion. The reversal potential of Na current (open squares), the zero-current Na conductance (open circles), and the maximum Sr current (filled circles) were plotted against the time after rupture. The insets in the upper (F⁻) and lower (Cl⁻) figures in Fig. 11 are sample current records in response to step changes in potential to +20 mV. Since no condi-tioning depolarization was applied, the recorded trace shows both initial fast Na and later slow Sr currents. Within 1 to 2 min after the initiation of perfusion, the reversal potential of Na current was usually above +40 mV, suggesting that in this initial period the intracellular medium is still almost the same (exchange of less than 20%) as in the intact egg. In this initial period, the records for F⁻ and Cl⁻ perfusates show a similar shape, consisting of initial Na and later Sr currents. With the progress of exchange, as indicated by the reversal potential change, the Sr current was abolish-ed in F⁻ perfusate, while the Na conductance doubled. However, in Cl⁻ perfusate, both Na con-ductance and the maximum Sr current stayed relatively constant. Fifty to 100 mM F⁻ ions seems to be necessary to abolish the Ca current, because the reversal potential at the time indicated a 30

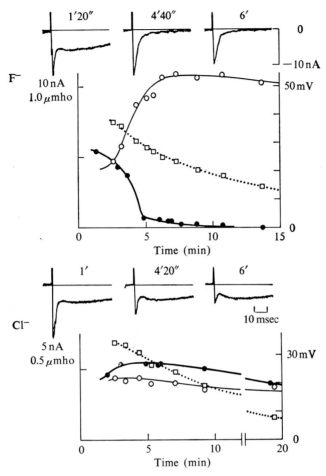

Fig. 11. The changes of Na reversal potential ($E_{r \cdot Na}$, open squares), peak amplitude of, Ca current (I_{Ca}, filled circles) at +17 mV, and Na conductance at zero current level (G_{Na}, open circles) during the transient phases of F^- (upper figure) and Cl^- (lower figure) perfusions. Internal solutions were F and Cl. Ordinate: nA for I_{Ca} and μmho for G_{Na}. Abscissa: the perfusion time after the rupture or initiation of perfusion. Insets are sample current records at +17 mV. Since no conditioning depolarization was carried out initially, both initial fast Na and later slow Ca currents were observed. The number on each trace indicates the perfusion time at which the record was obtained. (From Takahashi, K., and Yoshii, M., *J. Physiol.*, 279 (1978) 519–549.)

to 50% exchange and the F^- concentration in the perfusate was 170 mM in this case. The time course of reversal potential change for F^- perfusate was almost identical with that for Cl^- perfusate, suggesting that intracellular diffusion is similar with the two perfusates.

Differential effect of intracellular free Ca ions upon Na and Ca channels in the egg cell membrane

It is known that intracellular Ca ions have an inhibitory effect upon the Ca current through Ca channels.[19] In our experiments on egg internal perfusion, the effect was also tested by perfusing Ca ion-buffered solution intracellularly. Fig. 12 illustrates an experiment in which the egg was perfused with a solution containing a relatively high concentration of free Ca ions (3.3×10^{-5} M) and another experiment with control solution containing zero free Ca ions. The external solution contained 400 mM Na and 100 mM Ca and this was kept constant throughout the experiment. The time course of the perfusion is shown in the inset; the perfusion was started at zero time and the records a and b were obtained at the indicated times. The triangles indicate the time at which current at -20 mV was induced (to observe the maximum Na current) and the open triangles indicate the times at which current was induced at $+17$ mV (to observe the maximum Ca current). Within the initial 1 min, when record a was obtained, the observed Na and Ca currents in high Ca perfusate were identical to those in the control perfusate with zero Ca (Fig. 12A and B). A few minutes after the initiation of perfusion with high Ca perfusate, the holding current suddenly increased by a factor of three to five (inset in Fig. 12A), whereas the Na current nearly doubled and the Ca current was reduced to one-half. In the zero Ca perfusate, the holding current, the Na and the Ca currents were not significantly different from those observed within the initial 1 min. The time courses of the increased Na and decreased Ca currents in the high Ca perfusate were not significantly different from those observed during the initial few min or in the control perfusate. Thus, it seems likely that the chord conductance, but not the gating mechanism, was affected. The holding current, having once increased, stayed at a relatively high level and often started to increase

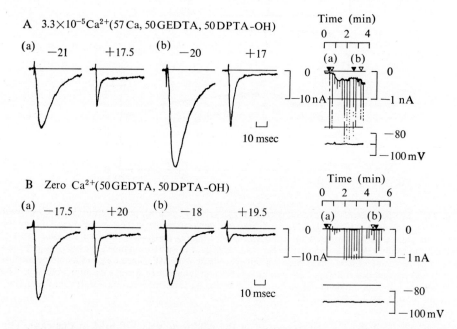

Fig. 12.   Effects of internal Ca ions upon Na and Ca currents. A illustrates current traces immediately after rupture (a) and 2.7–3.2 min later (b) in the presence of 3.3×10^{-5} M Ca ions in the internal perfusate. The external solution contained 400 mM Na and 100 mM Ca. The number above each current trace indicates its membrane potential in mV. The inset shows DC records of current (upper) and potential (lower). The zero time on the time scale indicates the time of rupture, and the times at which the illustrated current traces were obtained are also indicated (▼; -20 mV trace; ▽; $+17$ mV trace). B shows a control experiment on another egg in the absence of Ca ions in the internal perfusate. The external solution was the same as in A. Symbols, numbers and scales have the same meaning as in A. (From Takahashi, K., and Yoshii, M., *J. Physiol.*, 279 (1978) 519–549.)

further after 5 to 10 min. The later increase was probably due to greater fragility of the membrane in the high Ca perfusate.

Fig. 13A and B show collected data on the maximum Ca current (I_{Ca}) and the zero-current Na conductance (G_{Na}) from 23 egg cells which were perfused with different solutions containing various free Ca concentrations. I_{Ca} and G_{Na} were plotted against the Ca ion concentration in the buffered perfusate. The results showed that I_{Ca}, which was 2 to 3 nA in the zero Ca perfusate, decreased as the Ca concentration was increased above 10^{-6} M and fell to one-fifth at 8×10^{-4} M. By contrast, G_{Na} began to increase at Ca concentrations above 10^{-6} M and reached a maximum at around 5×10^{-5} to 10^{-4} M. G_{Na} became about twice that of the zero Ca solution. G_{Na} appeared to decrease slightly above 10^{-4} M Ca. Therefore, it can be concluded that intracellular free Ca in the range from 10^{-6} to 10^{-3} M has reciprocal effects upon the Na and Ca channels. The open circles in Fig. 13A and B indicate data from eggs which showed a small I_{Ca} of less than 1 nA in zero Ca or 8×10^{-7} M Ca perfusate. These eggs always showed a relatively large G_{Na} in comparison with eggs which gave I_{Ca} of 2 to 3 nA. Although there is no definite evidence, it is possible that the eggs with small I_{Ca} may have had a higher internal concentration of free Ca, possibly because of an increased Ca influx or spontaneous Ca release from the intracellular stores. In some experi-

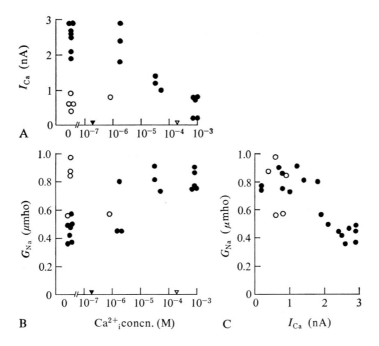

Fig. 13.   The relationships of peak Ca current I_{Ca} (A) and zero current Na conductance G_{Na} (B) when intracellular free Ca concentrations were determined by means of various Ca buffer solutions. Each point in the figures was obtained from one egg preparation. A total of 23 eggs is illustrated. Filled and open triangles on the abscissa indicate apparent binding constants for GEDTA and DPTA-OH, respectively, at pH 7.0. Open circles indicate the egg preparations which showed small I_{Ca} values of less than 1.0 nA. C shows the reciprocal relationship between I_{Ca} (abscissa) and G_{Na} (ordinate). Each point was obtained from one egg. The open circles have the same meaning as in A and B. (From Takahashi, K., and Yoshii, M., *J. Physiol.*, 279 (1978) 519–549.)

ments, in which the internal perfusate contained more than 10 mM Ca ions and no chelating agents, both Na and Ca currents were abolished irreversibly.

In Fig. 13C, G_{Na} is plotted against I_{Ca} of the same egg perfused with various concentrations of intracellular Ca ions, from the data illustrated in Fig. 13A and B. There is a clear reciprocal relationship between G_{Na} and I_{Ca}. It is interesting that an egg which showed a relatively low Ca current, even during the perfusion of low levels of intracellular Ca, tended to have larger G_{Na}, as indicated by open circles in Fig. 13C.

Discussion

Analysis of the membrane current by the voltage-clamp technique indicated that the Na inward current of the egg membrane was essentially identical with that of other excitable membranes. The reasons for this conclusion can be summarized as follows. (1) The egg Na current showed both activation and inactivation processes and the kinetic parameters were correlated with the membrane potential in the same way as in other excitable membranes. (2) Li could replace the Na component of the inward current but neither Tris nor choline could. The selectivity ratios for the Na channels were found to be Na : K : Rb : Cs = 1.0 : 0.088 : 0.045 : 0.027 by changing the cationic composition of the external solution[44] and 1.0 : 0.14 : 0.05 : 0.04 by changing that of the internal perfusate[51]. The ratios were similar to those obtained for the Na channels of other excitable membranes[6,8,22]. (3) Ca ions could also permeate through the egg Na channels, as has been found in squid axons[2,35,53]. (4) A specific inhibitor of the Na channel, tetrodotoxin, had no effect upon the egg Na current. It has been reported that Na spikes in the denervated muscle[47] or the embryonic heart muscle[26,50] or in clone-cultured rat myotube[29] are all tetrodotoxin-resistant. It is not strange that the undifferentiated egg cell membrane had tetrodotoxin-insensitive Na channels. Although tetrodotoxin did not have any effect upon egg Na channels, a polypeptide toxin, (a purified scorpion venom), prolonged the falling phase of egg Na current selectively as in the case of myelinated axon and the squid axon[42]. It was also found that binding of the toxin with egg Na channels was on a one-to-one basis, as in the case of myelinated axons with saxitoxin[22]. (5) The Q_{10} of the maximum chord conductance of the egg Na channels was about two, while the Q_{10} of the time constant for the activation or inactivation process was much larger and in the range of 3 to 4, just as in the case of other Na channels[44]. The difference between the two Q_{10}'s suggests that the permeation gating processes are quite independent of each other, as proposed in the channel hypothesis for excitable membrane.

The minor component of the inward current was distinctly different from the major component, showing a much less critical level of -10 mV in standard ASW and a slower time course. The following findings indicate that the minor component was a Ca current through the "Ca" channels, the existence of which has been established in the crustacean striated muscle[48]. (1) The minor component was independent of the presence of Na in the external medium, while elimination of Ca from ASW abolished this component. (2) The current intensity at a fixed potential level, at which the minor component was supposed to be fully activated, was a monotonically increasing function of the external Ca concentration. (3) Co^{2+} and La^{3+} inhibited the minor component selectively. (4) The results of previous studies indicate that the kinetics of the Ca current are quite slow in comparison with those of the Na current[14,28], the rise time at room temperature being of the order of 10 msec, and fast inactivation being absent. In this egg membrane of the tunicate, the absence of or the highly positive critical level of K outward current allowed us to analyze precisely the kinetics of the Ca current[45]. The activation time constant of the Ca current was at least 2.5 times that of the egg Na current, which was in the same range as that of the barnacle muscle fiber. The inactivation of the egg Ca current was also slow and incomplete. (5) Sr or Ba could replace Ca in the minor component.

The selectivity ratio of the egg Ca channels was found to be Ca : Sr : Ba = 1.0 : 1.7 : 1.1 by measurement of the maximum peak current under voltage-clamp conditions. Ca current in the giant muscle fiber of the barnacle has also been studied by the voltage-clamp technique[14,15,28]. The separation of Ca current from K current has been attempted by using tetraethyl-ammonium or Cs perfused outside or inside the muscle membrane to block the latter current[14,28]. The permeability ratio obtained in the muscle was Ca : Sr : Ba = 1.0 : 1.05 : 1.30[14] and apparently differs for Ba from that found in the egg experiments. Our comparative studies on the membrane excitability of various oocytes demonstrated that Ca channels existed in mouse and sea urchin oocytes as well.[43] The existence of Ca channels may therefore be a general characteristic of the egg membrane. A comparison of egg Ca channels indicated some differences in channel properties among the oocytes of three different species: the mouse, the tunicate and the sea urchin. The selectivity ratios among alkaline earth cations, Ca : Sr : Ba, for egg "Ca" channels were 1.0 : 1.4 : 0.7 in the mouse, 1.0 : 1.7 : 1.1 in the tunicate and 1.0 : 1.7 : 0.5 in the sea urchin, comparing the maximum peak currents. The critical membrane potential of Ca channels in the tunicate was about −10 mV in 30 Ca ASW and was markedly positive in comparison with the other two. Different sequences of stabilizing effects of Ca, Sr and Ba upon the Ca channels among the three species were found: Ca > Sr ≫ Ba in the tunicate, Ba ≫ Ca > Sr in the mouse, and Ba ≫ Sr > Ca in the sea urchin. According to the channel hypothesis for the ionic current in an excitable membrane[1,22], the selectivity ratios of the channels for permeating cations are considered to be due to intrinsic properties of the negatively charged sites within the channels, and not to the properties of the sites which are responsible for the stabilizing effect. Therefore, the differences in the selectivity ratios of Ca channels for Ca, Sr and Ba observed in the oocyte membranes of these three species may indicate that the Ca channels are specific to animal species. However, recent studies of the stabilizing effect on the ionic channels in the tunicate egg membrane have confirmed that apparent conductance changes of channels do occur in direct relation to the shifts of the *I-V* curves along the voltage axis[41]. The results suggest that the accumulation of the permeating cations at the orifices of channels is also regulated by the negativity of the surface double-layer potential. Therefore, the different sequences of the stabilizing effects of alkaline earth cations upon Ca channels among the three species could produce apparent differences in the selectivity ratios of Ca channels for these cations. When the current density through Ca channels is corrected for the critical levels for Ca channels, the revised selectivity sequences all become Ca > Sr > Ba, being common to all three species.

Tasaki and his colleagues have demonstrated that Ca in Na-free media can evoke the tetrodotoxin-sensitive action potential in the squid giant axon[55,56,58,59]. Ca influx analyzed in terms of the luminescence of aequorin suggests that Ca is able to flow through "Na" channels[2-4], although Tasaki and his colleagues have considered the appearance of tetrodotoxin-sensitive bi-ionic potentials on the basis of the phase transition theory of macromolecules in the membrane[52]. The membrane current under controlled voltage of the CsF-perfused axon in Na-free media is a transient inward current which is dependent upon the external Ca level and is tetrodotoxin-sensitive.[35] The Ca-sensitive photosubstance aequorin revealed two types of Ca influx, one tetrodotoxin-sensitive and the other tetrodotoxin-insensitive, during membrane depolarization[2]. Tetrodotoxin-insensitive Ca influx is considered to flow through the "Ca" channels, which are closely related to those of crustacean muscle membrane and to the Ca influx at the nerve terminal, which triggers transmitter release.[3,4] In this egg cell membrane, two types of Ca currents were clearly separated from each other on the basis of critical levels, time courses and the relations of inactivation to the membrane potential. In particular, the current with the more negative critical level in the Na-free ASW was proved to be the one through egg Na channels. One noteworthy feature of Ca current through egg Na channels is the difference of permeability ratios of Ca : Sr : Ba from those through Ca channels, for Ca through Na channels could scarcely be replaced by Sr or Ba.

Internal perfusates containing F^- ions were found to be the best for reducing the leakage current and keeping the amplitude of Na current large[54]. This effect of F^- ions is well known with squid axons[54], *Myxicola* axons[8] and snail neurons[32]. In the tunicate egg, internal F^- ions not only enhanced the Na current but also shifted its current-voltage relation along the voltage axis in a negative direction as compared with internal Cl^- ions. It may be inferred that the increase in Na conductance is derived from the lowered threshold for Na channel-gating. According to the theory of the diffuse double layer[13,41], a negative shift in the current-voltage relation corresponds either to an increase in negative charges or negative surface potential at the outer surface or to a decrease of either at the inner surface. Thus, in order to explain the present results in terms of a change in the surface potential, one would have to conclude that there is a specific binding of Cl^- ions but not of F^- ions to the inner membrane or alternatively, that Cl^- ions somehow extract a positive charged substance from the internal membrane surface, this substance being unaffected by F^- ions. In the tunicate egg, about 100 mM F^- ions in the perfusate abolished Ca or Sr current completely, whereas it doubled Na current. This suppressive effect of internal F^- ions upon Ca current has also been found in snail neurons[32]. The reciprocal effect on Na and Ca currents can hardly be explained only by uniform changes in the surface potential at either side of the membrane.

An internal free Ca concentration ($[Ca^{2+}]_i$) of more than 10^{-6} M was inhibitory for Ca spike generation in barnacle muscle fibers[19]. Kostyuk *et al.* have reported that $[Ca^{2+}]_i$ over 2×10^{-8} M abolishes Ca current in internally perfused snail neurons[31]. The present experiments indicate that, at $[Ca^{2+}]_i$ greater than 10^{-6} M, reduction of Ca current occurred, and its complete abolition would probably require $[Ca^{2+}]_i$ of more than 1 mM. It seems, therefore, that the egg membrane is slightly less sensitive to internal Ca ions than the barnacle muscle and considerably less than the snail neuron, which might be of some developmental significance in view of the undifferentiated stage of the egg membrane. Recent studies on Ca-accumulating and -releasing structures, such as the sarcoplasmic reticulum, have shown the existence of Ca-induced Ca release inside the cell[10,57]. If this mechanism is also applicable to the barnacle muscle and snail neuron, the intracellular Ca in these experiments might have been much higher than that prescribed by the buffer solution used. Since high concentrations of Ca-chelating agents as well as pH buffers were used[51], an unregulated rise in the Ca ion concentration was less likely to occur. However, very localized enhancement of Ca ion concentration might still be possible inside the egg cell[49].

A facilitatory effect of internal Ca ions upon the Na current has not previously been found. There have been some reports which suggest that there is no effect or even a suppressive effect of internal Ca ions up to 10 mM in squid giant axons[5,55], although Begenisich and Lynch[5] have reported an enhancement of Na current in one axon of the squid perfused with 10 mM Ca solution. Yamagishi[62] also suggested the possibility with increase of intracellular Ca ions in squid giant axons. The facilitatory effect in the egg membrane may also be related to these findings. However, the specific inductory effect of intracellular Ca ions cannot be neglected at the initial stage of development, such as in the uncleaved egg or the early blastula.

During an attempt to determine the appearance of excitability on presumptive muscle cells in the tunicate embryo[36,37], we found that the egg cell membrane itself was excitable[37], having ionic channels identical with those found in other excitable membranes, as described above. By utilizing cell differentiation in cleavage-arrested embryo treated with cytochalasin B, the ionic currents of the egg were directly compared with those of differentiated excitable membrane, such as nerve or muscle membranes, in the tunicate larva using the voltage-clamp technique (Takahashi and Yoshii, in preparation). The results indicate that the channel properties, such as kinetics and potential dependence of the time courses, did not change during development, though the threshold potentials and channel densities were altered. The changes in the density or in the threshold usually occurred at critical stages of development and showed close time relations with the initial fertilization or with the appearance of other properties, ACh receptors or synapse formation on the muscle membrane. In the muscle cell, Na channels were reduced and Ca channels were increased, while in the nerve cell, the situation seemed to be reversed. Some aspects of such reciprocal changes in the channel densities were mimicked by increase in the level of intracellular Ca ions, as discussed above.

The mechanisms of alteration in channel densities by differentiation or by intracellular Ca ion perfusion are not well understood at present. Considering that the replacement of Cl^- with F^- in the internal perfusate doubled Na conductance as the intracellular Ca increased, it may be suggested that there are immediately available reserves of Na channels in the intracellular membranous structures and that the channel molecules are in a state of equilibrium between the intracellular structures and the surface plasma membrane. In this case, some agents, such as intracellular free Ca ions or fluoride ions, may shift the equilibrium toward the plasma membrane side, assuming that the initial amount of the reserves is comparable to that of the Na channels in the surface membrane. It is also possible that the Ca channels themselves are the reserves of Na channels, because the effects of free Ca or F ions were reciprocal. The abolition of Ca current by high intracellular free Ca is not accompanied by enhancement of the Na current in the barnacle muscle membrane, in which no Na component has been observed[19], and the enhancement of Na current by internal F^- ions is not followed by the abolition of Ca current in squid axons, in which very few Ca channels exist[55]. Thus, direct interconversion between Na and Ca channels seems unlikely to occur. However, this mechanism cannot be ruled out at the highly inductive stage of the initial egg cell membrane or the initial presumptive excitable membrane. Interconversion between inactive and active forms of the channels may also be possible.

REFERENCES

1. Armstrong, C.M., Ionic pores, gates, and gating currents, *Q. Rev. Biophys.*, 7 (1975) 179–210.
2. Baker, P.F., Hodgkin, A.L. and Ridgway, E.B., Depolarization and calcium entry in squid giant axons, *J. Physiol.*, 218 (1971) 709–755.
3. Baker, P.F., Meves, H. and Ridgway, E.B., Effects of manganese and other agents on the calcium uptake that follows depolarization of squid axons, *J. Physiol.*, 231 (1973a) 511–526.
4. Baker, P.F., Meves, H. and Ridgway, E.B., Calcium entry in response to maintained depolarization of squid axons, *J. Physiol.*, 231 (1973b) 527–548.
5. Begenisich, T. and Lynch, C., Effects of internal divalent cations on voltage-clamped squid axons, *J. gen Physiol.*, 63 (1974) 675–689.

6. Campbell, D.T., Ionic selectivity of the sodium channel of frog skeletal muscle, *J. gen. Physiol.*, 67 (1976) 295–307.

7. Chandler, W.K. and Meves, H., Voltage clamp experiments on internally perfused giant axons, *J. Physiol.*, 180 (1965) 788–820.

8. Ebert, G.A. and Goldman, L., The permeability of the sodium channel in *Myxicola* to alkali cations, *J. gen. Physiol.*, 68 (1976) 327–340.

9. Fatt, P. and Ginsborg, B.L., The ionic requirements for the production of action potentials in crustacean muscle fibres, *J. Physiol.*, 142 (1958) 516–543.

10. Ford, L.E. and Podolsky, R.J., Regenerative calcium release within muscle cells, *Science*, 167 (1970) 58–59.

11. Frankenhaeuser, B. and Moore, L.E., The specificity of the initial current in myelinated nerve fibres of *Xenopus laevis*, *J. Physiol.*, 169 (1963) 438–444.

12. Geduldig, D. and Junge, D., Sodium and calcium components of action potentials in the *Aplysia* giant neurone, *J. Physiol.*, 199 (1968) 347–365.

13. Gilbert, D.L., Fixed surface charges. In *Biophysics and Physiology of Excitable Membranes*, Van Nostrand Reinhold Co., Amsterdam, 1971, pp. 359–378.

14. Hagiwara, S., Fukuda, J. and Eaton, D.C., Membrane currents carried by Ca, Sr and Ba in barnacle muscle fiber during voltage clamp, *J. gen. Physiol.*, 63 (1974) 564–578.

15. Hagiwara, S., Hayashi, H. and Takahashi, K., Calcium and potassium currents of the membrane of a barnacle muscle fibre in relation to the calcium spike, *J. Physiol.*, 205 (1969) 115–129. .

16. Hagiwara, S. and Kidokoro, Y., Na and Ca components of action potential in *Amphioxus* muscle cells, *J. Physiol.*, 219 (1971) 217–232.

17. Hagiwara, S. and Naka, K., The initiation of spike potential in barnacle muscle fibers under low intracellular Ca^{2+}, *J. gen. Physiol.*, 48 (1964) 141–162.

18. Hagiwara, S. and Nakajima, S., Differences in Na and Ca spikes as examined by application of TTX, procaine and manganase ions, *J. gen. Physiol.*, 49 (1966) 793–806.

19. Hagiwara, S. and Nakajima, S., Effects of the intracellular Ca ion concentration upon the excitability of the muscle fiber membrane of a barnacle, *J. gen. Physiol.*, 49 (1966) 807–818.

20. Hagiwara, S. and Takahashi, K., Surface density of calcium ions and calcium spikes in the barnacle muscle fiber membrane, *J. gen. Physiol.*, 50 (1967) 583–601.

21. Hille, B, The permeability of the sodium channel to metal cations in myelinated nerve, *J. gen. Physiol.*, 59 (1972) 637–658.

22. Hille, B, Ionic channels in nerve membranes, *Prog. Biophys. molec. Biol.*, 21 (1970) 1–32.

23. Hodgkin, A.L., Ionic movements and electrical activity in giant nerve fibres, *Proc. R. Soc. B*, 148 (1958) 1–37.

24. Hodgkin, A.L. and Huxley, A.F., A quantitative description of membrane current and its application to conduction and excitation in nerve, *J. Physiol.*, 117 (1952) 500–544.

25. Hodgkin, A.L. and Katz, B., The effect of sodium ions on the electrical activity of the giant axon of the squid, *J. Physiol.*, 108 (1949) 37–77.

26. Ishima, Y., The effect of tetrodotoxin and sodium substitution on the action potential in the course of development of the embryonic chicken heart, *Proc. japan. Acad.*, 44 (1968) 170–175.

27. Iwasaki, S. and Satow, Y., Sodium and calcium dependent spike potentials in the secretory neuron soma of the X-organ of the crayfish, *J. gen. Physiol.*, 57 (1971) 216–238.

28. Keynes, R.D., Rojas, E., Taylor, R.E. and Vergara, J., Calcium and potassium systems of a giant barnacle muscle fibre under membrane potential control, *J. Physiol.*, 229 (1973) 409–455.

29. Kidokoro, Y., Development of action potentials in a clonal rat skeletal muscle cell line, *Nature New Biol.*, 241 (1973) 158–159.

30. Koketsu, K. and Nishi, S., Calcium and action potentials of bullfrog sympathetic ganglion cells, *J. gen. Physiol.*, 53 (1969) 608–623.

31. Kostyuk, P.G. and Krishtal, O.A., Effects of calcium and calcium-chelating agents on the inward and outward current in the membrane of mollusc neurones, *J. Physiol.*, 270 (1977) 569–580.

32. Kostyuk, P.G., Krishtal, O.A. and Pidoplichko, V.I., Effect of internal fluoride and phosphate on membrane currents during intracellular dialysis of nerve cells, *Nature (Lond.).*, 257 (1975) 691–693.

33. Lee, K.S., Akaike, N. and Brown, A.M., Trypsin inhibits the action of tetrodotoxin on neurones, *Nature (Lond.).*, 265 (1977) 751–753.

34. Meves, H., The ionic requirements for the production of action potentials in *Helix pomata* neurones, *Pflügers Arch. ges. Physiol.*, 304 (1968) 215–241.

35. Meves, H. and Vogel, W., Calcium inward currents in internally perfused giant axons, *J. Physiol.*, 235 (1973) 225–265.

36. Miyazaki, S., Takahashi, K. and Tsuda, K., Calcium and sodium contributions to regenerative responses in the embryonic excitable cell membrane, *Science.*, 176 (1972) 1441–1443.

37. Miyazaki, S., Takahashi, K. and Tsuda, K., Electrical excitability in the egg cell membrane of the tunicate, *J. Physiol.*, 238 (1974) 37–54.
38. Moore, J.W., Anderson, N.C., Blaustein, M.P., Takata, M., Letivin, J., Pickard, W.F., Bernstein, T. and Pooler, J., Alkali cation specificity of squid axon membrane, *Ann. N. Y. Acad. Sci.*, 137 (1966) 818–829.
39. Nakamura, Y., Nakajima, S. and Grundfest, H., The action of tetrodotoxin on electrogenic components of squid giant axons, *J. gen. Physiol.*, 48 (1965) 985–996.
40. Narahashi, T., Moore, J.W. and Scott, W.R., Tetrodotoxin blockage of sodium conductance increase in lobster giant axons, *J. gen. Physiol.*, 47 (1964) 965–974.
41. Ohmori, H. and Yoshii, M., Surface potential reflected in both gating and permeation mechanisms of sodium and calcium channels of the tunicate egg cell membrane, *J. Physiol.*, 267 (1977) 429–463.
42. Okamoto, H., Takahashi, K. and Yamashita, N., One-to-one binding of a purified scorpion toxin to Na channels, *Nature (Lond.)*, 266 (1977) 465–468.
43. Okamoto, H., Takahashi, K. and Yamashita, N., Ionic currents through the membrane of the mammalian oocyte and their comparison with those in the tunicate and sea urchin, *J. Physiol.*, 267 (1977) 465–495.
44. Okamoto, H., Takahashi, K. and Yoshii, M., Membrane currents of the tunicate egg under the voltage-clamp condition, *J. Physiol.*, 254 (1976) 607–638.
45. Okamoto, H., Takahashi, K. and Yoshii, M., Two components of the calcium current in the egg cell membrane of the tunicate, *J. Physiol.*, 255 (1976) 527–561.
46. Overton, E., Beitrage zur allgemeinen Muskel- und Nervenphysiologie, *Pflügers Arch. ges. Physiol.*, 92 (1902) 346–386.
47. Redfern, P. and Thesleff, S., Action potential generation in denervated rat skeletal muscle. II. The action of tetrodotoxin, *Acta physiol. Scand.*, 82 (1971) 70–78.
48. Reuter, H., Divalent cations as charge carriers in excitable membranes. *Progr. Biophys. molec. Biol.*, 26 (1973) 3–43.
49. Ridgway, E.B., Gilkey, J.C. and Jaffe, L.E., Free calcium increases explosively in activating *Medaka* eggs, *Proc. nat. Acad. Sci. (Wash.)*, 74 (1977) 623–627.
50. Shigenobu, K. and Sperelakis, N., Development of sensitivity to tetrodotoxin of chick embryonic hearts with age, *J. molec. cell. Cardiol.*, 3 (1971) 271–286.
51. Takahashi, K. and Yoshii, M., Effects of internal Ca upon the Na and Ca channels in the tunicate egg analysed by the internal perfusion technique, *J. Physiol.*, 279 (1978) 519–549.
52. Tasaki, I., *Nerve Excitation: A Macromolecular Approach*, Thomas, Springfield, 1968.
53. Tasaki, I., Lerman, L. and Watanabe, A., Analysis of excitation process in squid giant axons under bi-ionic conditions, *Amer. J. Physiol.*, 216 (1969) 130–138.
54. Tasaki, I., Singer, I. and Takenaka, T., Effects of internal and external ionic environment on excitability of squid giant axons. A macromolecular approach, *J. gen. Physiol.*, 48 (1965) 1095–1123.
55. Tasaki, I., Watanabe, A. and Lerman, L., Role of divalent cations in excitation of squid giant axons, *Amer. J. Physiol.*, 213 (1967) 1465–1474.
56. Tasaki, I., Watanabe, A. and Singer, I., Excitability of squid giant axons in the absence of univalent cations in the external medium, *Proc. nat. Acad. Sci. (Wash.)*, 56 (1966) 1116–1122.
57. Thorens, S. and Endo, M., Calcium-induced calcium release and "depolarization"-induced calcium release: Their physiological significance, *Proc. japan. Acad.*, 51 (1975) 473–478.
58. Watanabe, A., Tasaki, L. and Lerman, L., Bi-ionic action potentials in squid giant axons internally perfused with sodium salts, *Proc. nat. Acad. Sci. (Wash.)*, 58 (1967) 2246–2252.
59. Watanabe, A., Tasaki, I., Singer, I. and Lerman, L., Effect of tetrodotoxin on excitability of squid giant axons in sodium free media, *Science* 158 (1967) 95–97.
60. Werman, R. and Grundfest, H., Graded and all-or-none electrogenesis in arthropod muscles. II. The effects of alkali earth and onium ions on lobster muscle fibers, *J. gen. Physiol.*, 44 (1961) 997–1027.
61. Yamagishi, S., Manganese-dependent action potentials in intracellularly perfused squid giant axons, *Proc. japan. Acad.*, 49 (1973) 218–222.
62. Yamagishi, S., Effect of intracellularly perfused Ca ions on the membrane properties of squid giant axons, *Proc. int. Union physiol. Sci.*, 13 (1977) 824.

Three dimensional observations of neurons and glia cells by means of the high voltage electron microscopy

KIYOSHI HAMA AND TOSHIO KOSAKA

Department of Fine Morphology, Institute of Medical Science, University of Tokyo, Minato-ku, Tokyo 108, Japan

The high voltage electron microscope has three major advantages: the higher penetration power of electrons, lower specimen damage, and higher resolution. Among these, the first property, the higher penetration power of electrons, has been most effectively utilized in the field of biology[1-4]. At 1000 KV, sections even up to 5 μm in thickness can be observed with reasonable resolution.

In conventional electron microscopy of thin specimens, the information gained about biological structures tends to be rather fragmental although the two dimensional resolution is extremely high. On the other hand, thick specimen observation by means of high voltage electron microscopy permits integration of information over the depth of the specimen. Thus, especially with the aid of stereoscopy, the biological fine structure can be observed as an entity. This feature of high voltage electron microscopy is well suited to neurological research since the neuron and glia cell have highly complicated configurations with elaborate fine processes. It is extremely difficult, if not impossible, to reconstruct the three dimensional image of a neuron or glia cell from thin section images even when using many serial sections. High voltage electron microscopic observations of relatively thick Golgi preparations can thus be expected to permit more accurate correlation between light microscope and conventional electron microscope images.

Goldfish olfactory bulb, rat cerebellum and rat cerebrum were fixed by perfusion with a fixative consisting of 4% paraformaldehyde, 0.8% glutaraldehyde and Millonig's phosphate buffer. The specimens were post-fixed with 1% OsO_4 in the same buffer for 1 hr, and then treated by a modified rapid Golgi method[5]. The impregnated materials were embedded in Epon after dehydration through an ethanol series. Thick sections (100 μm) were cut and examined under the light microscope. The impregnated cells were recorded using either camera lucida drawing or photomicrography. Serial sections (1–5 μm) of the recorded area were then cut and mounted on a copper grid. The specimens were examined under a high voltage electron microscope at 1000 KV. Stereo pair pictures were prepared by tilting the specimen stage by $\pm 8°$.

Fig. 1 shows a light micrograph of a pyramidal cell in the rat cerebrum as seen in a 100 μm thick Golgi preparation. The dendrites are covered by numerous spines, however, their detail cannot be resolved. Fig. 2 is a stereo pair of high voltage electron micrographs of 5 μm thick serial sections cut from the same specimen showing part of the basal dendrite which has slender tortuous spines. Some of the spines are over 5 μm long and less than 0.1 μm in diameter. They run in various directions, sometimes branch, and form bulbous terminals. The detail of the three dimensional organization of these slender spines on the basal dendrites of the pyramidal cells was first detected by high voltage electron microscopy of a thick Golgi preparation.

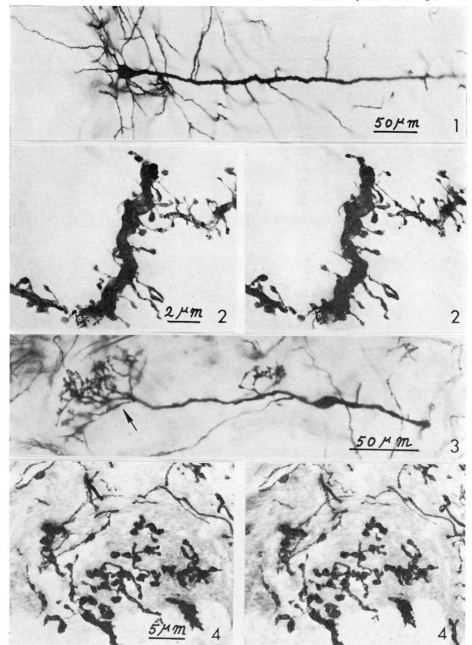

Fig. 1. Light micrograph of a pyramidal cell in the rat cerebrum (100 μm thick Golgi preparation.)
Fig. 2. A stereo pair showing spines on the basal dendrite of the pyramidal cell (Golgi preparation; 1000 KV electron micrographs).
Fig. 3. Light micrograph of a mitral cell in the goldfish olfactory bulb (100 μm thick Golgi preparation). The arrow indicates a glomerulus.
Fig. 4. A stereo pair of high voltage electron micrographs showing a glomerulus in the goldfish olfactory bulb.

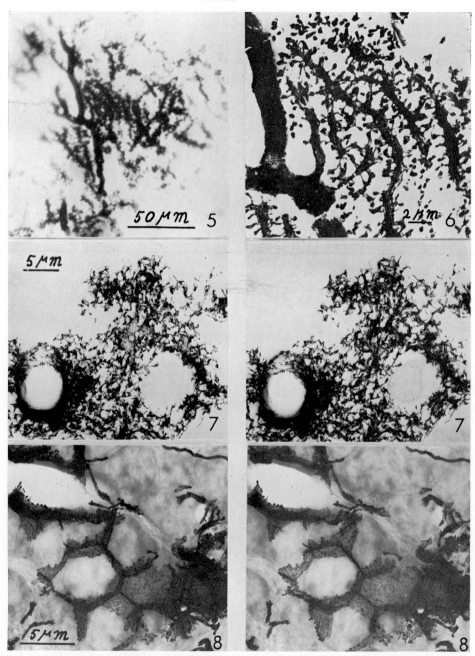

Fig. 5.   Light micrograph showing part of a Purkinje cell dendrite (5 μm thick Golgi preparation).
Fig. 6.   High voltage electron micrograph showing spines in the dendrites from the area shown in
Fig. 5.
Fig. 7.   A stereo pair of high voltage electron micrographs showing the sponge-like meshwork
formed by an astrocyte in the rat cerebrum.
Fig. 8.   A stereo pair showing lamellar astrocyte processes in the granular layer of the rat cerebellum.

Fig. 3 shows a light micrograph of a mitral cell in the goldfish olfactory bulb as seen in a 100 μm thick Epon section. The primary dendrite of the mitral cell branches to form several glomeruli (arrow). Fig. 4 is a stereo pair of high voltage electron micrographs of a glomerulus. The terminal branches in the glomerulus display many irregular varicosities and run a tortuous course. The primary afferent fibers from the olfactory epithelium can easily be distinguished from the mitral cell dendrites by their smaller size and smooth outlines.

The Purkinje cell of the cerebellum exhibits an enormous dendritic arborization which is well visualized by the Golgi impregnation method. Fig. 5 shows part of the dendritic branches as seen in a 2 μm thick Epon section mounted on a copper grid. The surface of the dendrites displays an irregular outline reflecting the spines attached to it. Fig. 6 is a high voltage electron micrograph of the area shown in Fig. 5. The dendrites are surrounded by numerous short spines about 1 μm long, which sprout in many directions from them. Each spine has a bulbous end and a thin stalk of less than 0.1 μm in diameter.

The configuration of the terminal arborization and shape of the spines seen in Golgi preparations have been used as criteria for the classification of neurons in the central nervous system. The fine structural details of the synapses as revealed by electron microscopy have also been used as criteria for identification of the type of neurons. However, it is difficult to correlate electron microscopic images with light microscopic images because of the thinness of the sections used in conventional electron microscopy. Moreover, it seems that accurate three dimensional reconstruction of the dendritic branches and spines is barely possible using thin serial sections due to the complexity and thinness of these structures as demonstrated in the present study. High voltage electron microscopic observations of thick Golgi preparations clearly provide detailed information on the three dimensional organization of the dendritic terminal arborization and spines of neurons in the central nervous system.

High voltage electron microscopy of thick Golgi preparations has also shown that astrocyte processes atenuate into thin lamellae and interpose between the neuronal elements constituting a sponge-like meshwork (Fig. 7). In the granular layer of the rat cerebellum, honeycomb-like compartments are formed by flattened lamellae of the astrocyte processes (Fig. 8). A nucleus or group of nculei of the granule cell are seen in the compartment.

The lamellar nature of the glial cell process has been pointed out by many investigators. However, its three dimensional organization was first demonstrated by high voltage electron microscope stereoscopy using thick Golgi preparations[4]. This finding was further confirmed by the present investigations.

REFERENCES

1. Cosslett, V.E., High voltage electron microscopy and its application in biology, *Phil. Trans. ryo. Soc. (Lond.) Ser. B Biol. Sci.*, 261 (1971) 35.
2. Hama, K. and Hirosawa, K., High voltage electron microscopy: A study of autoradiography, *J. Electron Microsc. (Tokyo)*, 126 (1977) 187.
3. Hama, K. and Porter, An application of high voltage electron microscopy to the study of biological materials. *J. Microscopic.* (1969), 8, 149.
4. Palay, V.C. and Palay, S.L., The form of velate astrocytes in the cerebellar cortex of monkey and rat: High voltage electron microscopy of rapid Golgi preparations, *Z. Anat. Entwickl.-Gesch.*, 138 (1972) 1.
5. Stell, W.K. and Lightfoot, D.O., Color-specific interconnections of cones and horizontal cells in the retina of the goldfish, *J. Comp. Neur.* (1975) 159, 473.

Kinetics of the inhibitory postsynaptic current in crayfish muscle

KAYOKO ONODERA AND AKIRA TAKEUCHI

Department of Physiology, School of Medicine, Juntendo University,
Bunkyo-ku, Tokyo 113, Japan

The kinetic properties of transmitter action have been most extensively studied at the excitatory synapses. However, relatively little is known about the time course of transmitter action at the inhibitory synapses. There are several difficulties in measuring the conductance changes produced by the transmitter, particularly at the inhibitory synapses. Among these difficulties are: a) the inhibitory postsynaptic current (IPSC) is usually small and it is necessary to record the IPSC at membrane potentials some distance from the resting potential; b) the inhibitory synapses are distributed diffusely over the cell surface or are located at points distant from the cell body where voltage-clamp is applied. In spite of these difficulties the IPSC has been recorded in several synapses: spinal motoneurons of the frog[2], *Onchidium* neurons[5] and *Aplysia* neurons[1].

Opener muscle of the claw dactylpodite in the crayfish was cannulated with a stainless steel wire of 70 μm diameter. This electrode was connected to the negative phase of a feedback amplifier and the membrane potential was voltage-clamped[6,7]. With this technique the space-clamp condition along the muscle fiber was usually satisfied. The inhibitory and excitatory axons were dissected at the melopodite and stimulated separately with a pair of silver electrodes. In some cases, dantrolene sodium was added to the solution to reduce the contraction. The experiments were performed at room temperature (23°C).

After cannulation with a longitudinal electrode, the membrane potential was clamped at the resting potential. Stimulation of the inhibitory nerve produced IPSC. The size and direction of the IPSC depended on the value of the resting potential. When the resting potential was relatively low, e.g. −60mV, the IPSC was outwardly directed, while if the resting potential was −70mV or more negative, the IPSC was almost zero or inwardly directed. The reversal potential was about −70 mV. The IPSC rose to a peak in 3 – 4 msec and thereafter decayed approximately exponentially, lasting for 30 – 40 msec. The time course of excitatory postsynaptic current (EPSC) recorded from the same muscle was short compared to that of IPSC, the peak time of EPSC being 1.5 – 2.0 msec and the total duration being less than 10 msec at 23°C. Therefore, the time course of IPSC was about five times longer than that of EPSC.

When the membrane was hyperpolarized the time course of IPSC became shorter, and it was prolonged in the case of depolarization[4,7]. When the time constant of the declining phase was measured, the time constant (τ) depended on the voltage (V) according to the relation $\tau = a \exp(AV)$, with $a = 18.6$ msec and $A = 0.0065$ mV^{-1}. The voltage dependence of the decay time constant was the reverse of that in frog end-plate and IPSC in *Aplysia*, but it was in the same direction as that of EPSC in the crayfish muscle[3,8]. This result suggests that the charge distribution in the transmitter-receptor complex is opposite in direction to those in frog end-plate and *Aplysia* ganglia.

There are several factors which change the time course of IPSC: for instance, temperature, pH and permeant foreign anions. When the temperature was changed between 12.5° C and 22.6° C the value of Q_{10} was 2.4. This value was the same as that observed in other synapses, including frog and toad end-plates and EPSC of the crayfish neuromuscular junction. Decrease in the pH of the bath solution also prolonged the time course of IPSC. When the pH was decreased from 7.2 to 5.5, the decay time constant increased by about 50%. In these cases the voltage dependence of the decay time constant was not changed. Increase in the pH to 9 caused no appreciable change in the time course.

A most remarkable change in the time course was observed when the chloride in the bath solution was replaced with iodide. The rise and fall of IPSC were prolonged in iodide solution; in particular the decay time constant was increased by a factor of 3. When chloride in the bath solution was replaced with bromide, the decay time constant increased by about 50%. In these cases the voltage dependence of the decay time constant was not changed. There are several possibilities that can account for the prolongation of the time course by foreign anions. Since these anions can permeate, iodide or bromide ions may enter the ion channels and affect the channel macromolecules, thereby changing the time course of conformational change of the ion channels. Another possibility is that foreign anions may affect the receptor molecules and change their binding and unbinding properties with respect to the transmitter.

When the peak amplitude of IPSC was measured at various membrane potentials, it varied almost linearly as the membrane was depolarized. However, when the membrane was hyperpolarized beyond the reversal potential, the amplitude deviated from linearity and became almost saturated at −100 mV or beyond. This non-linearity was not attributable to insufficient voltage-clamping, because the EPSC recorded from the same muscle fiber under the same clamping conditions was almost linear between −120 mV and 0 mV[8]. Although IPSC is carried by chloride, the non-linearity is not due to a change in the internal chloride concentration.

In the case of the inhibitory synapse, the principle may be the same as that in the excitatory synapse. However, there are some differences between IPSC and EPSC. For example, the inhibitory synaptic membrane or the anion channel may have a rectifying property. The effect of permeant anions on the time course of IPSC and the permeability changes of the ion channels may provide important information on the basic mechanism of ion permeation.

REFERENCES

1. Adams, D.J., Gage, P.W. and Hamill, O.P., Voltage sensitivity of inhibitory postsynaptic currents in *Aplysia* buccal ganglia, *Brain Research.*, 115 (1976) 506–511.
2. Araki, T. and Terzuolo, C.A., Membrane currents in spinal motoneurons associated with action potential and synaptic activity, *J. Neurophysiol.*, 25 (1962) 772–789.
3. Dudel, J., Nonlinear voltage dependence of excitatory synaptic current in crayfish muscle, *Pflügers Arch., ges. Physiol.*, 352 (1974) 227–241.
4. Dudel, J., Voltage dependence of amplitude and time course of inhibitory synaptic current in crayfish muscle, *Pflügers Arch. ges. Physiol.*, 371 (1977) 167–174.
5. Hagiwara, S. and Kusano, K., Synaptic inhibition in giant nerve cell of *Onchidium verruculatum, J. Neurophysiol.*, 24 (1961) 167–175.
6. Onodera, K. and Takeuchi, A., Ionic mechanism of the excitatory synaptic membrane of the crayfish neuromuscular junction, *J. Physiol. (Lond.)*, 252 (1975) 295–318.
7. Onodera, K. and Takeuchi, A., Inhibitory postsynaptic current in voltage-clamped crayfish muscle, *Nature (Lond.)*, 263 (1976) 153–154.
8. Onodera, K. and Takeuchi, A., Effects of membrane potential and temperature on the excitatory post-synaptic current in the crayfish muscle, *J. Physiol. (Lond.)*, 276 (1978) 183–192.

Dopamine release in reconstituted synapses from rat cerebrum

MINORU TAKEDA, RYO TANAKA* AND KUNIO KONNO

*Department of Biochemistry, School of Medicine, Showa University,
Shinagawa-ku, Tokyo 142, Japan*

The biochemical mechanism of transmitter release in the central nervous system is not well understood, partly because of difficulty in establishing suitable experimental systems. In general, it has been accepted that catecholamines are released from synaptic vesicles into the extracellular space without being liberated into the nerve terminal cytosol. Heuser and Reese[3] reported that the stimulus–coupled release of transmitter is through exocytosis, based on their morphological observations of the frog neuromuscular junction. If this were the case with the central nervous system, then an interaction between synaptic vesicle membrane and synaptic plasma membrane would be required for transmitter release. In order to test this, we attempted to establish an experimental system by reconstituting synaptic components isolated from rat cerebrum, and sought to characterize the effects of interaction between subsynaptosomal components on the release of [^{3}H]dopamine from preloaded plain synaptic vesicles.

Plain synaptic vesicle fractions were isolated from 25 male Sprague–Dawley rats according to the method of Kadota and Kadota[4] with a minor modification as described previously[7]. An electron microscopic picture of the vesicles is shown in Fig. 1a. The enzymological properties of this fraction were reported elsewhere[7,9]. The method of Abood *et al.*[1] was employed to prepare a synaptic membrane fraction from rat cerebrum; an electron micrograph of the preparation is shown in Fig. 1b. The specific activities of the enzymes were as follows: Na$^+$, K$^+$-dependent ATPase, 4.5; 5′-mononucleotidase, 2.1; Mg^{2+}–ATPase, 4.7; Ca^{2+}–ATPase, 4.5 μmol Pi/mg protein/30 min, at 37°. No activities of monoamine oxidase and succinate dehydrogenase were detected in the fraction. Synaptic junctions were isolated from rat cerebrum by the method of Cotman *et al.*[2] The final pellet was washed with 50 mM Tris, pH 7.4, and resuspended in the same buffer. An electron micrograph of the junction is shown in Fig. 1c. Myelin was prepared from rat cerebrum by the method of Norton and Poduslo[5]. Heavy microsomal fractions were isolated from rat brains as described elsewhere[6].

Plain synaptic vesicles (100 to 150 μg protein) were loaded at 25° for 5 min with [^{3}H]dopamine in the standard reaction medium containing 156 mM KCl, 5 mM Nacl, 10 mM Tris, pH 7.4, 2 mM MgCl$_2$, 0.2 mM CaCl$_2$, 2 mM ATP, and 10 μM (1 μCi) [^{3}H]dopamine in a final volume of 200 μl. After loading, a 50 μl suspension of subsynaptosomal fraction was added and mixed thoroughly, and incubation was continued for a further 5 min to examine the effects on radioactivity release from the vesicles. The reaction was terminated by the addition of 1.7 ml of ice-cold K, Na buffer[7]. The radioactivity in 150,000 $\times$ g pellets was measured. As a control system, 50 μl of 50 mM Tris, pH 7.4, was added instead of subsynaptosomal fraction to the reaction mixture to measure the total radioactivity incorporation into the plain synaptic vesicles during the entire

---

* Present address: Center for Brain Research, University of Rochester, Rochester, New York, U.S.A.

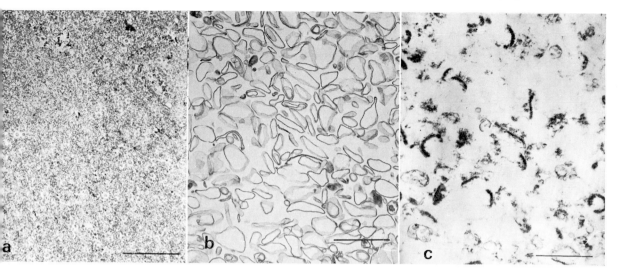

Fig. 1. Electron microscopic pictures of synaptic components. Specimens for microscopic examination were fixed in dilute Karnovsky solution, postfixed in 2% osmium tetroxide in cacodylate buffer, dehydrated in ethanol and embedded in Spurr's plastic mixture. a, Plain synaptic vesicle fraction; b, synaptic membrane; c, synaptic junction. The bar represents 1 μm.

incubation period. In order to examine [³H]dopamine binding to subsynaptosomal fractions, 50 μl aliquots of the fractions were incubated in the standard medium without vesicles for 5 min (subsynaptosomal fraction system). The degree of release is expressed as a percentage, defined by the following equation:

$$\text{Degree of release } (\%) = \left[100 - \left(\frac{\text{Experimental system (cpm)} - \text{Subsynaptosomal fraction system (cpm)}}{\text{Control system (cpm)}} \times 100 \right) \right]$$

When [³H]dopamine-loaded plain synaptic vesicles (120 μg protein) interacted with synaptic membranes (30 μg protein), approximately 50% of the incorporated radioactivity was found to be released. This membrane-dependent release was proportional to the amount of the added synaptic membrane protein (data not shown). Since EDTA markedly inhibited the radioactivity release, as illustrated in Fig. 2, divalent cations are required for release from the vesicles in the reconstituted system.

Several types of subsynaptosomal fractions were tested for their effects on the release (Fig. 3). Approximately 65% of incorporated radioactivity was released by synaptic junctions; and the value was twice that obtained in the presence of synaptic membranes. The biomolecules required for transmitter release are probably concentrated in the synaptic junction. The myelin sheath is not the site of transmitter release; indeed, the release effect of myelin was less than one–seventh of that of synaptic junctions. The heavy microsomal fraction, which is known to contain synaptic membranes[8], exerted the same effects as synaptic membranes. The amounts of [³H]dopamine bound to the same amount of protein of subsynaptosomal fractions do not differ much (Table 1). Consequently, the different effects of each subsynaptosomal fraction on radioactivity release were

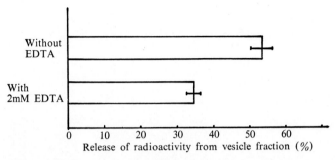

Fig. 2. Effects of EDTA on synaptic membrane-dependent [³H]dopamine release. EDTA was added to the incubation medium simultaneously with synaptic membrane in the releasing phase of the reaction.

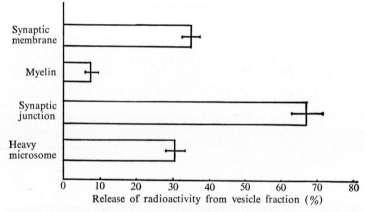

Fig. 3. Effects of subsynaptosomal fractions on [³H]dopamine release from the vesicles. The amounts of protein of added subsynaptosomal fractions were kept constant (18 μg/tube).

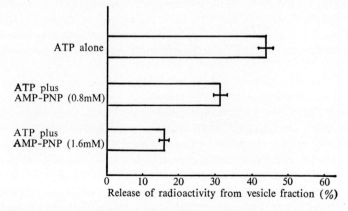

Fig. 4. Effects of AMP-PNP on the membrane-dependent release. Various concentrations of AMP-PNP were added to the reaction medium at the releasing phase of the reaction.

TABLE 1. Binding of [³H]dopamine to the subsynaptosomal fractions. Each subsynaptosomal fraction (26 μg protein) was incubated with [³H]dopamine in the standard reaction mixture for 5 min at 25°. After termination of the reaction, the fraction was precipitated by centrifugation at 150,000 $\times$ g for 45 min, and the radioactivity of the pellet was measured. Under the same conditions, the radioactivity incorporated in plain vesicles (150 μg protein) was approximately 9,800 cpm.

Subsynaptosomal fraction	Amounts of [³H]dopamine binding (cpm)
Synaptic membrane	3,218 ± 156
Synaptic junction	3,400 ± 157
Myelin	3,005 ± 135
Heavy microsomes	3,012 ± 133.

Values are averages ± S.E., $n = 7$.

not due to decrease in the [³H]dopamine concentration in the medium as a result of dopamine binding to subsynaptosomal fractions.

The addition of 1.6 mM adenyl imidodiphosphate (AMP-PNP) inhibited by 55% the radioactivity release from vesicle fraction (Fig. 4). Therefore, hydrolysis of adenosine triphosphate may well be involved in the release process of dopamine from vesicles upon interaction with synaptic membranes. Although ATP-hydrolyzing activity was found in our subsynaptosomal fractions[7,9], it has not yet been proved that the release process is coupled with an energy-consuming reaction.

REFERENCES

1. Abood, L.G., Hong, J.S., Takeda, F. and Tometsko, A.M., Preparation and characterization of calcium-binding and other hydrophobic proteins from synaptic membranes, *Biochim. Biophys. Acta,* 443 (1976) 412–427.
2. Cotman, C.W. and Taylor, D., Isolation and structural studies on synaptic complexes from rat brain, *J. Cell Biol.,* 55 (1972) 696–711.
3. Heuser, J.E. and Reese, T.S., Evidence for recycling of synaptic vesicle membrane during transmitter release at the frog neuromuscular junction, *J. Cell Biol.,* 57 (1973) 315–344.
4. Kadota, K. and Kadota, T., Isolation of coated vesicles, plain synaptic vesicles, and flocculent material from a crude synaptosome fraction of guinea-pig whole brain, *J. Cell Biol.,* 58 (1973) 135–151.
5. Norton, W.T. and Poduslo, S.E., Myelination in rat brain: Method of myelin isolation, *J. Neurochem.,* 21 (1973) 749–757.
6. Takeda, M. and Tanaka, R., Changes in nucleoside triphosphate sensitivity of bovine brain 5'-mononucleotidase by solubilization, *Fed. Proc.,* 34 (1975) 596.
7. Tanaka, R., Asaga, H. and Takeda, M., Nucleoside triphosphate and cation requirement for dopamine uptake by plain synaptic vesicles isolated from rat cerebrums, *Brain Research,* 115 (1976) 273–283.
8. Tanaka, R. and Strickland, K.P., Role of phospholipid in the activation of Na⁺, K⁺-activated adenosine triphosphatase of beef brain, *Arch. Biochim. Biophys.,* 111 (1965) 583–592.
9. Tanaka, R., Takeda, M. and Jaimovich, M., Characterization of ATPases of plain synaptic vesicle and coated vesicle fractions isolated from rat brains, *J. Biochem. (Tokyo),* 80 (1976) 831–837.

Acetylcholine synthesis in a stretch receptor cell of crayfish *in vivo*

HIROYUKI KOIKE AND KAZUKO TSUDA

Department of Neurophysiology, Tokyo Metropolitan Institute for Neurosciences, Fuchu, Tokyo 183, Japan

The crustacean stretch receptor cell contains acetylcholine (ACh) in the cell body[3], and also contains the ACh-synthesizing enzyme, choline acetyltransferase[4]. Its cholinergic synaptic nature has been investigated[1]. It seems likely the stretch receptor cell synthesizes the presumed transmitter substance (ACh) in the cell, as do other cholinergic neurons. We have attempted to confirm this by looking for radioactive ACh formation in the cell after injecting radioactive choline (a precursor of ACh) into a single stretch receptor cell of crayfish[6].

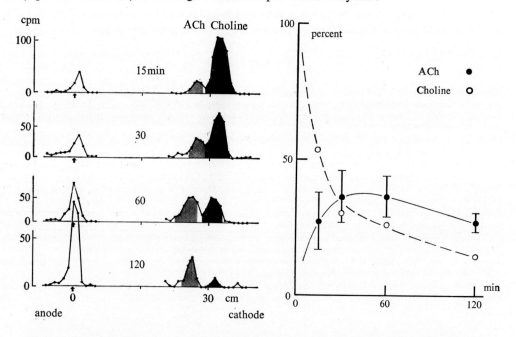

Fig. 1. Paper electrophoresis results from homogenates of 4 stretch receptor cells, cultured for 15 min to 2 hr after injection as indicated. The homogenates were applied at the upward arrows. The ordinates show the measured radioactivity in each 1 cm length of the paper. Cold choline and ACh were added as markers and were visualized by treatment with iodine vapor. Choline travelled about 30 cm and is indicated by dark shading. ACh was slightly less mobile and is indicated by light shading. *(left)*

Fig. 2. Time course of [³H]ACh formation (dots) in the stretch receptor cell following the injection, expressed as a percentage of the injected amount of [³H]choline. Each point is the mean of 3 to 10 experiments with the standard deviation. The remaining free [³H]choline in the cell is also plotted as open circles (mean only). *(right)*

36

[³H]Choline was injected into the cell by air pressure[5,6], and the cell was cultured for various periods at 15° C. Typical results from four experiments are shown in Fig. 1. The injected [³H] choline was converted to [³H] ACh and to non-charged substances in the cell. Although we did not analyze the latter materials, they are presumably phospholipids, as in the case of *Aplysia* cholinergic neuron[2]. The amounts of [³H]ACh formed after the injection are plotted in Fig. 2. The amount increased rapidly in the initial 15–30 min and then tended to saturate. After 1 hr, both [³H]ACh and [³H]choline decreased concomitant with an increase in the radioactivity of non-charged substances, as shown in Fig. 1 (120 min). The maximum amount of choline injected in this experiment corresponds to 6×10^{-13} mol, calculated from the specific radioactivity of the [³H]choline used. The conversion ratio to [³H]ACh was relatively constant for injection of amounts up to this level. The initial velocity of [³H]ACh formation corresponded to about 120% of the injected [³H]choline in 1 hr. Therefore ACh formation amounted to about 7×10^{-13} mol per hr in a stretch receptor cell.

REFERENCES

1. Barker, D.L., Herbert, E., Hildebrand, J.G. and Kravitz, E.A., Acetylcholine and lobster sensory neurones, *J. Physiol.*, 226 (1972) 205–296.
2. Eisenstadt, M.L. and Schwartz. J.H., Metabolism of acetylcholine in the nervous system of *Aplysia californica*, III. Studies of an identified cholinergic neuron, *J. gen. Physiol.*, 65 (1975) 293–313.
3. Florey. E. and Biederman. M.A., Studies on the distribution of factor I and acetylcholine in crustacean peripheral nerve, *J. gen. Physiol.*, 43 (1960) 509–522.
4. Hildebrand, J.G., Barker, D.L., Herbert, E. and Kravitz, E.A., Screening for neurotransmitters: A rapid radiochemical procedure, *J. Neurobiol.*, 2 (1971) 231–246.
5. Koike, H., Eisenstadt, M. and Schwartz, J.H., Axonal transport of newly synthesized acetylcholine in an identified neuron of *Aplysia*, *Brain Research*, 37 (1972) 152–159.
6. Koike, H. and Tsuda, K., Transmitter identification of crustacean sensory cells by means of intracellular injection of labelled precursors, *Proc. int. U. physiol. Sci.*, 11 (1974) 152.

Cholinergic agents and synaptic transmissions in the striatum

MASAHARU TAKAGI AND CHOSABURO YAMAMOTO

*Department of Physiology, University of Kanazawa Medical School,
Kanazawa, Ishikawa 920, Japan*

The striatum contains high concentrations of acetylcholine (ACh)[4], of choline acetylase[2] and of acetylcholinesterase[1]. Therefore, ACh has been assumed to function as a transmitter in the striatum[3,5]. However, the mode of action of ACh in the striatum is not clear. In the present experiments, the effects of ACh and carbamylcholine (CCh) on synaptic transmissions were studied both *in vitro* in thin sections of the striatum and *in vivo* in anesthetized animals.

For *in vitro* experiments, sections of 0.2 mm thickness were prepared from the anterior portion of the striatum of the rat by means of a Vibrotome. After incubation for more than 40 min, these sections were transferred one by one into an observation chamber, then stimulated with a bipolar silver electrode and potentials were recorded with glass pipette electrodes inserted into the tissue adjacent to the site of stimulation. ACh or CCh were administered electrophoretically or added to the perfusing medium at known concentrations. Details of procedures for the preparation of sections, incubation, and stimulation have been reported elsewhere[6].

For *in vivo* experiments, rats anesthetized with alphachloralose were clamped in a stereotaxic apparatus. Two- or three-barrel electrodes were used for recording electrical activity and for electrophoretic administration of chemicals. The striatum was stimulated with a bipolar electrode consisting of a pair of thin silver wires near the site of recording. The substantia nigra and the motor cortex were stimulated with a concentric electrode and a bipolar silver electrode, respectively.

In response to stimuli applied to striatal sections, two negative waves, N_1 and N_2, were recorded with latencies of about 0.5 and 3 msec, respectively (Fig. 1A, record 1). The N_1 and N_2 waves reflected summated action potentials elicited in striatal neurons directly and through synapses by electric pulses, respectively. Since atropine or tubocurarine did not suppress the N_2 wave appreciably, generation of this potential did not seem to be mediated by Ach. When Cch (more than 1 μM) or ACh (more than 20 μM) was added to the perfusing medium or administered electrophoretically, the N_2 wave was reversibly suppressed (Fig. 1A, record 2). This action of CCh was blocked by atropine (record 5) but not by tubocurarine. Single cell discharges superimposed on the N_2 wave were also suppressed by CCh. This means that CCh had a strong suppressing action on the synaptically induced firing of striatal neurons. On the other hand, CCh had a weak or negligible effect on the firing of striatal neurons induced by electrophoretic administration of glutamate. Only when CCh was administered at concentrations 10–100 times that needed to block synaptic activation of neurons were striatal cells excited consistently or changed in firing pattern.

In the experiments *in vivo*, observations obtained in *in vitro* experiments were confirmed and extended. A single stimulus delivered to the striatum induced a negative wave of about 10 msec duration (Fig. 1B, record 1). When CCh was administered electrophoretically, the negative wave was markedly depressed (record 2). Single cell discharges elicited by electric stimulation disappeared with a reduction of the negative wave. In contrast to this, firing induced by glutamate was

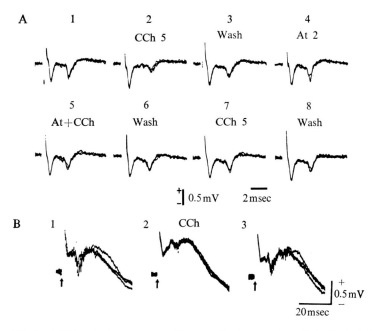

Fig. 1. A: Effects of CCh and atropineon the N_2 wave (*in vitro* experiment). 1, Control: 2, 3.5 min after perfusion with a medium containing CCh in 5 μM; 3, 5 min after washing the section with the standard medium: 4, 5 min after perfusion with a medium containing 2 μM atropine: 5, 4 min after perfusion with a medium containing 2 μM atropine and 5 μM CCh: 6, 7 min after washing: 7, 4 min after perfusion with a medium containing 5 μM CCh: 8, 5 min after washing.
B: Effects of CCh (*in vivo* experiment). CCh suppressed negative field potentials evoked by local striatal stimulation. 1, control: 2, 15 sec after CCh administration for 15 sec with a current of 80 nA: 3, recovery of field potentials 3 min after record 2 was taken.

not affected significantly by CCh. Stimuli applied to the cerebral cortex or the substantia nigra evoked firing of striatal neurons. Though CCh suppressed firing induced by stimulation to the cerebral cortex, it was without effect on the activation of striatal neurons elicited by substantia nigra stimulation.

In conclusion, cholinergic agents block synaptic transmissions in the striatum without causing any appreciable hyper- or depolarization in postsynaptic neurons.

REFERENCES

1. Burgen, A.S.V. and Chipman, L.M., Cholinesterase and succinic dehydrogenase in the central nervous system of the dog, *J. Physiol. (Lond.)*, 114 (1951) 296–305.
2. Hebb, C.O. and Silver, A., Choline acetylase in the central nervous system of man and some other mammals, *J. Physiol. (Lond.)*, 134 (1956) 718–728.
3. Herz, A. and Zieglgansberger, W., The influence of microelectrophoretically applied biogenic amines, cholinomimetics and procaine on synaptic excitation in the corpus striatum, *Int. J. Neuropharmacol.*, 7 (1968) 221–230.
4. MacIntosh, F.C., The distribution of acetylcholine in the peripheral and the central nervous system, *J. Physiol. (Lond.)*, 99 (1941) 436–442.
5. McLennan, H. and York, D.H., Cholinergic mechanisms in the caudate nucleus, *J. Physiol. (Lond.)*, 187 (1966) 163–175.
6. Yamamoto, C., Activation of hippocampal neurons by mossy fiber stimulation in the thin brain sections *in vitro*, *Exp. Brain Res.*, 14 (1972) 423–435.

Development of acetylcholine sensitivity in cultured embryonic chick atrium

KUNIHIKO OBATA AND MOMOKO OIDE

Department of Pharmacology, School of Medicine, Gunma University,
Maebashi, Gunma 371, Japan

Receptors are produced and distributed in the postsynaptic cells during the development of synaptic connections in both the central and peripheral nervous system. In skeletal muscle the appearance of acetylcholine (ACh) receptors precedes neuromuscular junction formation and the localization of the receptors is under the control of innervation and muscle activity[3]. Using 1- to 2- day culture of atrial cells, Fänge, Persson and Thesleff[2] have demonstrated cardio-inhibitory action of ACh only in chick embryos older than 6 days. Parasympathetic innervation occurs in the embryonic hearts at about 5 days old and an intimate relationship has been suggested between the development of ACh receptors and the innervation in the cardiac muscle.[4] To investigate the neural (neurotrophic) influence on induction of ACh receptors, we have examined the ACh sensitivity of cultured atrium and the effect of tissue extract.

ACh usually suppressed beating of the atrium excised from 6-day-old chick embryo, as reported previously,[2] but was definitely ineffective with 4-day-old atrium. The following experiments, therefore, were carried out on the 4-day-old embryo. Whole atria (not divided into the left and right sides) were placed in collagen-coated Petri dishes (Falcon, 3001) and cultured at 37°C with Eagle's MEM (Nissui Co.) containing fetal calf serum and chick serum (5% each by volume, both from Flow Labs.). Crude extracts were obtained from the spinal cord, liver and whole body of 6-, 8-, 10- and 12-dayold embryos and added to the medium at concentrations of 0.6–2.0 mg protein/ml.

After incubation for 2 hr to 6 days, the culture was mounted on the stage of an inverted microscope (Nikon, MTD), kept at a constant temperature of 37°C and superfused continuously with MEM (without sera) at a rate of 0.5 ml/min (volume of the bath, 1 ml). Beating was counted with a stopwatch or recorded with an ink recorder via a TV camera (Ikegami, CTC6000) and a phototransistor device. ACh was supplied to the bath. An atrium was judged to be "sensitive" to ACh when it stopped beating at 0.5 mM. It resumed beating after several minutes of perfusion without ACh. Atropine antagonized ACh immediately. "Insensitive" atria were also insensitive to 5.0 mM ACh. Thus, the difference was quite clear-cut. The experiments were performed under sterile conditions and tests on the same culture were repeated on different days.

As shown in Table 1, ACh sensitivity was very low even after 2 days in culture, but increased markedly thereafter. Embryo extracts significantly facilitated the increase in ACh–sensitive atria. There was no noticeable difference between the spinal cord and others and between embryos of different age as sources of the extract, so the results are arranged according to the presence or absence of the extract in Table 1. ACh–sensitive atria remained so when the culture was maintained for a few days in the absence of the extract.

Beating rates decreased gradually with culture age but were not affected by the extracts (Table 1). The tissue became flattened and fibroblasts migrated out in culture, but the general

TABLE 1.   Beating rate and acetylcholine (ACh) sensitivity of embryonic chick atrium cultured with or without embryo extract (0.6–2.0 mg protein/m*l*).

Culture age	Extract in medium	No. of atria	Beating rate (beats/min)	ACh sensitivity[†] (%)
2–10 hr	(+)	11	112 ± 27[†2]	0
2 days	(−)	3	121 ± 1	0
	(+)	24	119 ± 27	4.2
3	(−)	11	104 ± 35	18.2
	(+)	28	99 ± 28	64.3
4	(−)	17	90 ± 46	53.0
	(+)	23	95 ± 38	78.3

[†] Percentage of atria which stopped beating in the presence of 0.5 mM ACh.   [†2]Mean ± S.D.

TABLE 2.   Total protein content and acetylcholinesterase (AChE) activity of embryonic chick atrium before and after organ culture for 3–4 days with or without embryo extract (0.26–0.32 mg protein/m*l*).

Culture age (days)	Extract in medium	Protein content (μg/atrium)	AChE activity [†] (nmol thiocholine formed/ min/mg protein)
0		8.8 (1)	0.4 ± 0.4 (3)
3–4	(−)	13.3 (1)	7.5 ± 1.2 (2)
	(+)	13.3 ± 0.9 (2)	8.4 ± 3.4 (4)

[†] Determination was done with pooled samples of 8 atria. Number of determinations in parentheses. Values are mean ± S. D.

appearance and total protein content in an atrium (Table 2) did not change in the presence of the extract. The activity of acetylcholinesterase (AChE) increased markedly after 3 days of culture (Table 2). AChE activity in chick atria increases with embryonic age and the value for 3-day culture corresponds to that for a 10-day-old embryo *in ovo*. The activity was not affected by the extracts.

In conclusion, ACh sensitivity in embryonic chick atria appeared after 2–4 days of organ culture, and tissue extract facilitated the development of ACh sensitivity without any effect on growth, beating or AChE activity. The effect was not specific to the nervous tissue extract. The culture medium contained chick serum because its removal impeded the survival of the atria. As ACh-sensitive atria were found in the culture without tissue extract, it is possible that the chick serum itself might promote the appearance of ACh receptors. Further investigations are required to elucidate the mechanism of receptor induction in the cardiac muscle.

REFERENCES

1. Ellman, G.L., Courtney, D., Andres, V. Jr. and Featherstone, R.M., A new and rapid colorimetric determination of acetylcholinesterase activity, *Biochem. Pharmacol.*, 7 (1961) 88–95.
2. Fänge, R., Persson, H. and Thesleff, S., Electrophysiologic and pharmacological observation on trypsin-disintegrated embryonic chick hearts cultured in vitro, *Acta physiol. scand.*, 38 (1956) 173–183.
3. Rosenthal, J., Trophic interactions of neurons. In J. M. Brookhart *et al.* (Eds.), *Handbook of Physiology, Section 1, The Nervous System*, Vol. I, American Physiological Society, Bethesda, 1977, pp. 775–801.
4. Pappano, A. J., Ontogenic development of autonomic neuroeffector transmission and transmitter reactivity in embryonic and fetal hearts, *Pharmacol. Rev.*, 29 (1977) 3–33.

The GABA receptor and GABA-induced anion permeability in mammalian primary afferent neurons

SYOGORO NISHI AND HIDEHO HIGASHI

Department of Physiology, School of Medicine, Kurume University,
Kurume, Fukuoka 830, Japan

Evidence has been accumulated to suggest that γ-aminobutyric acid (GABA) is the transmitter mediating presynaptic inhibition. Recent studies have revealed that GABA also depolarizes the somata of primary afferent neurons and autonomic ganglia. Nishi *et al.*[2], using bullfrog spinal ganglion cells, found that GABA was the most effective depolarizing substance among its closely related compounds, and that the GABA-induced depolarization was due to an increase in chloride conductance of the cell membrane. Their findings and also those of others[1] suggested that the cell-body of primary afferent neurons is endowed with GABA receptors which may be similar, if not identical, to the ones at the afferent terminals. The present study is concerned with the specificity of the GABA receptor on mammalian primary afferent neurons, and also the ionic mechanism underlying the GABA depolarization of these neurons.

Cats were anesthetized with α-chloralose and the L-7 or S-1 spinal ganglion was carefully excised with its attached dorsal rootlet. The ganglion preparation was superfused with a modified Krebs solution gassed with 95% O_2 and 5% CO_2 at 37°C. Cells were impaled with glass microelectrodes filled with 2 M potassium citrate and having tip resistances of 20 to 40 MΩ. GABA was applied either by superfusion as an addition to the superfusion solution or by iontophoresis. The electrodes used for iontophoresis had resistances of 60 to 100 MΩ and were filled with 1 M GABA adjusted to pH 4.5. During the iontophoresis experiments, a sufficient bias voltage was applied to the GABA-containing electrode to prevent continuous leakage onto the cell and possible desensitization. Extracellular substitution for anions or cations was performed isoosmotically. The modified Krebs solution had the following composition (in mM): NaCl, 117; KCl, 4.7; $CaCl_2$, 2.5; $MgCl_2$, 1.2; NaH_2PO_4, 1.2; $NaHCO_3$, 25; glucose, 11.5.

GABA in concentrations greater than 1×10^{-4} M caused a slow depolarization of the ganglion cell membrane. The GABA depolarization was associated with a reduction in membrane resistance as indicated by a decreased amplitude of the simultaneously recorded electrotonic potentials. Even when the depolarization by GABA was nullified by delivering a continuous inward current across the cell membrane through the recording electrode, there was a definite reduction in membrane resistance which amounted 10 to 40% of the control. This suggests that the interaction of GABA with its receptor causes an increased membrane conductance for certain ions.

The membrane currents elicited by the compounds structurally related to GABA were compared with the GABA-induced current in the same cells. Of the 15 compounds tested, GABA was found to be the most potent. Some general principles may be derived from the data with respect to the chemical structure required to activate the GABA receptor, as follows. (1) The distance between the external amino-N and the carboxyl-C is very critical; for example, reduction of only one carbon between the terminals eliminates the depolarizing action. (2) The terminal amino and carboxyl groups are essential for combination with the GABA receptor; substitution of either group with a different one abolishes the depolarizing activity. (3) Substitutions on the carbon chain of GABA invariably reduces the depolarizing action; it is evident therefore that a terminal amino and carboxylmoiety must be separated by three unsubstituted methylene groups to achieve optimum GABA-like activity.

A detailed dose-response relationship was obtained for the response to GABA as a basis for determining the kinetics of the GABA-GABA receptor interaction. Analysis of data from the superfusion experiments suggested that at least two molecules of GABA are required to activate the GABA receptor. This estimate is in agreement with the results of Takeuchi and Takeuchi[3,4] who used a similar technique to estimate the cooperativity of GABA for its receptor at the crayfish neuromuscular junction. However, when GABA was applied iontophoretically the relationship between the GABA-induced currents and iontophoretic current intensities indicated that three rather than two GABA molecules react with the receptor. It is difficult at present to determine which estimate (two or three) is the essential number for cooperativity. Analysis of dose-response curves in the presence of bicuculline or picrotoxin (10^{-7}–10^{-5} M) suggested that both these compounds act as non-competitive antagonists in depressing the membrane current generated by activation of the GABA receptor. This may indicate that the antagonists combine at a site different from the recognition site, i.e., an allosteric site, and thereby reduce the necessary combination of GABA with the recognition site, and this inhibits the activation process.

The GABA depolarization was reversed in polarity at approximately -25 mV; the mean reversal level in 23 neurons was -23.5 ± 6.1 mV (S.E.). Replacement of external sodium with Tris or choline, removal of external potassium or elevation of external potassium to 10 mM, did not affect the reversal level (E_{GABA}). Intracellular injection of 11 different anions including ClO_3^- and those smaller in hydrated size than ClO_3^- greatly augmented the GABA response and shifted the E_{GABA} value to a more positive level. On the other hand, injection of cations or 8 larger anions including BrO_3^- did not affect the amplitude, time course or equilibrium potential of the GABA response. When the NaCl of the perfusion solution was replaced stepwise with sucrose, there was a shift in E_{GABA} dependent on the external chloride concentration. Plots of E_{GABA} versus external chloride concentration yielded a line with a slope of approximately 59 mV for 10-fold change in external chloride concentration. The above results indicate that the ionic mechanism whereby GABA produces an increased conductance in cat primary afferent somata involves primarily chloride ions and that the activated GABA receptor membrane becomes permeable to anions having a hydrated size equal to or less than that of ClO_3^-, 5.7 Å. If it is assumed that the chloride equilibrium potential is equal to E_{GABA}, then the intracellular chloride concentration would appear to be 53 mM. This relatively high chloride concentration could be explained only by a metabolically dependent, inwardly directed chloride pump, which must be present in these neurons.

REFERENCES

1. Feltz, P. and Rasminsky, M., A model for the mode of action of GABA on primary afferent terminals: Depolarizing effects of GABA applied iontophoretically to neurons of mammalian dorsal root ganglia, *Neuropharmacology*, 13 (1974) 553–563.
2. Nishi, S., Minota, S. and Karczmar, A.G., Primary afferent neurons: the ionic mechanism of GABA-mediated depolarization, *Neuropharmacology*, 13, (1974) 215–219.
3. Takeuchi, A. and Takeuchi, N., Anion permeability of the inhibitory post-synaptic membrane of the crayfish neuromuscular junction, *J. Physiol. (Lond.)*, 191 (1967) 575–590.
4. Takeuchi, A. and Takeuchi, N., A study of the action of picrotoxin on the inhibitory neuromuscular junction of the crayfish, *J. Physiol. (Lond.)*, 205 (1969) 377–391.

Calcium measurement in axons with a fluorescent probe

KATSUO AIZAWA AND SHIZUKO IWASAKI

Department of Physiology, Tokyo Medical College,
Shinjuku-ku, Tokyo 160, Japan

The important role of calcium ions in the functions of various membranes, including excitable ones, has been known for many years. Reviews have been published on excitable membranes by Tobias[4] and Baker.[2] In the present work, changes in the amount of calcium bound to the axonal membrane of the crayfish were detected by means of a fluorescent probe. It has been found that the complex [mitochondrial membrane–Ca–chlorotetracycline] emits characteristic fluorescence.[3] In order to obtain information about calcium ions at the neural membrane of the crayfish, chlorotetracycline (CTC) was adopted as a fluorescent probe. Emission from the complex [axonal membrane–Ca–CTC] was detected with a high speed micro-fluorospectrometer devised by Aizawa *et al.*[1] Excitation light was derived from a high-voltage xenon lamp (Xe), as shown in Fig. 1. After passage through a monochromater (MC), excited light at 385 nm (16 μm in diameter in the present experiment) was applied to the sample (S) and its emission was dispersed by a polychromater (PC) and projected on a silicon target visicon tube (V). High-speed detection (32.8 msec) data on the emission were stored at A. The emission from the medium in which CTC and calcium ions were present was stored at B, and A minus B was taken as the sample emission.

The abdominal nerve cord between the 2nd and 3rd ganglion of a crayfish was mounted on slide glass and immersed in modified Harreveld solution (NaCl 205 mM, KCl 5.4 mM, CaCl$_2$ 1 mM, MgCl$_2$ 2.6 mM, EGTA 1 mM, HEPES 4 mM, pH 7.4). The emission from the 16 μm spot was detected at the nerve surface in a solution containing 1 mM CTC (Fig. 2 A). With excitation at 385 nm, the emission showed a maximum at 504 nm. In this [axon–Ca–CTC] system, the emission maximum shifted to 515 nm when medium [Ca^{++}] was increased from 1.4×10^{-5} M to 1.1×10^{-2} M (Fig. 2 B). Taking the integrated emission from 518 to 536 nm as the intensity (striped area in Fig. 2 B), it increased with calcium ion concentration, as shown in Figs. 2 and 3 A. The log intensities are plotted against log concentration of [Ca^{++}] of the medium in Fig. 3 B. The intensity increased with calcium concentration at levels over 1×10^{-6} M. Since [Ca–CTC] emission is subtracted by memory B, this increase in the emission intensity is entirely attributable to the increase of calcium ions associated with the axonal membrane and bound to CTC. In other words, the intensity is a measure of the amount of calcium ions in the [axon–Ca–CTC] system.

When the K ion concentration of the medium was raised to 100 mM in medium containing 3 mM CaCl$_2$, the emission intensity decreased, indicating a significant decrease of calcium ions on the axon membrane. The recovery was not complete in some cases. Since an increase of potassium concentration depolarizes the axon membrane, the decrease in membrane calcium concentration in the presence of high potassium levels seems to endorse the view of Tobias[4] that calcium ions move out of the membrane in advance of initiation of membrane excitation.

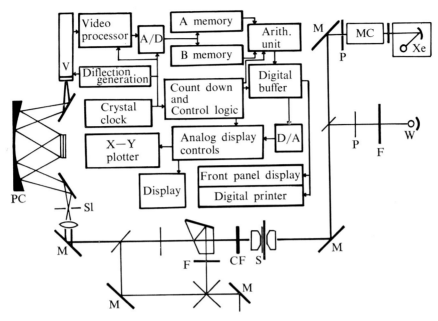

Fig. 1. Diagram of the high-speed fluoromicrospectrometer. Monochromatic light was passed through a pin hole able to produce a spot on the sample (S) as small as 1 μm. The emission from the sample (S) as small as 1 μm. The emission from the sample was dispersed by a polychromater to project on a visicon tube. The sweep time on the visicon surface was 32.8 msec. Several to 100 sweeps were performed to reduce the signal/noise ratio in the present experiments.

Xe, Xenon lamp; MC, monochromater; M, mirror; P, pin hole; F, filter; W, tungsten lamp; S, sample; CF, cut filter; Sl, slit; PC, polychromater; V, visicon tube; A, A memory; B, B memory.

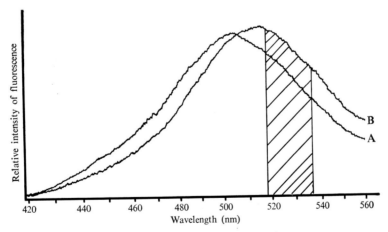

Fig. 2. Emission shift by calcium ions in the axon of the crayfish.

A: In medium containing 1mM CTC with excitation at 385 nm the emission peak was 504 nm when [Ca^{++}] was 1.4×10^{-5} M.

B: It shifted to 515 nm when [Ca^{++}] was increased to 1.1×10^{-2} M.

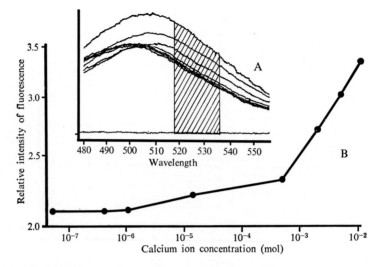

Fig. 3.   Emission intensity on the crayfish axon membrane *vs.* [Ca^{++}].
A (Inset): A red shift in emission was apparent when [Ca^{++}] was over 1.4×10^{-5} M. The emission increased with [Ca^{++}].
B: The integrated intensities at 518–536 nm (striped area in the inset, ordinate) were plotted *vs.* Ca ion concentration of the medium (abscissa).

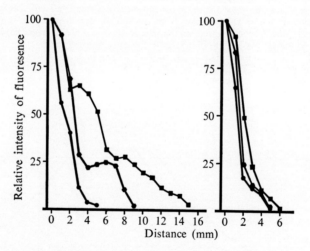

Fig. 4.   Axonal transport of the emission.
Left: The intensity dependent on [Ca^{++}] was plotted along the crayfish neuron. CTC-containing solution was applied at 0 mm. The emission was measured 30 min (circle), 60 min (hexagon), and 90 min (square) after application of CTC. Each plot is from one nerve cord which was dried on the slide glass to measure the emission.
Right: Emission intensity along the axon length as above; however, the axon was previously immersed in medium containing 0.1 mM colchicine.

When the cut end of the central part of the axon was immersed in standard solution containing 1 mM CTC, transportation of the fluorescence dependent on calcium was detected moving along the axon at a velocity of 0.17 mm/min (Fig. 4, left). On application of 0.1 mM colchicine, no detectable fluorescence was observed at the peripheral part of the axon (Fig. 4, right). It can be inferred that the complex [neural substance (possibly protein)–Ca–CTC] can be transported along the axon by a system which is blocked by colchicine.

The present experiments clearly show that chlorotetracyclin emits characteristic fluorescence in combination with calcium ions and the axon of crayfish, and that this increases with the calcium ion concentration of the medium. Calcium-dependent emission was also detected along the axon length, suggesting axonal transport of neural substance. This fluorescent probe, chlorotetracyclin, should facilitate further analytical studies on the role of calcium ions in excitable tissue.

REFERENCES

1. Aizawa, K. and O'hata, S., Analysis of intracellular substance by high speed micro-fluorospectrometer, *Proc. Japan. Biophys. Soc.*, 14 (1975) 60 (in Japanese).
2. Baker, P. F., Transport and metabolism of calcium ions in nerve, *Progr. Biophys. mol. Biol.*, 24 (1972) 177–223.
3. Caswell, A.H., The migration of divalent cations in mitochondria visualized by fluorescent probe, *J. Memb. Biol.*, 7 (1972) 345–364.
4. Tobias, J.M., A chemically specified molecular mechanism underlying excitation in nerve: A hypothesis, *Nature (Lond.)*, 203 (1964) 13–17.

A study of the mechanism of synaptogenesis in the inner ear and cerebellar cortex of chick embryo through chronic treatment and immunocyochemistry with β-bungarotoxin

NOBUTAKA HIROKAWA AND JUNNOSUKE NAKAI

Department of Anatomy, Faculty of Medicine, University of Tokyo,
Bunkyo-ku, Tokyo 113, Japan

One of the most characteristic features of the nervous system is the high degree of precision with which nerve cells are connected to each other and to the peripheral target cells, such as receptor cells and skeletal muscles. The developing nerve cell recognizes its target cell and makes synaptic contact with a certain area of the target cell. At most synaptic regions the presynatpic elements show presynaptic membrane specializations with associated vesicles and postsynaptic elements represent postsynaptic membrane specializations. The precise mechanisms of synaptogenesis are, however, largely unknown. In the present study we have attempted to investigate the mechanism of synaptogenesis between hair cells and dendrites of acoustic ganglion cells in the inner ear and between parallel fibers and dendritic spines of Purkinje cells in the cerebellar cortex, with special reference to the problems of whether target cells (hair cells) are able to develop synaptic specializations (synaptic bodies and presynaptic membrane specializations) without contact with growing nerve tips (dendrites of acoustic ganglion cells) and whether the growing nerve tips (parallel fibers) are able to differentiate synaptic specializations (presynatpic vesicular grids composed of presynaptic dense projections and associated vesicles) in the absence of the target cells (Purkinje cells).

The present author's previous study demonstrated that β-bungarotoxin (β-BT) has cytotoxic effects on specific nerve cells upon chronic treatment in chick embryos, and the affected nerve cells were found to have binding sites for β-BT through immunocytochemistry using horseradish peroxidase-labeled anti β-BT guinea-pig IgG[5]. β-BT has thus been proved to be an effective chemical denervator in developmental studies[5].

Forty μg of β-BT was injected into yolk sacs of chick embryos at 3-day intervals beginning on the 4th day of incubation. The inner ears and cerebellar cortices of the treated embryos and control embryos were observed electron microscopically at various stages in the present study.[3,4,6] It was demonstrated that the neurons affected by β-BT were acoustic ganglion cells in the inner ears and Purkinje cells in the cerebellar cortices of the chick embryos by a direct immunocytochemical method using HRP-labeled anti β-BT IgG.[5,6]

Inner Ear

In a normal developmental study[4] synaptic bodies associated with presynaptic membrane specializations are first observed in the differentiating hair cells on the 10th day and about either supporting cells or afferent nerve processes where slight membrane thickenings are occasionally found. Thus the primary event initiating the formation of a synapse is the differentiation of synaptic bodies with presynaptic specializations. It is important to note that virgin synaptic bodies

48

associated with presynaptic membrane thickenings but not in contact with nerve processes are present at the time synaptogenesis is first recognized, and are often still present at the 14th day, while almost all synaptic bodies associated with presynaptic specializations are in contact with afferent nerve tips at the 21st day. In the β-BT-treated embryos most of the acoustic ganglion cells have degenerated and disappeared by the 14th day, and the majority of the hair cells lack synaptic contacts with nerve terminals, but their presynaptic specializations remain intact and show evidence of continuing differentiation till the 21st day.[3] These results suggest that the precise location of synaptic sites on hair cells is determined by the hair cells themselves. The synaptic bodies and presynaptic specializations are able to differentiate even when they cannot make synaptic contact with afferent nerve processes.

Cerebellar cortex

The cerebella of β-BT-treated chick embryos are markedly reduced in size and most of the Purkinje cells as well as nerve fibers in the white matter disappear from the 18th day to the 21st day of incubation. At the 21st day, despite the absence of the bulk of the Purkinje cells, the majority of the inner granule cells of treated cerebellar cortices are developed well, as in the case of the controls. In the molecular layer some of the parallel fibers representing presynatic vesicular grids make synaptic contact with stellate cells and dendritic spines of the few surviving Purkinje cells. On the other hand, in most of the molecular layer, there are neither dendrites of Purkinje cells, nor parallel fibers displaying presynaptic vesicular grids devoid of contact with post synaptic elements. Most of the molecular layers are occupied by parallel fibers of rather constant diameter, which contain occasional accumulations of vesicles, but never display presynaptic dense projections. In the control cerebellar cortices, however, synaptogenesis between dendritic spines of Purkinje cells and parallel fibers is most marked on the 21st day and numerous synapses are observed in the molecular layer. The present study[6] suggests that parallel fibers may be able to represent only accumulations of vesicles but may not be able to develop completely the presynaptic vesicular grids associated with presynaptic dense projections devoid of contact with target cells.

In the lateral line organs of salamander, in spite of dissection of afferent nerves at the early developmental stages, hair cells can develop fully and grow synaptic bodies with presynaptic specializations.[7] In the agranular cerebellar cortices induced by mutation[2] and under various experimental conditions[1] Purkinje dendritic spines are able to develop postsynaptic specializations despite the absence of the presynaptic elements. Thus in many synapses, the synaptic specializations of target cells (defined only as cells towards which the nerve processes grow), which are presynaptic specializations in the hair cells of the inner ears[3,4] and lateral line organs[7], but postsynaptic specializations of dendritic spines of Purkinje cells[1,2], are evolved in the absence of growing nerve tips. In this way, during normal synaptogenesis the synaptic sites of the target cells may develop first and then the growing nerve processes seek out and recognize the preexisting synaptic specializations to establish final synaptic contacts. As shown in the present study, the growing nerve tips may be able to completely differentiate their synaptic specializations, which are the presynaptic vesicular grids of the parallel fibers in the cerebella, only after they have touched target cells.

REFERENCES

1. Hirano, A., Dembitzer, H.M. and Jones, M., An electron microscopic study of cycasin-induced cerebellar alteration, *J. Neuropath. exp. Neur.*, 31 (1972) 113–125.
2. Hirano, A., and Dembitzer, H.M., Cerebellar alterations in the weaver mouse, *J. Cell Biol.*, 56 (1973) 478–486.
3. Hirokawa, N., Disappearance of afferent and efferent nerve terminals in the inner ear of the chick embryo after chronic treatment with β-bungarotoxin, *J. Cell Biol.*, 73 (1977) 27–46.
4. Hirokawa, N., Synaptogenesis in the basilar papilla of the chick, *J. Neurocytol.*, 7 (1978) 283–300.
5. Hirokawa, N., Characterization of various nervous tissues of the chick embryos through responses to chronic application and immunocytochemistry of β-bungarotoxin, *J. Comp. Neurol.*, (1978) (in press).
6. Hirokawa, N., A study of the synaptogenesis in the cerebellar cortex through chronic treatment and immunocytochemistry of β-bungarotoxin, (1978) (manuscript in preparation).
7. Jorgensen, J.M. and Flock, Å., Non-innervated sense organs of the lateral line: Development in the regenerating tail of the salamander *Ambystoma mexicanum*, *J. Neurocytol.*, 5 (1976) 33–41.
8. Nakai, J. and Kawasaki, Y., Studies on the mechanism determining the course of nerve fibers in tissue culture, *Z. Zellforsch.*, 51 (1959) 108–122.

Interpeduncular nucleus: multiple innervation by fibers of the fasciculus retroflexus Meynerti

KIYOSHI KATAOKA[*1], KOSAKU SUNAYASHIKI[*1], CHIYE NAKATA[*1],
HIROKI YOSHIMI[*2], SHIGERU MATSUKURA[*2], AND YASUO IMURA[*2]

[*1] *Department of Physiology, Ehime University School of Medicine, Onsen-gun, Ehime 791 – 02, Japan*
[*2] *Department of Internal Medicine, Kobe University School of Medicine, Ikuta-ku, Kobe 650, Japan*

The interpeduncular nucleus receives afferent inputs principally from the habenular nuclei. The habenulo-interpeduncular tract, the fasciculus retroflexus Meynerti, may be composed of fibers of at least two different types with respect to transmitter substance contained, viz. acetylcholine[1,3,4,5,6,8] or substance P[2,9]. On the other hand, our recent findings on the content of β-endorphin, an analgesic endogenous cerebral peptide[7,10], in discrete brain areas of the Japanese monkey revealed that, although large amounts were present in the pituitary gland, insofar as the brain regions examined were concerned and the present antiserum specimen was used for the assay, the interpeduncular nucleus contained the greatest amount of immunoreactive β-endorphin (in preparation). This led us to analyze the origin of the interpeduncular β-endorphin. We now report that the fibers, at least in part, of the fasciculus retroflexus Meynerti contain immunoreactive β-endorphin.

Bilateral electrolytical lesions were formed in the habenula of male rats under Nembutal anesthesia. After allowing survival for one week in good condition, the operated animals were decapitated after ether anesthesia. The whole brains were rapidly removed and the interpeduncular nucleus as well as the head of the caudatoputamen were dissected, weighed and immediately frozen in liquid nitrogen. The portions of the brains containing the lesions were immersed in 10% formaldehyde and processed for histological evaluation of lesion placement.

Radioimmunoassay for β-endorphin of the dissected tissues was carried out as described previously.[11] Since the serum showed a 5% crossreactivity with β-lipotropin, prior fractionation of the extract on a Sephadex G-50 column was performed in some experiments. Although the values presented were referred to as β-endorphin content, some contribution from β-lipotropin was highly probable.

As shown in Fig. 1, the β-endorphin content of the interpeduncular nucleus after habenular lesion was found to be marked and significant, with decrement related to the relative success of lesion placement. This result indicates that most of the β-endorphin in the interpeduncular nucleus is present in axons and nerve terminals originating from the habenula. To provide evidence that the effect is specific to the interpeduncular nucleus, the β-endorphin content in the head of the caudatoputamen was also analyzed. There was no significant alteration by the habenular lesion. Thus, the present findings for the fasciculus retroflexus Meynerti may be the first demonstration of the efferent fiber connection of central β-endorphin neurons.

Based on the present data, together with earlier findings on the cholinergic nature as well as content of substance P, the complexity of the fibers in the fasciculus retroflexus should be emphasized. It represents a subject for further analysis, including the question of whether this complexity reflects a real selectivity of chemical transmission in the respective fibers.

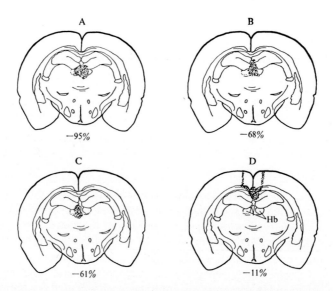

Fig. 1.   Four of the rat brains used for β-endorphin assay: individual habenular lesions (shaded portions) in frontal sections. A, Almost complete destruction of the habenula; B and C, the habenula partially escaped being damaged; D, the habenula was almost unaffected. The values preceded by minus signs indicate the percentage decrease in immunoreactive β-endorphin in the interpeduncular nucleus compared to the controls (193 $\pm$ 21 pg/mg tissue, $N = 10$). Hb, Habenula.

REFERENCES

1. Hattori, T., McGeer, E.G., Singh, V.K. and McGeer, P.L., Cholinergic synapse of the interpeduncular nucleus, *Exp. Neurol.*, 55 (1977) 666–679.
2. Hökfelt, T., Johansson, O., Kellerth, J.O., Ljungdahl, Å., Nilsson, G., Nygårds, A. and Pernow, B., Immuno-histochemical distribution of substance P. In U.S. von Euler and B. Pernow (Eds.) *Substance P*, Raven Press, New York, 1976, pp. 117–145.
3. Kataoka, K., Nakamura, Y. and Hassler, R., Habenulo-interpeduncular tract. A possible cholinergic neuron in rat brain, *Brain Research*, 62 (1973) 264–267.
4. Kataoka, K., Sorimachi, M., Okuno, S. and Mizuno, N., Cholinergic and GABAergic fibers in the stria medullaris of the rabbit, *Brain Res. Bull.*, 2 (1977) 461–464.
5. Kuhar, M.J., DeHaven, R.N., Yamamura, H.I., Rommelspacker, H. and Simon, J.R., Further evidence for cholinergic habenulo-interpeduncular neurons: pharmacologic and functional characteristics, *Brain Research*, 97 (1975) 265–275.
6. Léránth, C.S., Brownstein, M., Záborszky, L., Járányi, Z.S. and Palkovits, M., Morphological and biochemical changes in the rat interpeduncular nucleus following the transection of the habenulo-interpeduncular tract, *Brain Research*, 99 (1975) 124–128.
7. Ling, N. and Guillemin, R., Morphinomimetic activity of synthetic fragments of β-lipotropin and analogs, *Proc. nat. Acad. Sci (Wash.)*, 73 (1976) 3308–3310.
8. Mata, M.M., Schrier, B.K. and Moore, R.Y., Interpeduncular nucleus: Differential effects of habenula lesions on choline acetyltransferase and glutamic acid decarboxylase, *Exp. Neurol.*, 57 (1977) 913–921.
9. Mroz, E.A., Browstein, M.J. and Leeman, S.E., Evidence for substance P in the habenulo-interpeduncular tract, *Brain Research*, 113 (1976) 597–599.
10. Tseng, L.-F., Loh, H.H. and Li, C.H., β-Endorphin as a potent analgesic by intravenous injection, *Nature*, 263 (1976) 239–240.
11. Yoshimi, H., Matsukura, S., Sueoka, S., Fukase, M., Yokota, M., Hirata, Y. and Imura, H., Radioimmunoas-say of β-endorphin: presence of immunoreactive (big-big β-endorphin) and (big β-endorphin) in human and rat pituitary, *Life Sci.* (in press).

Fluorographic and quantitative analyses of slowly migrating axonal polypeptides in bifurcating axons

MASANORI KUROKAWA, YOSHIAKI KOMIYA AND HIROSHI MORI

Department of Biochemistry, Institute of Brain Research, Faculty of Medicine, University of Tokyo,
Bunkyo-ku, Tokyo 113, Japan

The rate of slow transport of proteins in the central branch of dorsal root ganglion cell axons is significantly lower than that in the peripheral branch.[2] Slowly migrating axonal polypeptides were labelled with L-[^{35}S] methionine, subjected to SDS-polyacrylamide slab gel electrophoresis, and visualised by flourography[4] (Fig. 1). Three polypeptides with molecular weights of 200,000, 160,000 and 68,000 daltons are collectively referred to as the slow component triplet, and are tentatively associated with neurofilaments (10 nm filaments).[1,3] In addition, two polypeptides with molecular weights of 59,000 and 55,000 daltons have the same electrophoretic mobilities as α- and β-tubulins from porcine brain, and a 43,000 dalton polypeptide has the same mobility as skeletal muscle actin.

Quantitative analyses of radioactivities in the triplet polypeptides, tubulins and actin at weeks 2,3 and 4 after labelling indicate that each of these three polypeptide groups migrates more slowly in the central as compared with peripheral axons, and also that the central axons are relatively more enriched with the triplet polypeptides, which migrate at the lowest rate among the three polypeptide groups.

REFERENCES

1. Hoffman, P.N. and Lasek, R.J., The slow component of axonal transport: identification of major structural polypeptides of the axon and their generality among mammalian neurons, *J. Cell Biol.*, 66 (1975) 351–366.
2. Komiya, Y. and Kurokawa, M., Asymmetry of protein transport in two branches of bifurcating axons, *Brain Research*, 139 (1978) 354–358.
3. Lasek, R.J. and Hoffman, P.N., The neuronal cytoskeleton, axonal transport and axonal growth. In R. Goldman, T. Pollard and J. Rosenbaum (Eds.), *Cell Motility*, Cold Spring Harbor Laboratory, 1976, pp. 1021–1049.
4. Mori, H., Komiya, Y. and Kurokawa, M., Slow axoplasmic transport: its asymmetry in two branches of bifurcating axons, *Proc. japan. Acad.* 53, Ser. B (1977) 252–256.

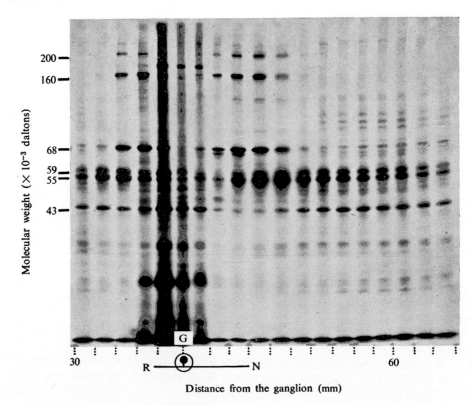

Fig. 1. Fluorographic analysis of polypeptides slowly migrating in the central and peripheral axons of the dorsal root ganglion neurons of the adult rat.

L-[35S]Methionine (200 μCi in 0.4 μl) was injected into the L$_5$ ganglion after its exposure by partial laminectomy, and animals were killed 1, 2, 3, 4, 5, 6 and 8 weeks thereafter. Consecutive 6 mm segments of the dorsal root (R; central branch) and sciatic nerve (N; peripheral branch), and the ganglion (G) were each ground in a total volume of 400 μl of the medium, which contained (final concentrations) sodium dodecyl sulfate (2.3%, w/v), β-mercaptoethanol (5 mM), glycerol (10%, v/v) and Tris-HCl (62.5 mM), pH 6.8. After brief centrifugation, the supernatant was heated, and a 30 μl portion of the extract from each segment was applied to a slot of the gel. Electrophoresis and fluorography were carried out as described elsewhere[4]. The fluorogram shown here is for the nerve obtained from an animal at week 2 of the postlabelling period.

Scanning electron microscopic studies on developing brain of mouse and man

SETSUYA FUJITA AND SHINJI FUSHIKI

Department of Pathology, Kyoto Prefectural University of Medicine,
Kamigyo-ku, Kyoto 602, Japan

In studying the cytoarchitectural characteristics of the developing brain wall, the usefulness of the fractographic technique[1] employing a scanning electron microscope has been recognized. We report here the cytoarchitectural features of diencephalic portions of developing brain in conjunction with the developing cerebral cortex.

The materials used for this study were fetal mice at 13 to 14 days after mating and human embryos at 12 weeks of gestation. They were fixed in 10% formalin or Bouin fixative. Small pieces of tissue containing developing brain were then dissected out. The tissue was washed in phosphate buffer and dehydrated through graded ethanol solutions. The alcohol was substituted by graded solutions of isoamyl acetate and the specimens were dried by the critical point method. Each piece of dried tissue was folded in two, or fractured with needles until the brain wall became split. Pieces of the tissue fractured in this way were mounted, with the fractured surface uppermost, onto specimen stubs with silver glue, coated under vacuum with carbon and gold, and observed at an accelerating voltage of 10 KV in a JEOL-S1 scanning electron microscope.

The cerebral wall from human embryo at about 12 weeks of gestation, when viewed on a fractograph, consisted of four distinctive layers: a matrix layer, a transitional layer, a cortical plate and a marginal layer (Fig. 1). The future neurons in the cortical plate were arranged in a vertical cell column along the bundle formed by the processes of the matrix cells. The future hypothalamic region of the fetal mouse at embryonic day 13 appeared to comprise a type of pseudostratified epithelium (Fig. 2). Most of the matrix cells were bipolar with spindle-shaped soma and processes. Just beneath the pial surface, unipolar cells with a large spherical soma were occasionally encountered. These cells are thought to be the neuroblasts into which matrix cells differentiate. At the base of the third ventricle in the 14–day-old fetal mouse, stage II of cytogenesis was terminated and the tissue consisted mainly of neuroblasts which were grouped together along the bundles formed by the processes of the ependymal cells (Fig. 3).

In previous studies[2] it was found that, with thickening of the brain wall, the matrix cells extend their outer processes through the overlying layers, keeping their somata confined to within the matrix layer. At stage II of cytogenesis, the processes of the matrix layer becomes sufficiently thinned and elongated to span the entire thickness of the developing brain wall. These processes appear to form a bundle, along which the neuroblasts migrate out from the matrix layer. It was suggested that the bundle of processes of the matrix cells may serve as a guideline for cell migration resulting in columnar organization of the cerebral cortex. However, there appears to be no definite columnar organization of neurons at either the thalamus or hypothalamus in the adult brain. In our present study, however, confined to the early stage of morphogenesis of the brain at least, it was found that processes of matrix cells did also exist in these regions and neuroblasts migrated out from the matrix layer along bundles of these processes. However, it still remains to

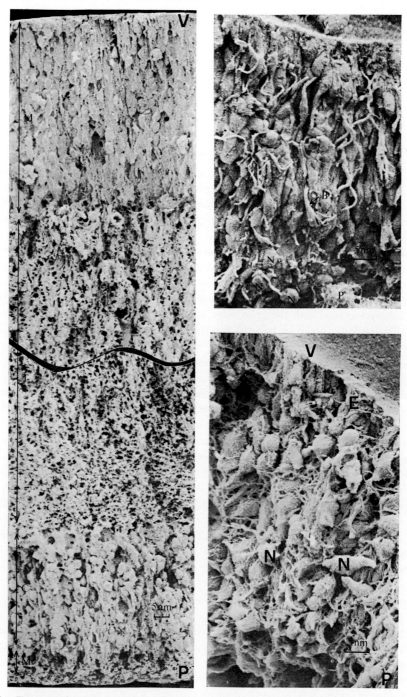

Fig. 1.   Fractograph of the cerebral wall of a 12-week-old human fetus. M, Matrix layer; T, transitional layer; C, cortical plate; Mr, marginal layer; V, ventricular surface; P, pial surface. A part of the transitional layer is omitted. *(left)*

Fig. 2.   Fractograph of the future hypothalamus of a 13-day-old fetal mouse. B, Bundle of processes of matrix cells; N, neuroblast; V, ventricular surface; P, pial surface. *(above right)*

Fig. 3.   Fractograph at the base of the third ventricle of a 14-day-old fetal mouse. N, Neuroblast; E, ependymal cell layer; V, ventricular surface; P, pial surface. *(below right)*

be studied how the cytoarchitecture of the above regions is modified regionally with further development of the brain.

REFERENCES

1. Hattori, T.: On cell proliferation and differentiation of the fundic mucosa of the golden hamster, *Cell Tissue Res.*, 148 (1974) 213–226.
2. Hattori, T. and Fujita, S.: Scanning electron microscopic studies on morphology of matrix cells, and on development and migration of neuroblasts in human and chick embryos, *J. Electron Microsc. (Tokyo)*, 23 (1974) 269–276.

A search for neurogenetic genes among behavioral and lethal mutations in *Drosophila melanogaster*

YOSHIKI HOTTA

Department of Physics, Faculty of Science, University of Tokyo, Bunkyo-ku, Tokyo 113, Japan

To study genetic mechanisms of brain functions, a method is to look for mutations which perturb the system. Indeed, several genetic disorders of central nervous system (CNS) are known which affect neuronal differentiation; eg. abnormal wiring in the visual system of Siamese cats and hereditary cerebellar diseases in mice. It is, therefore, important to obtain a number of such genes in a more systematic manner. We chose *Drosophila* as an experimental organism, since it has a brain which is complex enough to be interesting and yet simple enough for such a study. Another obvious advantage of using *Drosophila* is in the fact that many useful methods of genetic manipulations are readily available.

Since such mutations would cause behavioral anomalies, efforts have been made to isolate a large number of behaviorally defective mutations. Some of the results were already summarized as reviews.[1,2] For further analyses, however, a difficulty arrises since it is not uncommon to find a single mutation causing a complex series of syndromes among which causality is hard to establish. We overcome this difficulty by identifying a "primary focus" for each gene by means of genetic mosaic technique (see a review[3] for technical details). A primary focus is a structure (or a set of structures) in which malfunction of the gene initiates a chain of events which leads to the mutant character in question. This is made possible by making composite individuals (genetic mosaics) of which a part is mutant but the rest is normal. Primary focus is identified as a structure whose genotype always coincides with behavioral phenotype of each mosaic fly. Even without knowing the internal mosaicism pattern, focus in the brain, thoracic ganglion, mesoderm or surface receptors can be inferred by correlating cuticular mosaic pattern with presence or absence of behavioral anomaly in each mosaic fly by means of blastoderm fate map technique[5] (Fig. 1A). Once focus is identified, electronmicroscopic[7] or microbiochemical[4] analyses on the focus structure are carried out for some of these mutations, and will eventually clarify the link between gene and behavior.

However, not all relevant genes could be uncovered as behavioral mutations. There will be a number of genes, whose malfunctions in the nervous system causes lethality. Thus we are also looking for neurogenetic genes among lethals by identifiying their primary foci with the blastoderm fate map technique. Among about 100 X-linked lethals induced with an alkylating agent, ethyl methanesulfonate, about 40 were found unable to survive even as a part in mosaic flies. Since it suggests that their primary foci must extend practically to all the blastoderm cells (including primordial nervous system), these genes are called systemic lethals. They must be supporting basic cellular functions common to all cell types. Among the rest (focal lethals), ten genes were found to have their lethal foci in entire or a part of CNS (see Fig. 1B). Many other lethals were found to have their foci in other structure such as mesoderm, intestine and imaginal discs.

Since the lethal genes studied can be regarded as a random sample from an entire lethal ensemble which constitutes a majority of a genome, the results can be interpreted to mean that about

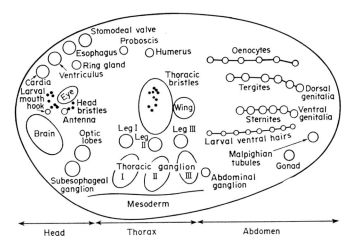

Fig. 1 A: Summary of *Drosophila* blastoderm fate map determined by the genetic mosaic technique, showing a right hemisphere seen from inside. Primordia for various larval and adult structures are placed in the map under the assumption that any pair of structures is separated by mosaic boundary with a probability proportionate to the distance between their primordia on the blastoderm. Note that all the CNS structures are localized along the ventral midline (the lower surround) of the map. For more details about construction of the fate map, see our previous papers[5,6].

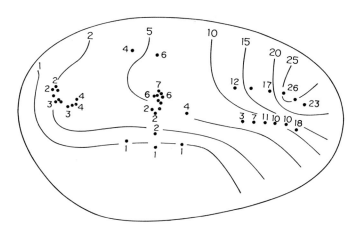

B: An example of focus mapping for an X-linked lethal mutation called EI 103. About 1000 genetic mosaics for the mutation initiated their development, among which 9% could survive as adults. Numbers attached to each surface landmark are proportionate to the frequency with which each structure was of lethal genotype among the survivors, whose primary focus ought to be of normal genotype. The low values along the anteroventral midline indicate that the primary focus of EI 103 gene is in entire CNS.

10% of all genes are specifically vital to CNS; their mutations causing death primarily due to its malfunction in the nervous system.

We are currently investigating how these mutations induce CNS disturbances by using both histological and microbiochemical techniques.

REFERENCES

1. Benzer, S., Genetic dissection of Sehavior, *Sci. Amer.*, 229 (1973) 24–37.
2. Grossfield, J., Behavioral mutants of *Drosophila*, In R. C. King (Ed.) Handbook of Genetics Vol. 3, Plenum Press, New York, 1975. pp. 679–702.
3. Hall, J. C., Gelbart, W. M. and Kankel, D. R., Mosaic Systems, In M. Ashburner and E. Novitski (eds.) The Genetics and Biology of Drosophila, Vol. la, Academic Press, London, New York, San Francisco, 1976, pp. 265–314.
4. Hotta, Y., A biochemical analysis of visual mutations in *Drosophila melanogaster*—Changes in major eye proteins, In J.D. Ebert and T.S. Okada (eds.), Mechanism of Cell Change, John-Wiley & Sons, 1978 (in the press).
5. Hotta, Y. and Benzer, S., Mapping of behavior in *Drosophila* mosaics, In F.H. Ruddle (ed.) Genetic Mechanisms of Development, Academic Press, New York, 1973, pp. 129–167.
6. Hotta, Y. and Benzer, S., Courtship in *Drosophila* mosaics: Sex-specific foci for sequential action patterns, *Proc. Natl. Acad. Sci. USA,* 73 (1976), 4154–4158.
7. Koana, T. and Hotta, Y., Isolation and characterization of Flightless Mutants in *Drosophila melanogaster, J. Embryol. exp. Morph,* 45 (1978), 123–143.

PART II

NEURAL MECHANISMS OF SENSATION AND ITS DISORDERS

KYOJI TASAKI

*Department of Physiology, Tohoku University School of Medicine,
Sendai, Miyagi, 980, Japan*

Sensory physiology deals with the functions of the sensory systems, including such problems as, how receptors are excited by various kinds of natural stimuli, how afferent impulses are initiated and transmitted into the central nervous system, and finally how in the brain the sensory informations are perceived as sensations. In the past the major interests in sensory physiology were in the peripheral mechanisms, and relatively little attention has been paid to the central processes until recently. This is particularly true in this country, although sensory physiology is one of the most advanced fields in Japanese physiology. The purpose of the present project is to consider the neural mechanism of sensation, and a group of leading investigators in different disciplines has been brought together, with more emphasis being placed on the central mechanisms. The research areas covered by this group are vision, audition, taste, olfaction, and somatic sensation.

In the frog muscle spindle Ito and Komatsu, studying the abortive spike potential, suggested that these abortive spikes may be a kind of non-overshooting spike evoked at the axon terminal. These investigators further suggested that similar mechanisms may be involved in the generation of spike-like responses in the central nervous system. Furukawa, reviewing his 10 years' studies on the goldfish ear, discussed the role of hair cell-afferent fiber synaptic transmission in encoding the auditory impulses.

In the retina of the fish Kaneko and his associates have been using a refined technique of intracellular dye injection to study the synaptic connections between the retinal cells. They have shown that in mixed ON bipolar cells the spectral sensitivity curve depends on the state of adaptation, and in mixed OFF bipolar cells a shift of λ max was readily observed on changing the state of adaptation (Purkinje shift), demonstrating the convergence of inputs from rods and cones to bipolar cells.

In the relay cells of the rat lateral geniculate nucleus Fukuda *et al.* carried out an extensive analysis of the receptive field properties in relation to conduction velocities of the retinal afferents. The cells recorded were classified into two main types; common and uncommon types. The former consists of OFF-phasic, ON-phasic, ON-tonic and ON-OFF types. ON-inhibited, moving-sensitive, ON-OFF-cell-like cells were included in the latter type.

One of the most interesting and challenging subjects in the physiology of vision is the neural circuitry which produces the selective responsivenss of the cortical cells to an appropriately oriented line. Although two basic connections are present between the visual cortex and the lateral geniculate nucleus (monosynaptic excitation and disynaptic inhibition in layersIII-V, and disynaptic excitation and trisynaptic inhibition in layers II and VI), the importance of the intracortical connections was pointed out by Toyama. By means of simultanuous recordings from two neighboring cells and cross-correlation analysis of impulses of these two cells, three types of synaptic interactions were found to operate between the visual cortical cells; common excitation, monosynaptic excitation, and monosynaptic inhibition. Based on their different functions, Toyama made the important suggestion that the determining factor for the response type is the intracortical connection rather than afferent inputs from the lateral geniculate nucleus.

Following their previous study on the input pathway to the vestibulocerebellum Purkinje cells from the optic nerve through climbing and mossy fibers, Maekawa and Takeda have sought the origins of visually activated climbing fibers which project to the flocculus by using the horseradish peroxidase tracing technique combined with electrophysiological methods. Ogawa and Takemori also studied visual input to the nucleus centralis lateralis from which the motor cortex receives axonal projection.

In the gustatory system the afferent pathway between the solitary tract nucleus and the ventral posteromedial nucleus of the thalamus was studied electrophysiologically (Ogawa et al.). A newly developed intracellular staining technique with a fluorescence dye, Procion Yellow, was employed in rabbit olfactory bulb neurons to study the structure-function relationship.

In the field of somatic sensation Iwamura and his associate have carried an extensive study on the receptive field properties of somatosensory cortical neurons. They demonstrated the presence of a stimulus feature extraction mechanism and an integration mechanism for complex stimuli. Iwamura also emphasized that the functional organization of the cortical receiving areas and the method of information processing reflect the behavioral characteristics of the animals.

In studying the neural mechanism of pain, the pattern of trigeminal field projection was investigated by Yokota at various parts of the primary relay nucleus, the caudal medulla oblongata, since the trigeminal system is convinient for studying pain. In the rabbit spinal dorsal horn Takagi carried out an important study on the physiological role of enkephalin in the pain-controlling mechanism, demonstrating that this naturally occurring pentapeptide in the mammalian brain showed an agonistic effect only when nociceptive stimuli were applied but no effect for non-nociceptive, such as tactile, stimuli.

Takaori and his associates adopted a different approach to the study of the sensory system and found an inhibitory effect of electrical stimulation of the locus coeruleus upon afferent transmission at the two relay nuclei, the spinal trigeminal nucleus and coclear nucleus, both nuclei being innervated by noradrenergic nerves originating from the locus coeruleus. Since the inhibitory effect could be produced by iontophoretically applied noradrenaline, the effect is apparently mediated by this substance.

Histological studies were carried out by two groups. By using horseradish peroxidase as a neuronal marker for electron microscopy, Mizuno et al. made an extensive search of the spinothalamic pathway. Malformation of the visual system was studied histologically by Otani in anophthalmic rats, and an electrophysiological investigation is in progress. Another interesting approach to an understanding of the central mechanisms of color and pattern vision is that of Okuma and Takahashi, who have been conducting an extensive survey of epileptic patients.

Interneuronal connectivity in cat visual cortex: studies by cross-correlation analysis of the responses of two simultaneously recorded neurons

KEISUKE TOYAMA

Department of Physiology, Faculty of Medicine, University of Tokyo,
Bunkyo-ku, Tokyo 113, Japan

Structure-function problem in visual cortex

Visual cortical cells exhibit a variety of responses which are highly selective to some features of patterned light stimuli.[1-3] The question of how the neuronal circuitry in the visual cortex yields the selective responsiveness to the light stimuli provides a challenging problem in vision physiology. To this end, numerous studies have been made to determine the neuronal connectivity specific to each response type of visual cortical cells[10].

Two basic organizations have been demonstrated in the synaptic connections of the visual cortex with the lateral geniculate body[12,14]. These are (1) monosynaptic excitation and disynaptic inhibition of cells in layers III-V, and (2) disynaptic excitation and trisynaptic inhibition in layers II and VI. The first type of synaptic connectivity is common in three response types, i.e., a simple cell, a complex cell, and a cell with exclusively ON or OFF area[6,8-11,13]. The second type is common in a complex cell and a hypercomplex cell[9]. It was also shown that each response type was characterized by a specific spatial pattern of connectivity with the retinal receptive area[9,11]. To answer the question of structure-function relationships, however, more information is required on the intracortical connectivity among visual cortical cells.

Cross-correlation analysis provides a new approach to the problem. It reveals the interaction working between two cells, and thereby identifies the synaptic connectivity and the activities that proceed there[4,5].

Simultaneous recording from two visual cortical neurons and cross-correlation analysis of their activities

Impulse discharges were recorded simultaneously from two visual cortical cells using two glass microelectrodes, each of which was double-barreled. One barrel was filled with 2 M NaCl and used for extracellular recording of neuronal impulses. The other was filled with 0.2 M sodium glutamate and used for ejecting glutamate ions electrophoretically (see below). A pair of these microelectrodes was inserted into the visual cortex of the cat (area 17), one perpendicularly to the cortical surface and the other obliquely at 10° to the first (Fig. 1A). The tips of the electrodes were set about 200μ apart on the cortical surface, so that they approached each other to within a few tens of microns at 1 mm below the cortical surface[4].

The responses of the pair of neurons were studied simultaneously using stationary and moving light stimuli. In the majority of pairs, two cells shared the same ocular dominance and preference, and their receptive fields overlapped each other. These neurons were thus classified into four response types: a simple cell, a complex cell, a hypercomplex cell, and a cell with exclusively ON or OFF area. The interaction working between the paired cells was determined by computing a cross-correlogram for their impulse discharges. Visual cortical cells usually exhibited low spontaneous discharges (0.2–5 impulses/sec), so that continuous recording over a relatively long period was required to obtain a reliable correlogram. This difficulty was overcome by increasing the impulse discharges of the visual cortical cells in two ways: (1) by electrophoretic ejection of glutamate ions, a potent chemical activator of nerve cells, or (2) by photic stimulation of their receptive area.

Fig. 1 illustrates impulse trains (I_1 and I_2) that occurred in two cells (c_1 and c_2) during photic and chemical stimulations. Electrophoretic application of glutamate ions to c_1 facilitated impulse discharges at a frequency a few times (C) that of the spontaneous impulse discharges with no

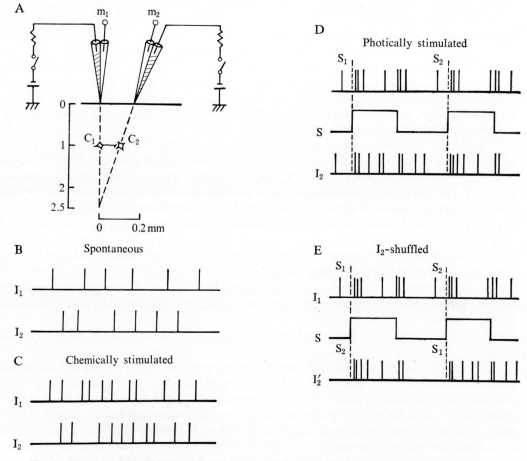

Fig. 1. Experimental arrangement for cross-correlation studies of two visual cortex neurons. A, Schematic diagram for simultaneous recording from a pair of neurons (c_1 and c_2) using two double barreled microelectrodes (hatched barrel filled with sodium glutamate; blank one with NaCl). B, Impulse trains recorded from c_1 (I_1) and from c_2 (I_2) with no stimulus. C, As B but with chemical stimulation of c_2. D, As B and C but with repetitive photic stimulation (S_1 and S_2). E, As D but with I_2 shuffled (see text).

stimulus (B). There was also a facilitatory effect on c_2. This might be due either to excitatory synaptic action exerted by c_1 on c_2 (see below), or to diffusion of glutamate ions to c_2.

Photic stimulation activated the two cells conjointly (D). In this case, the cross-correlogram of the responses should represent the sum (gross correlogram) of the correlation due to their coincidental activation (stimulus-coordinated correlogram) and that due to their interaction though synaptic connections (neurally-coordinated correlogram). The stimulus-coordinated correlation can be obtained in isolation by shuffling the impulse train of c_2 fractionated at each moment of photic stimulation. The neurally-coordinated correlogram is determined by subtracting the stimulus-coordinated correlogram from the gross correlogram.

Interneuronal interactions

Cross-correlation was studied in 80 pairs of cells by employing the two methods of stimulation. Cross-correlation analysis revealed three types of interactions.

Common excitation: The first type of interaction was the conjoint activation of two cortical neurons due to the common excitatory inputs. Fig. 2A represents the total extent of the receptive area for a pair of complex cells, c_1 and c_2. It is apparent that their individual receptive areas largely overlapped each other. A cross-correlogram of impulse trains of c_1 and c_2 obtained with no stimulus is shown in Fig. 2B. A slight positivity is observed around zero time. This positivity was greatly enhanced by photic stimulation. Fig. 2C shows a gross correlogram obtained during photic stimulation with a stationary light slit exposed in the receptive area, and Fig. 2D gives the stimulus-coordinated correlogram. In the neurally-coordinated correlogram (E) determined as the difference between the former two correlograms, the positivity was greater and was sharply distributed around zero time (extending for only 0.9 msec). This precise coincidence of activities could be due to simultaneous activation of the two cells by the common excitatory inputs which are presumably transmitted through monosynaptic connections from the lateral geniculate cells.

The number of conjoint impulses (N_c) which were locked to each other within an interval of 1.2 msec ($\pm$ 0.6 msec from zero time) was determined from the positiviy in the cross-correlogram, and the locking rate was calculated as the ratio of N_c to the total number of impulses in the impulse trains in c_1 (N_1) and c_2 (N_2). With no stimulus (B), the locking rates for c_1 ($R_1 = N_c/N_1$) and c_2 ($R_2 = N_c/N_2$) were very small ($R_1 = 17/418$, $R_2 = 17/197$), but they were increased several times during photic stimulation ($R_1 = 122/620$, $R_2 = 122/523$). Thus, a significant part of the excitatory inputs to these two cells should be transmitted through the common afferent pathway from the lateral geniculate body.

A similar sharp positivity around zero time ($\pm$ 0.6 msec) was found in about half of the neuron pairs ($n = 42$) which shared the same ocular dominance and optimum orientation of light stimulus. The locking rate was moderate (0.2–0.5) in most of these pairs ($n = 38$), extremely high (0.6–0.9) in a few pairs ($n = 4$), but weak or null (0–0.1) in the remaining half ($n = 38$).

Monosynaptic excitation: The second type of interaction was excitation monosynaptically exerted from one cortical cell to the other. The cross-correlogram of two complex cells (c_1 and c_2 in Fig. 3A) revealed no significant interaction, when no stimulus was applied (B). When c_2 was chemically stimulated, a positivity appeared (C). The positivity was even greater in the neurally-coordinated correlogram obtained during photic stimulation (D). A similar positivity was found in 7 neuron pairs. The positivity usually started at about –0.6 msec, attained a maximum at –2 msec and declined gradually for about 10 msec. This positivity signifies that impulse discharges in c_1 were faci-

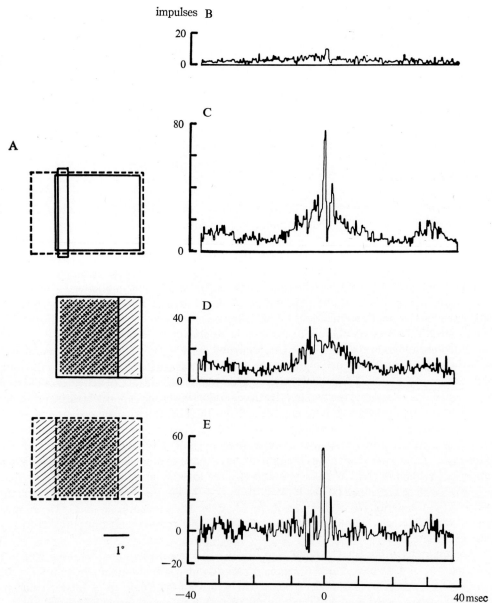

Fig. 2. Cross-correlogram of common excitation between two complex cells. A, Schematic diagram representing the receptive areas of two complex cells (c_1 and c_2). Thin solid line indicates the total extent of the receptive area of c_1 and broken line that of c_2. Thick line indicates a stationary light slit exposed on part of the receptive areas of c_1 and c_2. Spatial arrangement of ON (stippled) and OFF areas (hatched) is shown below. B, Cross-correlogram with no stimulus. C, Gross correlogram with photic stimulation. D, Stimulus-coordinated correlogram. E, Neurally-coordinated correlogram.

litated after those in c_2 with a time lag comparable to a monosynaptic delay. This excitatory interaction is explained by assuming an excitatory synaptic connection from c_2 to c_1. The time cour-

A

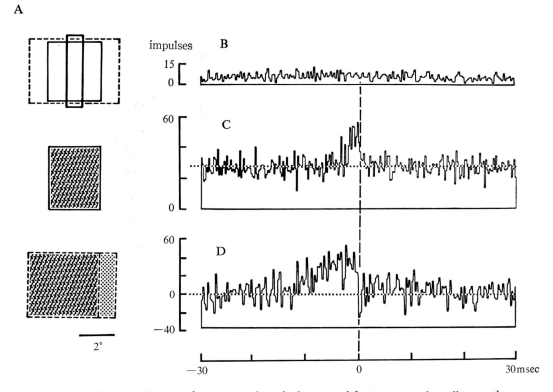

Fig. 3. Cross-correlogram of monosynaptic excitation exerted from one complex cell to another. A, Similar diagram to Fig. 2A, representing the receptive areas of two complex cells. B, Correlogram with no stimulus. C, Correlogram with chemical stimulation. D, Neurally-coordinated correlogram with photic stimulation.

se of the positivity might reflect that of an excitatory postsynaptic potential (EPSP) produced in c_1 by impulses in c_2.

Since the number (N_p) of impulses composing the positivity (area circumscribed by an envelope of the correlogram and a base-line) represents the impulses initiated from c_1 during the excitatory action, the contribution of this excitatory action to the photic responses in c_1 is given by the ratio between N_p and N_1 ($C_e = N_p/N_1$). The contribution of the excitatory action thus determined for 7 pairs was fairly large (0.2–0.4). A considerable part of the photic response in the target cell of excitation (c_1) should therefore be produced through the monosynaptic excitation exerted from the source cell (c_2).

Monosynaptic inhibition: The third type of interaction was an inhibition exerted monosynaptically from one cortical cell to the other. As illustrated in Fig. 4A, the OFF area (hatched part) of a simple cell (c_1) overlaps on the ON area (stippled part) of a cell with exclusively ON area (c_2). The correlogram obtained during chemical stimulation (Fig. 4B) reveals a small negativity starting at about –0.9 msec (downward arrow) and continuing up to –40 msec. A comparable negativity also occurred in the neurally-coordinated correlogram, although it was associated with a sharp negativity at zero time (Fig. 4C).

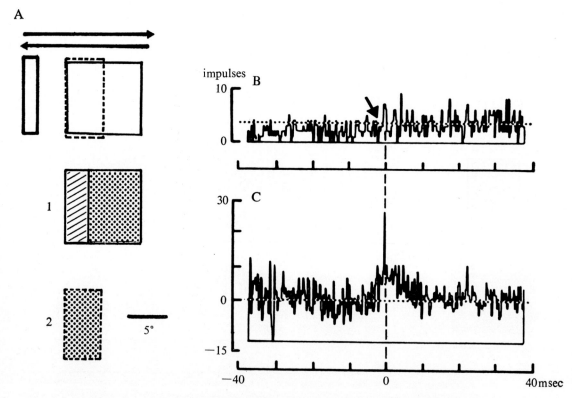

Fig. 4.   Cross-correlogram of monosynaptic inhibition exerted from a cell with exclusively ON area onto a simple cell A, Diagram of the receptive areas. c_1, Simple cell; c_2, Cell with exclusively ON area. B, Correlogram with chemical stimulation. C, Neurally-coordinated correlogram with photic stimulation.

A similar negativity was found in 9 pairs. In a correlogram obtained from these cells with chemical stimulation, the negativity started at about −0.6 msec and lasted for about 100 msec. The early onset of the negativity indicates that the impulse discharges in c_2 depress those in c_1 with a monosynaptic delay. The long duration of the negativity presumably represents the long time course of the inhibition exerted from c_2 to c_1[13]. A similar negativity was found in the neurally-coordinated correlogram obtained with photic stimulation, but it was frequently associated with a sharp positivity around zero time. The source (c_2) and target (c_1) cells of the inhibition should therefore share common excitatory inputs from the lateral geniculate cells. For the 9 pairs, the contribution of the inhibitory interaction was determined as the ratio between the total number of impulses involved in the negativity (N_i) and that of the target cell (c_1) of the inhibition ($E_i = N_i/N_1$). The contribution determined for inhibition was of the same magnitude (0.1–0.4) as that for excitation.

Factors relevant to intercellular interactions

The above three types of interactions were related with the following two factors: response type and location of the cells.

Response type: The relationship of the neuronal interaction with the response type of the cortical cells was demonstrated by constructing interaction tables. Table 1 indicates the numbers of sampled neuronal pairs for each combination of response types. Similarly, Table 2 shows the numbers of pairs which exhibited the common excitation. It can be seen that the common excitation occurred frequently in all combinations of response types except those involving a hypercomplex cell. In contrast, as shown in Table 3, the monosynaptic excitation was specifically exerted from one response type to another (i.e., from a complex cell to a complex cell or to a hypercomplex cell). The monosynaptic inhibition was also found in only two combinations (i.e., from a cell with exclusively ON or OFF to a simple cell, and from a simple cell to a complex cell) (Table 4).

Table 1. Combination of response types

Between	S	C	E	H
S	9	—	—	—
C	17	12	—	—
E	12	5	14	—
H	3	3	3	2

Table 2. Common excitation

Between	S	C	E	H
S	7	—	—	—
C	7	7	—	—
E	10	3	8	—
H	0	0	0	0

Table 3. Monosynaptic excitation

To From	S	C	E	H
S	0	0	0	0
C	0	4	0	3
E	0	0	0	0
H	0	0	0	0

Table 4. Monosynaptic inhibition

To From	S	C	E	H
S	0	5	0	0
C	0	0	0	0
E	4	0	0	0
H	0	0	0	0

S, Simple cell; C, Complex cell; E, Cell with exclusively ON or OFF area; H, Hypercomplex cell.

Cellular location: The three types of interactions were also related with the location of the neuron pair. Common excitation was found between neuron pairs located in layers III-V. There was a tendency for common excitation to be stronger for a neuron pair with a shorter intercellular distance: the locking rate was greater for a pair with a shorter intercellular distance. Monosynaptic excitation was exerted from cells in layers III and IV (0.3–1.0 mm from the cortical surface) onto those in layer II (0.1–0.3 mm). Monosynaptic inhibition was exerted from cells in layers IV onto those in layers III–IV.

Conclusion

Cross-correlation analysis revealed three types of synaptic interactions working between visual cortex neurons, i.e., (1) common excitation, (2) monosynaptic excitation, and (3) monosynaptic inhibition. Common excitation was shared by different response types of visual cortex cells, while excitatory and inhibitory interactions were specifically exerted from one response type onto another. It is suggested therefore that the primary determinant of the response type is the intracortical interaction rather than the afferent inputs from the lateral geniculate cells. Quantitative analysis of cross-correlation indicates that the interaction between two cortical cells accounts for a considerable part of their responses to light stimuli (5–30%). The characteristic responsiveness of a cortical cell may therefore be determined through interactions with a relatively small number of other cortical cells.

References

1. Bishop, P.O., Coombs, J.S. and Henry, G.H., Responses to visual contours: spatio-temporal aspects of excitation in the receptive fields of simple striate neurones, *J. Physiol. (Lond.)*, 219 (1971) 625—657.
2. Hubel, D.H. and Wiesel, T.N., Receptive fields, binocular interaction and functional architecture in the cat's visual cortex, *J. Physiol. (Lond.)*, 160 (1962) 106–154.
3. Hubel, D.H. and Wiesel, T.N., Receptive fields and functional architecture in two nonstriate visual areas (18 and 19) of the cat, *J. Neurophysiol.*, 28 (1965) 229–289.
4. Kimura, M., Tanaka, K. and Toyama, K., Interneuronal connectivity between visual cortical neurones of the cat as studied by cross-correlation analysis of their impulse discharges, *Brain Research*, 118 (1976) 329–333.
5. Perkel, H., Gerstein, G.L. and Moore, G.P., Neuronal spike trains and stochastic point processes. II. Simultaneous spike trains. *Biophys. J.*, (1967) 418–440.
6. Singer, W., Tretter, F. and Cynader, M., Organization of cat striate cortex: a correlation of receptive-field properties with afferent and efferent connections, *J. Neurophysiol.*, 38 (1975) 1080–1098..
7. Stone, J., A quantative analysis of the distribution of ganglion cells in the cat's retina, *J. comp. Neurol.*, 124 (1975) 337–352.
8. Stone, J. and Dreher, B., Projection of X- and Y-cells of the cat's lateral geniculate nucleus to areas 17 and 18 of visual cortex, *J. Neurophysiol.*, 36 (1973) 551–567.
9. Toyama, K., Kimura, M., Shiida, T. and Takeda, T., Convergence of retinal inputs onto visual cortical cells: II. A study of the cells disynaptically excited from the lateral geniculate body, *Brain Research*, 137 (1977) 221–231.
10. Toyama, K., Maekawa, K. and Takeda, T., An analysis of neuronal circuitry for two types of visual cortical neurones classified on the basis of their responses to photic stimuli, *Brain Research*, 61 (1973) 395–399.
11. Toyama, K. Maedawa, K. and Takeda, T., Convergence of retinal inputs onto visual cortical cells: I. A study of the cells monosynaptically excited from the lateral geniculate body, *Brain Research*, 137 (1977) 207–220.
12. Toyama, K., Matsunami, K., Ohno, T. and Tokashiki, S., An intracellular study of neuronal organization in the visual cortex, *Exp. Brain Res.*, 21 (1974) 45–66.
13. Toyama, K. and Takeda, T., A unique class of cat's visual cortical cells that exhibit either ON and OFF excitation for stationary light slit and are responsive to moving patterns, *Brain Research*, 73 (1974) 350–355.
14. Watanabe, S., Konishi, M. and Creutzfeldt, O., Postsynaptic potentials in the cat's visual cortex following electrical stimulation of afferent pathways, *Exp. Brain Res.*, 1 (1966) 272–283.

Neuronal mechanisms of active and passive touch

YOSHIAKI IWAMURA

Department of Physiology, Toho University School of Medicine,
Ota-ku, Tokyo 143, Japan

Introduction

Animals appear to perceive the outer world in a very specific manner, which is determined not only by the variety of sensory receptors,[1] but also by the central mechanisms which give meaningfulness to the sensory signals coded by receptors.

In studies of the central mechanism of the sensory systems, receptive field analysis of single units in unanesthetized animals has proved to be one of the most effective methods[6,7,18,19,22]. By examining the preferred stimulus of each unit in a neuronal population, experimenters can in effect ask neurons what they perceive, and the functional organization of the particular cortical site can thus be inferred. In the initial single unit studies of the somatosensory cortex in cats and monkeys, it was clear that clustering of cells with the same submodality and location occurred in vertical columns[18,22]. This led to the idea of submodality segregation and point-to-point representation of the peripheral receptor sheets in the cortical neurons. Indeed, it was confirmed in more recent investigations in unanesthetized monkeys that the sensory information encoded in the peripheral afferents is transmitted and reproduced in the SI with remarkable fidelity.[20] Many neurons of the SI were correlated with one receptor type, such as Meissner's corpuscles, Merkel's discs, Pacinian corpuscles, etc. They responded to relatively simple and punctate stimuli of the skin. However, these simple and sensitive neurons of the SI were mainly localized in area 3, which receives the heaviest projection from the ventrobasal complex of the thalamus. Recent single unit studies in unanesthetized animals have suggested the existence of the systematic integratory mechanism in the posterior part of the somatosensory cortex. The following is a brief review of such studies.

Functions of the SI suggested by lesion studies and clinical observations

In clinical observations of patients and lesion studies done in monkeys, it has been repeatedly stated that the ablation of the postcentral gyrus produced a long-lasting somesthetic defect, a disturbance of touch-pressure sensitivity, two-point discrimination, position sense, etc[2,21,26,30]. Orbach and Chow[21] showed that a lesion in the SI of the monkey disturbed the discrimination of size, form and roughness of tactile objects. Moreover, Roland[25] stated in a clinical study that astereognosis, a deficit in tactile object recognition by palpation, is correlated with lesions specifically placed on the postcentral hand area of human subjects.

The first somatosensory cortex (SI) of primates can be subdivided cytoarchitecturally into three subdivisions, Brodmann's areas 3, 1 and 2.

According to recent anatomical evidence[15,16], the thalamic projection is heaviest to area 3.

73

Areas 3, 1 and 2 are interconnected by cortico-cortical fibers[16,17,31], and the main stream of sensory signals could travel from area 3 to areas 1 and 2. On the basis of such anatomical arrangements, sequential processing of sensory signals has been proposed to occur within the SI, and consequently, one can assume that the function may differ in different cytoarchitectural subdivisions. This possibility was examined by selective ablation of areas 3, 1 and 2[24]. In these experiments ablation of area 3 impaired all somatosensory performance whereas ablation of area 1 impaired performance involving discrimination of texture, and ablation of area 2 that of angles. Discrimination of angles would require complex integratory processes of sensory messages originating from both cutaneous and deep tissues. On the other hand, the indispensability of area 3 shown in these experiments supports the hypothesis of the sequential flow of sensory messages in the somatosensory cortex.

Receptive field analysis in the monkey SI

Recent single unit studies[8,13,14] on the monkey SI have offered more direct evidence of sequential processing. The receptive field tended to increase in size as the recording site was shifted posteriorly.

At the same time, the number of cells activated by simple skin indentation decreased posteriorly within the SI and a corresponding increase in the number of more "complex" cells occurred instead. In the posterior part of the SI, units with submodality convergence were also observed.

Fig. 1 illustrates the receptive fields of SI neurons collected in areas 3b, 1 and 2 of rhesus monkeys. The RFs were smaller and more fragmentary in area 3b on both the volar and dorsal surfaces of the hand. The RFs of areas 1 and 2 neurons were larger in size and involved several RFs of area 3b neurons. Furthermore, it was noted that in area 2 the increase in RF size is not a result of mere convergence but occurs in such a way as to cover functionally significant regions often independent of dermal order, as described earlier. For example, a unit in area 2 which covered the tips of three fingers may be significant for the recognition of single tiny objects picked up with three fingers. Similarly, another large RF of area 2 neurons may correspond to the area of the volar surface which may come into contact with the object when the monkey grasps it. The RF configuration was similar but not identical among sequentially recorded units in relation to the vertical columnar organization of the cortex. Moreover, several adjacent vertical columns contained neurons with similar RF and some mutually interrelated receptive characteristics.

In addition, within the same or adjacent vertical organization, non-skin units as well as skin-and-deep units were intermingled, and their preferred stimuli were often self-initiated behavior of the monkey's hand. For example, one unit which had the disjunctive skin receptive field on the second to fourth finger tips with directional selectivity towards the radial side also responded to passive flexion of the fingers. However, the preferred stimulus for this unit was the complex pattern of stimulus produced by natural movements of the hand such as scratching the surface of the table with the hand. In certain other units, finger joint position (either extended or flexed) was critical for eliciting the response to finger or palm skin stimulation. It is suggested that area 2 of the monkey SI is an aggregate of multiple clusterings of vertical columns and that each clustering represents a functional fragment for processing complex sensory information concerning special features of tactile objects, motion of the hand and fingers, etc.

Area 3b   Area 1   Area 2

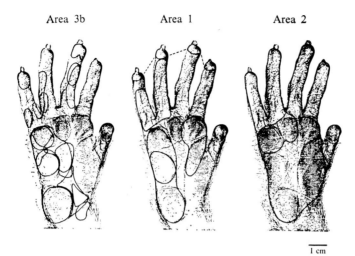

1 cm

Fig. 1. Cutaneous receptive fields of areas 3b, 1 and 2 neurons of the hand region of the monkey SI. Note that the RF in the finger tips involves the same neuron in area 1, as indicated by the dotted line (Source: ref. 27. Reproduced by kind permissions of the Pergamon Press Ltd., Oxford).

Stimulus feature extraction in the monkey SI

As is well known in the visual cortex, feature-detecting neurons signal stimulus properties of different degrees of complexity.[6] This complexity increases with the projection from the striate to prestriate cortex along with increase of receptive field size.[7,34] Prestriate neurons thus signal the occurrence of an adequate stimulus with increasing independence from the actual site of stimulus impingement on the retina.

In the somatic sensory cortex, a similar increase of complexity of stimulus features occurs: some neurons in somatic sensory areas 1 and 2 signal the direction of stimulus motion over circumscribed cutaneous receptive fields.[29,32,33] There are neurons in area 2 which respond to edges placed on the receptive field in a particular orientation.[8,23] Some other neurons found in area 2 responded to elongated narrow objects when they were in passive contact with the monkey's hand (Fig. 2). These neurons may be interpreted as also responding to an "edge". However, the neurons described in the following section give examples of a remarkable specificity of stimulus.

Neurons possibly related to form discrimination of tactile objects

As described previously, Randolf and Semmes[24] concluded from their lesion study that area 2 was concerned with the discrimination of angles. Detection of angles may be one of the most important cues for discriminating three-dimensional tactile objects. Identification of objects by palpation is based on the sensory information from both cutaneous touch and articular position since palpation includes the shaping of the hand to grasp the object. On the other hand, area 2 of the monkey SI is known to receive both skin and deep submodality inputs[19].

Thus, the possibility exists that there are certain neural mechanisms in area 2 for discriminating objects by palpation. Iwamura and Tanaka[13] recently found peculiar neurons in the postcentral area 2 possibly related to form discrimination by palpation. A total of 155 units recorded in area 2 were classified into simple skin units (26.4%), complicated skin units (25.8%), joint mani-

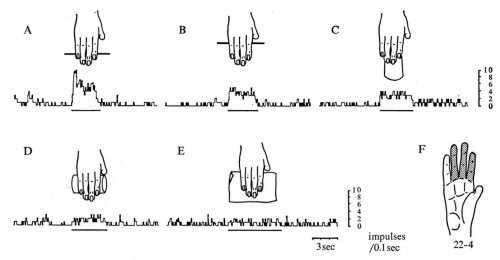

Fig. 2. The response histograms of unit 22–4 to topical application of various objects to the finger skin receptive field as indicated in F. A, a piece of thin metal wire (2 mm dia.) to the distal phalanges; B, the same object to the proximal phalanges; C, the flat bottom of a glass bottle (3 cm dia.); D, the cylindrical surface of the bottle; E, a piece of felt (Iwamura and Tanaka, 1978c).[13]

pulation units (11.6%), joint and skin units (23.9%), and undrivable units (12.3%). In the category of complicated skin units were included those responding to a moving probe over the skin and those for which narrowness of the stimulated area was most important, as described in the previous section. Fig. 3 shows the most peculiar type of units found in area 2, which were driven when the monkey grasped objects. These units did not respond to ordinary cutaneous stimuli with the probe nor to simple manipulation of wrist or finger joints and thus were different from any others described above. The unit shown in Fig. 3A was driven when the monkey grasped a rectangular block of wood or a straight-edged ruler in its hand. However, no response was obtained when a small cylindrical bottle was grasped instead. In contrast, the unit shown in Fig. 3B was activated by the grasping of round objects such as a cylindrical bottle, or a small apple of about 5 cm diameter, but not by a rectangular block.

It was not driven by mere contact of palm skin on a flat surface, nor by bending the fingers to make a hand pose similar to grasping. It appears that the grasping of objects with particular forms was the only effective mode of stimulus for the units shown in Fig. 3. Grasping objects must yield complex patterns of activity in both skin and deep receptors in the hand. However, these units seem to utilize the information of both cutaneous and deep sources only in particular combinations. Gibson[3] emphasized the superiority of "active" over "passive" touch in discriminating tactile objects. Only by active exploration can an organism get enough information about the environment.

Receptive field analysis in cat SI

By a systematic study of the sizes and shapes of receptive fields (RF), Iwamura and Tanaka[10,11,12] demonstrated that cutaneous RFs of SI neurons in unanesthetized cats were integrated into functionally significant areas of skin surface. They compared the RFs in the coronal region

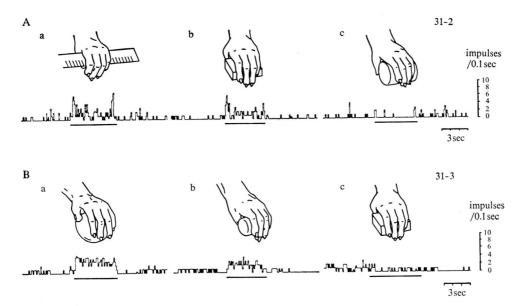

Fig. 3. The response histograms of unit 31–2 (A) and unit 31–3 (B) during grasping of different objects. Aa, a straight-edged ruler; b, a rectangular block; c, a small cylindrical bottle; Ba, an apple of about 5 cm dia.; b, a small cylindrical bottle; c, a rectangular block (Iwamura and Tanaka, 1978c).[13]

(area 3b) and the ansate region (areas 1 and 2) of the cat SI. In the former, most of the RFs were small, focal, and confined to single digits or pads, whereas in the latter, most of the unit RFs covered two or three digits, or the entire dorsal or ventral forepaw surface including digit tips.

RFs of the coronal neurons were more-or-less similar to the RFs of thalamic ventrobasal (VB) neurons. On the other hand, if the RFs of ansate neurons are compared with those of VB neurons in the same region of the body, it is clear that the RFs of the cortical neurons are not only larger in size, but also more uniform in shape (Fig. 4). The results suggest the presence of an integratory mechanism for molding and sculpturing the RF configuration within the SI. Moreover, some SI neurons had inhibitory RFs. These inhibitory areas were found to be adjacent to the excitatory fields, and their configurations resembled those of excitatory fields of neighboring neurons. These inhibitory RFs also suggest a specific processing for discrimination of particular skin regions from neighboring ones. In a similar sense, some of the inhibitory RFs of subcortical somatosensory neurons may be interpreted as serving for the discrimination of one RF configuration from another when they are found to be present side-by-side with the excitatory RFs[4,5,9].

The functional significance of the RF integration

The functional significance of this mode of integration becomes more apparent through observation of the natural behavior of the cat. The shapes of the relatively large receptive fields resembled corresponding skin areas which come into contact with objects or other parts of the body when the animal sits or assumes some characteristic pose.

Examples of such correspondence are shown in Fig. 5. Large RFs on the ulnar and ventral sides of the forearm cover the area which comes into contact with the ground (A and B) when

A   B

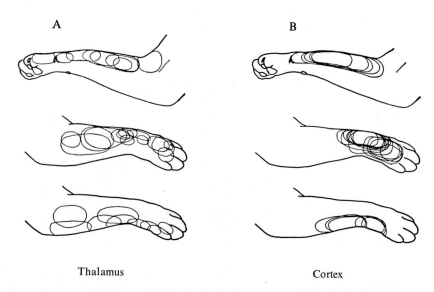

Thalamus   Cortex

Fig. 4. Samples of receptive fields in thalamic ventrobasal neurons (A), and in cortical SI neurons (B) in corresponding forearm regions. Thalamic RFs were calculated from anesthetized cat preparations.[8] Note the smaller size of the RFs in the thalamic neurons (Iwamura and Tanaka, unpublished).

the cat lies down as illustrated, and each corresponds to a subtle difference in pose. RFs in the dorsal forepaw surfaces (C and D) come into contact with the ground when the cat assumes the characteristically feline crouching position. Typical long RFs on the radial side of the forearm (E) may be correlated with the grooming behavior in cats when they wipe their face with their forelimbs. Thus, each of these integrated types of RFs found is considered to represent a "functional surface". This leads to an important conclusion that the increase in the size of RFs within the SI is also a process of data reduction to extract meaningful information about somatotopic locations of stimuli. The results suggest that the cat SI is organized as a mosaic of sub-areas divided on the basis of the afferent inputs, the mode of integration, efferent output, etc.

In the ansate region, the mode of activation of units was not as simple as in the coronal region. Some units required rapidly moving stimuli with or without directional selectivity. Light rubbing or tapping instead of light touching on the hair tips, or stimuli covering broad areas instead of punctate stimuli were more effective.

A few units displayed inhibitory effects as a result of different modes of stimulation on the same receptive areas. The temporospatial characteristics of these units could be the result of combined activation of various types of peripheral receptors. Furthermore, the responses of certain units were characteristically influenced by both skin and deep submodalities. The preferred deep stimuli for these units have been found to be organized movements of the limb rather than simple movements of single joints. For example, for a unit with its RF on the forearm skin, the effects of skin stimulation were dependent on shoulder position: it was effective only when the forelimb was held in the forward position. Similar submodality convergence has been interpreted in the monkey as serving a purpose in the recognition of limb movements and position[28].

As described in the monkey SI[28,29], directionally selective units were frequently found in the cat SI. The functional significance of these units with directional preference can be understood

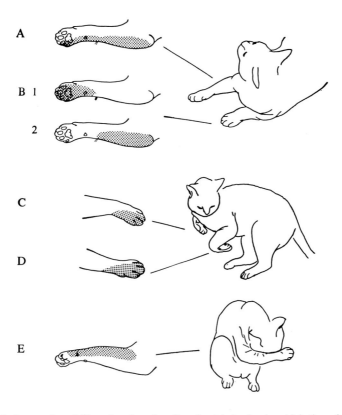

Fig. 5. Typical examples of "functional surfaces" and cat behavior in which these functional surfaces come into contact with the ground or other objects to be thereby stimulated. A full explanation is given in the text (Source: ref. 27. Reproduced by kind permission of Pergamon Press Ltd., England).

in the light of particular stimuli corresponding to the directional considerations of complex limb movements. The preferred direction of the unit shown in Fig. 6 and its tonic inhibition from possible deep receptors can be understood, for instance, if it is related to the feline crouching position illustrated (Fig. 6D). The initial movement to fold the paw will stimulate the skin receptors as it makes contact with the ground. Once the cat assumes the position, the paw will be pressed down by the body weight, and the unit would cease to fire as the crouching motion is completed. The detection or perception of the movement of a part of the body in connection with postural change and locomotion would then be achieved through the combination of information from both the skin and deep structures.

Summary

This brief review has described recent studies, mainly of our own, on neurons of the somatosensory cortex of both monkeys and cats aimed at seeking the mechanisms by which the animals perceive the somatosensory world. The most important conclusion so far drawn in these studies is that the functional organization of the somatic sensory receiving areas and their ways of informa-

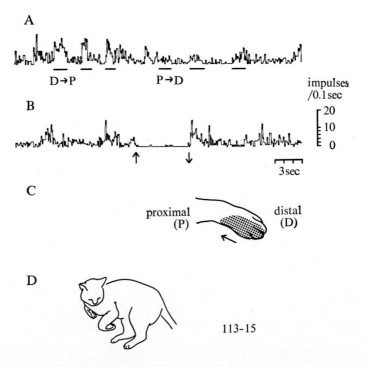

Fig. 6. A: Directionally selective response of unit 113–15 to the moving stimulus in the preferred direction (D → P) and in the reverse direction (P → D). B: Inhibition of background activity by gentle pressing of the receptive field. C: The receptive field of unit 113–15. D: A typical crouching position of the cat. A full explanation is given in the text (Iwamura and Tanaka, 1978b)[12].

tion processing reflect the behavioral peculiarities and uniqueness of each species of animal. It was suggested in the monkey that the hand region of the SI is organized for processing tactile information collected by active exploration with the hand. The somatic sensory function of the monkey, as an active perceiver, should thus be better understood when studied in combination with motor performance executed by the precentral gyrus.

It is proposed that the cat SI is organized as a mosaic of clusterings of neurons, each of which has behavioral correlates: some aspect of a cat's behavior, such as licking, grooming, crouching, etc. The functional significance of the submodality convergence and directional selectivity observed in the cat SI can thus be discussed in the light of these behavioral correlates.

References

1. Burgess, P.R. and Perl, E.R., Cutaneous mechanoreceptors and nociceptors. In A. Iggo (Ed.) *Handbook of Sensory Physiology, Vol. II, Somatosensory System,* Springer, Berlin, 1973, pp. 29–78.
2. Corkin, S., Milner, B. and Rasmussen, T., Somatosensory thresholds, *Arch. Neurol.*, 23 (1970) 41–58.
3. Gibson, J.J., *The Senses Considered as Perceptual Systems*, Houghton Mifflin Co., Boston, 1966, pp. 133.
4. Gordon, G. and Jukes, M.G.M., Dual organization of the exteroceptive components of the cat gracile nucleus, *J. Physiol. (Lond.)*, 173 (1964) 263–290.
5. Hongo, T., Jankowska, E. and Lundberg, A., Post-synaptic excitation and inhibition from primary afferents in neurons of the spinocervical tract, *J. Physiol. .(Lond.)*, 199 (1968) 569–592.

6. Hubel, D.H. and Wiesel, T.N., Receptive fields, binocular interaction and functional architecture in the cat's visual cortex, *J. Physiol. (Lond.)*, 160 (1962) 106–154.

7. Hubel, D.H. and Wiesel, T.N., Receptive fields and functional architecture in two nonstriate visual areas (18 and 19) of the cat, *J. Neurophysiol.*, 28 (1965) 229–289.

8. Hyvärinen, J., Cellular mechanisms in the parietal cortex in alert monkey, In Y. Zotterman (Ed.), *Sensory Functions of the Skin in Primates with Special Reference to Man*, Pergamon, Oxford, 1976. .

9. Iwamura, Y. and Inubushi, S., Regional diversity in excitatory and inhibitory receptive-fielded organization of cat thalamic ventrobasal neurons, *J. Neurophysiol.*, 37 (1974) 910–919.

10. Iwamura, Y. and Tanaka, M., Multiple representation of the forepaw skin area in the cat somatosensory cortex (SI), *Abstract for the 27th International Congress of Physiological Science*, 1977, pp. 349.

11. Iwamura, Y. and Tanaka, M., Functional organization of receptive fields in the cat somatosensory cortex I: integration within the coronal region, *Brain Research*, 151 (1978a) 49–60.

12. Iwamura, Y. and Tanaka, M., Functional organization of receptive fields in the cat somatosensory cortex II: second representation of the forepaw in the ansate region, *Brain Research*, 151 (1978b) 61–72.

13. Iwamura, Y., and Tanaka, M., Postcentral neurons in hand region of area 2: their possible role in the form discrimination of tactile objects, *Brain Research*, 150 (1978c) 662–666.

14. Iwamura, Y., Tanaka, M. and Hikosaka, O., Functional organization of neurons in area 2 of monkey somatosensory cortex (SI), *Abstract for the Annual Meeting of the Society for Neuroscience*, 1978.

15. Jones, E.G., Pattern of cortical and thalamic connections of the somatic sensory cortex, *Nature (Lond.)*, 216 (1967) 704–705.

16. Jones, E.G. and Powell, T.P.S., Anatomical organization of the somatosensory cortex, In A. Iggo (Ed.) *Handbook of Sensory Physiology, Vol. II, Somatosensory System*, Springer, Berlin, 1973, pp. 743–790.

17. Künzle, H., Cortico-cortical efferents of primary motor and somatosensory regions of the cerebral cortex in *Macaca fascicularis, Neuroscience*, 3 (1978) 25–39.

18. Mountcastle, V.B., Modality and topographic properties of single neurons of cat's somatic sensory cortex. *J. Neurophysiol.*, 20 (1957) 408–433.

19. Mountcastle, V.B. and Powell, T.P.S., Central nervous mechanisms subserving position sense and kinesthesis, *Bull. Johns Hopkins Hosp.*, 105 (1959) 173–200.

20. Mountcastle, V.B., Talbot, W.H., Sakata, H. and Hyvärinen, J., Cortical neuronalm echanisms in flutter-vibration studied in unanesthetized monkeys, neuronal periodicity and frequency discrimination, *J. Neurophysiol.*, 32 (1969) 452–484.

21. Orbach, J. and Chow, K.L., Differential effects of resection of somatic areas I and II in monkeys, *J. Neurophysiol.*, 22 (1959) 195–203.

22. Powell, T.P.S. and Mountcastle, V.B., Some aspects of the cortex of the postcentral gyrus of the monkey, a correlation of findings obtained in a single unit analysis with cytoarchitecture, *Bull. Johns Hopkins Hosp.*, 105 (1959) 133–162.

23. Pubols, L.M. and Leroy, R.F., Orientation detectors in the primary somatosensory neocortex of the racoon, *Brain Research*, 129 (1977) 61–74.

24. Randolf, M. and Semmes, J., Behavioral consequences of selective subtotal ablations in the postcentral gyrus of *Macaca mulatta, Brain Research*, 70 (1974) 55–70.

25. Roland, P.E., Astereognosis, tactile discrimination after localized hemispheric lesions in man, *Arch. Neurol.*, 33 (1976) 543–550.

26. Ruch, T.C., Fulton, J.F. and German, W.J., Sensory discrimination in monkey, chimpanzee and man after lesions of the parietal lobe, *Arch. Neurol. Psychiat.*, 39 (1938) 919–937.

27. Sakata, H. and Iwamura, Y., Cortical processing of tactile information in the first somatosensory and parietal association areas of the monkey, In G. Gordon and Y. Laporte (Eds.), *Active Touch*, Pergamon, Oxford, 1978.

28. Sakata, H., Takaoka, Y., Kawarasaki, A. and Shibutani, H., Somatosensory properties of neurons in the superior parietal cortex (area 5) of the rhesus monkey, *Brain Research*, 64 (1973) 85–102.

29. Schwarz, D.W.F. and Frederickson, J.M., Tactile direction sensitivity of area 2 oral neurons in the rhesus monkey cortex, *Brain Research*, 27 (1971) 397–401.

30. Semmes, J., A non-tactual factor in astereognosis, *Neuropsychologia*, 3 (1965) 295–315.

31. Vogt. B.A. and Pandya, D.N., Cortico-cortical connections of somatic sensory cortex (areas 3, 1 and 2) in the rhesus monkey, *J. comp. Neurol.*, 177 (1977) 179–192.

32. Werner, G., Neural information processing with stimulus feature extractors, In F.O. Schmitt and F.G. Worden (Eds.), *The Neurosciences, 3rd Study Program*, MIT Press, Cambridge, Mass., 1974, pp. 171–183.

33. Whitsel, B.L., Roppolo, J.R. and Werner, G., Cortical information processing of stimulus motion on primate skin, *J. Neurophysiol.*, 35 (1972) 619–717.

34. Zeki, S.M., The functional organization of projections from striate to prestriate visual cortex in the rhesus monkey, *Cold Spring Harb. Symp. Quant. Biol.*, 40 (1975) 591–600.

Rod and cone convergence to carp bipolar cells

AKIMICHI KANEKO, MASAO TACHIBANA AND EDWARD V. FAMIGLIETTI, Jr.*

*Department of Physiology, School of Medicien, Keio University,
Shinjuku-ku, Tokyo 160, Japan*

Most vertebrates have two kinds of photoreceptors, rods and cones. In Golgi-EM studies of cyprinid fish retina, Stell[7] has shown that bipolar cells of one morphological type (mixed bipolar cells) have connections with both rods and cones. The present study was undertaken to investigate,

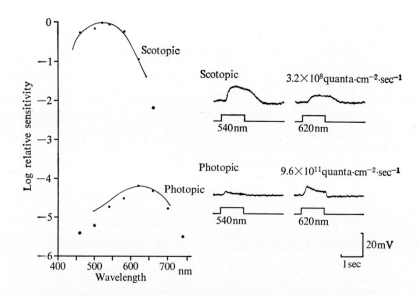

Fig. 1.   Spectral sensitivity of an ON type mixed bipolar cell under the scotopic and photopic conditions. After the scotopic sensitivity was determined, the retina was light-adapted by steady diffuse background illumination (white light, 118 μW· cm^{-2}) and the photopic sensitivity was measured. The sensitivity was calculated as the reciprocal of the light intensity yielding a criterion amplitude of 4 mV to a 240 μm spot, and normalized in reference to the scotopic peak. The continuous curve on the scotopic data indicates the absorption spectrum of porphyrhopsin[5]; that on the photopic data indicates the spectrum of the red-sensitive cones.[3] The insets show the responses of this cell to green (540 um) and red (620 nm) flashes of equal photon number under the two conditions. (Reprinted from Kaneko *et al*[8] by permission of John Wiley & Sons, Inc.)

* Present address: Department of Physiology and Biophysics, School of Medicine, Washington University, St. Louis, Missouri 63110, U.S.A.

on a physiological basis, how rods and cones connect with bipolar cells. To do this, bipolar cells were first studied in the scotopic condition. The same cells were then studied in the photopic condition. Recorded cells were morphologically identified by intracellular staining with Procion Yellow.[2,4] In the carp retina the population of ON and OFF bipolar cells is nearly equal.

Fig. 1 shows records obtained from a mixed ON bipolar cell, as an example of 10 such cells. In response to spot illumination in the receptive field center, this cell showed depolarizing responses to all parts of the spectrum. In the scotopic state, the response amplitude to a short wavelength (540 nm) was larger than that to a long wavelength spectrum (620 nm) of equal photon number. The spectral sensitivity curve showed good agreement with the absorption spectrum of the rod pigment, porphyrhopsin.[5] When the retina was made photopic with diffuse background illumination (white light, 118 μW·cm^{-2}), the same cell also exhibited a depolarizing response to spot illumination. However, under the new condition, the response amplitude was larger to 620 nm than to 540 nm. The spectral sensitivity under the photopic condition peaked at about 620 nm and the points fell close to the spectral absorption curve of the red-sensitive cone.[3] We obtained similar results also with 5 OFF type mixed bipolar cells. These cells responded with hyperpolarization under the scotopic and photopic conditions and the wavelength evoking the maximal response amplitude shifted from 520 nm in the scotopic to 620 nm in the photopic condition (Purkinje shift).

The present results show that the mixed bipolar cell received mixed inputs both from rods and red-sensitive cones with the same response polarity. In goldfish ganglion cells,[1,6] the response polarity of rod signals is the same as that from red-sensitive cones. As shown schematically in Fig. 2, the first stage of rod and cone convergence was found to be at the bipolar cells. The synaptic connection between photoreceptors and individual mixed bipolar cells appears to be unimodal in both cone-bipolar and rod-bipolar cell pairs, producing either ON or OFF responses. Both presynaptic neurons (photoreceptors) are hyperpolarized by illumination, so that the response

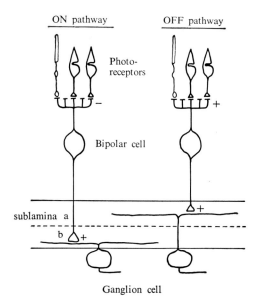

Fig. 2. Schematic drawing illustrating separate ON and OFF pathways from bipolar to ganglion cells in carp retina and the convergence of rods (having rod-shaped outer segments) and cones (having conical outer segments) to bipolar cells. Plus signs indicate that the response polarity of the presynaptic cell is preserved in the postsynaptic cell, and the minus sign indicates a synapse where the response polarity is reversed.

polarity is evidently determined by the type of postsynaptic elements, not by the input. Separation of the ON and OFF pathways from bipolar to ganglion cells has been demonstrated.[2]

References

1. Beauchamp, R.D. and Daw, N.W., Rod and cone input to single goldfish optic nerve fibers, *Vision Res.* 12, (1972) 1201–1212.
2. Famiglietti, E.V.Jr., Kaneko, A. and Tachibana, M., Neuronal architecture of ON and OFF pathways to ganglion cells in carp retina, *Science*, 198 (1977) 1267–1269.
3. Harosi, F.I. and MacNichol, E.F.Jr., Visual pigments of goldfish cones. Spectral properties and dichroism, *J. gen. Physiol.*, 63 (1974) 279–304.
4. Kaneko, A., Physiological and morphological identification of horizontal, bipolar and amacrine cells in goldfish retina, *J. Physiol. (Lond.)*, 207 (1970) 623–633.
5. Munz, F.W. and Schwanzara, S.A., A nomogram for retinene$_2$-based visual pigments, *Vision Res.*, 7 (1967) 111–120.
6. Raynauld, J.-P., Goldfish retina: sign of the rod input in opponent color ganglion cells, *Science*, 177 (1972) 84–85.
7. Stell, W.K., The structure and relationships of horizontal cells and photoreceptor-bipolar synaptic complexes in goldfish retina, *Amer. J. Anat.*, 121 (1967) 401–424.
8. Kaneko, A., Famiglietti, E.V.Jr. and Tachibana, M., Physiological and morphological identification of signal pathways in the carp retina, In *Neurobiology of Chemical Transmission* (eds., M. Otsuka and Z.W. Hall), John Wiley & Sons, Inc., N.Y. (in press).

Some relations between receptive-field properties and afferent conduction velocities in relay cells of the rat lateral geniculate nucleus

YUTAKA FUKUDA, ICHIJI SUMITOMO, MICHIO SUGITANI AND KITSUYA IWAMA

Department of Neurophysiology, Institute of Higher Nervous Activity, Osaka University Medical School, Kita-ku, Osaka 530, Japan

Previously, Fukuda[1] established that ganglion cells of the rat retina can be classified into three groups according to the size of the cell soma and the axonal conduction velocity. As an extension of this work, studies were made with relay cells of the rat lateral geniculate nucleus (LGN) to determine whether their receptive-field properties were related to the conduction velocities of the retinal afferents, in the way that is found in the Y-, X- and W-type relay cells of the cat LGN.[2]

Under urethane anesthesia (1.2–1.5 g/kg), adult albino rats were fixed to a stereotaxic apparatus and immobilized with Flaxedil. Single unit activities were recorded from the left LGN with microelectrodes filled with 3 M KCl. Based on the response properties to single electrical shocks to the optic chiasm (OX), units were identified as relay cells. For each of them, the OX-latency was determined by averaging 10 consecutive responses. Receptive fields were plotted by projecting light spots or dark disks of 0.5–5° onto a tangent screen placed 30 cm in front of the right eye. The cornea was protected from drying with a contact lens of zero power.

A total of 273 relay cells were sampled. According to the receptive-field properties, they were classified into two main types: Common ($N = 243$) and Uncommon (30). The Common type consists of the OFF-phasic, ON-phasic, ON-tonic and ON-OFF-phasic types, while the Uncommon type includes the ON-inhibited, Moving-sensitive, ON-OFF-inhibited, Simple-cell-like and Complex-cell-like types. The numbers of samples with these cell types are listed in the second

TABLE 1. OX-latencies and receptive-field sizes of various classes of receptive-field type

Receptive-field type	Sampling number	OX-latency (msec)	Receptive-field size (deg)
Common types			
OFF-phasic	74 (27.1%)	1.94 ± 0.8 (57)[†]	7.05 ± 2.6 (57)[†]
ON-phasic	86 (31.5%)	2.35 ± 0.8 (57)	6.45 ± 2.7 (59)
ON-tonic	32 (11.7%)	2.78 ± 1.1 (21)	5.87 ± 1.8 (18)
ON-OFF-phasic	51 (18.6%)	3.04 ± 0.8 (32)	6.97 ± 2.8 (38)
Uncommon types			
ON-inhibited	10 (3.7%)		
Moving-sensitive	9 (3.2%)		
ON-OFF-inhibited	3 (1.1%)	3.18 ± 1.3 (18)	11.33 ± 8.4 (22)
Simple-cell-like	7 (2.6%)		
Complex-cell-like	1 (0.4%)		
Total	273 (100%)	185	194

†No. of cells studied.

column of Table 1. Fig. 1 shows typical records of the visual responses of certain classes of relay cells. The cells so classified were also distinguished as regards OX-latency. The average OX-latency increased in the order of OFF-phasic, ON-phasic, ON-tonic, ON-OFF-phasic and Uncommon types (Table 1, column 3). With regard to receptive-field size, the four classes of the Common type were not distinguishable from each other. The average receptive-field size of the Uncommon type cells was about twice that of the Common type cells (Table 1, column 4).

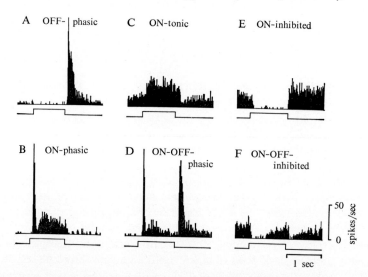

Fig. 1.   Sample responses of relay cells to stationary light spots flashing at the receptive-field center. A–D are representatives of the four Common types, while E and F are representatives of the two Uncommon types. For the peristimulus time histograms 10 responses were added, using a bin width of 10 msec and an analysis time of 2560 msce. The trace below the histograms represents the luminance of the activated region. The trace rises as the luminance increases and falls as it decreases. The size of the centered light spot was adjusted so as to cover the center of each receptive field: 8.6°(A), 9.1°(B), 5.1°(C), 7.2°(D), 5.9°(E), and 12.5°(F).

The Uncommon type cells and the ON-OFF-phasic cells of the rat LGN are innervated by the slowest group of retinal afferents and their visual properties are more complex than any others. In view of this, these two types of cells are taken together as corresponding to the W-type cells of the cat LGN. Since rat OFF-phasic and ON-phasic cells are characterized by short OX-latencies, they would be homologized with cat Y-type cells whose retinal afferents are faster than for others. Concerning the ON-tonic cells of the rat, some probably correspond to X-type cells and others to ON-tonic, W-type cells of the cat. In conclusion, it is said that in the rat LGN the Y- and W-systems predominate over the X-system.

References

1. Fukuda, Y., A three-group classification of rat retinal ganglion cells: histological and physiological studies, *Brain Research*, 119 (1977) 327–344.
2. Wilson. P.D., Rowe, M.H. and Stone, J., Properties of relay cells in cat's lateral geniculate nucleus: A comparison of W-cells with X- and Y-cells, *J. Neurophysiol.*, 39 (1976) 1193–1209.

Unitary responses in the nucleus centralis lateralis to electrical stimulation of the visual pathways in chloralose-anesthetized cat

TETSURO OGAWA AND TOORU TAKIMORI

*Department of Physiology, Akita University School of Medicine,
Hondo, Akita 010, Japan*

It has been well documented that neurons in the pericruciate cortex of the cat are responsive not only to somesthetic but also to visual and auditory stimulation[1,3–5,7,12,14]. For this reason, this cortical area has been regarded as one of the polysensory or non-primary response areas.[3] However, which structures are involved in the neural pathways from the retina to the motor cortex has not yet been determined, although there have been suggestions that the medial thalamic nuclei and the brain stem reticular formation may be involved[2,13]. In a previous report, we showed that in cat precruciate cortex some PT-and Non PT cells, as classified on the basis of their antidromic responsiveness to stimulation of the bulbar pyramid, could respond to electrical stimulation of the visual pathway at a latency of not more than 10 msec[10]. In this context we suggested that some subcortical structures might be responsible for the mediation of visual responses to the motor cortex in view of the fact that ablation of the primary visual cortex did not affect the responsiveness of the motor cortical neurons to visual stimulation.

Recent anatomical and physiological studies have established the projections of the nucleus centralis lateralis (CL) to the motor cortex[6,8,9]. The present experiments were undertaken to ascertain whether neurons in the CL sending their axons to the motor cortex are responsive to visual stimulation.

Twenty-two adult cats anesthetized with α-chloralose (70mg/kg, i.v.) were used. The anesthetic level was adjusted throughout the experiment by administering an additive dose of α-chloralose at regular intervals to the degree that no jerky movements were elicited by pinching the skin on the back. Stimulating bipolar needle electrodes were placed in the optic chiasm (OX), optic tract (OT), superior colliculus (SC), visual areas (VC) and precruciate cortex (MC) ipsilateral to the explored CL and also in the brachium conjunctivum (BC) contralateral to the CL. A tungsten microelectrode was guided stereotaxically into the CL for recording unitary discharges of neurons. Action potentials were amplified by a conventional RC amplifier and displayed on a dual beam oscilloscope. They were also fed into a signal processor (San'ei, Co.) and processed to construct PST histograms for responses to flash light delivered through a glow modulator tube (Sylvania R 1131C). In the present experiments, mapping of receptive fields of CL neurons was not attempted. Only the responsiveness of CL neurons to flash light and electrical stimulation of the above-mentioned structures was studied.

The present study was based on a total of 37 units which were located within the CL as verified histologically.

Fig. 1 illustrates unitary responses to flash light delivered to either eye and to electrical stimulation of OX, OT, SC, VC, and MC of neurons encountered while the microelectrode was inserted through the caudal part of the CL which histological investigations have indicated to

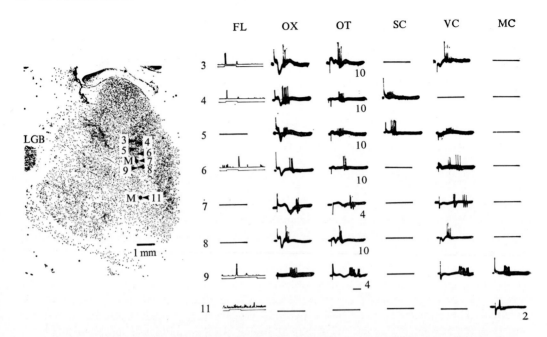

Fig. 1.   Unitary responses in the nucleus centralis lateralis (CL). A tungsten microelectrode was advanced vertically through the CL. In the course of penetration, units 3 through 11 were obtained. Their responses to flash light (FL) and to electrical stimulation of the optic chiasm (OX), optic tract (OT), superior colliculus (SC), visual cortex (VC) and precruciate cortex (MC) are displayed on the right. The responses to FL of 500 msec duration given to the contralateral eye 50 times at a repetition rate of 1/2.5 sec were compiled and displayed as PST histograms (bin width, 10 msec; full scale of horizontal axis, 2 sec except for 9 where it is 1 sec). Stepwise deflection of the trace below each PST histogram indicates the presentation of flash light. The same vertical scale is applied to all histograms, the largest peak in 3 standing for 50 imp/bin. The time calibration for each trace representing five superimposed responses is given numerically in msec below each trace in the OT and MC columns, the short horizontal bar just below the unit 9 OT trace showing the calibrated time scale. On the left, the electrode track with two lesions (marked with asterisks) is shown in a frontal section through the left half of the dorsal thalamus of the cat at 8.5 mm anterior. LGB, lateral geniculate nucleus.

project to the precruciate cortex[8,9]. The position of each neuron recorded successively during the advance of the microelectrode is indicated by an arrow head with a number on the photograph of a cresyl violet stained histological section with reference to two electrocoagulations (marked with asterisks) which were made at sites where responses of units 7 and 11 were recorded. Units 3 through 8 were located within the CL and unit 9 was just at the border of the CL. Units 10 (not indicated in Fig.1) and 11 were outside the CL. Units 3 through 9 responded to OX and OT stimulation in a similar fashion: the responses consisted of either single or a burst of impulses and their latencies ranged from 4 to 22 msec. These figures are comparable to those described by Schlag-Rey and Schlag[11]. No neurons within the CL responded to MC stimulation, but unit 9 responded with a burst of impulses after a latency of about 4.6 msec. This failure might be attributable to the penetration having been made through the middle of the CL as opposed to the medial or lateral border of the CL which has been shown to project to the precruciate cortex[8]. However, this may not be the case, since in no experiment were we able to show antidromic activation of border-lying CL neurons by MC stimulation. Unit 11 located in the nucleus ventralis lateralis (VL) did not respond to electrical stimulation of the visual pathway, but it was activated antidromically by MC stimulation. In other experiments most VL neurons located adjacent to the CL were found to be antidromically activated by MC stimulation, some of which were also driven by flash light.

The present results indicate that CL neurons have binocular inputs through polysynaptic routes. The question of whether CL neurons which send their axons to the precruciate cortex receive visual input remains to be solved.

REFERENCES

1. Batuev, A.S., Lenkov, D.N. and Pirogov, A.A., Postsynaptic responses of motor cortex neurons of cats to sensory stimulation of different modalities, *Acta neurobiol. exp.*, 34 (1974) 317–321.
2. Buser, P., Subcortical controls of pyramidal activity. In D.P. Purpura and M. D. Yahr (Eds.), *The Thalamus*, Columbia Univ. Press, New York, 1966, pp. 323–347.
3. Buser, P. and Bignall, K.E., Non primary sensory projections on the cat neocortex, *Int. Rev. Neurobiol.*, 10 (1968) 111–165.
4. Buser, P. and Imbert, M., Sensory projections to the motor cortex in cats: A microelectrode study. In W.A. Rosenblith (Ed.), *Sensory Communication*, Wiley, New York, 1961, pp. 607–626.
5. Chu, N.-S. and Rutledge, L.T., Multisensory activation of pyramidal tract neurons in the cat, *Exp. Neurol.*, 30 (1971) 352–361.
6. Endo, K., Araki, T. and Ito, K., Short latency EPSPs of pyramidal tract cells evoked by stimulation of the striatum with reference to those by intralaminar nuclei of the thalamus, *Brain Research*, 132 (1977) 547–552
7. Garcia-Rill, E. and Dubrovsky, B., Responses of motor cortex cells to visual stimuli, *Brain Research*, 82 (1974) 185–194.
8. Itoh, K. and Mizuno, N., Topographical arrangement of thalamocortical neurons in the centrolateral nucleus (CL) of the cat, with special reference to a spino-thalamo-motor cortical path through the CL, *Exp. Brain Res.*, 30 (1977) 471–480.
9. Macchi, G., Bentivoglio, M., D'Atena, C., Rossini, P. and Tempesta, E., The cortical projections of the thalamic intralaminar nuclei restudied by means of the HRP retrograde axonal transport, *Neurosci. Lett.*, 4 (1977) 121–126.
10. Ogawa, T., Visual input to the cat's motor cortex, *J. Physiol. Soc. Japan*, 37 (1975) 369–370.
11. Schlag-Rey, M. and Schlag, J., Visual and presaccadic activity in thalamic internal medullary lamina of cat: A study of targeting, *J. Neurophysiol.*, 40 (1977) 156–173.
12. Teyler, T.J., Shaw, C. and Thompson, R.F., Unit responses to moving visual stimuli in the motor cortex of the cat, *Science*, 176 (1972) 811–813.
13. Thompson, R.F., Johnson, R.H. and Hoopes, J., Organization of auditory, somatic sensory and visual projections to association fields of cerebral cortex in the cat, *J. Neurophysiol.*, 26 (1963) 343–363.
14. Voronin, L.L. and Ezrohki, V.L., Convergence of impulses on neurons of the motor cortex in cats anesthetized with chloralose, *Bull. exp. Biol. Med.*, 73 (1972) 494–497.

Vestibular and visual influences on superior colliculus neurons in the cat

MINORU MAEDA[*1], TOHRU SHIBAZAKI[*2] AND KAORU YOSHIDA[*3]

[1] *Department of Neurosurgery, School of Medicine, Juntendo University, Bunkyo-ku, Tokyo 113, Japan*

[2] *Department of Neurophysiology, Institute of Brain Research, University of Tokyo, Bunkyo-ku, Tokyo 113, Japan*

[3] *Department of Physiology, Institute of Basic Medical Sciences, Univeristy of Tsukuba, Niihari-gun, Ibaragi 300–31, Japan*

The tectospinal tract, as well as the vestibulospinal tract, is one of the major descending pathways of the extrapyramidal motor system in mammals. It has been suggested that the superior colliculus plays an important role in the coordination of eye and head movements during gaze[11]. In fact, the spike discharge recorded in the superior colliculus increased in frequency prior to saccadic eye movement[9,12]. Electrical stimulation of the superior colliculus leads to movement not only of the eye (see refs. 4, 8 and 9) but also of the neck and body.[1] Disturbances of visually guided behavior after destruction of the superior colliculus have been reported[10,13]. On the other hand the vestibular system has also been found to regulate eye and head movement[6,7,11]. In this respect studies of the neuronal organization between the vestibular and retino-tectal systems and the interaction between them are required for elucidating the mechanism for gaze control.

Experiments were performed on 24 cats under α-chloralose anesthesia. The animals were paralyzed with gallamine triethiodide and ventilated artificially. The surface of the superior colliculus was exposed by removal of the occipital lobe, and glass micropipettes filled with 2 M potassium citrate or 3 M KCL were used for intracellular recording from tectal neurons. Bipolar electrodes were implanted in the ipsi- and contralateral labyrinths to stimulate the vestibular nerve. Bipolar electrodes were also used for stimulation of the optic disk on both sides. The projection areas of the neurons impaled were identified by their antidromic responses to stimulation of the contralateral abducens nucleus, the contralateral prepositus hypoglossi (tecto-reticular neurons) or the C_2-segment (tecto-spinal neurons) with bipolar tungsten electrodes. In several experiments, pairs of sharpened tungsten needles were used for bipolar stimulation of the contralateral superior colliculus and the vestibular nucleus. The location of the neurons recorded intracellularly was reconstructed from the reference points (2–3 fast green dye marks made during and at the end of the experiment).

Single-shock stimulation of the contralateral optic disk (ODc) typically caused depolarizations in tecto-spinal (TS) neurons. They were increased in amplitude by passing a hyperpolarizing current and decreased by depolarization, and were therefore, EPSPs. Their amplitude varied with stimulus strength and with the number of stimuli. Stimulation of the ipsilateral optic disk (ODi) evoked very slowly rising depolarizations. Single shocks to the contralateral vestibular nerve (Vc) induced EPSPs and occasionally generated action potentials. The response could be followed by a later, larger depolarization. In a few cases mixed effects, i.e., depolarization-hyperpolarization sequences, were also obtained. The most common potential changes induced from the ipsilateral vestibular nerve (Vi) were slow-rising small EPSPs. Multiple stimuli were usually necessary to elicit PSPs and the responses to successive shocks were markedly facilitated. In short tecto-spinal neurons were influenced most consistently and strongly from the contralateral optic disk and vestibular nerve.

The latencies of the EPSPs evoked in TS neurons showed the following ranges: ODc, 2.2–7.2 msec (median 3.0 msec); ODi, 4.0–12.0 msec (7.0 msec); Vc, 2.4–12.0 msec (3.6 msec); Vi, 4.0–13.0 msec (7.0 msec).

The characteristics and patterns of synaptic potentials evoked in tecto-reticular (TR) neurons were very similar to those obtained in TS neurons. They were also influenced predominantly from ODc and Vc. In a few TR- neurons, IPSPs were evoked from Vi. The latencies of the EPSPs induced in tecto-reticular neurons showed the following ranges: ODc, 2.1–9.0 msec (median 2.8 msec); ODi, 3.2–11:0 msec (7.0 msec); Vc, 2.2–10.0 msec (3.6 msec); Vi, 2.4–12.0 msec (5.4 msec). TR- and TS-neurons were located in both the intermediate and deep layers. In the case of neurons in the superficial layer, which have been known to send their axons to the deeper layers, stimulation of ODc induced monosynaptic EPSPs with latencies of 1.4–1.9 msec and usually generated action potentials shortly after EPSP onset. Addition to these values of about 0.4 msec for synaptic delay in the superior colliculus gives an expected shortest latency range of 1.8–2.3 msec for a disynaptic pathway between the contralateral retina and neurons located in the intermediate or deep layer. Clearly then, the early EPSPs recorded in TS- or TR- neurons indicated disynaptic transmission. ODi-induced EPSPs had a latency of more than 3.2. msec, suggesting that these EPSPs were evoked via a pathway containing more synapses.

Stimulation of the contralateral vestibular nucleus induced EPSPs in TS- and TR- neurons with latencies ranging from 1.8 to 2.5 msec, and clear temporal summation was observed. This indicates the existence of disynaptic connections between them or, in other words, trisynaptic pathways linking the vestibular nerve to tectal neurons.

In three experiments, the cochlear nerve was cut on one side in the internal auditory meatus. This cut exerted no effect on the Vc-evoked potentials.

Stimulation of the contralateral superior colliculus (the intermediate or deep layer) evoked IPSPs in TS- and TR- neurons, which were easily reversed by Cl⁻ ion injection. The latencies ranged from 0.7 to 1.4 msec, indicating mostly monosynaptic IPSPs. These IPSPs may participate in the production of tecto-tectal inhibition as was suggested from lesion experiments in the rat[3] and the cat[5].

The interaction of vestibular and visual effects upon TS- or TR-neurons was tested (see ref. 2), Stimulation of Vc and ODc produced trisynaptic EPSPs. When conditioned by Vc stimulation which was adjusted so as to produce only a small EPSP, the same test ODc volley induced a larger trisynaptic EPSP than the algebraic summation. This finding indicates that the Vc volleys converge on and facilitate interneurons that mediate trisynatpic excitation from the ODc. These interneurons may play an important role in the control of gaze—a saccade accompanied by head movement. The precise locations of these interneurons remain to be studied.

REFERENCES

1. Anderson, M.E., Yoshida, M. and Wilson, V.J., Influence of the superior colliculus on cat neck motoneurons, *J. Neurophysiol.*, 34 (1971) 898–907.
2. Bisti, S., Maffei, L. and Piccolino, M., Visuovestibular interactions in the cat superior colliculus, *J. Neurophysiol.*, 37 (1974) 146–155.
3. Goodale, M.A., Cortico-tectal and intertectal modulation of visual responses in the rat's superior colliculus, *Exp. Brain Res.*, 17 (1973) 75–86.
4. Grantyn, A.A. and Grantyn, R., Synaptic actions of tectofugal pathways on abducens motoneurons in the cat, *Brain Research*, 105 (1976) 269–285.
5. Hoffmann, K.P. and Straschill, M., Influences of corticotectal and intertectal connections on visual responses in the cat's superior colliculus, *Exp. Brain Res.*, 12 (1971) 120–131.
6. Lorente De Nó, R., Vestibulo-ocular reflex arc, *Arch. Neurol. Psychiat. (Chic.)*, 30 (1933) 245–291.
7. Maeda, M., Magherini, P.C. and Precht, W., Functional organization of vestibular and visual inputs to neck and forelimb motoneurons in the frog, *J. Neurophysiol.*, 40 (1977) 225–243.
8. Precht, W., Schwindt, P.C. and Magherini, P.C., Tectal influences on cat ocular motoneurons, *Brain Research*, 82 (1974) 27–40.
9. Schiller, P.H., and Stryker, M., Single-unit recording and stimulation in superior colliculus of the alert rhesus monkey, *J. Neurophysiol.*, 35 (1972) 915–924.
10. Sprague, J.M. and Meikle, T.H. Jr., The role of the superior colliculus in visually guided behavior, *Exp. Neurol.*, 11 (1965) 115–146.
11. Wilson, V.J. and Maeda, M., Connections between semicircular canals and neck motoneurons in the cat, *J. Neurophysiol.*, 37 (1974) 346–357.
12. Wurtz, R.H. and Goldberg, M.E., Activity of superior colliculus in behaving monkey. III. Cells discharging before eye movements, *J. Neurophysiol.*, 35 (1972) 575–586.
13. Wurtz, R.H. and Goldberg, M.E., Activity of superior colliculus in behaving monkey. IV. Effects of lesions on eye movements, *J. Neurophysiol.*, 35 (1972) 587–596.

Origin of the mossy fiber projection to the cerebellar flocculus from the optic nerves in rabbits

KYOJI MAEKAWA AND TOSHIAKI TAKEDA

*Department of Physiology, Jichi Medical School,
Kawachi-gun, Tochigi 329–04, Japan*

Purkinje cells in the vestibulocerebellum were activated from the optic nerves not only through the climbing fibers[5] but also through the mossy fibers input.[6] The origin of the visually activated climbing fiber projections to the flocculus has been identified as the dorsal cap of the inferior olive[1,7]. In order to identify the origin of the mossy fiber (m.f.) projection to the flocculus activated from the optic nerves, both a histochemical tracing study using horseradish peroxidase (HRP) (six cases) and electrophysiological studies by stimulation threshold mapping and destruction experiments of the brain stem (15 cases) were carried out on rabbits.

Albino rabbits were anesthetized with alpha-chloralose plus urethane or with a mixture of N_2O–O_2. A glass microelectrode filled with 2M NaCl solution was inserted dorsoventrally into the right flocculus. As reported previously[6], the m.f. responses evoked from the optic nerves usually predominated in the rostromedial part of the dorsal folia of the flocculus. After confirming the site of large m.f. responses from the optic nerves in the flocculus (Fig. 1A), the microelectrode was replaced with a micropipette filled with 10% HRP (Toyobo Grade-I-C) in Tris-HCl buffer solution (pH 8.0). HRP was iontophoresed into the granular layer of the flocculus by passage of 2–4 μA positive DC current for 20 min. After a survival time of 24 hr, the rabbits were deeply anesthetized with alpha-chloralose plus urethane and the brains were perfused with 1% paraformaldehyde-2.5% glutaraldehyde-2% formaline-2.5% sucrose solution with phosphate buffer (pH 7.4). The brain stem and cerebellum were frozen and cut into 50 μm thick serial sections, then treated as described previously[9].

In all six cases, the brown-stained HRP injection areas were confined to the rostro-medial part of the dorsal-most folium of the right flocculus (Fig. 1B). Cells filled with HRP-postitive granules found in eight of the 50 μm thick serial sections (400 μm) were superimposed and dotted on line drawings of the transverse section (Fig. 1C). Labelled cells were found mainly in the nucleus reticularis tegmenti pontis (Bechterew) (Nrt), including the processus tegmentosus lateralis[3] on both sides and a few were found also in the pontine nucleus itself.

Fig. 2 shows an example of the stimulation threshold mapping experiments. Two stimulating electrodes 1.5mm apart mediolaterally were inserted stereotaxically into the pons (Fig. 2B). The depth of the electrodes was measured from the level of the rostral edge of the posterior commissure exposed by aspiration of the overlying cortex. Fig. 2C shows the relation between the electrode positions and the threshold currents in mA (pulse width, 0.05 msec) necessary to evoke the m.f. responses in the dorso-rostral flocculus. The threshold currents were lowest at a depth of around 10 mm, which corresponds well with Nrt (horizontal arrow). Fig. 2A shows the m.f. responses evoked in the flocculus by 100 μA current pulses from the stimulating sites indicated in B by arrows. Two characteristic features should be noted in this figure. First, the latencies of the m.f. responses evoked from the pontine region decreased gradually from 4.5 msec (A, 9.0) to 3.0

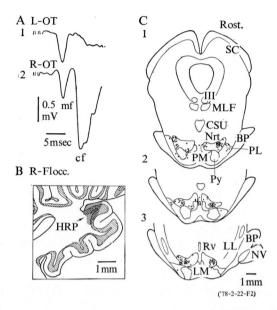

Fig. 1. HRP-labelled cells in the nucleus reticularis tegmenti pontis (Bechterew) (Nrt) after HRP injection into the dorso-rostral part of the right flocculus. A: Field potentials in the molecular layer of the dorsal-most folium of the right flocculus. The m.f. response (mf) from the left (L-OT, A_1) and the mossy and climbing fiber (cf) responses from the right optic tract (R-OT, A_2) are illustrated. HRP was iontophoresed into the granular layer just beneath this molecular layer. B: Line drawing of a transverse section of the right flocculus, showing the HRP injection site (shaded). C: Line drawings of the transverse sections of the pons. In each drawing, dots represent HRP-labelled cells found in 8 adjacent 50 μm serial sections. Rost, rostral; SC, superior colliculus; III, third nucleus; MLF, medial longitudinal fasciculus; CSU, nucleus centralis superior; PM, PL, medial and lateral pontine nucleus; Py; cerebral peduncle; BP, brachium pontis; Rv, ventral raphe; LM, LL, medial and lateral lemniscus; NV, the fifth nerve.

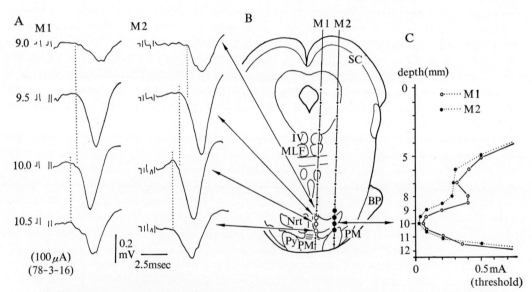

Fig. 2. Stimulation threshold mapping at the pontine region for evoking m.f. responses in the ipsilateral flocculus. A: Sample records elicited in the molecular layer of the dorsorostral flocculus by two stimulating electrodes (M_1 and M_2) using 100 μA pulses. B: Line drawing of a transverse section of the pons indicating stimulated sites (dots) along the two electrode tracks. Open circles and large closed circles indicate the sites of low threshold (less than 100 μA). C: Relation between the depth of the electrode (in mm, ordinate) and the threshold current (in mA, abscissa). A horizontal arrow at a depth of 10 mm indicates the corresponding site in B of the lowest threshold.

msec (A, 10.0), which may indicate that nuclear delays occurred around the Nrt. Second, the threshold currents abruptly increased in the pontine nucleus (C), which suggests that the pontine nucleus may not be involved in the visual m.f. activation of the flocculus.

Further, the m.f. responses evoked from the optic nerves and from the Nrt not only occluded each other but also were mutually inhibitory for 30–50 msec. In addition, a small, restricted destruction of the Nrt ipsilateral to the flocculus eliminated the m.f. response evoked from the optic nerves (three cases). These findings strongly suggest that the optic activities are transferred, at least partly, through the Nrt to the flocculus as m.f. activation.

The stimulation threshold mapping experiments on the surface of the meso-diencephalon demonstrated that the optic activities evoking the m.f. responses in the flocculus could be traced along the brachium of the superior colliculus (SC) to the dorsal part of the accessory optic tract and then appeared to enter the lateral pretectal region just before reaching the SC itself, thus confirming the results of the destruction experiments previously reported.[6] These findings are also consistent with the anatomical studies showing ipsilateral pretectal projections to the Nrt[2,4,8].

REFERENCE

1. Alley, K., Baker, R. and Simpson, J.I., Afferents to the verstibulo-cerebellum and the origin of the visual climbing fibers in the rabbit, *Brain Research*, 98 (1975) 582–589.
2. Berman, N., Connections of the pretectum in the cat, *J. comp. Neur.*, 174 (1977) 227–254.
3. Brodal, A. and Brodal, P., The organization of the nucleus reticularis tegmenti pontis in the cat in the light of experimental anatomical studies of its cerebral cortical afferents, *Exp. Brain Res.*, 13 (1971) 90–110.
4. Graybiel, A., Some efferents of the pretectal region in the cat, *Anat, Rec.*, 178 (1974) 365.
5. Maekawa, K. and Simpson, J.I., Climbing fiber responses evoked in vestibulocerebellum of rabbit from visual system, *J. Neurophysiol.*, 36 (1973) 649–666.
6. Maekawa, K. and Takeda, T., Mossy fiber responses evoked in the cerebellar flocculus of rabbits by stimulation of the optic pathway. *Brain Research*, 98 (1975) 590–595.
7. Maekawa, K., Climbing and mossy fiber visual pathways to the cerebellar flocculus, *J. physiol. Soc. Japan*, 37 (1975) 366–367.
8. Mizuno, N., Mochizuki, K., Akimoto, C. and Matsushima, R., Pretectal projections to the inferior olive in the rabbit, *Exp. Neurol.*, 39 (1973) 498–506.
9. Takeda, T. and Maekawa, K., The origin of the pretecto-olivary tract. A study using the horseradish peroxidase method, *Brain Research*, 117 (1976) 319–325.

High amplitude photic driving evoked by red-flicker and flickering-pattern

TAKEO TAKAHASHI AND TERUO OKUMA

Department of Neuropsychiatry, Tohoku University School of Medicine,
Sendai, Miyagi 980, Japan

Photic driving (PD) or photic following is a physiological response which is recorded from the occipital regions and is synchronized with the flicker frequency. In studying PD, intermittent stroboscopic white light has been widely used since the early work of Walter *et al.*[5] However, we found in a previous study that a red-flicker (RF) and a flickering-dot-pattern (FDP) were superior to intermittent photic stimulation for evoking high amplitude PD.[3] Since the data in our previous study were obtained from a limited number of subjects, it was considered necessary to repeat the experiment on a larger scale and with a greater variety of subjects. In the present study, therefore, a total of 713 subjects (356 females, 357 males) were tested for RF and FDP stimulation, including normal subjects and patients with various neuropsychiatric disorders. Particular attention was paid to an analysis of high amplitude PD. The subjects were divided into a "normal EEG group" (180; 25 were normal healthy persons), "epilepsy with abnormal EEG group" (430), and neuropsychiatric patients with abnormal EEG group ("abnormal EEG group" (103)). The ages of the subjects ranged from 5 to 70 yr.

FDP and RF were provided by the methods described previously[2-4] and the stimuli were given to the subject in a sitting position. The apparatus yielded an approximately sine-wave output of light intensity. After 2 to 3 min dark adaptation, the subjects were instructed to look through a small window at the center of a tangent screen set 25 cm from the eyes, and the stimuli were projected onto the screen (12 × 18 cm). When the pattern was projected onto the screen, the visual angle of a single dot was 0.80. Examinations were performed in the following order: (1) dark adaptation for 2 to 3 min, (2) RF for 7 sec, (3) dark adaptation for 10 sec, (4) FDP for 7 sec.

The amplitude of the fundamental PD recorded from the occipital area was expressed by that of the maximal PD during each 7 sec recording. The PD was arbitrarily classified into one of the following three groups based on amplitude: (1) low amplitude PD ($< 25 \mu V$) including cases of unidentified PD, (2) medium amplitude PD ($25-50 \mu V$), and (3) high amplitude PD ($> 50 \mu V$). The RF occasionally evoked PD of the second and third harmonics mixed with fundamental PD, whereas only fundamental PD was evoked by the FDP.

As shown in Fig. 1, high amplitude PD evoked by RF and FDP could generally be seen in the 0–10 yr age-group in all three groups of subjects. In this age-group in the "normal EEG group", high amplitude PD evoked by RF and FDP was found in 33% and 17%, respectively. When the incidences of high amplitude PD evoked by RF and FDP in the 0–10 yr age-group in the "epilepsy with abnormal EEG group" and "abnormal EEG group" were compared with those in the "normal EEG group", no statistically significant difference was observed. This may be due to the small number of cases in all groups. In the age-group of 11 yr old or above in the "normal EEG group", neither RF nor FDP evoked high amplitude PD. In the same age range of the "epilepsy with abnormal EEG group" and "abnormal EEG group", high amplitude PD was more frequent-

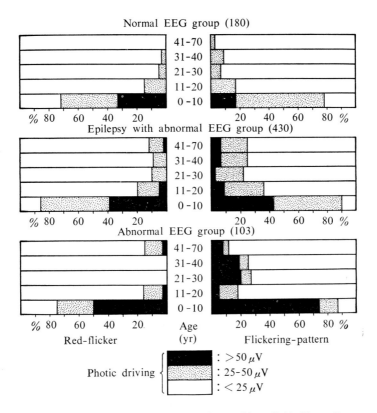

Fig. 1. Photic driving (PD) in a total of 713 subjects divided into a "normal EEG group" (180), "epilepsy with abnormal EEG group" (430), and "abnormal EEG group" (103). The incidences of PD of high amplitude ($> 50 \mu$V), medium amplitude (25–50 μV) and low amplitude ($< 25 \mu$V) evoked by red-flicker (left) and flickering-dot-pattern (right) are expressed in percent in each group.

ly evoked by FDP than by RF: high amplitude PD evoked by RF was found in 3% and 2% of these groups, respectively, whereas high amplitude PD evoked by FDP amounted to 7% and 11%, respectively. When the incidences of high amplitude PD in the "epilepsy with abnormal EEG group" and "abnormal EEG group" were compared with that in the "normal EEG group", only the incidences of high amplitude PD evoked by FDP in both groups were significantly high (in the "epilepsy with abnormal EEG group": $\chi^2 = 10.63$, $p < 0.005$; in the "abnormal EEG group": $\chi^2 = 15.04$, $p < 0.005$).

The following conclusions can be drawn from these results. (1) High amplitude PD is more frequently evoked by either RF or FDP in children irrespective of diagnostic group. (2) When high amplitude PD is evoked by FDP in adult patients, the presence of some kind of brain disturbance in the occipital area (visual cortex) is suggested.

Our previous studies on the photoconvulsive response have demonstrated that geometric patterns could selectively activate the epileptic focus in the occipital area of the brain.[1] Therefore, studies of PD using pattern stimuli should provide further valuable information not only for the diagnosis of brain dysfunction but also for determining the detailed functions of the visual cortex of the human brain.

References

1. Takahashi, T. and Tsukahara, Y., Generalized paroxysmal discharges induced by visual stimuli and eye movements, *Tohoku J. exp. Med.,* 115 (1975) 1–10.
2. Takahashi, T. and Tsukahara, Y., Influence of color on the photoconvulsive response, *Electroenceph. clin. Neurophysiol.,* 41 (1976) 124–136.
3. Takahashi, T. and Tsukahara, Y., Influence of red light and pattern on photic driving. *Tohoku J. exp. Med.,* 126 (1978) in press.
4. Tsukahara, Y. and Takahashi, T., Visual stimulator for EEG activation, *Electroenceph. clin. Neurophysiol.,* 35 (1973) 333–335.
5. Walter, W.G., Dovey, V.J. and Shipton, H., Analysis of the electrical response of the human cortex to photic stimulation, *Nature (Lond.),* 158 (1946) 540–541.

Morphology of the eye and brain in anophthalmic rats

KATSUMI OTANI, KENJI KOBAYASHI AND GUNSHIRO KATO

*Department of Anatomy, School of Medicine, Chiba University,
Inohana, Chiba 280, Japan*

Anophthalmia or microphthalmia has been reported in all classes of vertebrates, including man.[5] It has been shown that eyelessness in the embryonic stages generally occurs as a result of various agencies such as environmental, chemical, and physical factors, or according to genetic constitution. Although the inheritance of certain kinds of anophthalmia and microphthalmia in mice seems to be fairly well understood[3,4,6], there are few reports on the maldevelopment of eyes[1,2] and especially malformation of the brain resulting from eyelessness in the rat. The present paper describes the maldevelopment of eyes and resulting malformation of the brain in an anophthalmic strain of rats.

The animals were offspring of genetically anophthalmic rats supplied by Dr. M. Saito, Central Institute for Experimental Animals. These animals had already undergone 3 generations by means of sib inbreeding by the time they were used. The anophthalmic expression of these rats varied widely from severely anophthalmic to a range of microphthalmia including almost normal. Among a total of 30 rats from 4 to 7 generations, 18 exhibited anophthalmia on one side with microphthalmia on the other, 6 showed bilateral anophthalmia, and the remaining 6 had bilateral small eyes or microphthalmia on one side with almost normal-sized eyes on the other. For histological studies of the malformation of the brain, serial sections at 20 μm were cut from the brain of adult rats and stained by the Pal-carmine and Klüver-Barrera techniques. In the developmental study, embryos were obtained at daily intervals from day 10 to 20 of gestation and their embryonic stages were scored, taking the day when sperm was first detected in the maternal morning smear as day 0. Control embroys were obtained from the original Donryu strain rats from which the hereditary anophthalmic strain had separated mutantly. All embryos were fixed in 10% formalin solution. Complete serial sections at 5 μm were made from paraffin embedded materials and 15 μm serial sections from celloidin embedded blocks. For routine staining, Hematoxylin-eosin was used.

Maldevelopment of eyes: By day 10 of gestation, optic vesicles had not yet formed in the litter of the anophthalmic strain. However, seemingly, they budded off normally from the brain vesicles at day 11 and were well developed by day 12, without contacting with a single layer of the head ectoderm. At day 13, the optic vesicles differentiated into the optic cups, inducing the lens vesicles. In the control embryos with normal eyes, mitotic activity increased in the neuroblastic layer at the 14th day and development of the primitive optic nerve fibers began. Also, the chorioid fissure was obliterated. In anophthalmic animals at the same stage, however, differentiation of the neuroblastic cell layer was seriously affected and its thickness was attenuated to only about half of that in the control. Differentiation of the lens epithelia seemed to be arrested and the lens failed to develop normally. Moreover, the chorioid fissure still remained open. At day 16, differentiation of the neuroblastic layer in the anophthalmic fetus had completely stopped giving a degenerative appearance, and the pigment layer with a single nuclear row showed strong folding in some parts.

The lens epithelia were maldeveloped and their arrangement was irregular, although they continued to grow progressively in size. By the 20th day in anophthalmic cases, it was difficult to detect the neuroblastic layer which was reduced to debris. Cavities of various sizes were found to arise from the pigment layer and the debris of the lens showed a severely degenerated appearance.

Malformation of the optic nerves: In anophthalmic animals, optic nerve fibers were not detected during the embryonic and adult stages. In microphthalmic animals, which exhibited very small to almost normal-sized eyes, the optic nerves were found to show a great variety corresponding roughly to the size of the eyes.

Malformation of the brain: In anophthalmic cases, the primary terminal nuclei of the optic nerve as a rule seemed to be in hypoplasia, whereas the secondary terminal nuclei such as the visual area and others receiving projection fibers from the former, appeared to have grown normally in size and form. Hypoplasia of the primary terminal nuclei was of various grades: the main terminal nuclei such as the dorsal and ventral nuclei of the lateral geniculate body, and the superficial three layers including the stratum opticum of the superior colliculus were moderately reduced in size, whereas the small terminal nuclei such as the nucleus tractus peduncularis transversus and the nucleus tractus opticus lateralis exhibited rather severe hypoplasia, and the nucleus suprachiasmaticus receiving the retinohypothalmic tract appeared to be almost normal. In microphthalmic animals, malformation of the primary terminal nuclei of the opric nerve appeared to be variable in extent, corresponding roughly to the development of the eyes and optic nerves. However, the hypoplasia of these nuclei was generally milder than that in anophthalmic animals. The motor nuclei for the eye movements, i.e., the occulomotor, trochlear, and abducent nuclei in cases of anophthalmia, showed a tendency to be almost normal or to be mildly hypoplastic in some nuclei, corresponding roughly to the size of the developed eye muscles.

REFERENCES

1. Browman, L.G., Microphthalmia and maternal effect in the white rat, *Genetics*, 39 (1954) 261–265.
2. Browman, L.G., Microphthalmia and optic blood supply in the rat, *J. Morph.*, 109 (1961) 37–55.
3. Chase, H.B. and Chase, E.B., Studies on an anophthalmic strain of mice, *J. Morph.*, 68 (1941) 279–301.
4. Kimura, I., Morphogenetic studies on a microphthalmic strain (mc) in the mouse, *Cong. Anom.*, 9 (1969) 75–86.
5. Sassani, J.W. and Yanoff, M., Anophthalmos in an infant with multiple congenital anomalies, *Amer. J. Ophthal.*, 83 (1977) 569–576.
6. Truslove, G.M., A gene causing ocular retardation in the mouse, *J. Embryol. exp. Morph.*, 10 (1962) 652–660.

How are optic impulses transferred to the cerebellum?

KOKI KAWAMURA

Department of Anatomy, School of Medicine, Iwate Medical University, Morioka, Iwate 020, Japan

Since Snider and Stowell[18] recorded optically evoked impulses from the midvermal region of the cerebellum, lobules VI–VIII have been taken as visual receptive fields of the cerebellum. Recent physiological and anatomical investigations have shown, however, that the pathways concerned in the transmission of optic inputs to the cerebellum are multiple and more complexly organized than previously assumed.

Following injections of horseradish peroxidase (HRP) in lobules VI–VIII, Hoddevik et al.[10] found many labeled cells in four areas of the pontine nucleus situated in the dorsolateral, peduncular, lateral and paramedian nucleus (referred to as columns A, B, C and D, respectively). Available data from the literature show that columns A, D and the rostral part of B may be involved in the transmission of optic afferents from the superior colliculus[7,13], the lateral geniculate body[5], the pretectal region[12] and the visual cortex[3]. Our autoradiographic findings indicate in addition that these pontine areas send fibers to the ansiform lobule, particularly crus II, the dorsal paraflocculus and probably the paramedian lobule.

Pathways for visual inputs to the vermal area via the inferior olive likewise exist, since the medial portion of the caudal half of the medial accessory olive, which receives fibers from the superior colliculus[4], projects onto vermal lobules VI-VII.[11]

With the Nauta and Fink-Heimer methods, Mizuno et al[16]. in the rabbit and Itoh[12] in the cat found olivary projections from the pretectal region to the dorsal cap and the nucleus β, and the latter author found, in addition, the termination to the rostral portion of the dorsal accessory olive. The pretecto-olivary pathway in the rabbit has been studied physiologically by Maekawa and Simpson[15]. In further studies with the HRP method, it was concluded that the nucleus of the optic tract and the dorsal and lateral terminal nuclei of the accessory optic tract project to the dorsal cap[19]. The above three olivary areas send fibers to the flocculonodular lobe,[9] the uvula[1] and parts of zones C_1 and C_3 of the anterior lobe[2], respectively. These projections have also been confirmed in our and other[6] autoradiographic studies.

Furthermore, there will be other minor routes for optic impulses to the cerebellum from the superior colliculus via the nucleus reticularis tegmenti pontis (N.r.t.), the lateral reticular and the paramedian reticular nuclei (see Figs. 2 and 3 of ref. 14). In our autoradiographic studies, evidence has been obtained for a mossy fiber projection from the N.r.t. to extensive cerebellar regions, including the midvermal portion and the flocculus, bilaterally. This is in agreement with the HRP-findings obtained by others.[8] However, pathways involving the other two reticular nuclei have not so far been studied in detail.

Observations of visually evoked climbing and mossy fiber responses obtained in extensive areas in the cerebellar cortex, e.g., by Mortimer,[17] can in part be explained by the above morphological findings.

It appears from our present knowledge that optic inputs can be transmitted to the cerebellum by way of both *mossy* and *climbing* fibers. The mossy fiber route is from the pontine nuclei and the N.r.t. to the midvermal area as well as to the hemisphere. The inputs may reach the pons from the superior colliculus, the lateral geniculate body, the visual cortex and the pretectal region. The climbing fiber route goes via the olive and reaches lobules VI-VII, the flocculus, noculus, uvula and parts of the anterior lobe. The olivary inputs may come from the superior colliculus and the pretectum (the nucleus of the optic tract) and the terminal nuclei of the accessory optic tract.

REFERENCES

1. Brodal, A., The olivocerebellar projection in the cat as studied with the method of retrograde axonal transport of horseradish peroxidase. II. The projection to the uvula, *J. comp. Neurol.*, 116 (1976) 417–426.
2. Brodal, A. and Walberg, F., The olivocerebellar projection in the cat studied with the method of retrograde axonal transport of horseradish peroxidase. IV. The projection to the anterior lobe, *J. comp. Neurol.*, 172 (1977) 85–108.
3. Brodal, P., The corticopontine projection from the visual cortex in the cat. I. The total projection and the projection from area 17, *Brain Research*, 39 (1972) 297–317.
4. Graham, J., An autoradiographic study of the efferent connections of the superior colliculus in the cat, *J. comp. Neurol.*, 173 (1977) 629–654.
5. Graybiel, A.M., Visuo-cerebellar and cerebello-visual connections involving the ventral lateral geniculate nucleus, *Exp. Brain Res.*, 20 (1974) 303–306.
6. Groenewegen, H.J. and Voogd, J., The parasagittal zonation within the olivocerebellar projection. I. Climbing fiber distribution in the vermis of cat cerebellum, *J. comp. Neurol.*, 174 (1977) 417–488.
7. Hashikawa, T. and Kawamura, K., Identification of cells of origin of tectopontine fibers in the cat superior colliculus: an experimental study with the horseradish peroxidase method, *Brain Research*, 130 (1977) 65–79.
8. Hoddevik, G.H., The projection from nucleus reticularis tegmenti pontis onto the cerebellum in the cat. A study using the methods of anterograde degeneration and retrograde axonal transport of horseradish peroxidase, *Anat. Embryol.* 153 (1978) 227–242.
9. Hoddevik, G.H. and Brodal, A., The olivocerebellar projection studied with the method of retrograde axonal transport of hoseradish peroxidase. V. The projections to the flocculonodular lobe and the paraflocculus in the rabbit, *J. comp. Neurol.*, 176 (1977) 269–280.
10. Hoddevik, G.H., Brodal, A., Kawamura, K. and Hashikawa, T., The pontine projection to the cerebellar vermal visual area studied by means of the retrograde axonal transport of horseradish peroxidase, *Brain Research*, 123 (1977) 209–227.
11. Hoddevik, G.H., Brodal, A. and Walberg, F., The olivocerebellar projection in the cat studied with the method of retrograde axonal transport of horseradish peroxidase. III. The projection to the vermal visual area, *J. comp. Neurol.*, 169 (1976) 155–170.
12. Itoh, K., Efferent projections of the pretectum in the cat, *Exp. Brain Res.*, 30 (1977) 89–105.
13. Kawamura, K. and Brodal, A., The tectopontine projection in the cat: an exerpimental anatomical study with comments on pathways for teleceptive impulses to the ceebellum, *J. comp. Neurol.*, 149 (1973) 371–390.
14. Kawamura, K., Brodal, A. and Hoddevik, G.H., The projection of the superior colliculus onto the reticular formation of the brain stem. An experimental anatomical study in the cat, *Exp. Brain Res.*, 19 (1974) 1–19.
15. Maekawa, K. and Simpson, J.I., Climbing fiber activation of Purkinje cells in the flocculus by impulses transferred through the visual pathway, *Brain Research*, 39 (1972) 245–251.
16. Mizuno, N., Mochizuki, K., Akimoto, C. and Matsushima, R., Pretectal projections to the inferior olive in the rabbit, *Exp. Neurol.*, 39 (1973) 498–506.
17. Mortimer, J.A., Cerebellar responses to teleceptive stimuli in alert monkeys, *Brain Research*, 83 (1975) 369–390.
18. Snider, R.S. and Stowell, A., Receiving areas of the tactile, auditory, and visual systems in the cerebellum, *J. Neurophysiol.*, 7 (1944) 331–358.
19. Takeda, T. and Maekawa, K., The origin of the pretecto-olivary tract. A study using the horseradish peroxidase method, *Brain Research*, 117 (1976) 319–325.

Role of the hair cell-afferent fiber synapse in the coding of afferent impulses

TARO FURUKAWA

Department of Physiology, School of Medicine, Tokyo Medical and Dental University, Bunkyo-ku, Tokyo 113, Japan

Although a wealth of information exists on the activity of single auditory afferent fibers, the mode of action of the hair cell-afferent fiber synapse remains generally unclarified. According to a simplified view, the hair cell-afferent fiber synapse faithfully conveys information received by hair cells to afferent fiber terminals where the amount of depolarization is converted to the frequency of afferent impulses. Although many important aspects of the activity of auditory fibers may conform to this picture, the detailed mechanisms underlying it remain to be elucidated. Moreover, other features in the activity of auditory fibers, such as the partial synchrony of the firing (phase-locking) and adaptation, lie outside the scope of the above-mentioned simplified view. The present paper discusses the possible role of the hair cell-afferent fiber synapse in patterning auditory afferent discharges.

Our group has been working on goldfish ear (the sacculus) for about 10 years, by recording potentials intracellularly from the vicinity of afferent fiber terminals[2]. It was found that each sound wave served as an independent stimulus and evoked an excitatory postsynaptic potential (EPSP) which in turn elicited a spike potential when the threshold was reached. This enabled us to analyze the mechanisms of transmission at the hair cell-afferent fiber synapse in more detail than by extracellular records of afferent impulses. Moreover, the virtual absence of temporal dispersion by the propagation of the travelling wave rendered it easy to study the temporal factors involved in the synaptic processes. For example, the presence of a synaptic delay of about 0.5 msec was very clearly demonstrated[3].

One finding of note in our study was the brief time course of the EPSPs evoked in afferent fiber terminals[3]. This certainly forms the basis for the precise phase-locking phenomenon. We also demonstrated that the release of transmitter from the sensory hair cells took place on a quantal basis. The unitary miniature EPSP had a time course of an equilateral triangle whose half-width was only 0.4 msec or so. The temporal changes in the probability of release of transmitter quanta are apparently responsible for an interesting property of the cochlear nerve fibers, viz., that the frequency of occurrence of phase-locked impulses rather closely mimics the half-rectified wave form of the sound.[5]

The other phenomenon in which involvement of the afferent synapse has been proven is adaptation. Although adaptation in the rate of afferent discharges has been demonstrated in the cochlea and in vestibular organs, its site and mechanism have remained unclaified. In goldfish sacculus, EPSPs evoked in afferent fibers by each sound wave exhibit a successive rundown in their size. We have shown that the rundown in size of the EPSPs is attributable to depletion of the readily available store of transmitter quanta in the hair cells. In this work, we analyzed the actual process of EPSP rundown[4] and also studied it on the basis of the quantal release theory.[1] Interestingly, however, the manner in which the available quanta were depleted was found to be closely related to the mechanism of a graded release of transmitter quanta from the sensory hair cells. Our study led to the conclusion that the release sites within the single sensory cell had to be sorted out into different classes according to the threshold for release. In other words, on stimulation with a weak sound, release would occur only from a small number of the most sensitive release sites, while more and more release sites would be recruited on stimulation with a stronger sound. It then follows that on stimulation with a weak sound, only quanta associated with the most sensitive release sites would be depleted, leaving intact the quanta associated with less sensitive release sites. This is a rough outline of our multicompartment model.[4]

Although our study was limited to goldfish sacculus, the results of Smith[6] appear to indicate that his short-term adaptation in the rate of afferent discharges in the cochlear nerve may have an origin similar to the adaptation in our preparation. In his experiment, tones of constant sound intensity served as an adapting background or pedestal on which increments and decrements in sound intensity were superimposed. He found that the incremental responses were equal before and after adaptation even though the steady-state response to the pedestal was substantially less than the onset response. Moreover, the rate of recovery from the adapted state after cessation of the stimulus sound roughly coincides in the two preparations. It seems reasonable to assume therefore that a fundamental similarity may exist in the mode of action of the hair cell-afferent fiber synapse between fish sacculus and cochlea, insofar as the mechanisms of graded transmitter release and adaptation are concerned. That is to say, our multicompartment model is probably applicable also to the release of transmitter from cochlear hair cells.

REFERENCES

1. Furukawa, T., Hayashida, Y. and Matsuura, S., Quantal analysis of the size of the excitatory postsynaptic potentials at synapses between hair cells and afferent eighth nerve fibres in goldfish, *J. Physiol. (Lond.)*, 276 (1978) 211–226.
2. Furukawa, T. and Ishii, Y., Neurophysiological studies on hearing in goldfish, *J. Neurophysiol.*, 30 (1967) 1377–1403.
3. Furukawa, T., Ishii, Y. and Matsuura, S., Synaptic delay and time course of postsynaptic potentials at the junction between hair cells and eighth nerve fibers in the goldfish, *Jap. J. Physiol.*, 22 (1972) 617–635.
4. Furukawa, T. and Matsuura, S., Adaptive rundown of excitatory post-synaptic potentials at synapses between hair cells and eighth nerve fibres in the goldfish, *J. Physiol. (Lond)*, 276 (1978) 193–209.
5. Rose, J.E., Kitzes, L.M., Gibson, M.M. and Hind, J.E., Observations on phase-sensitive neurons of the anteroventral cochlear nucleus of the cat: nonlinearity of the cochlear output, *J. Neurophysiol.*, 37 (1974) 218–253.
6. Smith, R.L., Short-term adaptation in single auditory nerve fibers: some poststimulatory effects, *J. Neurophysiol.*, 40 (1977) 1098–1112.

An electron microscopic study of spinothalamic fibers which end at the centrolateral nucleus neurons sending their axons to the motor cortex in the cat and monkey: the use of horseradish peroxidase as a neuronal marker for electron microscopy

NOBORU MIZUNO, AKIRA KONISHI, KAZUO ITOH AND SAKASHI NOMURA

Department of Anatomy, Faculty of Medicine, Kyoto University,
Sakyo-ku, Kyoto 606, Japan

In the previous study[4,5] a spino-thalamo-motor cortical path through the centrolateral nucleus (CL) of the thalamus was found to exist in the cat by means of the combined horseradish peroxidase (HRP) and Fink-Heimer method[2]. The present paper offers electron microscopic evidence showing the termination of spinal fibers at CL neurons sending their axons to area 4 of the cerebral cortex in the cat and monkey.

Experiments were performed with 8 cats and 2 Japanese monkeys. Under pentobarbital anesthesia hemicordotomy was performed in the upper cervical segments (CI-C4), and 2–6 days after this operation, 40–50% HRP (Toyobo Grade-I-C, RZ: 3.4) dissolved in sterile 0.9% saline was injected ipsilaterally into area 4 of the cerebral cortex under direct vision by slow pressure through a 1 μl Hamilton syringe. After a survival period ranging from 30–40 hr, the cats were perfused transcardially with a mixture composed of 2.5% paraformaldehyde, 1.0% glutaraldehyde and 0.002% calcium chloride in Millonig's buffer (pH 7.4). Upper brain stems were removed immediately and sectioned transversely at 100 μm thickness on a vibratome, floated on a bath of Millonig's buffer, and then treated for the HRP reaction as described by Graham and Karnovsky[3], Streit and Reubi[8] or Adams.[1] The coupled oxidation reaction described by Lundquist and Josefsson[6] was also applied (details to be published). Subsequently, small tissue slices containing CL neurons labeled with HRP were cut, using razor blades under a dissecting microscope, and postfixed for 40 min in a chilled 2% solution of osmium tetroxide in Millonig's buffer. Embedding was done in an epoxy resin after dehydration in a graded series of ethanol. The location of CL neurons labeled with HRP injected into area 4 was verified in semithin sections which were cut from each block (Fig. 1). Ultrathin sections unstained or stained with lead acetate or lead citrate were examined with a Hitachi HU-12 electron microscope.

In both cats and monkeys electron-dense degenerated axon terminals were seen in the CL areas containing many neurons labeled with HRP injected into area 4 of the cerebral cortex. All of the degenerated axon terminals found so far were in contact with small or medium-sized dendritic profiles and appeared to be filled with spherical synaptic vesicles (Fig. 2).

The spinothalamic fibers were reported to end within the CL in the cat and monkey (for reviews, see refs. 2 and 7), and the locus and extent of the caudal CL areas in the cat were shown to correspond to those of the terminal sites of the spino-CL fibers.[4,5] The present study has confirmed that the spino-CL fibers of the cat and monkey made synaptic contacts upon dendrites of CL neurons sending their axons to area 4 of the cerebral cortex.

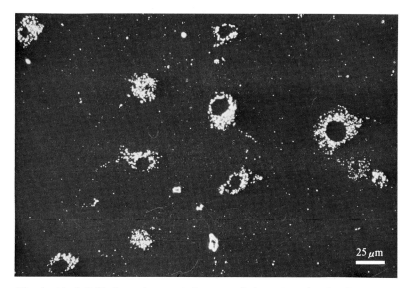

Fig. 1. Dark-field photomicrograph from a semithin section, showing CL neurons labeled with HRP injected ipsilaterally into area 4 of the cerebral cortex in a cat; 40 hr after injection. The scale bar represents 25 μm.

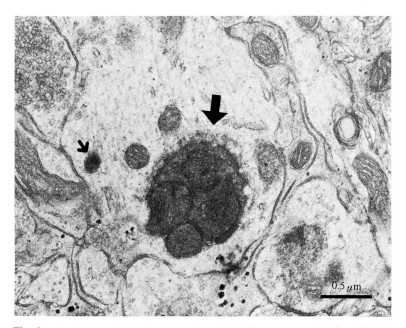

Fig. 2. An electron-dense degenerated axodendritic axon terminal found in the CL after hemisection of the second cervical cord segment in a cat; 4 days survival. The larger arrow points to the synaptic active zone. The smaller arrow indicates an electron-dense granule labeled with HRP injected ipsilaterally into area 4 of the cerebral cortex 40 hr before sacrifice. The scale bar represents 0.5 μm.

References

1. Adams, J.C., Technical considerations on the use of horseradish peroxidase as a neuronal marker, *Neuroscience*, 2 (1977) 141–145.
2. Boivie, J., The termination of the spinothalamic tract in the cat. An experimental study with silver impregnation methods, *Brain Research*, 12 (1971) 331–353.
3. Graham, R.C. and Karnovsky, M.J., The early stages of absorption of injected horseradish peroxidase in the proximal tubules of mouse kidney: ultrastructural cytochemistry by a new technique, *J. Histochem. Cytochem.*, 14 (1966) 291–302.
4. Itoh, K. and Mizuno, N., Topographical arrangement of the centrolateral nucleus (CL) neurons projecting directly to the motor cortex in the cat, with special reference to the spino-thalamo-cortical projection system through CL, *Anat. Rec.*, 187 (1977) 768.
5. Itoh, K. and Mizuno, N., Topographical arrangement of thalamocortical neurons in the centrolateral nucleus (CL) of the cat, with special reference to a spino-thalamo-motor cortical path through the CL, *Exp. Brain Res.*, 30 (1977) 471–480.
6. Lundquist, I. and Josefsson, J. -O., Sensitive method for determination of peroxidase activity in tissue by means of coupled oxidation reaction, *Analyt. Biochem.*, 41 (1971) 567–577.
7. Mehler, W.R., Some neurological species differences —— *a posteriori. Ann. N.Y. Acad. Sci.*, 167 (1969) 424–468.
8. Streit, P. and Reubi, J.C., A new and sensitive method for axonally transported horseradish peroxidase (HRP) in the pigeon visual system, *Brain Research*, 126 (1977) 530–537.

Somatotopic trigeminal projection onto the caudal medulla oblongata. Part. I. Tactile representation within the pars magnocellularis of the trigeminal subnucleus caudalis

TOSHIKATSU YOKOTA, NOZOMU NISHIKAWA AND YASUO NISHIKAWA

Department of Physiology, Medical College of Shiga,
Otsu, Shiga 520–21, Japan

Previous electrophysiological studies in a variety of animal species indicated that the trigeminal brain-stem sensory nuclear complex was dominated by a somatotopically arranged collection of low threshold mechanoreceptive neurons throughout its rostrocaudal axis[1,2]. Recently, segregation of nociceptive and thermosensitive neurons was found in the marginal layer surrounding the substantia gelatinosa of the trigeminal subnucleus caudalis[4,6,7], and trigeminal neurons similar to lamina 5 neurons in the spinal dorsal horn were identified in the bulbar lateral reticular formation immediately adjacent to the trigeminal subnucleus caudalis[5,6,8]. Lamina 5 type neurons have a graded response to brush, touch and pressure in the center of the receptive field but respond only to pressure applied to the edge of the receptive field[3]. Apparently, neurons of this type were included in the previous studies on the somatotopic organization of tactile representation within the trigeminal subnucleus caudalis[1,2]. It has recently been established that trigeminal neurons with a restricted low threshold mechanoreceptive field are exclusively located within the pars magnocellularis of the trigeminal subnucleus caudalis in the caudal medulla oblongata[6,9]. In the present study, therefore, the pattern of projection of the trigeminal tactile field onto the pars magnocellularis of the trigeminal subnucleus caudalis was investigated.

Experiments were carried out on adult cats anesthetized with urethane-chloralose at an intravenous dose of 3.5 ml/kg (urethane 125 mg/ml; chloralose 10 mg/ml). Single unit recording was done using glass micropipette electrodes filled with Fast Green FCF in 1 M sodium acetate. At two sites of recording units in each microelectrode track, dye marks were made by electrophoretic extrusion of Fast Green FCF from the microelectrode. Frozen sections at 40 μ were prepared from the caudal medulla oblongata of the microelectrode penetrations. Sections containing the dye marks were counterstained with cresyl violet.

As shown in Fig. 1, units with a restricted low threshold mechanoreceptive field falling within the mandibular distribution were found in the dorsomedial portion of the pars magnocellularis, units with maxillary fields were next to these, and units with ophthalmic fields were situated ventrolaterally. All the fields were strictly ipsilateral even in midline areas such as the tongue.

Along the rostrocaudal axis of the brain-stem, a differentiation was found: the center of the face had its major projection just behind the obex, whereas the more peripheral part of the face was better represented more caudally. For example, near the rostral end of the subnucleus caudalis, only the intraoral, perioral and paranasal areas were represented as shown in Fig. 1. These findings are in agreement with the rostrocaudal differentiation maintained by Darian-Smith *et al.*,[1] but disagree with the view of others[2] that each zone of the facial skin was represented by a string of cells oriented in the rostrocaudal axis.

According to previous reports[1,2,10], the pattern of tactile representation within any transverse plane through the subnucleus caudalis approximated to an inverted face with circumoral structure being placed in the dorsomedial part of the subnucleus, as exemplified by the felliculus illustrated in Fig. 1C. In contrast, the present results could be interpreted in a different way. At each transverse plane of the pars magnocellularis, the most rostral segment of the represented trigeminal integument projected onto the marginal part of the pars magnocellularis adjacent to the substantia gelatinosa, while the most peripheral segment projected towards the core of the quasi-semicircular pars magnocellularis. In the previous scheme, for example, the paranasal-area must be represented in the ventromedial part of the subnucleus caudalis. In the transverse plane shown in Fig. 1, however, the paranasal area was represented dorsolaterally. Therefore, the scheme illustrated in D of the figure fits the results in A and B better than the previous one illustrated in C. A schematic representation of the distorted projection of the trigeminal integument in the cat in various transverse planes of the pars magnocellularis is given in Fig. 2.

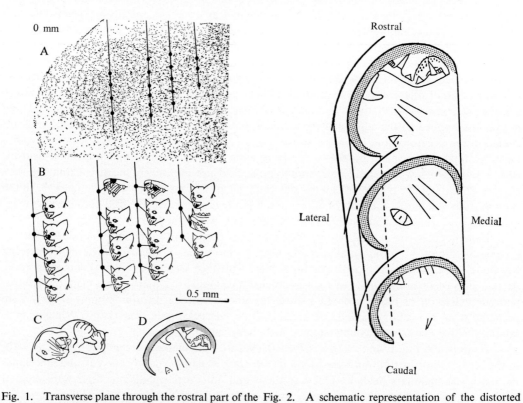

Fig. 1.   Transverse plane through the rostral part of the subnucleus caudalis, showing the positions and tactile receptive fields of pars magnocellularis units isolated in a series of four microelectrode penetrations. A, Positions of units; B, receptive fields of individual units; C, a previous scheme of tactile representation within the subnucleus caudalis; D, a modified scheme based on the results shown in A and B.

Fig. 2.   A schematic represeentation of the distorted projection of the trigeminal nerve territory of the cat in the pars magnocellularis of the subnucleus caudalis.

REFERENCES

1. Darian-Smith, I., Proctor, R. and Ryan, R.D., A single-neurone investigation of somatotopic organization within the cat's trigeminal brain-stem nuclei, *J. Physiol. (Lond.)*, 168 (1963) 147–157.
2. Kruger, L. and Michel, F., A morphological and somatotopic analysis of single unit activity in trigeminal sensory complex of the cat, *Exp. Neurol.*, 5 (1962) 139–156.
3. Hillman, P. and Wall, P.D., Inhibitory and excitatory factors influencing the receptive fields of lamina 5 spinal cord cells, *Exp. Brain Res.*, 9 (1969) 284–306.
4. Mosso, J.A. and Kruger, L., Receptor categories represented in spinal trigeminal nucleus caudalis, *J. Neurophysiol.*, 36 (1973) 472–488.
5. Nord, S.G. and Ross, G.S., Responses of trigeminal units in the monkey bulbar lateral reticular formation to noxious and non-noxious stimulation of the face: experimental and theoretical considerations, *Brain Research*, 58 (1973) 385–399.
6. Price, D.D., Dubner, R. and Hu, J.W., Trigeminothalamic neurons in nucleus caudalis responsive to tactile, thermal and nociceptive stimulation of monkey's face, *J. Neurophysiol.*, 39 (1976) 936–953.
7. Yokota, T., Excitation of units in marginal rim of trigeminal subnucleus caudalis elicited by tooth pulp stimulation, *Brain Research*, 95 (1975) 154–158.
8. Yokota, T., Two types of tooth pulp units in the bulbar lateral reticular formation, *Brain Research*, 104 (1976) 325–329.
9. Yokota, T. and Nishikawa, N., Somatotopic organization of trigeminal neurons within caudal medulla oblongata. In D.J. Anderson and B. Matthews (Eds.), *Pain in the Trigeminal Region*, Elsevier/North Holland, Amsterdam-New York, 1977, pp. 243–257.
10. Young, D.W. and Iggo, A., Neurones in the spinal trigeminal nucleus of the cat responding to movement of the vibrissae, *Exp. Brain Res.*, 28 (1977) 457–567.

Central monoaminergic neurons in sensory transmission ——An electrophysiological study——

SHUJI TAKAORI, MASASHI SASA, YOSHINORI CHIKAMORI AND IZURU MATSUOKA*

*Department of Pharmacology, Faculty of Medicine, Kyoto University,
Sakyo-ku, Kyoto 606, Japan*

The locus coeruleus (LC) is composed of noradrenaline-containing neurons and sends fibers to various parts of the brain. Noradrenaline-mediated inhibition from LC of transmission of relay neurons in the spinal trigeminal nucleus (STN) has been reported in our previous papers.[2,3] The existence of noradrenergic nerve terminals has been histochemically demonstrated in the cochlear nucleus (CN), but not in the vestibular nucleus (VN).[1] A comparison of the effect of LC stimulation on CN and VN neurons was therefore made to determine whether or not noradrenaline from LC acts on the neurons as an inhibitory transmitter.

Cats weighing 2.5–3.5 kg were anesthetized with α-chloralose (30 mg/kg i.v.) and immobilized with gallamine triethiodide (5 mg/kg/hr i.v.). A pair of silver wire electrodes was twined round the inferior alveolar nerve for stimulation of the trigeminal nerve. The round window in the middle ear cavity was exposed under a ventral approach, and a bipolar electrode for stimulation of the VIIIth nerve was inserted into the lateral ampulla. All wound edges and pressure points were locally anesthetized with 8% lidocaine spray. A glass-insulated silver wire microelectrode was inserted into the STN (P: 9.0, L: 5.5, H: −5.0 to −6.0), lateral VN (P: 8.0, L: 4.0, H: −2.8) and dorsal CN (P: 7.5, L: 8.0, H: −5.0). Conditioning stimuli of 4 train pulses (0.1 msec, 250 Hz, 2–20 V) were applied to the ipsilateral LC (P: 2.0, L: 2.0, H: −2.0) at various intervals preceding the test stimulus to the peripheral nerve (C–T interval). The responses were amplified and displayed on an oscilloscope (Nihon Kohden, VC–9).

STN: The field potential in the STN elicited by inferior alveolar nerve stimulation consisted of pre- and postsynaptic components. The postsynaptic component was significantly inhibited by LC conditioning stimulation, as previously reported.[2] The inhibition was maximum at a 30-msec C–T interval, and lasted for 150 msec of the C–T interval. Therefore, when the reduction in the height of the postsynaptic component exceeded 20%, the electrode was considered to be properly positioned in the LC. The inhibitory effect of LC conditioning stimulation on the spike generation of STN relay neurons was reconfirmed. Fig. 1 represents the reduction in spike number in the STN neurons elicited by alveolar nerve stimulation during 30–100 msec of the C–T interval.

VN: The field potential in the VN evoked by VIIIth nerve stimulation was composed of pre-, mono- and polysynaptic components. The mean peak latencies were approximately 0.5, 1.0 and 2.4 msec, respectively. These components were not altered by LC conditioning stimulation. In addition, the spike number of monosynaptic neurons in the VN following stimulation of the VIIIth nerve remained unaffected with LC conditioning stimulation (Fig. 1). Even when the stimulus to LC was increased to 30 V, the spike generation by VIIIth nerve stimulation remained

---

* Present address: Department of Otorhinolaryngology, Faculty of Medicine, Kyoto University, Kyoto 606, Japan

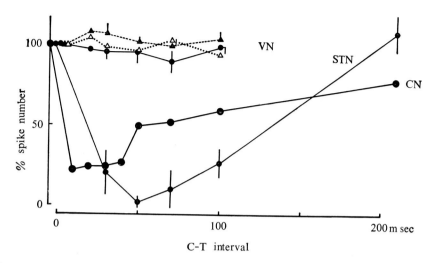

C-T interval

Fig. 1. Effects of conditioning stimulation of the locus coeruleus on the number of spikes of neurons in the spinal trigeminal nucleus (STN), lateral vestibular nucleus (VN) and dorsal cochlear nucleus (CN). Abscissa: C-T interval. Ordinate: mean percent change in spike number. Three different intensities of stimulus were used for the conditioning, viz. ●——●: 10 V, ▲----▲: 20 V, and △····△: 30 V. The vertical bar at each point indicates the standard error.

the same. Inhibition of spike generation of VN neurons, however, was observed with the conditioning stimulus to the cerebellar nodulus.

CN: The field potential in the CN elicited by VIIIth nerve stimulation consisted of pre- and postsynaptic components, and the mean peak latencies were 0.5 and 1.1 msec, respectively. When conditioning stimuli were applied to LC, there was an inhibition in the height of the postsynaptic component. The spike number of the CN neurons on VIIIth nerve stimulation was also reduced by LC conditioning stimulation during 10–200 msec of the C–T interval (Fig. 1).

Our finding of an LC-induced inhibition on the CN but not the VN neurons coincided well with the histochemical evidence which shows that noradrenergic nerve terminals exist in the former but not the latter. Since the inhibition of spike firing in the STN neurons induced by LC conditioning stimulation was considered to be due to noradrenaline originating in the LC[2,3], it can be concluded that the inhibitory effect of LC on the CN neurons is also probably mediated by noradrenaline. In conclusion, it can be said that the inhibitory effect of LC stimulation was specific for the neurons of nuclei where noradrenergic nerve terminals are located. Such findings add support to the idea that noradrenaline from the LC acts as an inhibitory transmitter.

REFERENCES

1. Fuxe, K., Evidence for the existence of monoamine neurons in the central nervous system. IV. Distribution of monoamine nerve terminals in the central nervous system, *Acta physiol. scand.*, 64 Suppl. (1965) 39–85.
2. Sasa, M., Munekiyo, K., Ikeda, H. and Takaori, S., Noradrenaline-mediated inhibition by locus coeruleus of spinal trigeminal neurons, *Brain Research*, 80 (1974) 443–460.
3. Sasa, M. and Takaori, S., Influence of the locus coeruleus on transmission in the spinal trigeminal nucleus neurons, *Brain Research*, 55 (1973) 203–208.
4. Yamamoto, C., Pharmacological studies of norepinephrine and related compounds on neurons in Deiters' nucles and cerebellum, *J. Pharmacol. exp. Ther.*, 156 (1967) 39–47.

Selective action of enkephalins on lamina V neurons of the spinal dorsal horn: a microelectrophoretic study

MASAMICHI SATOH, SHIN-ICHI KAWAJIRI, MASAKI YAMAMOTO AND HIROSHI TAKAGI

Department of Pharmacology, Faculty of Pharmaceutical Sciences, Kyoto University, Sakyo-ku, Kyoto 606, Japan

Leucine-enkephalin (Leu-enk) and methionine-enkephalin (Met-enk) are naturally occurring pentapeptides in mammalian brains and have agonistic activity at opiate receptors[5]. These peptides have been shown to produce a definite analgesic effect when directly injected into several regions of the central nervous system[9,12]. Recent immunohistochemical studies indicate that the density of enkephalin-containing neurons varies in different regions with moderate to high levels in the spinal dorsal horn[4,11]. Among six laminae of the spinal dorsal horn, laminae I and V cells play an important role in the transmission and integration of nociceptive inputs at the spinal cord, while lamina IV cells receive mostly low-threshold cutaneous input[3]. It is of interest to determine the physiological roles of endogenous pentapeptides in pain control mechanisms. In the present experiments, we studied the actions of Leu- and Met-enk on the responses of laminae IV and V neurons of lumbar dorsal horn to non-noxious and noxious stimuli, using a microelectrophoretic method. Morphine was also used as a reference drug

Experiments were performed on unanesthetized male albino rabbits, weighing 2.5–3.5 kg. The spinal cords of all animals were transected at the L2 level under ether anesthesia, immobilized with gallamine triethiodide and artificially ventilated. The method for preparing the twin electrode assembly, which consisted of a tungsten electrode for recording extracellularly and a bent 4-barrelled multipipette for phoresis was as described elsewhere.[8] Solutions for microelectrophoresis were: monosodium-L-glutamate (1 M), Leu- and Met-enk (kindly supplied by Prof. H. Yajima, Kyoto University, Kyoto; 10 mM in 165 mM NaCl), morphine HCl and naloxone HCl (a kind gift from Endo Laboratories, Garden City, N.Y.; 50 mM in 165 mM NaCl). An NaCl-filled barrel (3 M) was employed for current compensation. The pHs of these solutions were about 5.0. Glutamate was passed as an anion, while the other compounds were passed as cations. The laminae IV and V neurons were selected and distinguished according to the electrophysiological properties described by Wall[10] and Kitahata *et al*[6]. Single injections of bradykinin (0.1–1.0 µg) into the femoral artery were used as noxious stimulation. The method for such injections has been described elsewhere[7]. Bradykinin-induced activation was encountered only at lamina V neurons. A light touch on the center of the receptive field was used as non-noxious stimulation. The two types of stimuli were applied at regular intervals (5 min in most cases) and reproducible responses were obtained throughout the recording period. Only units excitable by phoretically applied glutamate were selected.

The excitatory response following bradykinin injection was depressed by Leu-enk in 15 out of 19 neurons tested, by Met-enk in 10 out of 12 and by morphine in 10 out of 21, when each of these substances was microelectrophoretically applied from 30 or 60 sec before the bradykinin injection until 90 sec after it (for 120 or 150 sec) at 100–300 nA (Table 1). The depressant effects of Leu–enk, Met–enk and morphine were antagonized by naloxone simultaneously phoretically applied (100–200 nA) or intravenously administered (0.1–0.3 mg/kg), indicating that the effects were mediated by specific opiate receptors. A facilitation of the bradykinin-induced response by morphine was seen in 2 out of 21 neurons (Table 1). On the other hand, the excitatory response following non–noxious stimulation was hardly affected in most neurons tested with Leu–enk (all of 11 neurons), Met–enk (7 out of 9) and morphine (all of 14), when each of them was phoretically applied at 100–300 nA for 150 sec (Table. 1). The compounds used in the above experiments produced no changes in spike height or duration when phoretically ejected at up to 300 nA.

TABLE 1.   The effects of Leu–enk, Met–enk and morphine on the activities of dorsal horn laminae IV and V cells induced by noxious and/or non-noxious stimuli in spinal cords of rabbits.

	Leu-enkephalin		Met-enkephalin		Morphine		
	Inhibition	No effect	Inhibition	No effect	Inhibition	No effect	Facilitation
Nox. stim. (bradykinin)-induced activity (Lamina V cells)	15†	4	10†	2	10†	9	2
Non-nox. stim. (light touch)-induced activity (Laminae IV and V cells)	0	11	2	7	0	14	0

†Inhibitory effects were antagonized by naloxone applied microelectrophoretically or administered intravenously.

Recently Duggan et al.[1,2] reported that morphine and Met-enkephalinamide, a derivative of Met-enk, administered in the substantia gelatinosa caused a selective inhibition of nociceptive responses of laminae IV and V neurons. It should be pointed out, however, that the latencies of onset for the depressant action of morphine on nociceptive activation were quite long (4–35 min)[1] and that naturally occurring Met–enk itself did not produce any inhibition of the nociceptive response in most neurons tested (6 out of 8).[2] On the other hand, the present experiments demonstrated that in the lamina V of lumbar dorsal horn, Leu–enk and Met–enk as well as morphine selectively inhibited the neuronal responses to noxious stimulation through specific opiate receptors. The inhibitory actions of these substances appeared within 1 min after the beginning of phoresis. Judging from the nature of the tips of electrodes used (the recording electrode protruded beyond the tip of the micropiptete by about 20 μm), the substances ejected from the pipette may not have been reached the substantia gelatinosa. If the results of this study are considered together with the immunohistochemical findings[4,11], it is suggested that endogenous Leu- and Met-enk in the spinal dorsal horn act on the lamina V neurons as pain control substances. It remains to be determined how these endogenous substances are released from the neurons containing them.

REFERENCES

1. Duggan, A.W., Hall, J.G. and Headley, P.M., Suppression of transmission of nociceptive impulses by morphine: Selective effects of morphine administered in the region of the substantia gelatinosa, *Br. J. Pharmacol.*, 61 (1977) 65–76.
2. Duggan, A.W., Hall, J.G. and Headley, P.M., Enkephalins and dorsal horn neurones of the cat: Effects on responses to noxious and innocuous skin stimuli, *Br. J. Pharmacol.*, 61 (1977) 399–408.
3. Heavner, J.E., Jamming spinal sensory input: Effects of anesthetic and analgesic drugs in the spinal cord dorsal horn, *Pain*, 1 (1975) 239–255.

4. Hökfelt, T., Ljungdahl, A., Terenius, L., Elde, R. and Nilsson, G., Immunohistochemical analysis of peptide pathways possibly related to pain and analgesia: Enkephalin and substance P, *Proc. nat. Acad. Sci.* (Wash.), 74 (1977) 3081–3085.
5. Hughes, J., Smith, T.W., Kosterlitz, H.W., Fothergill, L.A., Morgan, B.A. and Morris, H.R., Identification of two related pentapeptides from the brain with potent opiate agonist activity, *Nature (Lond.)*, 258 (1975) 577–579.
6. Kitahata, L.M., Taub, A. and Sato, I., Lamina-specific suppression of dorsal horn unit activity by nitrous oxide and by hyperventilation, *J. Pharmacol. exp. Ther.*, 176 (1971) 101–108.
7. Satoh, M., Nakamura, N. and Takagi, H., Effect of morphine on bradykinin-induced unitary discharges in the spinal cord of the rabbit, *Europ. J. Pharmacol.*, 16 (1971) 245–247.
8. Satoh, M., Zieglgänsberger, W. and Herz, A., Actions of opiates upon single unit activity in the cortex of naive and tolerant rats, *Brain Research*, 115 (1976) 99–110.
9. Takagi, H., Satoh, M., Akaike, A., Shibata, T., Yajima, H. and Ogawa, H., Analgesia by enkephalins injected into the nucleus reticularis gigantocellularis of rat medulla oblongata, *Europ. J. Pharmacol.*, 49 (1978) 113–116.
10. Wall, P.D., The laminar organization of dorsal horn and effects of descending impulses, *J. Physiol. (Lond.)*, 188 (1967) 403–423.
11. Watson, S.J., Akil, H., Sullivan, S. and Barchas, J.D., Immunocytochemical localization of methionine enkephalin: Preliminary observations, *Life Sci.*, 21 (1977) 733–738.
12. Yaksh, T.L., Huang, S.P., Rudy, T.A. and Frederickson, R. C.A., The direct and specific opiate-like effect of Met[5]-enkephalin and analogues on the spinal cord, *Neuroscience*, 2 (1977) 593–596.

Morphology of mitral cell dendrites in the rabbit olfactory bulb: intracellular Procion Yellow injection

KENSAKU MORI, MASAHIKO SATOU and SADAYUKI F. TAKAGI

Department of Physiology, School of Medicine, Gunma University,
Maebashi, Gunma 371, Japan

The relations between morphological and physiological properties of a neuron have been investigated in several regions of the mammalian brain using an intracellular staining technique with Procion Yellow.[1,5,6,8] Since the physiological properties of neurons in the rabbit olfactory bulb have been studied intensively by many investigators[4,10–13,18] (see Shepherd[15] for a review), we considered it desirable to apply this technique to the analysis of the structure-function relationship in the olfactory bulb neurons. As a first step for the morphological identification of physiologically identified neurons, we tried to stain mitral cells of the olfactory bulb, because it is relatively easy to record the activities of the cells intracellularly and to identify them physiologically.

Experiments were performed on adult albino rabbits anesthetized with urethane. The general experimental procedures are described elsewhere[10]. The micropipettes used for recording and dye injection were filled with 5% solution of Procion Yellow MX-4R. After the physiological identification of mitral cells (Fig. 1B), they were stained by passing a hyperpolarizing current pulse (1–5 nA, 300 msec duration) at a frequency of 2/sec for 1–20 min.

To date, we have found 12 successfully stained mitral cells. Fig. 1A shows two examples of well-stained cells. They were identified physiologically as mitral cells by the antidromic spikes and subsequent large and long-lasting IPSPs following lateral olfactory tract stimulation (Fig. 1B).

The mitral cells had a primary dendrite which extended peripherally to the glomerular layer and terminated within a single glomerulus, showing an extensive ramification (Fig. 1A and C). Under a fluorescent microscope, the glomeruli in the olfactory bulb could be easily recognized by their relatively clear and uniform background fluorescence. In some mitral cells, the terminal arborizations of the primary endrite were distributed through almost the entire region of a single glomerulus. In addition to the primary dendrite, several secondary dendrites were found to develop laterally from the mitral cell soma. They branched a few times both at the vicinity of the cell body and at the peripheral parts (Fig. 1A and D). As can be seen in Fig. 1A, these secondary dendrites were found to develop mainly in the deeper half of the external plexiform layer. Though it was not possible to measure the entire lengths of the secondary dendrites because of the gradual weakening of the intensity of fluorescence at the peripheral parts of the dendrites, we could trace them over a distance of 900μ from the soma of the mitral cell. In six mitral cells, the axons could be seen to run toward the granule cell layer.

These features of the mitral cell dendrites are in agreement with those reported in morphological investigations using the Golgi-staining method[2,3,14,17]. It seems necessary to identify morphologically the other neurons in the olfactory bulb (e.g., tufted cells and granule cells).

The response types of the olfactory bulb neurons to odor stimulation have been investigated (e.g., Kauer and Shepherd[7]). Since the Procion Yellow-staining method makes it possible to trace

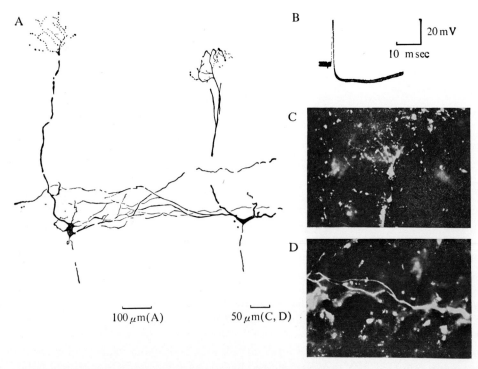

Fig. 1.   A. Reconstruction of dendrites and axons of two Procion Yellow-stained mitral cells. B: Intracellular potentials of the left mitral cell in A evoked by lateral olfactory tract stimulation. C and D: Photomicrographs showing the arborization of the primary dendrite of the left mitral cell and branchings of the secondary dendrite of the right mitral cell in A, respectively.

the primary dendrite of a stained mitral cell up to the glomerular layer, it may be possible to correlate the response pattern of the mitral cell to odor stimulation with the location of a glomerulus in which the primary dendrite of the mitral cell terminates. This kind of experiment may play an important role in testing the hypothesis that the glomerulus is a functional unit[9,16].

REFERENCES

1. Barrett, J.N. and Graubard, K., Fluorescent staining of cat motoneurons *in vivo* with beveled micropipettes, *Brain Research*, 18 (1970) 565–568.
2. Cajal, S.R., *Studies on the Cerebral Cortex* (Translated by L.M. Kraft) Lloyd Luke, London, 1955.
3. Freeman, W.J., Depth recording of averaged evoked potential of olfactory bulb, *J. Neuorphysiol.*, 35 (1972) 780–796.
4. Getchell, T.V. and Shepherd, G.M., Short-axon cells in the olfactory bulb: dendrodendritic synaptic interactions, *J. Physiol. (Lond.)*, 251 (1975) 523–548.
5. Jankowska, E. and Lindström, S., Morphological identification of physiologically defined neurons in the cat spinal cord, *Brain Research*, 20 (1970) 323–326.
6. Jankowska, E. and Lindström, S., Morphological identification of Renshow cells, *Acta physiol. scand.*, 81 (1971) 428–430.
7. Kauer, J.S. and Shepherd, G.M., Analysis of the onset phase of olfactory bulb unit responses to odour pulses in the salamander. *J. Physiol. (Lond.)*, 272 (1977) 495–516.

8. Kelley, J. and Van Essen, D., Cell structure and function in the visual cortex of the cat, *J. Physiol. (Lond.)*, 238 (1974) 515–548.
9. Leveteau, J. and MacLeod, P., Olfactory discrimination in the rabbit olfactory glomerulus, *Science*, 153 (1966) 175–176.
10. Mori, K. and Takagi, S.F., An intracellular study of dendrodendritic inhibitory synapses on mitral cells in the rabbit olfactory bulb, *J. Physiol. (Lond.)*, 279 (1978) (in press).
11. Mori, K. and Takagi, S.F., Activation and inhibition of olfactory bulb neurones by anterior commissure volleys in the rabbit, *J. Physiol. (Lond.)*, 279 (1978) (in press).
12. Nicoll, R.A., Inhibitory mechanisms in the rabbit olfactory bulb: dendrodendritic mechanisms, *Brain Research*, 14 (1969) 157–172.
13. Phillips, C.G., Powell, T.P.S. and Shepherd, G.M., Response of mitral cells to stimulation of the lateral olfactory tract in the rabbit, *J. Physiol. (Lond.)*, 168 (1963) 65–88.
14. Price, J.L. and Powell, T.P.S., The mitral and short axon cells of the olfactory bulb, *J. Cell Sci.*, 7 (1970) 631–651.
15. Shepherd, G.M., Synaptic organization of the mammalian olfactory bulb, *Physiol. Rev.*, 52 (1972) 864–917.
16. Shepherd, G.M., The olfactory bulb: a simple system in the mammalian brain. In J.M. Brookhart and V.B. Mountcastle (Eds.) *Handbook of Physiology—The Nervous System*, Williams and Wilkins, Baltimore, 1977, pp. 945–968.
17. Valverde, F., *Studies on the Piriform Lobe*, Harvard University Press. Cambridge, 1965.
18. Yamamoto, C., Yamamoto, T. and Iwama, K., The inhibitory system in the olfactory bulb studied by intracellular recording, *J. Neurophysiol.*, 26 (1963) 403–415.

Neurons in the solitary tract-parabrachial nucleus pathway

HISASHI OGAWA, TAKETOSHI AKAGI, HIROSUMI ITO AND MASAYASU SATO*

*Department of Physiology, Kumamoto University Medical School,
Honjyo, Kumamoto 860, Japan*

After the early work of Allen[1], it was assumed that gustatory impulses in neurons of the solitary tract nucleus, evoked by primary qustatory afferents, travelled to a part of the ventrobasal complex of the thalamus (i.e., ventral posteromedial nucleus, VPM) contralaterally via the lamina medialis with terminal projections to the cerebral cortex. However, Norgren et al.[3] recently demonstrated in the rat that the ipsilateral parabrachial nucleus was interposed between the solitary tract nucleus and VPM of the thalamus, and that the projections from the parabrachial nucleus to the VPM were almost bilateral. Ogawa and Akagi[1] have also shown that neurons in the parabrachial nucleus were labeled by injecting horseradish peroxidase type VI into the VPM but those in the solitary tract nucleus on either side were not.

The aim of the present experiment was to study the physiological characteristics of the solitary tract nucleus neurons projecting to the ipsilateral parabrachial nucleus.

About 30 albino rats (SD strain) of either sex and weighing 200–300 g were employed. After anesthesia with amobarbital sodium (60 mg/kg body wt), the trachea and left femoral vein were cannulated, and three lingual afferents (the lingual nerve, chorda tympani, and glossopharyngeal nerve) were then isolated for electrical stimulation at the left lower jaw. The rats were mounted on a stereotaxic instrument, and cerebellectomized to expose the dorsal surface of the medulla. While stimulating one of the lingual afferents, a pair of tungsten electrodes were inserted into the dorsal pons and positioned at a point where the evoked field potentials could be recorded maximally. Before stimulation was applied to the nerves, the animals were given gallamine (0.4 ml) and artificially ventilated. Anesthesia was maintained by additional intravenous injections of amobarbital (20 mg/kg body wt) if necessary. Neuronal activities were recorded in or around the ipsilateral solitary tract nucleus with glass microelectrodes filled with fast green FCF saturated in 2 M NaCl (10 MΩ), and the responses of these neurons to stimulation of the parabrachial nucleus (pulse duration, 0.2 msec; intensity, < 1mA) were studied.

The body temperature of the animals was maintained at around 37°C with an electric blanket, and EKG was monitored to check the general condition of the animals.

At the end of the experiment, the brain was perfused with 10% formalin in physiological saline, and both the recording sites in the solitary tract nucleus and the neighboring structures, and the stimulating sites in the dorsal pons were identified histologically.

A total of 130 neurons responding to electrical stimulation of the lingual afferents was recorded. Among them, 78 units were identified histologically as solitary tract nucleus neurons. The solitary tract nucleus neurons discharged 1–2 spikes with a latency of 3–6 msec in response to electrical stimulation of one of the three lingual afferents, but could not follow repetitive stimulation

* Present address: Tokyo Metropolitan Institute for Neurosciences, Fuchu city, Tokyo 183, Japan

120

of the nerves at 10 Hz. The response latency obtained here is in good agreement with that reported by Blomquist and Antem[2] from multiunit recordings. Neurons outside the solitary tract nucleus responded with several spikes and with a longer latency to electrical stimulation of the lingual afferents.

The thresholds of each of the lingual afferents to evoke a spike in single neurons were measured, and expressed relative to those (T) to produce field potentials on the dorsal surface of the medulla. The threshold of the chorda tympani was $1 \sim 10 \times T$ and relatively low compared with those of the other lingual afferents (2–$1000 \times T$). This difference may be ascribable to the fact that the threshold of the whole chorda tympani to evoke field potentials on the dorsal surface of the medulla is higher than those of the other lingual afferents since in the chorda tympani there are no fibers histologically[5] larger than 8 μ in diameter.

The responsiveness of 42 solitary tract nucleus neurons to electrical stimulation of the ipsilateral parabrachial nucleus was studied. They were classified into the following three types: type I neurons ($n = 17$), which responded with a fixed latency to over 3 or more stimulations; type II neurons ($n = 18$) which responded with variable latencies; and type III neurons ($n = 7$) which showed no responses at all. In some of the type I neurons, spikes evoked by nerve stimulation were shown to collide with those evoked by stimulation of the parabrachial nucleus. Some of the type I neurons might, therefore, project to the ipsilateral parabrachial nucleus or neighboring structures. Most of the neurons (including type I neurons) could not follow repetitive stimulation of the parabrachial nucleus at 10 Hz.

The differences in physiological characteristics between type I and type II neurons were examined. Nine of 11 type I neurons received inputs from all three lingual afferents and the remainder responded to stimulation of two of the lingual afferents. On the other hand, 8 of 14 type II neurons received projections from three lingual afferents, 2 from two lingual afferents, and the remainder from only one of the lingual afferents. Otherwise, no difference was detected in either response latency, discharge pattern or response threshold between the two types of neurons.

The present finding that most of the neurons responded to electrical stimulation of three lingual afferents might possibly derive from a tendency for the microelectrodes used to pick up responses selectively in bigger neurons receiving inputs from three lingual afferents.

References

1. Allen, W.F., Origin and destination of the secondary visceral fibers in the guinea pig, *J. comp. Neurol.*, 35 (1923) 275–311.
2. Blomquist, A.J. and Antem, A., Localization of the terminals of the tongue afferents in the nucleus of the solitary tract, *J. comp. Neurol.*, 124 (1965) 127–130.
3. Norgren, R. and Leonard, C., Ascending central gustatory pathways, *J. comp. Neurol.*, 150 (1973) 217–237.
4. Ogawa, H. and Akagi, T., Location of pontine relay neurons projecting to VPMm in the rat by means of horseradish peroxidase. In J. LeMagnen and P. MacLeod (Eds.), *Olfaction and Taste VI*, Information Retrieval Ltd., London, 1978, pp. 289.
5. Zotterman, Y., Action potentials in the glossopharyngeal nerve and in the chorda tympani, *Skand. Arch. Physiol.*, 72 (1935) 73–77.

Electrophysiological studies of gustation in the honeybee (*Apis mellifica* L.)

KIYOSHI AOKI AND MASUTARO KUWABARA

Life Science Institute, Sophia University,
Chiyoda-ku, Tokyo 102, Japan

The problem of the feeding behavior of the honeybee *Apis mellifica* L. can be explained in terms of taste thresholds.[2] The taste threshold can be observed in terms of proboscis extension during feeding in response to stimulation by sugars on the tarsus of the honeybee. The taste threshold during a period of sugar feeding rises to a high level; in contrast, a low taste threshold is found during a period of starvation.[3] The way in which elevation of the threshold might be brought about by feeding of a sugar solution is related to the central inhibition of the proboscis extension reflex. It was found that the proboscis extension was released from inhibition when we applied a simultaneous weak sugar stimulus to the tarsi of the 2nd leg pair of the honeybee. We could not observe proboscis extension response on application of a weak sugar stimulus to the tarsi of the 2nd leg. After applying an NaCl stimulus to the opposite tarsus, it was found that proboscis extension was inhibited even though a high sugar stimulus was given. It is suggested that the inhibitory system in the thoracic ganglion can account for these results.

This question was investigated by electrophysiological techniques to clarify the mechanism of the central inhibition and the pathways of the nervous system involved in proboscis extension during feeding behavior. The 3rd leg pair of the honeybee was fixed to the ventral side with beeswax, and the tarsi of the 2nd leg pair were used for the application of sugar and NaCl stimuli. A fine glass microelectrode was inserted into the thoracic ganglion from a small hole on the ventral side of the thorax between the 1st and 2nd legs. For recording from the subesophageal ganglion, a glass microelectrode was inserted through the compound eye. We found the responding units for sugar stimulation of the tarsus. Only the recording from the unit in the 2nd thoracic ganglion showed a response to tarsal sugar stimulation. The latency of the response between the unit of the thoracic ganglion and the chemoreceptor is about 10 msec. The impulse frequencies for various concentrations of sucrose, fructose and glucose were recorded from 60 honeybees, each of which had been starved for 48 hr. Fig. 1 shows the effects of these responses on the tarsal sugar receptor. The sugar chemoreceptor shows the highest sensitivity for sucrose, and has almost the same sensitivities for fructose and glucose. These results from the thoracic ganglion units are the same as those for the threshold of feeding behavior. The response from the unit of the 2nd thoracic ganglion to sugar stimulation of the tarsi of both legs shows an increase of impulse frequency 1.5 times greater than that to sugar stimulation to the tarsus on one side only. It should be noted that the results show the summation of impulses from the sugar receptors of the two tarsi in the thoracic ganglion. There was no difference in the sugar responses from the units in the 2nd thoracic ganglion with starvation time. These results show no inhibition effect in the 2nd thoracic ganglion to sugar stimulation. In addition, no NaCl inhibition could be found in the thoracic ganglion tarsus for NaCl stimulation.[1]

The recording response from the units in the subesophageal ganglion showed an increase of

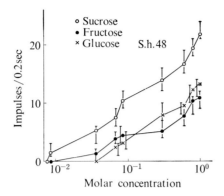

Fig. 1.   The relationship between the concentration of sugar and impulses frequencies after starvation for 48 hr.

impulse frequencies on sugar stimulation in proportion to the duration of the starvation period. The relationships between sucrose and NaCl were also investigated; it was found that the central inhibition by NaCl was related to tarsal stimulation by sugar. These results indicate central inhibition of feeding behavior in some parts of the brain after sugar feeding. At the same time, the convergence in the central nervous system of the two chemoreceptors was considered. After NaCl stimulation to the tarsus, sugar stimulation was applied to another tarsus, and conversely, after sugar stimulation, an NaCl stimulation was applied. The results indicated inhibition of the response in the central nervous system.

Further studies are in progress to clarify the mechanisms of inhibition of the proboscis extension response in the central nervous system.

REFERENCES

1. Aoki, K. and Kuwabara, M., The proboscis extension reflex in honeybee, *Apis mellifica.*, *Zool. Mag.* 81 (1972) 387 (in Japanese).
2. Evans, D.R. and Dethier, V.G., The regulation of taste thresholds for sugars in the blowfly, *J. Ins. Physiol.*, 1 (1957) 3–17.
3. Shiraishi, A. and Tanabe, Y., The proboscis extension response and tarsal and labellar chemosensory hairs in the blowfly, *J. Comp. Physiol.* 92 (1974) 161–179.

The site of origin of the abortive spikes in terminals of the frog muscle spindle afferent nerve

FUMIO ITO AND YUKIO KOMATSU

*Department of Physiology, Nagoya University School of Medicine,
Showa-ku, Nagoya 466, Japan*

Katz[3] found a local response smaller than one–tenth of the amplitude of propagated impulses in the record of electrical responses from the spindle afferent terminal in the frog toe muscle and termed it an 'abortive spike'. He supposed that this abortive spike is caused by a failure in transmission of an impulse from a fine non-myelinated filament into the myelinated axon, as a sudden increase in diameter of the axon at the transmission point may cause a reduction of density of the afferent action currents. Later, Ito, Kanamori and Kuroda[1] demonstrated that the relative amplitudes of abortive and full-sized spikes recorded intracellularly from the axon terminal of the frog muscle spindle were almost the same as those recorded extracellularly across a paraffin gap upon the axon. This may imply either that an abortive spike represents an electrotonic spread of a full-sized spike generated in a thin non-myelinated filament further distal to the recording site, or that it corresponds to a non-overshoot spike generated at the recording site. In fact, an axon terminal emits several non-myelinated thin filaments of 1 μm or less in diameter and of 100 μm or more in length. These two possibilities can be differentiated by testing the effect of polarizing currents applied along the axon; these should be more effective in the latter than in the former case.

Single-type muscle spindles were isolated from the sartorius muscles in young frogs (*Rana nigromaculata*). Such spindles are innervated by an axon without any myelinated ramification (Ito and Komatsu[2]). The preparation was placed in a pool of Ringer's solution on a glass plate and the isolated axon was passed into another pool of Ringer's solution through an air gap. The gap was placed on the myelinated segment just outside the spindle capsule. Calomel electrodes inserted into both pools of Ringer's solution were connected to an arm of a bridge circuit which served for both recording electrical responses of the axon terminal and for application of polarizing currents to that axon terminal. The muscle spindle was stretched differentially by 1 mm from the *in situ* length at a rate of 2.5 mm/sec.

The axon was transected at the node just proximal to the gap and the proximal Ringer's solution was replaced with 100 mM KCl solution. The trans-gap resting potential then obtained was 20–25 mV if the trans-gap resistance was relatively high, approximately 20 MΩ. Action potentials of 10–30 mV in amplitude occurred spontaneously at a frequency of 0.5–1 impulses/sec, while abortive spikes were scarcely observed (Fig. 1A). Application of depolarizing currents of 1 nA or more to the receptor pool depressed the spontaneous discharges and diminished the number of discharges during stretching, presumably due to cathodal depression of the terminal membrane. On the other hand, application of hyperpolarizing currents of more than 1 nA caused an increase in the discharge rate, presumably by restoration of the resting membrane potential. During application of currents of 3 nA or more, abortive spikes occurred between full-sized discharges (Fig. 1B). The amplitude of the abortive spikes varied from 0.5 to 3 mV. Discharges of both full-sized and abortive spikes were depressed during excessive hyperpolarization with 10 nA or more.

124

A   B

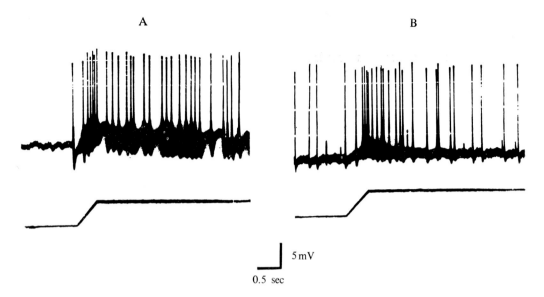

5 mV

0.5 sec

Fig. 1.   Discharges from a spindle terminal intact (A) and during application of a hyperpolarizing current of 3 nA (B). In record B, the slow deflection resembling a generator potential was eliminated by using a CR coupling amplifier. Upper traces: discharges. Lower traces: displacement in stretching.

These results favor the view that the abortive spike is a non-overshoot spike generated at the axon terminal. A similar mechanism might be considered for the partial spike responses observed in various nerve cells.

References

1. Ito, F., Kanamori, N. and Kuroda, H., Structural and functional asymmetries of myelinated branches in the frog muscle spindle, *J. Physiol. (Lond.)*, 241 (1974) 389–405.
2. Ito, F. and Komatsu, Y., Frog muscle spindles with unbranched myelinated afferent axons: The response to stretch and the length of the first myelinated segment, *J. Physiol. (Lond.)*, 264 (1977) 881–891.
3. Katz, B., Action potentials from a sensory nerve ending, *J. Physiol. (Lond.)*, 111 (1950) 248–260.

Statocyst-driven interneurons in crayfish circumesophageal commissure

MITUHIKO HISADA AND MASAKAZU TAKAHATA

Zoophysiological Laboratory, Zoological Institute, Faculty of Science, Hokkaido University, Kita-ku, Sapporo 060, Japan

Crayfish show various equilibrium reactions when they are tilted.[1] These reactions consist of compensatory eye movements and other appendage movements including those of uropods. The role of statocysts in these reactions has been extensively investigated. However, although the neuronal and muscular organization in the oculomotor reflex pathway has been partially established[2,3,5], the central connections between the statocyst afferents and the motoneurons remain undetermined. We investigated the central mechanism for uropod movements during body tilting, and identified four statocyst-driven interneurons in the circumesophageal commissure of the crayfish, *Procambarus clarki* (Girard).

The animal was fixed to a rotation apparatus with the anterior portion of the carapace removed. The commissure on one side was desheathed and divided into small bundles. Extracellular recordings were made from the proximal cut end of the bundles with a suction electrode affixed to the apparatus so that it could move with the animal as a unit. The other commissure was also severed in order to eliminate the effect of ascending pathways. Four statocyst-driven interneurons so found differed from each other in their location in the cross section, and each responded only to specific directions of body tilting. For example, interneuron C_1, located in Wiersma's[6] area 74, responded on head-up tilting around the transverse axis and on same-side-down tilting around the longitudinal axis. The location and direction of the responses of the four interneurons are given in Table 1. The statocyst input to each interneuron was studied by unilateral and bilateral statolith removal. Removal of the left statolith abolished the responses of interneuron I_2 in the left commissure and of interneurons C_1 and C_2 in the right commissure on tilting in any direction. Removal of both statoliths abolished the responses of all four interneurons. The inputs thus deduced are also shown in Table 1. These results have been further supplemented by direct stimulation of the statocyst sensory neurons. A pulse of 0.1 msec duration applied with a platinum electrode inserted into the statocyst lumen elicited a compound action potential in the sensory nerve. This stimulus also activated the statocyst-driven interneurons with certain latencies. Stimulation of the contralateral statocyst which provides the main input to interneuron C_1, activated it with both short (5–10 msec) and long (20–40 msec) latencies, while stimulation of the ipsilateral statocyst activated C_1 only with a short latency. The actual synaptic delay in the short-latency response may be less than 5 msec, suggesting monosynaptic transmission. Thus, interneuron C_1 is driven monosynaptically by both ipsi- and contralateral statocysts, and multisynaptically by contralateral statocyst. These two kinds of synaptic transmission were observed in all four interneurons. The functional meaning of the monosynaptic activation is not yet understood.

The directional responses of the interneurons appear to be attained primarily by selective connection of the interneurons with statolith hair receptors as in the directional mechanosensory interneurons in the abdominal cord.[7] These hair receptors are aligned in a crescent on the statocyst

TABLE 1. Location and direction of the responses of the four interneurons, C_1, C_2, I_1 and I_2

Interneuron	Input statocyst	Axis and direction around which the interneuron responds		Location[6]
		Horizontal transverse	Horizontal longitudinal	
C_1	contralateral	head up	same side down	L74
C_2	contralateral	head up and down	same side down	L66
I_1	ipsi- and contralateral	head up and down	same side up and down	L62
I_2	ipsilateral	head down	same side up	L68

floor and can be classified into two types according to their response characteristics to hair deflection: the phasic and tonic types.[4] The activity of the latter depends on the angle of hair deflection and becomes maximal when the hair is deflected towards the center of the crescent (Hisada and Takahata, in preparation). Hence, tilting of the statocyst in the head-up direction would activate the receptors whose hairs are located in the anterior region of the crescent. Thus, selective connection with the anterior hairs, for example, would render the interneuron responsive only to head-up tilting. In order to test this hypothesis, we carried out partial ablation experiments on interneuron C_1. Ablation of a small portion of the anterior region of the contralateral statocyst drastically reduced the response of C_1 to head-up tilting, and ablation of the remainder abolished the response completely. The effectiveness of ablation on the reduction of the C_1 response suggests that this fiber has a main functional connection with contralateral anterior receptors.

These statocyst-driven interneurons also responded to passive leg movements. All four interneurons showed either no spontaneous activity or, if any, a very low-frequency discharge while the animal was kept in the resting position. However, when the commissure other than the one severed for impulse recording was left intact, the interneurons showed spontaneous firing in the normal position. This indicates that these interneurons receive a large input from the leg proprioceptors through as yet unidentified ascending neurons. These statocyst-driven interneurons were also found to receive an input from the eye. This multimodality in the sensory input channels of the interneurons suggests that these interneurons may be commanding the uropod movements during tilting. This problem, together with sensory connections other than the statocyst, is currently being investigated.

REFERENCES

1. Davis, W.J., Lobster righting responses and their neural control, *Proc. roy. Soc. B*, 70 (1968) 435–456.
2. Hisada, M. and Higuchi, T., Basic response pattern and classification of oculomotor nerve in the crayfish, *Procambarus clarki*, *J. Fac. Sci. Hokkaido Univ. Ser. VI, Zool.*, 18 (1973) 481–494.
3. Mellon, DeF., The anatomy and motor nerve distribution of the eye muscles in the crayfish, *J. comp. Physiol.*, 121 (1977) 349–366.
4. Ozeki, M., Takahata, M. and Hisada, M., Afferent response patterns of crayfish statocyst with ferrite grain statolith to the magnetic field stimulation, *J. comp. Physiol.*, 123 (1978) 1–10.
5. Stein, A., Attainment of positional information in the crayfish statocyst, *Fortsch. Zool.*, 23 (1975) 109–117.
6. Wiersma, C.A.G., On the functional connections of single units in the central nervous system of the crayfish, *Procambarus clarkii* Girard, *J. comp. Neurol.*, 110 (1958) 421–471.
7. Wiese, K., Calabrese, R.L. and Kennedy, D., Integration of directional mechanosensory input by crayfish interneurons, *J. Neurophysiol.*, 39 (1976) 834–843.

Morphological study of a small nucleus in the posterolateral hypothalamus of the cat

MASAKO FUJII[*1], TOSHIO KUSAMA[*1], NOBUO YOSHII[*2] AND TORU MIZOKAMI[*2]

[*1] *Department of Neuroanatomy, Institute of Brain Research, School of Medicine, University of Tokyo, Bunkyo-ku, Tokyo 113, Japan*
[*2] *Division of Neurosurgery, 2nd Department of Surgery, Toho University Hospital, Ota-ku, Tokyo 143, Japan*

In our previous study in the cat[3] we found that a restricted area in the posterior part of the lateral hypothalamus received horseradish peroxidase (HRP) transport from the rostral part of the pulvinar-lp complex. This restricted area also showed such a clear border against the surroundings in sections of Nissl and myelin stains that it could be considered to be one of the hypothalamic nuclei. As a result of cytoarchitectural and myeloarchitectural investigations in this study using eight adult cats and two kittens the normal features of this nucleus have been more clearly defined. At the rostral-most level of the mamillary body this nucleus appears in the area between the fornix and the subthalamic nucleus and, as already reported,[3] has two parts: pars compacta and pars diffusa. The pars compacta is the small-celled part, which consists of densely packed small nerve cells (Fig. 1, c). In Heidenhein-Woelcke sections this part appears as a light myelin-poor area (Fig. 2, c). The pars diffusa is the rostral, ventral and lateral area surrounding the pars compacta (Fig. 1, d). Small and medium sized nerve cells in the pars diffusa are less dense than in the pars compacta, although a relatively compact cell assembly was noted in the pars diffusa lateral or ventrolateral to the pars compacta, where another myelin-poor area appears (Fig. 2). In addition to these histological characteristics, the bleached appearance of this nucleus due to light staining of individual nerve cells made it easy to draw the nuclear outline. The medial and lateral borders of this nucleus are often in contact with dorsomedially parallel-running blood vessels, although the lateral border sometimes occurs slightly beyond the laterally situated blood vessel. Ventrally this nucleus is delimited from the tuberomamillary nucleus by scattered and darkly stained nerve cells of medium size. In Golgi-Cox preparations of kittens, a well-outlined cell assembly is observed in a similar area (Fig. 3): the nerve cells are round, triangular or polygonal and emit a few short dendrites which are rather wavy and with poor arborization. The tip of the dendrites appears not to extend beyond the cytoarchitectural border of this nucleus. This neuronal pattern seems to be essentially the same as in the adult cat.

Lundberg[1] described two small nuclei (nuclei gemini) in the lateral hypothalamus and the rostral midbrain in the rabbit as the terminal portion of the medial forebrain bundle. Scott *et al.*[2] substantiated this result in other rodents. In the present study, the pars diffusa at least was observed to receive massive termination of a degenerating medial forebrain bundle caused by lesion of the olfactory tubercle (Fig. 4). This finding was confirmed in three cats, and further studies are in progress in our laboratories.

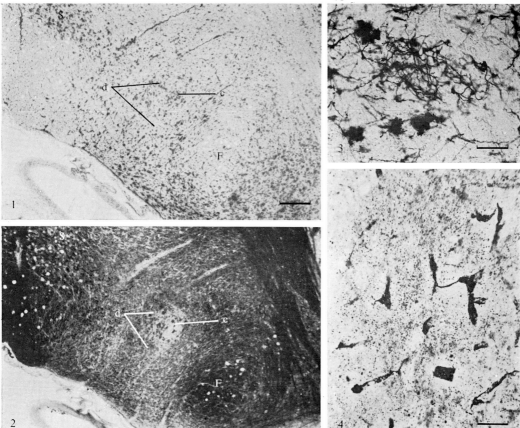

Fig. 1. (*Above left*) Frontal Nissl section through the rostral-most part of the mamillary body. c, pars compacta; d, pars diffusa; F, fornix; S, subthalamuc nucleus. Scale, 250 μm.

Fig. 2. (*Below left*) Section adjoining Fig. 1. Heidenhein-Woelcke stain. Symbols and magnification are as in Fig. 1.

Fig. 3. (*Above right*) Nerve cells in the pars compacta. Golgi-Cox stain. Frontal section through the rostral-most part of the mamillary body of a kitten weighing 260 g. Scale, 100 μm.

Fig. 4. (*Below right*) Degenerating fibers of the medial forebrain bundle, terminating in the pars diffusa. Fink-Heimer section. Scale 50 μm.

REFERENCES

1. Lundberg, P.O., The nuclei gemini: Two hitherto undescribed nerve cell collections in the hypothalamus of the rabbit, *J. comp. Neurol.*, 119 (1962) 311–316.
2. Scott, J.W. and Leonard, C.M., The olfactory connections of the lateral hypothalmus in the rat, mouse and hamster, *J. comp. Neurol.*, 141 (1971) 331–344.
3. Yoshii, N., Fujii, M. and Mizokami, T. Hypothalamic projection to the pulvinar-LP complex in the cat: a study by the HRP method, *Brain Research,* in press.

Brain-stem evoked potentials elicited by electrical stimulation of the vestibular and cochlear nerves: an animal experiment

NOBUHIKO FURUYA, AKIRA SAITO, MICHIO ISHIKAWA AND JUN-ICHI SUZUKI

Department of Otorhinolaryngology, School of Medicine, University of Teikyo, Itabashi-ku, Tokyo 173, Japan

Standard clinical tests of vestibular functions are important and useful for the evaluation and localization of brain-stem disorders[1,2,5,7-9,15]. These tests have some weaknesses, however. One is that they require the patient to be attentive and cooperative, which excludes the testing of comatose patients and infants. A second problem is that the tests, except the caloric tests, cannot generally assess the function of each ear alone. A third problem is that for evaluation of brain-stem function, the tests require intact labyrinths.

Auditory brain-stem evoked potentials are now being utilized successfully to evaluate brain-stem pathology in both comatose patients and infants[4,6,9-13]. This use of the auditory brain-stem potentials suggests an approach for solving the problems of the vestibular tests.

One diagnostic limitation of present methods of testing hearing is their inability to distinguish between sensory deafness and neural deafness. In the case of sensory deafness, some hearing could possibly be recovered through use of a cochlea implant.[3] However, such a procedure would not be appropriate in cases of neural deafness. The need for distinguishing between these two forms of deafness is thus evident. The present study attempts to test the feasibility of such an approach by recording potentials from the scalp associated with direct electrical stimulation of the vestibular and cochlear nerves of cats.

The experiments were performed on 15 adult cats with pentobarbital sodium anesthesia (initial dose 35 mg/kg, i.p.) under artificial respiration after immobilization with gallamine triethiodide (Flaxedil). For cochlear nerve stimulation, the bulla tympanica was opened on the ventral side, and the second turn of the cochlear was opened through a small hole cut in the modiolus with a sharp cutting burr. Bipolar 100 μm insulated Ag-AgCl stimulating electrodes were inserted into the modiolus. For vestibular nerve stimulation, the bipolar electrodes were placed on the utricular nerve through the oval window. When the electrodes were properly positioned, they were fixed in place with paraffin and acrylic resin cement. Body temperature was maintained at 37–38°C with a heating pad. The electrical stimulus was a rectangular pulse of 0.1 msec duration.

Evoked responses were recorded from the scalp using a pair of needle electrodes. One electrode was placed at the forehead and the other at the mastoid tip on the side of stimulation. After differential AC amplification, the response was averaged between 100 and 200 times with an averaging computer (7TO6 Sanei Instrument Co. Ltd.). Field potentials from the vestibular nucleus and cochlear nucleus were recorded with glass micropipettes filled with Ringer solutions. They were used for determining the threshold of each nerve. In most cases the stimulus strength was between threshold and twice threshold levels for each nerve[14]. Fig. 1 shows simultaneous evoked responses recorded from the scalp (upper trace) and the vestibular nucleus (middle trace)

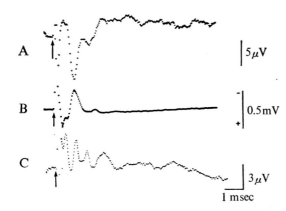

A

B

C

5 μV

0.5 mV

3 μV

1 msec

Fig. 1. Evoked potentials recorded from the scalp elicited by stimulation of the vestibular or cochlear nerve. A and B, Simultaneous recordings from the scalp and vestibular nucleus, respectively, after selective stimulation of the vestibular nerve. The recordings were averaged for 100–200 trials. C, Scalp evoked potentials after cochlear nerve stimulation.

following electrical stimulation of the vestibular nerve. The scalp responses consisted of 2 scalp-negative waves. The mean latency of the onset of the first downward deflection was 0.87 msec in 5 animals. The mean latency of the first negative peak (downward deflection) was 1.08 msec and that of the second negative peak was 1.84 msec. The latency and duration of the first peak were similar to those of the N1 field potential which was simultaneously recorded from the vestibular nucleus. When the stimulus strength was increased, the evoked response also increased in amplitude. This effect of stimulus strength paralleled that of N1 recorded from the vestibular nucleus. The thresholds of the N1 potential and the scalp response were virtually the same. It appears likely that most of the first negative deflection is attributable to the N1 field poetntials. The origin of the second negative deflection is less clear due to contemporaneous polysynaptic responses. Some part of the response may be attributable to the N2 vestibular field potential because of the similarity in latencies.

The bottom trace in Fig. 1 shows a scalp response following electrical stimulation of the cochlear nerve. It consists basically of 4 positive peaks (upward deflection). Occasionally, the first peak could not be differentiated from the stimulus artifact. These 4 positive waves were labeled P1, P2, P3, and P4 according to their mean latencies which were 0.45, 1.05, 1.65 and 2.46 msec, respectively. In the above experiments, a weak current was used to stimulate either the vestibular or cochlear nerve. However, the possibility remained that through current spread the other nerve was also stimulated. This possibility was excluded by two different experiments. In one, field potentials were recorded simultaneously from the vestibular and cochlear nuclei while stimulating either the vestibular or cochlear nerve. Within the stimulus range used, the field potentials evoked from each nerve were restricted to the corresponding nuclei. In the other experiment, the vestibular or cochlear nerve was selectively sectioned at the internal auditory canal under a binocular microscope after ablation of the flocculus and part of the paraflocculus. When the cochlear nerve was sectioned, stimulation of nerve VIII near the receptors produced scalp responses similar to those elicited during stimulation of the vestibular nerve. When the vestibular nerve was sectioned, the evoked response elicited by vestibular nerve stimulation disappeared, but the cochlear evoked response remained. These results confirmed that the stimulation of the vestibular or cochlear nerve was indeed selective.

Far-field potentials of the brain stem response were thus detected on the scalp following selective stimulation of the vestibular or cochlear nerve. The former stimulation produced 2 scalp-negative waves, whereas the latter produced a series of 4 waves resembling the typical response to click stimulation. These results indicate that the vestibular and cochlear nerves could be stimulated directly and selectively in cats. The stimulation procedure used in cats would be easily applicable to a patient during surgery. In terms of clinical tests, the present data therefore suggest that it may be feasible to solve the problems of testing non-cooperative patients, of unilateral evaluation, of receptor-independent stimulation, and of distinction between sensory and neural deafness, for the vestibular as well as the auditory systems.

Acknowledgements: We wish to express our thanks to Dr. Hink for his advice, and to Miss M. Ueno for her technical assistance.

References

1. Crosby, E.C., Relations of brain centers to normal and abnormal eye movements in the horizontal plane, *J. Comp. Neurol.*, 99 (1953) 437–479.
2. Goebel, H.A., Komatsuzaki, A., Bender, M.B. and Cohen, B., Lesions of the pontine tegmentum and conjugate gaze paralysis, *Arch. Neurol.*, 24 (1971) 431–440.
3. House, W.F., Cochlear implants, *Ann. Otol. Rhinol. Laryngol.*, 85 (1977) Suppl. 27.
4. Huang, C.M. and Buchwald, J.S., Interpretation of the vertex short-latency acoustic response: A study of single neurons in the brain stem, *Brain Research*, 137 (1977) 291–303.
5. Jacobs, L., Anderson, P.J. and Bender, M.B., The lesions producing paralysis of downward but not upward gaze, *Arch. Neurol.*, 28 (1973) 319–323.
6. Jewett, D.L., Romano, M.N. and Williston, J.S., Human auditory evoked potentials: Possible brain-stem components detected on the scalp, *Science*, 167 (1970) 1517–1518.
7. Komatsuzaki, A., Alpert, J., Harris, H. and Cohen, B., Effects of mesencephalic reticular formation lesions on optokinetic nystagmus, *Exp. Neurol.*, 34 (1972) 522–534.
8. Pasik, P., Pasik, T. and Bender, M.B., The pretectal syndrome in monkeys, I, *Brain*, 92 (1969) 521–534.
9. Pasik, T., Pasik, P. and Bender, M.B., The pretectal syndrome in monkeys, II, *Brain*, 92 (1969) 871–884.
10. Picton, T.W., Hillyard, S.A., Krauz, H.I. and Galambos, R., Human auditory evoked potentials. I. Evaluation of components, *Electroenceph. clin. Neurophysiol.*, 36 (1974) 179–190.
11. Starr, A. and Achor, L.J., Auditory brain stem responses in neurological disease, *Arch. Neurol. (Chic.)*, 32 (1975) 761–768.
12. Starr, A. and Hamilton, A., Correlation between confirmed sites of neurological lesions and abnormalities of far-field auditory brainstem response, *Electroenceph. clin. Neurophysiol.*, 41 (1976) 595–608.
13. Starr, A., Auditory brain stem responses in brain death, *Brain*, 99 (1967) 543–554.
14. Shimazu, H. and Precht, W., Tonic and kinetic responses of cat's vestibular neurons to horizontal angular acceleration, *J. Neurophysiol.*, 28 (1965) 991–1013.
15. Teng, P., Shanzer, S. and Bender, M.B., Effects of brain stem lesions on optokinetic nystagmus in monkeys, *Neurology (Minneap.)*, 8 (1958) 22–26.

PART III

MOTOR CONTROL AND ITS DISORDERS

HIROSHI SHIMAZU[*1] AND MITSUO YOSHIDA[*2]

[*1]*Department of Neurophysiology, Institute of Brain Research, School of Medicine, University of Tokyo, Bunkyo-ku, Tokyo 113, Japan*
[*2]*Department of Neurology, Jichi Medical School, Kawachi-gun, Tochigi 329-04, Japan*

Since Sherrington established the basic concept of the elementary reflex and its integration, a great deal of knowledge has accumulated on the role of reflex activity in the control of movements. Purposive movements adaptive to the environment are accomplished with the aid of external feedback arising from the muscle, joint and cutaneous receptors. On the other hand, the contribution of central patterning to the initiation of certain basic movements, such as locomotion, nystagmus, mastication, and so on, is also evident. Various internal feedback loops, i.e., the feedback arising from structures within the central nervous system, appear to be involved in the central patterning of sequential movement. Since corrective modification of centrally programmed motor output by external feedback is essential for animals to adapt to the environment, investigation of the interaction between external and internal feedback loops is crucial to an understanding of the mechanism of central control of movements. This can be approached in various ways; anatomical and electrophysiological analyses of neunal organization of basic circuitry, characterization of the dynamics of identified neurons in the circuitry during movement, and analyses of pathological conditions of the animal as well as of the neurological patients.

The studies described in Part III are directed to the following four major areas.

Motor cortex and spinal mechanism

It is well-known that the activity of pyramidal tract neurons in the motor cortex precedes muscle contraction in a behaving animal. The functional role of cortical neurons in the motor area and the supplementary motor area has been further investigated in task movements of the monkey (Matsunami, Tanji). To what extent a single corticospinal neuron can influence different muscles is an important but so far unanswered question. Electrophysiological analysis of axonal branching of single corticospinal neurons in the spinal cord is a first approach to this problem (Shinoda). Techniques of intracellular HRP injection make it possible to visualize axonal projection patterns of functionally identified single neurons and have been applied to spinal primary afferents (Mannen and Hongo).

Electrophysiological analyses of motoneuronal responses in the spastic state (Aoki) and in the tonic vibration reflex (Homma and Nakajima) and the study of human H-reflex elicited during voluntary contraction (Tanaka) are relevant to an elucidation of neurological disorders.

Functional organization of the cerebellar input and output systems

Now that the neuronal circuits interconnecting the cerebral cortex and the cerebellum have been increasingly clarified the concept of assigning to the cerebellum the role of a comparator or a site of interaction between internal and external feedback has become more accepted. There is evidence that a portion of the corticospinal axons transmits to the precerebellar nucleus the same signal as that conveyed to the spinal cord (Oshima), and that the afferent information transmitted from the spinal cord also reaches the cerebellum (Matsushita). The cerebellar output is sent back to the cerebral cortex (Sasaki), which makes use of the information to modify the cerebral output. The cerebello-rubro-olivo-cerebellar circuit forms another internal feedback loop (Oka). Another approach to the elucidation of cerebellar function is the comparative study of elementary circuits of the pathological cerebellum and the behavior of the animal (Ohno).

Basal ganglia and related structures

In spite of increasing knowledge of pharmacology and clinical interest in the basal ganglia, little is known about its function based on the neuronal organization. It is desirable to understand the function of the basal ganglia in connection with the thalamus and the cerebellum. In this regard, the physiology and pharmacology of pallido-thalamic and nigro-thalamic projections are areas of research interest (Uno, Yoshida). The human thalamus has been studied not only anatomically but also on the basis of broad experience of the stereotaxic thalamotomy for patients with neurological disorders such as tremor and rigidity (Ohye). It is expected to correlate clinical considerations of movement disorders with cerebellar function (Narabayashi) and comparative study of ocular, limb and truncal movements in the neurological patients (Shibazaki) with basic physiological, anatomical and pharmacological findings.

Brain stem organization and central patterning

Knowledge of neuronal circuits in the brain stem and related structures that underlie various reflex activities is required to understand the neural mechanism of central patterning. Visuo-vestibular interaction in the tecto-spinal and tecto-bulbar neurons (Maeda) should provide a neural basis for eye-head coordination. Identification of excitatory and inhibitory input to jaw motoneurons (Nakamura) is a clear step towards further understanding of the rhythmic mastication movement. Locomotor movements are considered to be an instance of centrally patterned motor output. Evidence is provided for a brain stem pathway activating the locomotion generator (Mori) and for cerebellar involvement in the control of locomotion (Udo). Comparative studies of the invertebrate nervous system (Hisada) should aid in understanding the command action in the central patterning.

Analyses of the human blink reflex (Hiraoka and Shimamura) and the far-field potential in response to stimulation of the vestibular and cochlear nerve (Suzuki et al.) are expected to be of clinical value.

Intraspinal multiple projections of single corticospinal neurons in the cat and monkey

YOSHIKAZU SHINODA

Department of Neurophysiology, Institute of Brain Research, School of Medicine, University of Tokyo, Bunkyo-ku, Tokyo 113, Japan

Introduction

The organization of the motor cortex and its effects on subcortical structures have been extensively reviewed by Allen and Tsukahara[3], Asanuma[8], Brooks and Stoney[17], Phillips[56], Porter[57], and Wiesendanger[77]. The present paper will therefore focus on only one aspect of this general problem; that is, whether single corticospinal (CS) neurons influence the activity of motoneurons innervating a number of different muscles.

Many pioneering studies since the original work of Fritsch and Hitzig[27] have concentrated on an analysis of the localization of outputs within the projection area of the motor cortex. For this purpose, electrical stimulation of the motor cortex has been employed and the effects of the outputs have been detected with increasingly refined methods; first, by inspection or palpation of muscle contraction[45], then myograms[21], recordings of monosynaptic reflexes[10], EMG[5,9] and recently, intracellular recordings from motoneurons[44].

The areas of origin of corticofugal projection to muscles were discussed in the early days and this projection included the cortico–rubrospinal, cortico–reticulospinal and other indirect corticomotoneuronal projections as well as the direct corticomotoneuronal projection. For understanding the function of the motor cortex, information is required about a localized cortical efferent zone from which corticofugal cells project to motoneurons mono- and polysynaptically as well as to other subcortical structures. However, physiological excitation by direct activation of cortical interneurons and afferent axons was inevitable when polysynaptic corticomotoneuronal effects were used for accurate mapping of outputs, since a single shock was not usually sufficiently strong to activate motoneurons through interneurons at a spinal or at a supraspinal level. Due to this uncertainty about the extent of intracortical physiological spread, we had to fall back on an analysis of the localization of CS neurons directly terminating upon motoneurons. The technique of intracellular recording from motoneurons was introduced[38,44] and monosynaptic postsynaptic potentials evoked from the cortex were utilized as a very sensitive indicator of responses. The limitations of this method derive from the fact that it is not easy to analyze connections mediated by fibers with slow conduction velocities, in a system where both slow and fast fibers run in parallel. This represents an unfortunate drawback, considering that about 90% of pyramidal tract fibers consist of fibers less than 3 μ in diameter in each of the species so far studied[75].

The main problem in mapping a projection area is to define the area in which CS neurons are fired directly. Surface-anodal stimulation has been known to activate CS neurons directly at the minimal stimulus of 0.2–0.3 mA[32]. However, surface stimulation with strong stimuli may overestimate the area, while stimulation with near–threshold stimuli may underestimate it. In addition, pyramidal cells have a large number of recurrent collaterals; they span up to 1.5 mm in the cortex[64]. These collaterals might be stimulated rather than the somata of CS neurons[11]. In the case of intracortical microstimulation, CS neurons can be excited at a stimulus intensity of the order of a few μA[72]. However, recent studies[11,37] have shown that the thresholds for direct and indirect activation of CS neurons are very close.

The important findings obtained by mapping with surface-anodal stimulation, can be summarized as follows: (1) CS neurons projecting to single motoneurons or single motoneuron pools, aggregate in a circumscribed area in the motor cortex, and (2) the areas of origin of cortical projections to different motoneuron pools overlap[38,43,44]. The results of experiments utilizing intracortical microstimulation led to the conclusion that "each efferent zone had a sharp boundary and frequently overlapped with another efferent zone which produced an opposite movement."[9] So far as the method of electrical stimulation (surface- or intracortical) of the motor cortex, is used, it is not possible to draw conclusions about the size, shape and arrangement of CS neurons of the cortical projection area of single muscles. The overlapping of projection areas is based on the assumption that single CS axons project to one species of motoneurons. In this model, the CS neurons for a particular muscle are distributed over a circumscribed area of the motor cortex which includes a considerable but undeterminable intermingling of the CS neurons which belong to the different projection areas. As an alternative to this model, it is possible that single CS axons terminate on motoneurons of more than one species. In this second model, the "overlapping" area, although the term "overlapping" is not really an adequate expression for this model, contains the CS neurons projecting to a particular group of motoneurons innervating different muscles. Between these two extreme models, a variety of intermediate structural forms including two types of CS neurons could be consistent with the experimental findings. To date, there have been no available experimental data about this basic relationship between CS neurons and motoneurons. A series of experiments[12,13,68,70] (Shinoda, Y., Zarzeckie, P. and Asanuma, H., in preparation) was therefore devoted to answering the question of whether a differentation of two projection patterns exists among CS neurons in the motor cortex.

Spinal axon collaterals of corticospinal axons

As a first step in the analysis of cortico-motoneuronal connections, an experiment was undertaken to determine whether single cortico-spinal neurons branch and project to separate levels of the spinal cord[13,68].

Cats were anesthetized with pentobarbital sodium (Nembutal) and the spinal cord was exposed from C3 to Th3 and also at L1, by laminectomy. The motor cortex was exposed by craniotomy and a chamber was installed on the skull over the craniotomy opening. The animals were then paralyzed by gallamine triethiodide (Flaxedil) and artificially ventilated. An array of 5–12 microelectrodes, 2–5 mm apart, was implanted in the cervical gray matter (C4–C8) contralateral to the recording site. Two large bipolar stimulating electrodes were inserted in the lateral column at the level of the caudal end of Th3 and at L1 to stimulate the lateral corticospinal tract contralateral to the cortical recording site. Microstimulation at an intensity of 50 μA or less was delivered through each microelectrode.

Whenever a CS neuron was activated antidromically by stimulation of the cervical gray matter, the corticospinal tract was stimulated at the thoracic and lumbar level to determine whether the same neuron sent axons to the lower levels of the spinal cord (Fig. 1). In the case of the neuron in Fig. 1, it was antidromically activated from both the cervical gray matter and the thoracic cord. To demonstrate the existence of axon collaterals from stem axons of CS neurons, it was essential to ascertain that cervical stimulation activated local axon branches in the gray matter rather than fibers within the corticospinal tracts. Several methods were used to exclude the possibility of direct activation of stem axons in the corticospinal tracts: these were estimation of current spread, measurement of the lowest threshold point along the tract, and calculation of the conduction time along axon collaterals (for details, see refs. 68, 69). The last method is very useful for distinguishing between a collateral projection and a passing fiber in a given structure. When a neuron was antidromically activated from the cervical gray matter, it was possible to study the collision of impulses initiated from the cervical gray matter and the thoracic cord by delivering a pair of stimuli in a conditioning-test fashion (Fig. 1)[68]. This procedure allowed us (1) to ascertain that both stimuli activate the same neuron, (2) to provide additional support that both responses were antidromic[22], and (3) to estimate the conduction time between the branching point of an axon collateral from a stem axon and the stimulated point.

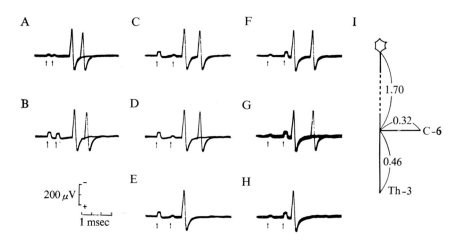

Fig. 1. A–I. Measurement of the conduction time along the branches of a corticospinal fiber. A–B: Measurement of refractory periods by double shock stimuli at cervical gray matter and thoracic cord. C–E: Measurement of collision time between thoracic and cervical branches. With the interval shown in D, the second spike appeared in 50% of the trials. F–H: As C–E, but with the sequence reversed. Six sweeps are superimposed in each case. I: Schematic drawing of branches and the conduction times along the branches obtained from the measurements shown in A–H. The latent periods for spike generation (about 0.2 msec) were subtracted from the measured conduction times. The same procedure was applied in Figs. 2 and 4. Further details are given in the text (Shinoda *et al.*, 1976)[68].

Among the CS neurons studied in the pericruciate cortex corresponding to area 4γ of Hassler and Muhs-Clement[31], about 30% sent axons not only to the cervical gray matter but also down to the thoracic spinal cord. The remaining neurons could be activated only from the cervical cord. The neurons activated only from the cervical cord were located in the "forelimb area" and the lateral border of the "trunk area"[6,10,78]. Most of the neurons projecting to both the cervical gray matter and the lower level of the spinal cord were located within the same area.

The existence of neurons projecting from the "forelimb area" of the motor cortex to the thoracic and lumbar cord was first described in the monkey by Sherrington[66] based on the Marchi method. This problem was reinvestigated in cats[20,52], and monkeys[42,46] using the Nauta method. More recently, Armand et al.[7] employing the HRP staining method, demonstrated an area in 4γ where there are neurons projecting to the cervical cord and to the lumbar cord. These anatomical studies, however, were unable to distinguish neurons projecting only to the thoracic or lumbar cord from neurons projecting to both the cervical gray matter and the lower level. The present study revealed the existence of CS neurons sending axon branches to both the cervical cord and the lower levels. The present methods, however, did not permit us to determine whether or not there exist neurons in the "forelimb area" of the cortex which terminate only at the thoracic or lumbar cord. This problem requires further experiments.

Branching pattern in the cervical cord

For detailed analysis of the branching pattern of individual CS neurons in the cervical cord, 8–12 microelectrodes implanted in the cervical gray matter were moved vertically over a distance of 1.5–2.5 mm and the effects of microstimulation from each electrode were examined at various depths. When several electrodes activated the same neuron antidromically, a collision test was performed between each possible pair. The conduction time along each axon branch was estimated using the values obtained from the collision experiments[68]. Fig. 2 shows an example of the longitudinal distribution of axon collaterals of a CS neuron in such an experiment. This neuron was activated antidromically from 4 electrodes arranged as shown in A. The dimensions of the axonal arborization of the neuron were determined as shown in C. This CS neuron sent at least four independent axon branches into the cervical gray matter over a distance of four segments (Fig. 2C). In this series of experiments, only 8–12 electrodes were implanted and the shortest distance between stimulating electrodes was 2 mm. The maximum current used (50 μA) is likely to have activated only those axon collaterals located within a radius of about 500 μm of the electrode tip. Hence, it is expected that the number of axon collaterals to the cervical cord in each CS neuron was underestimated. In spite of the wide interelectrode distance relative to the effective extent of the stimuli and the limited number of electrodes, a large number of CS neurons gave off multiple branches in the cervical cord[68]. The above experiment demonstrated the existence of CS neurons with multiple branches, but there were many CS neurons that could be activated only from one spinal segment. From a functional viewpoint, it is interesting to know whether neurons projecting to only a restricted area of the spinal cord exist or not.

Are there CS neurons projecting to restricted areas of the spinal cord?

The next series of experiments was undertaken to examine whether multiple branching of CS neurons in the cord is a common feature of all CS neurons or limited to only a small percentage of CS neurons[70]. For this purpose, antidromic spikes were extracellularly recorded from single CS neurons in the pericruciate cortex while stimulating the contralateral lateral corticospinal tract (LCST) at C2 with a pair of ball electrodes. Another pair of ball electrodes was moved on the surface of the contralateral dorso-lateral funiculus and the latencies of antidromically evoked spikes at each segment were measured. This pair of electrodes was fixed at the most caudal spinal level from which antidromic spikes for each neuron could be elicited. To detect axon collaterals for each neuron, a single movable microelectrode was inserted and moved vertically over 3 mm

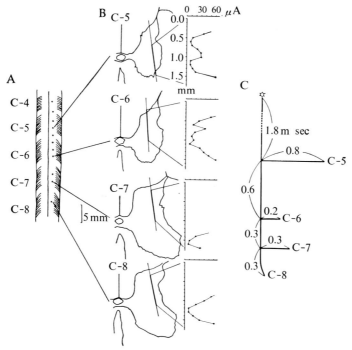

Fig. 2. Multiple branching of a corticospinal fiber in the cervical gray matter. The neuron was activated antidromically from C_5, C_6, C_7 and C_8. Stimulating electrodes were placed as shown in A. While recording from the same neuron, stimulating electrodes were moved vertically and the threshold currents at each position were determined. In B, threshold current (abscissa) is plotted against depth (ordinate). Electrode tracks were reconstructed from histological sections. Thin and thick lines represent an electrode track and the surveyed area in the track, respectively. The branching pattern of this neuron is shown in C. Numbers in the diagram indicate conduction times (msec) calculated from collision tests (Shinoda *et al.*, 1976)[68].

in the cervical gray matter. Stimuli with a pulse duration of 0.2 msec (maximum current, 150–200 μA) were delivered through the electrode. Similar tracks were made at 1 mm intervals along the longitudinal axis of the cord. All axon branches of single CS neurons could be detected in this way, because the minimum effective current spread of 150–200 μA well exceeds the 500 μm half interval distance. An example of such an experiment is given in Fig. 3. The neuron shown was located in the lateral gyrus of the pericruciate cortex and sent axons down to the first thoracic segment. The latencies of antidromic spikes from different levels of the LCST are plotted in B (open circles). The conduction velocity of this stem axon differed at different spinal levels, being 17.7 m/sec at the higher cervical level and becoming lower near the caudal end of the axon. In the same graph, the latencies of the antidromic spikes evoked from different sites in the gray matter (filled circles) are plotted relative to the distance along the cord. Comparing the latencies of the spikes evoked from the gray matter and from the LCST at the same spinal levels, it is evident that the axon collaterals were stimulated in the gray matter rather than the stem axon in the LCST due to current spread. Every occasion where effective stimulus points were found in the gray matter, collision of the impulses initiated from an axon collateral and the most caudal axon branch was studied by delivering a pair of stimuli in a conditioning-test fashion. Using this procedure, the conduction

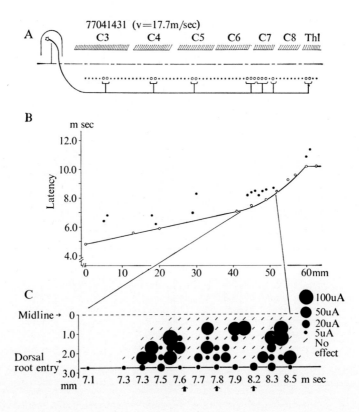

Fig. 3.   An example of the intraspinal branching pattern of a slow pyramidal tract neuron. The conduction velocity of the axon was 17.7 m/sec. A: Schematic diagram of the branching pattern. Dots and open circles indicate the non-effective and effective stimulating penetrations, respectively. B: The latencies of evoked spikes relative to the distance along the spinal cord. Dots and open circles represent the latencies of spikes evoked from the gray matter and LCST, respectively. C: Map of the current required for antidromic activation of the PT neuron around C_7 segment. The stimulus currents at threshold were measured at matrix points spaced at 500 μm and 100 μm intervals. The lowest threshold values at each penetration are indicated (dorsal view of the left cervical cord) (Shinoda *et al.*,1978)[70].

time from the branching point of an axon collateral to its stimulation site and the conduction time between that branching point and the most caudal branch of the stem axon could be calculated. The former value allowed it to be shown that the axon collaterals, not the stem axons, were stimulated in the gray matter. The latter value indicated whether the stimulated axon branches at different tracks belonged to the same terminal bush or to different bushes. The neuron in Fig. 3 gave off six different axon collaterals to C_3, C_4, C_5, C_6 and C_7 before terminating at Thl. As is evident from Fig. 3B, the conduction velocities on the axon collaterals are much lower than that on the stem axon. The validity of our calculation method was further confirmed in Fig. 3C. Our calculations revealed three independent axon branches at C_7 (Fig. 3A) but they were situated very close together. The axonal branches around C_7 were surveyed by mapping the effective stimulating sites systematically at matrix points spaced at 500 μm longitudinally and transversely and 100 μm in depth. The lowest threshold values at each stimulating track are indicated on the schematic map of the cord (dorsal view of the left cervical cord). Three groups of effective stimulating sites at adequate stimulus intensities of less than 100 μA were observed; there were ineffective zones between each of the effective zones. Taking the latencies of evoked spikes at each point into consideration, three independent axon collaterals were found to originate from the stem axon around C_7.

A total of 30 CS neurons were examined in the manner described above[70]. They were sampled in the "forelimb area" of the pericruciate cortex. All these CS neurons had 3 to 7 axonal branches and projected to widely separate levels of the cord. They included both slow and fast CS neurons projecting to the thoracic cord and those to the cervical cord. The maximum extent of distribution of all the axon branches in individual CS neurons observed was 8 segments.

Based on this study, it was concluded that intraspinal multiple branching of CS neurons is a common feature of all CS neurons. We were unable to find any CS neurons projecting to a restricted area of the spinal cord in the cat.

Do single CS neurons project to more than one motoneuron pool?

The results described so far were obtained from experiments using cats. Since it is generally accepted that pyramidal tract fibers do not terminate upon motoneurons, but upon interneurons in cats[17,47], it is difficult to correlate multiple axon terminals of single CS neurons with different motoneuron pools in cats. Anatomical studies indicate that axons from pyramidal tract neurons of cortical area 4 in the monkey terminate in both the ventral horn and intermediate zone of the spinal cord[40,46]. Physiological studies have confirmed a direct corticomotoneuronal connection in primates[15,38,43,58]. Taking advantage of this monosynaptic corticomotoneuronal connection in the monkey, we investigated the problem of whether individual CS neurons terminate in one and only one spinal motoneuron pool or in several motoneuron pools.

In this series of experiments, 6–10 microelectrodes were implanted in the forelimb motoneuron pools of adult capuchin monkeys (*Cebus* sp.)[12], (Shinoda, Y., Zarzecki, P. and Asanuma, H., in preparation). The stimulated sites were determined by observing the maximal antidromic field potentials on stimulation of the median, ulnar and deep radial nerve. About 200 CS neurons were recorded within the motor cortex, mainly in the "hand area[9]".

The same procedure as described above was used to determine the existence of spinal axon collaterals. A considerable fraction of CS neurons was found to have multisegmental branches in the monkey as in the cat. Since the purpose of this series of experiments was to examine the branching pattern of CS neurons to spinal motor nuclei, it was essential to differentiate fibers within motor nuclei from those in the neighboring gray matter. The extent of stimulus action was estimated from depth-threshold curves for many CS axons and the location of each stimulus site in a motor nucleus was determined histologically. Determination of whether an axon was activated from within a motor nucleus was made by comparing a motor nucleus demarcated histologically with the estimate of the spread of the threshold current for that axon. Of 210 CS neurons activated from electrodes in the cervical motor nuclei or in the white matter just ventral to the motor nuclei, 54 were classified as being activated from within the motor nuclei. The remaining 156 CS neurons could not be classified as being activated from motor nuclei since their activation required higher stimulus intensities and there was a possibility of current spread outside of the ventral horn. About 30% of the CS neurons projecting to the brachial motoneuron pools sent another axon branch to the thoracic cord. Unfortunately, we were unable to examine where in the thoracic cord these axons terminated. Six neurons were activated from motor nuclei of different segments; nine neurons terminated both in motor nuclei and unspecified regions of the cervical gray matter. The remaining neurons were activated from the motor nucleus in one segment. Although the sample size was small due to technical difficulties, the results showed that there were single CS neurons projecting to different motoneuron pools in the monkey. A larger proportion of these CS neurons than observed here must certainly exist since only a small portion of the brachial motor nuclei was examined. The present results also suggest that some single CS neurons send axon branches to both a motor nucleus and intermediate regions of the gray matter.

More recently, the branching pattern of CS neurons in the "hindlimb area" of the monkey motor cortex has been tested for projections to the lumbar and sacral cord (Asanuma, H., Zarzecki, P., Jankowska, E., Hongo, T. and Marcus, S., in preparation). Projections of single CS neurons to several motor nuclei in these levels were also confirmed. In this series of experiments, several motor nuclei were electrophysiologically identified and axon branches of single CS neurons were more extensively mapped using a single movable microelectrode.

Intraspinal branching of other long descending tract neurons

Since the corticospinal and rubrospinal systems have many features in common[28,41,65], we attempted to determine whether rubrospinal (RS) neurons had multiple axon collaterals in the spinal cord as do CS neurons in the cat[68]. An example of such an experiment is given in Fig. 4[69]. Electrodes were positioned as shown in Fig. 4A. The neuron was driven antidromically from 5 electrodes in the cervical gray matter. The branching pattern of the neuron was assessed using the spike-collision method described above (Fig. 4C). This particular neuron sent different axon branches to C_4, C_6 and C_8. Among 32 RS neurons projecting only to the cervical cord, five sent separate axon branches to two different cervical segments and five sent axon branches to three or more segments. Of 58 RS neurons projecting to the cervical cord, 26 sent axon branches to the thoracic cord, and five of these gave off two or more axon branches into the cervical gray matter.

It now appears that axons of all major long descending systems send axon collaterals to multiple levels of the spinal cord. This situation was first described by Abzug et al[1]. who found that 50% of vestibulospinal neurons which sent axon branches in C_6-Th_1 segments were also antidromically driven by stimulation of the lumbar vestibulosopinal tract. A similar percentage of reticulospinal neurons sent branches to the cervical gray matter as well as to the first lumbar segment[54]. In contrast, our data[68] indicated that 12 out of 193 (6%) corticospinal neurons activated from the cervical gray matter (C_4–C_8) also projected to the first lumbar segment. Similarly, only 2 out of 40 RS neurons (5%) projecting to the cervical gray matter (C_4–C_8) sent axon branches to the first lumbar level[69]. Although the branching patterns appear to be different in each descending system, it can be concluded that multisegmental branching of single axons is a common feature of long descending systems.

Discussion

In the present series of experiments, the problem of whether single CS neurons are able to control the activity of more than one motoneuron pool was investigated. Evarts[24] first proposed this possibility, but very few experimental studies had dealt with it previously. In discussing the "functional unit" of Jackson[35], Evarts schematized two extreme formulations, either of which could possess the necessary functional properties of Jackson's "unit". In one of the formulations,

Spinal Branches of Rubrospinal Neurons

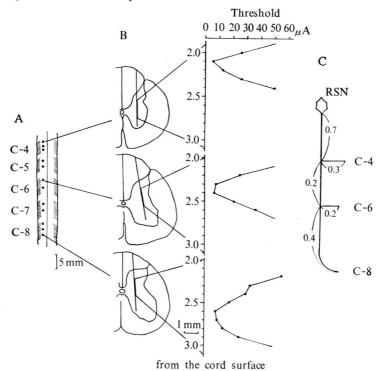

Fig. 4.   Multiple axon branching of a rubrospinal neuron in the cervical gray matter. Stimulating electrodes were implanted as shown in A. While recording from the same neuron, an array of the electrodes was moved vertically and the effects of stimulation were examined at each depth. In B, threshold current (abscissa) is plotted against depth (ordinate). Thin and thick lines represent electrode tracks reconstructed from the histological sections and the surveyed areas in each track, respectively. C: Branching pattern of this neuron. Numbers in the diagram indicate conduction times (msec) calculated from the values obtained from collision tests. The neuron was activated antidromically from Electrodes Nos. 1, 3, 6, 8 and 12 from top to bottom, but collision of evoked spikes from Electrodes 3 and 8 with those from the other electrodes could not be completed before the neuron died (Shinoda *et al.*, 1977)[69].

a single CS neuron was related to one and only one muscle. In the other, a single CS neuron had a divergent projection through its axon collaterals onto motoneurons innvervating a number of different muscles. Assuming that a single CS fiber directly influences spinal motoneurons of more than one muscle, it should have multiple axon branches and terminate at different sites in the spinal cord. This simple assumption formed our starting point. Axon collaterals of pyramidal tract neurons in the cortex[55,59,73], to the subcortical nuclei[2,23,76,79] have been well documented. The only available data on spinal branches were from the work of Scheibel and Scheibel[63] who reported that "most lateral corticospinal elements in the cat terminate over an area of 1 to 2 segments, via a series of collaterals and terminals turning sharply into the spinal gray." In the first series of experiments in the cat[13,68], the presence of CS neurons projecting to widely separate levels of the spinal cord was demonstrated. In the second series[70], it was confirmed that virtually all slow and fast CS neurons have multisegmental branches in the cord. Both anatomical and physiological evidence show that motoneurons innervating one muscle are aligned longitudinally in the spinal cord[18,60,62,71,74]. The distribution of one motor nucleus spreads over one to three segments[18,62,74]. The present data indicate that the projection area of a majority of CS neurons well exceeds the distribution area of any single motor nucleus. This finding suggests that single CS neurons may influence the activity of more than one motor nucleus.

This interpretation, however, requires further consideration since CS fibers terminate, not on spinal motoneurons, but rather on interneurons in the cat[17,77]. The terminal distribution of CS axons was found in laminae IV-VII of Rexed[20,52,61], and these axons exert their actions on primary afferents[4,19] and second-order neurons to the cerebellum along the dorsal spinocerebellar, rostral spinocerebellar and cuneocerebellar tracts[53]. They can thus moduluate sensory inputs to motoneurons, the cerebellum and the cerebral cortex. Besides this action on afferent inputs, CS neurons cause excitatory postsynaptic potentials in spinal motoneurons through interneurons[47]. The shortest connection between fast CS fibers and motoneurons is di-synaptic[33,34]. It must be considered therefore that there are at least three possible types of CS neurons with multiple axon branches which make some connection with motoneurons in the cat. In the first type, a single CS fiber has connections with more than one motor nucleus through different interneurons. In the second type, a single CS fiber may synapse on more than one interneuron terminating in one motor nucleus. In the third type, a single CS fiber has an indirect connection with one motor nucleus and is also related by other branches to a sensory system to modulate afferent and ascending signals. In the first case, individual corticospinal neurons are related to two or more different motoneuron pools and in the latter two, they are related to single motoneuron pools. Interneurons interposed between CS axons and the different motoneuron groups have been extensively investigated by Lundberg and his colleagues. Lundberg et al.[49]. found convergence of cutaneous and CS inputs on interneurons which intervene between these inputs and the motoneurons. In addition to interneurons involved in reflex arcs, there are also some interneurons which may not be activated by peripheral nerve stimulation[14,39]. These interneurons have been postulated to constitute a private pathway mediating cortical effects on motoneurons. More recently, Illert et al.[33,34]. reported propriospinal neurons at C_3 which are monosynaptically excited from the pyramidal tract and may have monosynaptic connections with motoneurons innervating the forelimb muscles in the cat. These propriospinal neurons are activated via collaterals from CS fibers which descend at least to C_6 segment. This finding agrees well with our observation that a majority of CS neurons in the "forelimb area" send at least one axon collateral to C_3 segment. Knowledge of the spatial arrangement of segmental interneurons related to a particular motor nucleus will help to interpret our result of multiple branching of single CS neurons in the cat.

Various other descending motor pathways in addition to CS fibers converge onto propriospinal neurons[34], and CS outputs modulate segmental reflex arcs[48]. These findings, together with the present finding of multiple projection of a given CS axon, suggest that CS descending signals are integrated at multisegmental levels through propriospinal and segmental interneurons. This would also hold true for other long descending motor pathways such as the vestibulo-, reticulo-, rubro- and tectospinal systems. These systems can no longer be viewed as simple "upper motor neuron" systems.

In experiments using monkeys[12] (Shinoda, Y., Zarzecki, P. and Asanuma, H, in preparation), we found that a small number of CS neurons existed whose axons projected to motor nuclei at different brachial segments. The proportion of these neurons must have been underestimated, judging from the wide interelectrode distances relative to the effective extent of the stimuli and the limited number of electrodes. A recent experiment by Asanuma et al. (Asanuma, H., Zarzecki,

P., Jankowska, E., Hongo, T. and Marcus, S., in preparation) has demonstrated more clearly that single CS neurons in the "hindlimb area" of the monkey motor cortex send branches to different motoneuron pools in the lumbar cord.

The motor nuclei contain a large number of small cells which do not send axons to the ventral roots[16]; there is a possibility that fibers of CS neurons activated from the ventral horn terminate on these interneurons. However, recent experiments employing horseradish peroxidase indicate that the majority of neurons in the lateral ventral horn are motoneurons[18]. It is highly possible therefore that individual CS neurons terminate on motoneurons of more than one pool.

Jankowska et al.[38]. mapped the projection area of the "hindlimb motor cortex" by surface-anodal pulses of 0.4 mA, monitoring monosynaptic EPSPs from hindlimb motoneurons. They found overlapping between the most effective spots (from which the largest EPSPs were evoked) for motoneurons of different muscle groups. In their paper, several possible neuronal structures were proposed to account for these findings. A CS axon projecting to different motor nuclei was carefully considered as one of the possible candidates. In this respect, some of the figures (Figs. 6, 7 and 9 in the paper of Andersen et al.[5].) are interesting. They mapped projection areas by intracortical microstimulation. In their depth-threshold curves for activating single units of different muscles, threshold minima for different muscles were often located very close together in the motor cortex. They suggested overlapping of different colonies of CS neurons projecting to respective, single motoneuron pools. However, it is also possible that the observed overlapping is attributable to an arrangement in which single CS neurons in a particular area send axon branches to different motoneuron pools.

Another line of experiments has provided evidence to suggest the existence of multiple projections of a single CS fiber to different motor nuclei. Fetz et al.[26]. recorded precentral unit activities and EMG from forelimb muscles in behaving monkeys. They examined corticomotoneuronal connections by using spike-triggered averages of EMG. Of 41 precentral units firing in synchrony with at least one of the recorded 5 wrist muscles, 10 units were found to be followed by facilitation in more than half of the recorded muscles. It was concluded that there were divergent terminal connections of single CS neurons to motoneurons of different muscles, based on the assumption that there is no cross-correlation between the spike activities of different CS neurons innervating different muscles (e.g. due to a common input from the thalamus or other cerebral structures to these neurons). If this assumption is confirmed experimentally, this experimental technique should be useful for the analysis of corticomotoneuronal relationships.

In primates, CS neurons may exist which exclusively target particular motoneurons without any collaterals. In fact, we observed CS neurons which were activated only from a single stimulating electrode in the cord. Since the whole area in the cervical gray matter was not surveyed by stimulation, it is at present difficult to draw any firm conclusions. Besides CS neurons sending divergent collaterals to a number of motor nuclei, there were several CS neurons activated from both a motor nucleus and the intermediate zone in the monkey. This finding suggests that single CS neurons may project to both a motoneuron and an interneuron. Jankowska et al.[36]. showed that CS neurons made synaptic contacts with Ia inhibitory interneurons in the monkey. Sherrington[67] found reciprocal relationships between muscles working antagonistically at hinge joints in response to stimulation of the monkey's motor cortex. Taken together, these observations suggest that single CS neurons send axons to both motoneurons and Ia inhibitory interneurons to antagonistic motoneurons.

The functional aspect of intraspinal multiple projections of single CS neurons has been viewed in various ways. Multiple branching to the cervical and lumbar cord has been observed in vestibulospinal[1] and reticulospinal axons[54]. These multisegmental "hard-wired" connections seem consistent with the role of these systems in postural control in which neural arrangements for the coordination of muscle contraction in a relatively stereotyped pattern of movement are required. In volitional or "less automatic" movement, selection of appropriate combinations of muscles occurs. In this process, suppression of the built-in reflex system at a spinal level must be important for the execution of complex or inexperienced movements. This "breaking-up of compounds already constructed by lower centers" may be attributed to one of the functions of the motor cortex[45]. Hammond[30] and Marsden et al.[50,51]. reported that stretch reflexes are modifiable by prior instructions in man. Evarts and Tanji[25] recently found that the stretch reflex response differed markedly depending upon prior instruction to the monkey; this instruction elicited marked alterations in discharge patterns of both PTNs and non-PTNs in the motor cortex. This finding suggests that PTNs preset spinal mechanisms by changing the excitability of α- and γ-motoneurons or of spinal interneurons, although a transcortical loop may also be involved[29]. This "presetting" as well as "setting" during movement of spinal mechanisms must occur at multisegmental levels in the performance of skilled movement. Multiple branching of CS axons may be a neural correlate for such multisegmental control.

To understand the relationship between single CS neurons and different muscles, it is necessary to have direct evidence that single CS neurons make direct synapses on motoneurons innervating different muscles. The question raised here is simply a question about structure, but its solution will provide an important clue for understanding the functional role of CS neurons in the control of movement.

References

1. Abzug, C., Maeda, M., Peterson, B.W. and Wilson, V.J., Cervical branching of lumbar vestibulospinal axons, J. Physiol. (Lond.), 243 (1974) 499–522.
2. Allen, G.I., Korn, H., Oshima, T. and Toyama, K., The mode of synaptic linkage in the cerebro-ponto-cerebellar pathway of the cat. II. Responses of single cells in the pontine nuclei, Exp. Brain Res., 24 (1975) 15–36.
3. Allen, G.I. and Tsukahara, N., Cerebrocerebellar communication system, Physiol. Rev., 54 (1974) 957–1006.
4. Andersen, P., Eccles, J.C. and Sears, T.A., Cortically evoked depolarization of primary afferent fibers in the spinal cord, J. Neurophysiol., 27 (1964) 63–77.
5. Andersen, P., Hangan, P.J., Phillips, C.G., Powell, F.R.S. and Powell, T.P.S.,Mapping by microstimulation of overlapping projections from area 4 to motor units of the baboon's hand, Proc. roy. Soc. Lond. B., 188 (1975) 31–60.
6. Armand, J., Padel, Y. and Smith, A.M., Somatotopic organization of the corticospinal tract in cat motor cortex, Brain Research, 74 (1974) 209–227.
7. Armand, J. and Aurenty, R., Dual organization of motor corticospinal tract in the cat, Neurosci. Lett., 6 (1977) 1–7.
8. Asanuma, H., Recent developments in the study of the columnar arrangement of neurons within the motor cortex, Physiol. Rev., 55 (1975) 143–156.
9. Asanuma, H. and Rosen, I., Topographical organization of cortical efferent zones projecting to distal forelimb muscles in the monkey, Exp. Brain Res., 14 (1972) 243–256.
10. Asanuma, H. and Sakata, H., Functional organization of a cortical efferent system examined with focal depth stimulation in cat, J., Neurophysiol., 30 (1967) 35–54.
11. Asanuma, H., Arnold, A. and Zarzecki, P., Further study on the excitation of pyramidal tract cells by intracortical microstimulation, Exp. Brain Res., 26 (1976) 443–461.
12. Asanuma, H., Shinoda, Y. and Zarzecki, P., Branching of cortico-spinal fibers in the monkey, Neurosci. Abstr., 2 (1976) 537.
13. Asanuma, H., Shinoda, Y., Arnold, A. and Zarzecki, P., Reexamination of functional arrangements of pyramidal tract neurons in the motor cortex of the cat, Exp. Brain Res., Suppl. I (1976) 440–444.

14. Bayev, K.V. and Kostyuk, P.G., Convergence of cortico- and rubrospinal influences on interneurons of cat cervical spinal cord, *Brain Research*, 52 (1973) 159–171.
15. Bernhard, C.G. and Bohm, E., Monosynaptic corticospinal activation of forelimb motoneurones in monkeys (*Macaca mulatta*), *Acta physiol. scand.*, 31 (1954) 104–112.
16. Brodal, A., *Neurological Anatomy in Relation to Clinical Medicine*, 2nd ed., Oxford University Press, London, New York, Toronto, 1969, 118 pp.
17. Brooks, V.B. and Stoney, S.D.K., Motor mechanisms: the role of the pyramidal system in motor control, *Ann. Rev. Physiol.*, 33 (1971) 337–392.
18. Burke, R.E., Strick, P.L., Kanda, K., Kimm, C.C. and Walmsley, B., Anatomy of medial gastrocnemius and soleus motor nuclei in cat spinal cord, *J. Neurophysiol.*, 40 (1977) 667–680.
19. Carpenter, D., Lundberg, A. and Norrsell, U., Primary afferent depolarization evoked from the sensorimotor cortex, *Acta physiol. scand.*, 59 (1963) 126–142.
20. Chambers, W.W. and Liu, C.N., Cortico-spinal tract of the cat, *J. comp. Neurol.*, 108 (1957) 23–55.
21. Chang, H.T., Ruch, T.C. and Ward, A.A. Jr., Topographical representation of muscles in motor cortex in monkey, *J. Neurophysiol.*, 10 (1947) 39–56.
22. Darian-Smith, I., Phillips, G. and Ryan, R.D., Functional organization in the terminal main sensory and rostral spinal nuclei in the cat, *J. Physiol. (Lond.)*, 168 (1963) 129–146.
23. Endo, K., Araki, T. and Yagi, N., The distribution and pattern of axon branching of pyramidal tract cells, *Brain Research*, 57 (1973) 484–491.
24. Evarts, E.V., Representation of movements and muscles by pyramidal tract neurons of the precentral motor cortex. In M.D. Yarr and D.P. Purpura (Eds.) *Neurophysiological Basis of Normal and Abnormal Motor Activities*, Raven Press, New York, 1967, pp. 215–251.
25. Evarts, E.V. and Tanji, J., Gating of motor cortex reflexes by prior instruction, *Brain Research*, 71 (1974) 479–494.
26. Fetz, E.E., Cheney, P.D. and German, D.C., Corticomotoneuronal connections of precentral cells detected by post-spike averages of EMG activity in behaving monkeys, *Brain Research*, 114 (1976) 505–510.
27. Fritsch, G. and Hitzig, E., Über die elektrische Erregbarkeit des Grosshirns, *Arch. Anat. Physiol. Wiss. Med.*, 37 (1870) 300–332.
28. Ghez, C., Input-output relationships of the red nucleus in the cat, *Brain Research*, 98 (1975) 93–108.
29. Ghez, C. and Shinoda, Y., Spinal mechanisms of the functional stretch reflex, *Exp. Brain Res.* (1978) in press.
30. Hammond, P.H., The influence of prior instruction to the subject on an apparently involuntary neuromuscular response, *J. Physiol. (Lond.)*, 132 (1956) 17.
31. Hassler, R. and Muhs-Clement, K., Architektonischer Aufbau des sensorimotorischen und parietalen Cortex der Katze, *J. Hirnforsch.*, 6 (1964) 377–420.
32. Hern, J.E.C., Landgren, S., Phillips, C.G. and Porter, R., Selective excitation of corticofugal neurones by surface-anodal stimulation of the baboon's motor cortex, *J. Physiol. (Lond.)*, 161 (1962) 73–90.
33. Illert, M., Lundberg, A. and Tanaka, R., Disynaptic corticospinal effects in forelimb motoneurones in the cat *Brain Research*, 75 (1974) 312–315.
34. Illert, M., Lundberg, A. and Tanaka, R., Integration in a disynaptic cortico-motoneuronal pathway to the forelimb in the cat, *Brain Research*, 93 (1975) 525–529.
35. Jackson, J.H., Observations on the localization of movements in the cerebral hemispheres, as revealed by cases of convulsion chorea, and "aphasia". In J. Taylor, G. Holmes and F.M.R. Walshe (Eds.) *Selected Writings of John Hughlings Jackson, Vol. I*, Basic Books, New York, 1958 ,pp. 77–89.
36. Jankowska, E. and Tanaka, R., Neuronal mechanism of the disynaptic inhibition evoked in primate spinal motoneurones from the corticospinal tract, *Brain Research*, 75 (1974) 163–166.
37. Jankowska, E., Padel, Y. and Tanaka, R., The mode of activation of pyramidal tract cells by intracortical stimuli, *J. Physiol. (Lond.)*, 249 (1975a) 617–636.
38. Jankowska, E., Padel, Y. and Tanaka, R., Projections of pyramidal tract cells to α-motoneurones innervating hindlimb muscles in the monkey, *J. Physiol. (Lond.)*, 249 (1975b) 637–667.
39. Kostyuk, P.G. and Vasilenko, D.A., Transformation of cortex motor signals in spinal cord, *Proc. Inst. elect. Engrs.*, 56 (1968) 1049–1058.
40. Kuypers, H.G.J.M., Central cortical projections to motor and somatosensory cell groups, *Brain*, 83 (1960) 161–184.
41. Kuypers, H.G.J.M., The descending pathways to the spinal cord, their anatomy and function. In J.C. Eccles and J.P. Schadé (Eds.), *Organization of the Spinal Cord, Progr. Brain Res., Vol. 11*, Elsevier, Amsterdam, 1964, pp. 178–202.
42. Kuypers, H.G.J.M. and Brinkman, J., Precentral projections to different parts of the spinal intermediate zone in the rhesus monkey, *Brain Research*, 24 (1970) 29–48.

43. Landgren, S., Phillips, C. and Porter, R., Minimal synaptic actions of pyramidal impulses on some alpha moto-neurones of baboon's hand and forearm, *J. Physiol. (Lond.)*, 161 (1962a) 91–111.

44. Landgren, S., Phillips, C. and Porter, R., Cortical fields of origin of the monosynaptic pyramidal pathways to some alpha-motoneurones of the baboon's hand and forearm, *J. Physiol. (Lond.)*, 161 (1962b) 112–125.

45. Leyton, A.S.F. and Sherrington, C.S., Observations on the excitable cortex of the chimpanzee, orang-tun and gorilla, *Q. J. exp. Physiol.*, 11 (1917) 135–222.

46. Liu, C.N. and Chambers, W.W., An experimental study of the corticospinal system in the monkey (*Macaca mulata*): The spinal pathways and preterminal distribution of degenerating fibers following discrete lesions of the pre- and postcentral gyri and bulbar pyramid, *J. comp. Neurol.*, 123 (1964) 257–284.

47. Lloyd, D.P.C., The spinal mechanisms of the pyramidal system in cats, *J. Neurophysiol.*, 4 (1941) 525–546.

48. Lundberg, A. and Voorhoeve, P., Effects from the pyramidal tract on spinal refelx arcs, *Acta physiol. scand.*, 56 (1962) 201–219.

49. Lundberg, A., Norrsell, U. and Voorhoeve, P., Pyramidal effects on lumbosacral interneurones activated by somatic afferents, *Acta physiol. scand.*, 56 (1962) 220–229.

50. Marsden, C.D., Merton, P.A. and Morton, H.B., Servo action in human voluntary movement, *Nature*, 238 (1972) 140–143.

51. Marsden, C.D., Merton, P.A. and Morton, H.B., Latency measurements comparable with a cortical pathway for the stretch reflex in man, *J. Physiol. (Lond.)*, 230 (1973) 58–59.

52. Nyberg-Hansen, R. and Brodal, A., Sites of termination of corticospinal fibers in the cat. An experimental study with silver impregnation methods, *J. comp. Neurol.*, 120 (1963) 369–391.

53. Oscarsson, O., Functional organization of the spino- and cuneo-cerebellar tracts, *Physiol. Rev.*, 45 (1965) 495–522.

54. Peterson, B.W., Maunz, R.A., Pitts, N.G. and Mackel, R.G., Patterns of projection and branching of reticulo-spinal neurons, *Exp. Brain Res.*, 23 (1975) 333–351.

55. Phillips, C.G., Actions of antidromic pyramidal volleys on single Betz cells in the cat, *Q. J. exp. Physiol.*, 44 (1959) 1–25.

56. Phillips, C.G., Cortical localization and "sensorimotor processes" at the "middle level" in primates, *Proc. roy. Soc. Med.*, 66 (1973) 987–1002.

57. Porter, R., Functions of the mammalian cerebral cortex in movement. In G.A. Kerkut and J.W. Phillips (Eds.), *Progress in Neurobiology, Vol. 1*, Pergamon, New York, 1973, part 1, pp. 1–51.

58. Preston, J.B. and Whitlock, D.G., Intracellular potentials recorded from motoneurons following precentral gyrus stimulation in primate, *J. Neurophysiol.*, 24 (1961) 91–100.

59. Ramon y Cajal, S., *Histologie de Système Nerveux de l'Homme et des Vertebres, Vol. 2*, Maloine, Paris, 1911.

60. Reed, A.F., The nuclear masses in the cervical spinal cord of *Macaca mulatta, J. comp. Neurol.*, 72 (1940) 187–206.

61. Rexed, B., A cytoarchitectonic atlas of the spinal cord in the cat, *J. comp. Neurol.*, 100 (1954) 297–380.

62. Romanes, G.J., The motor cell columns of the lumbosacral spinal cord of the cat, *J. comp. Neurol.*, 94 (1951) 313–358.

63. Scheibel, M.E. and Scheibel, A.B., Terminal axonal patterns in cat spinal cord. I. The lateral corticospinal tract, *Brain Research*, 2 (1966) 333–350.

64. Scheibel, M.E. and Scheibel, A.B., Elementary processes in selected thalamic and cortical subsystems–the structual substrates. In F.O. Schmitt (Ed.-in-Chief), *The Neurosciences Second Study Program*, The Rockefeller University Press, New York, 1970, pp. 443–457.

65. Shapovalov, A.I., Excitation and inhibition of spinal neurones during supraspinal stimulation. In R. Granit (Ed.), *Muscular Afferents and Motor Control, Nobel Symposium 1*, Almqvist and Wiksell, Stockholm, 1966.

66. Sherrington, C.S., On nerve-tract degenerating secondarily to lesions of the cortex cerebri. *J. Physiol. (Lond.)*, 10 (1889) 429–432.

67. Sherrington, C.S., *The Integrative Action of the Nervous System*, Yale University, 1906.

68. Shinoda, Y., Arnold, A. and Asanuma, H., Spinal branching of corticospinal axons in the cat, *Exp. Brain Res.*, 26 (1976) 215–234.

69. Shinoda, Y., Ghez, C. and Arnold, A., Spinal branching of rubrospinal axons in the cat, *Exp. Brain Res.*, 30 (1977) 203–218.

70. Shinoda, Y. and Yamaguchi, T., Intraspinal branching patterns of slow and fast pyramidal tract cells in the cat's pericruciate cortex, *J. Physiol. (Paris)* (1978) in press.

71. Sterling, P. and Kuypers, H.G.J.M., Anatomical organization of the brachial spinal cord of the cat. II. The motoneuron plexus, *Brain Research*, 4 (1967) 16–32.

72. Stoney, S.D., Thompson, W.D. and Asanuma, H., Excitation of pyramidal tract cells by intracortical micro-stimulation: Effective extent of stimulating current, *J. Neurophysiol.*, 31 (1968) 659–669.

73. Takahashi, K., Kubota, K. and Uno, M., Recurrent facilitation in cat pyramidal tract cells, *J. Neurophysiol.*, 30 (1967) 22–34.
74. Thomas, R.C. and Wilson, V.J., Recurrent interactions between motoneurons of known location in the cervical cord of the cat, *J. Neurophysiol.*, 30 (1967) 661–674.
75. Towe, A.L., Motor cortex and the pyramidal system. In J.D. Maser (Ed.), *Efferent Organization and the Integration of Behavior*, Academic Press, 1972, pp. 67–97.
76. Tsukahara, N., Fuller, D.R.G. and Brooks, V.B., Collateral pyramidal influences on the corticorubrospinal system, *J. Neurophysiol.*, 31 (1968) 467–484.
77. Wiesendanger, M., The pyramidal tract: recent investigations on its morphology and function, *Ergebn. Physiol.*, 61 (1969) 73–136.
78. Woolsey, C.N., Organization of somatic sensory and motor areas of the cerebral cortex. In C.N. Woosley and H.F. Narlow (Eds.), *Biological and Biochemical Bases of Behavior*, Univ. Wisconsin Press, Madison, Wisc., 1958, pp. 63–82.
79. Zagger, p. and Wiesendanger, M., Excitation of lateral reticular nucleus neurones by collaterals of the pyramidal tract, *Exp. Brain Res.*, 17 (1973) 144–151.

Anatomy and physiology of the thalamic nuculeus ventralis intermedius

CHIHIRO OHYE

Department of Neurosurgery, School of Medicine, Gunma University,
Maebashi, Gunma 371, Japan.

Introduction

In stereotactic thalamotomy for various kinds of extrapyramidal motor disturbances, a part of the ventrolateral mass of the thalamus, the nucleus ventralis lateralis (VL) and the nucleus ventralis intermedius (Vim) have been the targets of choice. The physiological as well as radiological identification of these nuclei in each individual case are important to ensure good results with minimal therapeutic lesions. Using a microelectrode technique, French and Canadian groups carried out pioneer work in this field: they discovered that rhythmic burst discharges time-locked with peripheral tremor were found mainly in the n. Vim, and this nucleus preferentially received kinesthetic afferents. Later, many investigators confirmed these findings, although the results were not fully established, because histological evidence was lacking.

The n. Vim develops only in higher primates, including man, and reports of animal experiments are still rare in the literature, except for anatomical studies.

The aim of this paper is to summarize present knowledge about the n. Vim and its position within the thalamus. Only studies on primates and humans are considered here; those on cats are not included. Readers should also refer to a review article by Lanoir and Schlag[20].

Definition of the n. Vim

Vogt[46] and Friedemann[12] were probably the first to distinguish myelo- and cytoarchitecturally an intermediate zone between the ventrooral and ventrocaudal thalamic nucleus in cercopithèque. Crouch[6] observed it in the macaque. In humans, the Vogts[47] recognized the n. ventrointermedius and Hassler[15] followed their classification in a stereotactic atlas of the human thalamus, which is now widely used in stereotactic surgery. Histologically, this area is characterized by the finding that there are large and darkly stained angular cells. According to van Buren and Borke[44], the size of the cells in humans is about 30 to 40 μm and these cells occur sparsely with occasional intervening paler, medium-sized fusiform cells.

Based on these cytoarchitectural characteristics, one can distinguish the n. Vim from the neighboring nuclei more clearly in sagittal or horizontal section, as pointed out by Andrew and Watkins[3] and van Buren and Borke[44] (Fig. 1). Van Buren and Borke[44] noted: "the transition from n. ventrointermedius to the ventrocaudalis is sharp because of the denser cell pattern and the addition of many smaller angular cells in the latter. The largest cells in the n. ventrocaudalis are about the same size as those in the n. ventrointermedius. Anteriorly the junction with the n. ventrooralis externus is marked by the abrupt change to the uniform smaller, somewhat paler and rounder cells of this nucleus. The superior margin with the n. dorsooralis and/or n. dorsocaudalis

152

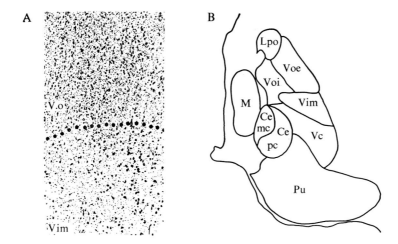

Fig. 1. A: Histological illustration of the n. Vo (VL) and Vim in sagittal section. Anterior above, posterior below. The line indicates the frontier between them (modified from Andrew and Watkins[3]). B: Horizontal plane of the human thalamus showing the anatomical location of the n. Vim. Lpo, n. lateropolaris; M, n. medialis; Voi, n. ventrooralis internus; Voe, n. ventrooralis externus; Vim, n. ventrointermedius; Cemc, n. centralis magnocellularis; Cepc, n. centralis parvocellularis; Vc, n. ventrocaudalis; Pu, n. pulvinaris (modified from van Buren and Borke[44]).

is again marked by the loss of the large dark cells of the n. ventrointermedius externus." They added that "the definition of the medial margin is difficult."

However, it is noteworthy, firstly, that the distinction of the n. Vim is marked only in higher primates, especially in the chimpanzee and man. Thus, the lower the animal on the phylogenetic scale, the more difficult is its separation from the surroundings. For example, Walker[48] stated that in the macaque "it (n. Vim) is a quite narrow, almost vertical, sheet of cells which are distinguished by their large size and deep staining." In a carnivore, it is even more difficult to distinguish the equivalent subdivision, although several anatomists have described it in the cat (see Angaut[4]). Secondly, although the definition (demarcation) of the n. Vim seems to be established, there are still many controversies in the nomenclature and classification of the thalamic nuclei in this particular area. In man, Hassler[15] adopted the most detailed scheme when he classified the ventro-lateral mass into dorsal, central, ventral dorsoventrally and oral, intermedius, caudal rostrocaudally in this order. His subdivision, however, has not been entirely accepted. Thus, typical variability was shown when Dewulf[10] attempted to standardize the normal human thalamic nomenclature. For instance, in Fig. 2, one can easily see how differently the same material is delineated and named by the different authorities. The n. Vim region in the standard atlas (Fig. 2E) is also named the n. lateralis thalami pars ventralis (Feremutsch and Simma, Fig. 2C), n. ventrointermedius pars externa (Hopf, Fig. 2B) or n. ventralis ventralis (Krieg, Fig. 2A). If we look for the equivalent or near equivalent of the human n. Vim in the current atlas of a laboratory animal (the monkey), the situation is further complicated. Van Buren and Borke[44] listed the following names:

N. ventrointermedius (their own)
N. ventralis intermedius (Walker[48])
N. ventralis posterior intermedius (Sheps[41])

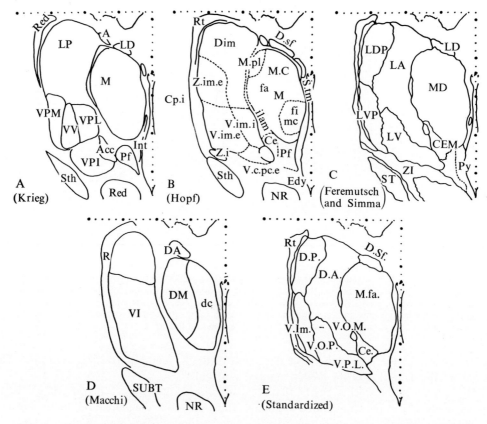

Fig. 2. Coronal sections of the human thalamus containing the n. Vim with standardized nomenclature (E), to illustrate how differently the same sections are delineated and named by different anatomists (A–D) (modified from Dewulf[10]).

N. ventralis posterior lateralis pars oralis (Olszewski[34])

Therefore, care is required with nomenclature and definitions in the literature.

Review of studies on afferent and efferent connections in the monkey

Vogt[46] also studied *the afferent input* to the n. Vim in the monkey. Following a small lesion of the dentate nucleus, degeneration was found by the Marchi method in the thalamus. According to Van Buren and Borke[43], this thalamic region designated as "n. ventral intermediaire" seems to be the n. Vim defined above. Crouch and Thompson[7] also used the Marchi method in the monkey and concluded that the n. Vim was the principal terminus of the brachium conjunctivum. Later, van Buren and his colleagues[43,45] reevaluated the earlier studies. Using chimpanzees as experimental material and using the silver technique, they found "degeneration crossing the brain stem through the red nucleus and its adjacent area of the brain stem following section of the superior cerebellar peduncle enters the n. ventrointermedius and adjacent regions of the n. ventrooralis externus most profusely. Scattered fibers run as far forward as the thalamic pole (n. lateropolaris) and posteriorly into the n. centralis-parafascicularis complex and the intralaminar nuclei. The

n. ventrocaudalis or posterior portion of n. ventralis posterior is avoided by these fibers." After reviewing the original histological preparations, they also confirmed[43] this finding in one of Walker's specimens "Babe" in which the superior cerebellar peduncle was sectioned. Kusama *et al.*[19], Mehler[23], and Mehler and Nauta[24] came to the same conclusion. The latter author also noted that some spinal and lemniscal fibers terminated in the Vim zone.

In this regard, Hassler's view was different[15]. On the basis of examinations of pathological changes in human material, he claimed that the cerebellar input to the thalamus terminated in his n. ventrooralis posterior, which was the caudal-most part of the ventrooral nucleus (n. VL) just anterior to the n. Vim. According to Hassler, the afferent connection to the n. Vim is via Forel's tegmental fascicles (fasciculus tegmenti dorsolateralis) which originates from the region of the vestibular nuclei, especially the lateral (Deiter's) nucleus. His view was based on the pathological finding that in four cases the degeneration in the lateral vestibular nucleus was associated with ipsilateral softening in the ventrolateral thalamic mass (n. ventrointermedius). To support the hypothesis of vestibular connection, he cited experiments in cats producing turning of the head or the whole animal to the side of stimulation on stimulation of this thalamic area.

This view was challenged later by many anatomists (see van Buren and Borke[44]). For example, Tarlov[42] examined by silver methods the thalamic degeneration following vestibular lesions in the monkey, baboon and chimpanzee, but he could not find degeneration above the posterior commissure. The vestibulothalamic connection, however, has been confirmed by electrophysiological studies, as will be described in the following section.

Concerning the *efferent connection* of the n. Vim, although it has not yet been confirmed anatomically, Hassler[15] stated that it projected to the central region of the cortex. More precisely, the cortical projection area would be area 3a of Brodmann and Vogt at the depth of the central sulcus, because in this region there is a vestibular projection to the cortex, according to him. He also cited the observations made by Penfield and Rasmussen in man, in which turning of the gaze to the same side was seen after stimulating the cortex in the central sulcus.

At present, no detailed experimental support for this is available. However, it might be relevant to recall an early study of Walker[48]. In an ablation study in the chimpanzee, he reported that "a small portion of the anterior layer of the n. ventralis posterior remains relatively normal and here scattered large cells characteristic of this nucleus are present." In this case, after complete ablation of the postcentral gyrus, the n. ventralis posterior was reported to be almost completely degenerated, with the exception of some retention of cells in a part of the n. ventralis posteromedialis and above mentioned rostral area of the n. ventralis posterolateralis. This result suggests that the cortical 3a area might have escaped ablation because it is located deeply in the bottom of the central sulcus and its medial portion was found even anterior to the latter (Powell and Mountcastle[37]).

Studying thalamic ascending and descending connections by means of the Nauta technique in the *Macaca* monkey, Jones and Powell[18] concluded that "the lateral and medial components of the ventroposterior nucleus had an organized projection to the SI and SII somatic sensory areas and to the transitional field 3a. The projection to area 3a is composed of thick fibers but terminal degeneration in it is sparse except when very large thalamic lesions are used." They thought that a specific part of the ventroposterior nucleus or some other nucleus also projected to area 3a.

In man, van Buren and Borke[44] observed degenerative changes of postmortem cases and concluded that the n. ventrointermedius externus was related to the most anterior parietal region.

Physiological studies in the monkey

In his extensive studies on the organization of the posterolateral part of the thalamus in the monkey, Mountcastle and his colleagues noted a tendency for modality-specific separation within the n. ventrolateral posterior (VB complex): neurons related to deep receptors were more common in the anterodorsal part and neurons activated by the skin were in the posteroventral part of the VB, but VI neurons showed a quite different pattern[36]. They also stated that this tendency for separation of submodalities occurred in blocks. Pubols[38] came to a similar conclusion in the spider monkey.

In chloralose-anesthetized monkey, Albe-Fessard and Lamarre[2] found an anteroposterior separation of naturally evoked responses in the thalamus. While pure tactile responses were obtained inferoposteriorly in the VPL_c (n. ventrocaudalis externus), the responses to deep sensation from joints and muscles were found anterosuperiorly, where pure tactile responses were lacking. This finding has been paralleled in the human thalamus, explored during the course of stereotactic surgery by several investigators. The details will be described in the next section.

Reexamining the body representation in the ventrobasal (VB) thalamus of the macaque in an awake state by single unit analysis, Loe *et al.*[22] showed that VB neurons are segregated according to submodality class along the anteroposterior dimension of the VB. They found that at levels near the anterior and posterior ends of the VB, mostly the VPL_o and VPI, and in the caudal end of the VPL_c of Olszewski, neurons with deep receptive fields predominate, whereas neurons with cutaneous receptive fields predominate at intermediate levels, mostly in the VPL_c.

Following the view of Hassler, who suggested a vestibular connection to the n. Vim as mentioned above, a German group investigated the vestibulothalamic relation by an electrophysiological method. In 1974, Deecke *et al.*[8] demonstrated in the rhesus monkey thalamic field potentials with maximal amplitude and minimal latency (2.5 msec) in the dorsal portion of the n. ventroposterior inferior (VPI) of Olszewski in reponse to vestibular nerve stimulation. According to Olszewski[34], the VPI is located just between the lower parts of the VPL and VPM nuclei, and its dorsal part "contains large well stained cells similar to VPL cells and the short horizontal fiber bundles." Further, they recorded[9] extracellular unit responses to vestibular stimulation (round–window polarization of either labyrinth) in the thalamic zone designated as VPI and in the n. ventroposterior lateralis pars oralis (VPL_o of Olszewski), where longer latency (4–5 msec) field potentials were found in their previous study. They stated that 95% of the cells responded to contralateral and 83% to ipsilateral labyrinth polarization with 78% receiving convergent input from both labyrinths. Half of the cells had a phasic response, 26% a tonic response and 24% a combination of tonic and phasic responses. Another important contribution was the finding that the great majority (80%) of those neurons responding to labyrinth polarization showed convergence with deep somatic input from joints and muscles of the vertebral column and limbs: 60% of these bimodal neurons responded to movement of the cervical joints. Cutaneous (6.6%), non-optokinetic visual or auditory (2.6% each) input was also seen. Receptive fields tended to be large, frequently involving more than one joint, and were sometimes bilateral. They discussed the functional importance of blending vestibular information into the somatic proprioceptive system. For the purpose of body orientation, the integration of neck and other proprioceptive afferents with the vestibular signals seems reasonable.

A somewhat different conclusion was reached as a result of thalamic unit analysis in awake squirrel monkey (Liedgren *et al.*[21]). Among 1174 units recorded in various thalamic areas, 167

(14.2%) responded to stimulation of the vestibular nerve. However, they claimed that these vestibular neurons were not confined to one cell group but were dispersed over wide areas of the various somatosensory nuclei. They found vestibular neurons not only in the VPL_c and VPL_o but also in the pulvinar, centre médian, centralis lateralis, zona incerta, lateralis posterior, reticularis and VPI (only two neurons). According to them, the shortest latencies in the total population pattern are caused by vestibular input to the n. posterior and VPL, particularly in the VL (VPL_o). As for the convergence pattern, they found that vestibular projection took place with the cells receiving deep sensation from the proximal part of the body, suggesting some functional significance. The differences from the previous view that the VPI is specialized for vestibular sensation are discussed in relation to the different thalamic organizations in the squirrel and rhesus monkey.

It is relevant to note here that the large afferent (Ia) from muscles to the cortical 3a area is now essentially confirmed by physiological studies in the monkey[40] and baboon[16,35]. Although the thalamic relay station was not considered in these studies, if we accept the large muscle afferent projection to the n. Vim, then it might be reasonable to deduce that this nucleus is the thalamic relay. Vestibular projection to the cortical 3a area has also been found in the squirrel monkey[26] by electrical stimulation of the vestibular nerve, and in rhesus monkey[40].

Neurophysiological observations on the n. Vim in man

The n. Vim has been studied by many investigators working in the field of stereotactic surgery in the human thalamus, since this nucleus is probably involved in the mechanism of tremor genesis[25].

In a continuation of the work in monkeys, Albe-Fessard *et al.*[1] described that in the human thalamus deep sensation also projected preferentially to the rostral-most part of the sensory nucleus (Vc). This particular area may correspond to the n. Vim, where they found rhythmic burst discharges apparently related to the peripheral tremor. These findings were mostly confirmed by Jasper and Bertrand[17]. They emphasized the possibility of separate distribution of deep kinesthetic sense in the n. Vim and not in the Vc nucleus, to which tactile sensation is projected.

Using a semimi croelectrode in the course of stereotactic surgery in cases of abnormal motor disturbances such as parkinsonism and various kinds of tremor cases in the awake state, we have been studying the unitary and multiunitary activities of the ventrolateral part of the human thalamus (see Ohye[27]). The results are briefly summarized below.

Approximate localization of the n. Vim: The n. Vim is located between the n. VL and n. Vc. According to the atlas of the human thalamus[39], it is a thin layer of about 3–4 mm thick and 10 mm height, being 5–7 mm anterior to the commissure posterior (CP) in its profile. It extends from 10–18 mm from the midline in the frontal section. In our frontal approach, the tentative target point was set at about 5 mm from the CP, on the IC-line and 15 mm lateral to the midline. In lowering the electrode, the Cd nucleus, the thalamic entrance and the border between the dorsal and ventral thalamus can be fairly well delineated by the characteristic neural noise pattern[13,29]. The n. Vim and Vc are distinguished by their high amplitude spikes on the high neural noise and background oscillation of 20–30 Hz. It was postulated that these findings reflected the clustering of large cells in this area, corresponding well to the anatomical findings mentioned above. Although no histological correlation is yet available, systematic studies of the neural noise in and around the ventrolateral area of the thalamus strongly support this view.

Unitary and multiunitary responses of the Vim neurons: Unitary or distinguishable multiunitary spikes can be selected from the high background neural noise with the aid of a remote-controlled hydraulic micromanipulator driven by a pulse-motor. It was shown that in our anteroposterior approach, the first neuron responsible for peripheral natural stimulation was activated without exception for the passive or active movement of the contralateral extremity[32]. The effective mode of stimulation comprised, for example, extension or flexion of a joint (Fig. 3A), compression of a muscle belly, small movement of a digit, etc. In studies on about 40 such neurons, two-thirds were activated by manipulation of the upper limb, and one-third by that of the lower limb. Stimulation of the distal part was more effective than at the proximal part. Dorsolateral to ventromedial organization of the lower to upper limb representation was also suggested. When all the thalamic points where the first kinesthetic neurons were recorded were reconstructed from x-ray film and superimposed on the atlas of the human thalamus with reference to the CP and IC-line, they were mostly distributed in the area defined as the n. Vim. We thus confirmed the previous finding of a large afferent projection to this area by the evoked potential method[14]. The tactile neurons were found more posteriorly, corresponding to the area of the n. Vc, having little overlap with the group of kinesthetic neurons.[5,30] In this regard, it is somewhat curious that Donaldson[11] is opposed to this notion of a separate distribution by submodality: his criticism is based on only one case in which the occurrence of "joint" units antero-inferior as well as postero-superior to "touch" units was seen in his posteroanterior approach from the posterior lobe. The double distribution of kinesthetic neurons in his case, being separated about 5 mm antero-posteriorly, is reminiscent of the recent findings in monkey thalamus described above.

On several occasions when a unitary spike corresponding to natural stimuli was found, the same spike was shown to respond to an electric stimulation of the appropriate peripheral nerve. A single electric shock, without causing peripheral muscle contraction or sensory effect, produced a group of 2–3 spikes superposed on a large positive slow wave of about 10 msec latency, almost comparable to that found by Goto *et al.*[14] The fastest spike latency was about 11–12 msec, no fluctuation being observed in any given case. Therefore, we postulated that some oligosynaptic pathway might exist. The ascending pathway responsible is still unclear. We did not try vestibular stimulation, which would be technically very difficult during the course of operative procedure in the awake state.

Evoked and spontaneous burst discharges in the n. Vim: As the neurons of the n. Vim receive kinesthetic afferents, it is not surprising that the neurons are involved in tremor movement, if it is present (Fig. 3B). In fact, it was very often the case that rhythmic burst discharges time-locked with the peripheral tremor were found in this area. In such cases, the receptive field could be determined by careful examination of the contralateral extremity. This kind of rhythmic burst discharges, therefore, is a reflection of the mechanical movement of the trembling extremity.

Often intermingling with the tremor time-locked burst discharge, two other types of burst discharges are recorded. One is rhythmic, but independent of tremor, and the other is non-rhythmic, being related to the sleep state. Characteristics of these burst discharges have already been reported[28,33].

It is interesting that evoked or spontaneous burst discharges are also found at almost the same thalamic area in non-parkinsonian cases without clinical manifestation of tremor. It seems that these burst discharges are more-or-less related to the tremor mechanism, though an integrative understanding is still difficult. The mechanism of burst discharges is another problem. For some reason, the Vim neurons readily produce bursts; deafferentation is a possible cause.

Electrical stimulation of the n. Vim: Electrical stimulation of the thalamic point at which the kinesthetic neurons were recorded demonstrated another characteristic of this nucleus[31]. Weak

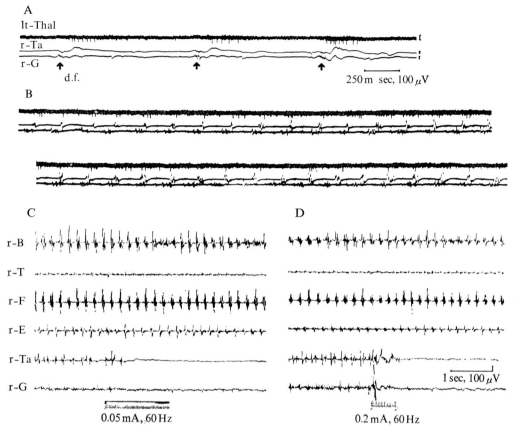

Fig. 3. Physiological observations during the course of stereotactic Vim thalamotomy in a case of parkinsonism. A: The left thalamic unit (lt-Thal) responded to passive dorsiflexion (d.f and arrow) of the right ankle joint. The lower two traces are EMGs from the right tibialis anterior (r-Ta) and gastrocnemius (r-G) muscles.

B: The same thalamic unit exhibits a rhythmic burst or single discharge time-locked to peripheral tremor.

C and D: EMGs showing arrest of tremor by stimulation of the thalamic point (60 Hz, 0.05 and 0.2 mA) at which the unit discharges shown in A and B were recorded. The effect is exerted only in the lower limb corresponding to the receptive field. Overall observations suggest that this point is the n. Vim. r, Right; B, biceps brachii; T, triceps brachii; F, forearm flexor; E, forearm extensor muscles.

stimulation (around 0.1–0.2 mA) induced sensation in the receptive field of these neurons. The correspondence was strict in some cases but it was generally the case that the sensation was induced in a larger area than the small receptive field This might be explained by the method of stimulation: constant current stimulation was applied with a bipolar electrode (interpolar distance, 0.3–0.5 mm), whereas the recording was made at the tip of the electrode referring to the second pole. Some patients used such expressions as paresthetic, burning or unpleasant sensation, the latter being induced only by high stimulus intensity.

When the intensity of stimulation was increased to 1.5 to 2 times the threshold to sensory response, slight motor response could be induced, again including the original receptive field. EMG recording showed irregular grouping discharge (Fig. 3C.) If tremor was present, it was suppressed (in about 60%) or exaggerated (in about 40%), without influencing the background muscle tone. These patterns of motor response contrast with those induced by capsular stimulation or thalamic VL stimulation, the former being characterized by jerky flexion and the latter by diffuse augmentation of muscle tone.

Effect of a coagulative lesion in the n. Vim: After these physiological observations, a small coagulation was made in this area of supposed n. Vim. In cases in which all or a part of the above physiological findings were obtained, a small thalamic lesion was made at the area including that kinesthetic neuron[31]. The volume of the lesion could not be estimated exactly but it was probably 2–3 mm in radius.

In several cases, mere impact of the coagulation needle was effective enough to arrest the tremor. It is noteworthy that the arrest of tremor occurs only in that extremity where the receptive field is found during the recording process. In cases in which insufficient physiological information was available, we depended on radiological measurements alone to decide the final target point. It seemed that in such cases, the therapeutic lesion tended to become larger than it was in physiologically well controlled cases. Details of the clinical evaluation will be described separately.

Selective Vim thalamotomy for the relief of tremor can thus be accomplished without sensory deficit. In fact, postoperative neurological examination revealed only transient slight cerebellar signs in a minority of the cases[49] and paresthesia due to involvement of the n. Vc has been experienced in only three cases among more than 400 Vim thalamotomy cases.

Summary and future problems

The thalamic n. Vim is defined histologically as a group of large, darkly stained cells, located between the n. VL and n. Vc. It develops only in the higher mammals, in which it can be distinguished from several adjacent nuclei by its morphological characteristics. In the lower animals, the problem of homology is controversial. For that reason, experimental studies are not well advanced in comparison with those of surrounding structures such as the n. VL and n. Vc. Studies in the monkey showed vestibular and kinesthetic afferents coming up to this nucleus, although their ascending pathways are not yet certain. It seems to be functionally significant that convergent neurons receiving both types of proprioceptive afferents are found in the majority of cases. The efferent connection is still obscure, cortical 3a projection being suggested by several indirect lines of evidence, and the connection from 3a is not known.

In the human thalamus, the n. Vim is one of the most interesting areas in relation to tremor, in the sense that tremor-dependent and -independent rhythmic burst discharges have been found, and a small coagulation of this area resulted in almost complete arrest of the tremor. Projection of kinesthetic afferents to this area is also established. Electrical stimulation of the n. Vim produced characteristic sensory and motor responses in the contralateral extremity. The vestibular projection to the n. Vim in the human thalamus is an interesting problem but has not yet been inevistigated, mainly because of the technical difficulty. At present, though we have no histological evidence, it appears that the physiological properties of the presumed n. Vim are sufficient to define it, at least in the course of stereotactic surgery.

Based on these anatomo-physiological observations, it seems likely that the n. Vim has, in fact, a character intermediate between those of sensory and motor systems, receiving proprioceptive, kinesthetic (sensation of movement) input and then sending these data to the cortical intermediate zone of the 3a area. In this sense, the n. Vim is quite distinct from the n. VL and n. Vc; the former receives cerebellar and pallidal inputs and projects to the precentral area, while the latter receives lemniscal input and projects to the postcentral area other than 3a (Fig. 4). Therefore, it is likely that this proprioceptive system functions, in part, in parallel with the classical cerebello-thalamo-cortical system and, in part, in parallel with the lemniscal system. The distinct separation is now evident as a result of experience in human stereotactic surgery, indicating that coagulation of the n. Vim does not bring about noticeable motor disturbance in any voluntary effort, nor sensory deficit, and moreover, it ameliorates almost every kind of tremor (resting and postural as well as intention tremor). As we find rhythmic or non-rhythmic, evoked or spontaneous burst discharges in this particular thalamic area including the n. Vim, but not in the n. VL, the impulses mediated through this accessory nucleus in pathological cases may be blended with these grouping discharges and finally come out as abnormal, uneven movement.

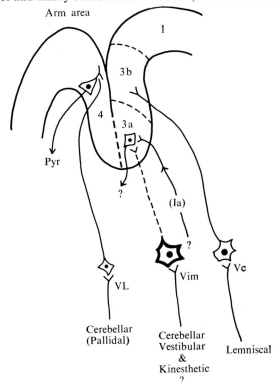

Fig. 4. Schematic illustration of three parallel thalamocortical relations through the n. VL, Vim and Vc. In the VL, pallidal input is not shown separately but is in parentheses. In the Vim, afferent pathways are not clear, and neither is the efferent cortical projection (dotted line). Ia projection to the 3a area seems to be established, though its thalamic relay is not. In the Vc, projections other than 3b are omitted. For details, see the text.

To test this hypothesis, better information is required about the ascending pathway sending proprioceptive sensations to the n. Vim and how and where these proprioceptive sensations are transmitted to play a role in the whole sensory-motor integration.

References

1. Albe-Fessard, D., Guiot, G., Lamarre, Y. and Arfel, G., Activation of thalamocortical projections related to tremorogenic processes. In D.P. Purpura and M.D. Yahr (Eds.) *The Thalamus*, Columbia University Press, 1966, pp. 237–253.
2. Albe-Fessard, D. and Lamarre, Y., Organization des projections somatiques dans le noyau ventral postérieur chez le singe, *J. Physiol. (Paris)*, 57 (1965) 539–540.
3. Andrew, J. and Watkins, E.S., Variability and probability studies of the thalamic nuclei (Chapter 5). In *A Stereotaxic Atlas of the Human Thalamus and Adjacent Structures. A Variability Study*, Williams and Wilkins, Baltimore, 1969, pp. 31–86.
4. Angaut, P., Bases anatomo-fonctionelles des interrelations cérébello-cérébrales, *J. Physiol. (Paris)*, 67 (1973) 53A–116A.
5. Bertrand, G., Jasper, H.H., Wong, A. and Mathews, G., Microelectrode recording during stereotactic surgery, *Clin. Neurosurg.*, 16 (1969) 328–355.
6. Crouch, R.L., The nuclear configuration of the thalamus of *Macacus* rhesus, *J. comp. Neurol.*, 59 (1934) 451–485.
7. Crouch, R.L. and Thompson, J.K., Termination of the brachium conjunctivum in the thalamus of the *Macacus* rhesus, *J. comp. Neurol.*, 69 (1938) 449–452.
8. Deecke, L., Schwarz, D.W.F. and Fredrickson, J.M., Nucleus ventroposterior inferior (VPI) as the vestibular thalamic relay in the rhesus monkey. I. Field potential investigation, *Exp. Brain Res.*, 20 (1974) 88–100.
9. Deecke, L., Schwarz, D.W.F. and Fredrickson, J.M., Vestibular responses in the rhesus monkey ventroposterior thalamus. II. Vestibulo-proprioceptive convergence at thalamic neurons, *Exp. Brain Res.*, 30 (1977) 219–232.
10. Dewulf, A., *Anatomy of the Normal Human Thalamus*, Elsevier, Amsterdam–London–New York, 1971.
11. Donaldson, I.M.L., The properties of some human thalamic units: Some new observations and a critical review of the localization of thalamic nuclei, *Brain*, 96 (1973) 419–440.
12. Friedemann, M., Die Cytoarchitektonik des Zwischenhirns der Cercopitheken mit besonderer Berüksichtigung des Thalamus opticus, *J. Phychol. Neurol.*, 18 (1912) 311–378.
13. Fukamachi, A., Ohye, C., Saito, Y. and Narabayashi, H., Estimation of the neural noise within the human thalamus, *Acta neurochir.*, Suppl. 24 (1977) 121–136.
14. Goto, A., Kosaka, K., Kubota, K., Nakamura, R. and Narabayashi, H., Thalamic potentials from muscle afferents in the human, *Arch. Neurol.*, 91 (1968) 302–309.
15. Hassler, R., Anatomy of the thalamus. In G. Schaltenbrand and P. Bailey (Eds.) *Introduction to Stereotaxis with an Atlas of the Human Brain, Vol. I*, Georg Thieme Verlag, Stuttgart, pp. 230–290.
16. Heath, C.J., Hore, J. and Phillips, C.G., Inputs from low threshold muscle and cutaneous afferents of hand and forearm to areas 3a and 3b of baboon's cerebral cortex, *J. Physiol. (Lond.)*, 257 (1976) 199–227.
17. Jasper, H.H. and Bertrand, G., Thalamic units involved in somatic sensation and voluntary and involuntary movements in man. In D.P. Purpura and M.D. Yahr (Eds.) *The Thalamus*, Columbia University Press, 1966, pp. 365–390.
18. Johnes, E.G. and Powell, T.P.S., Connexions of the somatic sensory cortex of the rhesus monkey. III. Thalamic connexions, *Brain*, 39 (1970) 37–56.
19. Kusama, T., Mabuchi, M. and Sumino, T., Cerebellar projections to the thalamic nuclei in monkeys, *Proc. Japan Acad.*, 47 (1971) 505–510.
20. Lanoir, J. and Schlag, J., Le thalamus de chat et du singe. Données anatomiques, hodologiques et fonctionnelles, *J. Physiol. (Paris)*, 72 (1976) 1–170.
21. Liedgren, S.R.C., Milne, A.C., Rubin, A.M., Schwarz, D.W.F. and Tomlinson, R.D., Representation of vestibular afferents in somatosensory thalamic nuclei of the squirrel monkey (Saimiri sciureus), *J. Neurophysiol.*, 39 (1976) 601–612.
22. Loe, P.R., Whitsel, B.L., Dreyer, D.A. and Metz, C.B., Body representation in ventrobasal thalamus of macaque. A single-unit analysis, *J. Neurophysiol.*, 40 (1977) 1339–1355.
23. Mehler, W.R., Idea of a new anatomy of the thalamus, *J. psychiat. Res.*, 8 (1971) 203–217.
24. Mehler, W.R. and Nauta, W.J.H., Connections of the basal ganglia and of the cerebellum, *Confin. neurol.*, 36 (1974) 205–222.
25. Narabayashi, H. and Ohye, C., Parkinsonian tremor and nucleus ventralis intermedius (Vim) of human thalamus. In J.E. Desmedt (Ed.) *International Symposium on Human Reflexes and Motor Disorders*, Brussels, (in press).
26. Ödkvist, L.M., Schwarz, D.W.F., Fredrickson, J.M. and Hassler, R., Projection of the vestibular nerve to the area 3a arm field in the squirrel monkey (*Saimiri sciureus*), *Exp. Brain Res.*, 21 (1974) 97–105.

27. Ohye, C., Depth microelectrode technique and study. Neurophysiological understanding of the ventrolateral thalamic mass in man. In G. Schaltenbrand and E.A. Walker (Eds.), *Textbook of Stereotaxy of the Human Brain*, Georg Thieme, Stuttgart (in press).
28. Ohye, C. and Albe-Fessard, D., Rhythmic discharges related to tremor in man and monkey. In N. Chalazonitis (Ed.), *Abnormal Neuronal Discharges*, Raven Press, New York (in press).
29. Ohye, C., Fukamachi, A., Miyazaki, M., Isobe, I., Nakajima, H. and Shibazaki, T., Physiologically controlled selective thalamotomy for treatment of abnormal movement by Leksell's open system, *Acta neurochir.*, 37 (1977) 93–104.
30. Ohye, C., Fukamachi, A. and Narabayashi, H., Spontaneous and evoked activity of sensory neurons and their organization in the human thalamus, *Z. Neurol.*, 203 (1972) 219–234.
31. Ohye, C., Maeda, T. and Narabayashi, H., Physiologically defined Vim nucleus. Its special reference to control of tremor, *Appl. Neurophysiol.*, 39 (1977) 285–295.
32. Ohye, C. and Narabayashi, H., Physiological observations of presumed ventralis intermedius neurons in the human thalamus (submitted for publication).
33. Ohye, C., Saito, Y., Fukamachi, A. and Narabayashi, H., An analysis of the spontaneous rhythmic and non-rhythmic burst discharges in the human thalamus, *J. neurol. Sci.*, 22 (1974) 245–259.
34. Olszewski, J., *The Thalamus of the Macaca mulatta. An Atlas for Use with the Stereotaxic Instrument*, S. Karger, Basel, 1952.
35. Phillips, C.G., Powell, T.P.S. and Wiesendanger, M., Projection from low threshold muscle afferents of hand and forearm to area 3a of baboon's cortex, *J. Physiol. (Lond.)*, 217 (1971) 419–446.
36. Poggio, G.F. and Mountcastle, V.B., The functional properties of ventrobasal thalamic neurons studied in unanesthetized monkeys, *J. Neurophysiol.*, 26 (1963) 775–806.
37. Powell, T.P.S. and Mountcastle, V.B., Some aspects of the functional organization of the cortex of the postcentral gyrus of the monkey: A correlation of finding obtained in a single unit analysis with cytoarchitecture, *Bull. Johns Hopkins Hosp.*, 105 (1959) 133–162.
38. Pubols, L.M., Somatic sensory representation in the thalamic ventrobasal complex of the spider monkey (*Ateles*), *Brain Behav. Evol.*, 1 (1968) 305–323.
39. Schaltenbrand, G. and Bailey P. (Eds.) *Introduction to Stereotaxis with Atlas of Human Brain*, Georg Thieme, Stuttgart, 1959.
40. Schwarz, D.W.F., Deecke, L. and Fredrickson, J.M., Cortical projection of group I muscle afferents to area 2, 3a and the vestibular field in the rhesus monkey, *Exp. Brain Res.*, 17 (1973) 516–526.
41. Sheps, J.G., The nuclear configuration and cortical connections of the human thalamus, *J. comp. Neurol.*, 83 (1945) 1–56.
42. Tarlov, E., The rostral projections of the primate vestibular nuclei: An experimental study in Macaque, baboon and chimpanzee, *J. comp. Neurol.*, 135 (1969) 27–56.
43. Van Buren, J.M. and Borke, R.C., A re-evaluation of the "nucleus ventralis lateralis" and its cerebellar connections. A study in man and chimpanzee, *Int. J. Neurol.*, 8 (1971) 155–177.
44. Van Buren, J.M. and Borke, R.C., The nuclei and cerebral connections of the human thalamus. In *Variations and Connections of the Human Thalamus*, Springer-Verlag, Berlin–Heidelberg–New York, 1972, pp. 119–123.
45. Van Buren, J.M., Borke, R.C. and Modesti, L.M., Sensory and nonsensory portions of the nucleus "ventralis posterior" thalami of chimpanzee and man, *J. Neurosurg.*, 45 (1976) 37–48.
46. Vogt, C., Le myéloarchitecture du thalamus du cercopithèque, *J. Psychol. Neurol. (Leipzig)*, 12 (1909) 285–324.
47. Vogt, C. and Vogt, O., Thalamusstudien I-III, *J. Psychol. Neurol. (Leipzig)*, 50 (1941) 32–152.
48. Walker, A.E., *The Primate Thalamus*, University of Chicago Press, Chicago, London, 1938.
49. Yasui, N., Narabayashi, H., Kondo, T. and Ohye, C., Slight cerebellar signs in stereotaxic thalamotomy and subthalamotomy for parkinsonism. *Appl. Neurophysiol.*, 39 (1977) 315–320.

The mode of tapering and distribution of nodes of Ranvier in group Ia fiber collaterals in the cat spinal cord

TOSHINORI HONGO*[1], NORIO ISHIZUKA*[2], HAJIME MANNEN*[2] AND SHIGETO SASAKI*[1]

*[1] *Laboratory of Physiology, Institute of Basic Medical Sciences, University of Tsukuba, Niihari-gun, Ibaraki 300–31, Japan*
*[2] *Third Department of Anatomy, Faculty of Medicine, Tokyo Medical and Dental University, Bunkyo-ku, Tokyo 113, Japan.*

Intracellular marking techniques have now made it possible to study various aspects of the intraspinal morphology of functionally identified, single primary afferent fibers[2,3,5,6]. The present study was aimed at clarifying the mode of tapering in relation to the spacing of nodes of Ranvier of the group Ia fibers during their intraspinal course towards the ventral horn, by means of intra-axonal staining with horseradish peroxidase (HRP). The data are derived from group Ia fibers innvervating hindlimb muscles in the cat. Methods of staining physiologically identified Ia fibers and the procedures of later analysis were as described previously[5,7].

Our observations concerned only the axon (axis cylinder) and did not cover the myelin sheath because of the staining technique (HRP) employed. Fig. 1A shows a transverse view of a reconstructed collateral bifurcated from a longitudinally running stem axon in the dorsal funiculus. The collateral passes ventrally through the dorsal horn without issuing terminal branches, and then passes ventrolaterally to reach the ventral horn, giving rise to terminal arborizations in Rexed's laminae VI, VII and IX during its course. Under the microscope, distinct constrictions of the axon (Fig. 1C) were observed to occur periodically, and they were recognized as sites of the nodes of Ranvier, since bifurcated branches always issued from such constrictions (Fig. 1D)[1,4,8]. The collateral in Fig. 1A is schematically redrawn in Fig. 1B, in which the locations of the constrictions, and hence most probably of the nodes, are indicated by open circles, axonal diameters by figures along the axons (in μm), and internodal distances by the lengths of the lines between two open circles (compare with the calibration mark).

Note the general tendency that both the diameter and the internodal length decrease progressively with the course towards the periphery, especially after bifurcation. Fig. 2A shows the relationship between the axonal diameter and the length of the corresponding internode, indicating an approximately linear relation between the two parameters with a slope of 100 in the regression line, which is close to the value obtained from cobalt-stained group Ia fibers in the spinal cord[6]. The number of nodes of Ranvier was counted along each axonal course to the ventral horn, i.e., from the stem axon in the dorsal funiculus to each terminal branch in the ventral horn, and was found to range from 8 to 19 with a mean of 12.1 (Fig. 2B, 103 measurements from three fibers). These morphological data, supplemented by information on the thickness of the meylin sheath, should be useful in developing a better understanding of intraspinal events occurring in collaterals of Ia fibers, such as the mode of impulse conduction to motoneurons and interneurons.

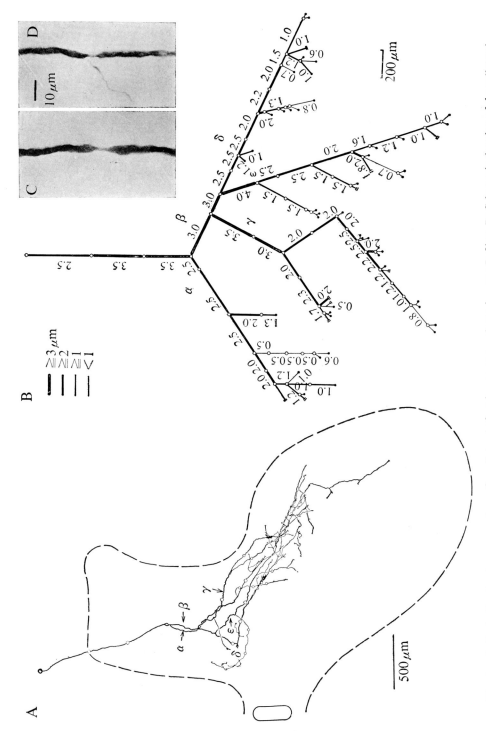

Fig. 1. A: Projection to a transverse plane of a collateral of a triceps surae—plantaris group Ia fiber. B: Schematic drawing of the collateral in A with locations of nodes, diameters and lengths of internodes indicated. The diameter given is the mean of several measurements, and the internodal length was obtained with corrections for undulations in the depth of the sections. No attempts were made to locate the node in terminal branches (indicated by a filled circle at the end) because of the uncertainties involved. Short double bars indicate the limit beyond which the stained axons could not be traced. C and D: Photomicrographs showing the nodes of Ranvier. See the text for further details.

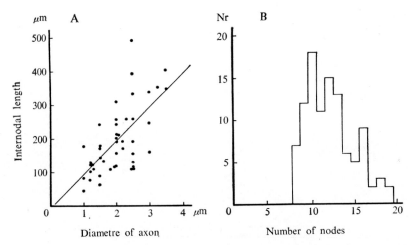

Fig. 2.   A: Relationship between the diameter and the internodal length. B: Frequency histogram showing the number of nodes contained in a collateral course reaching the ventral horn. See the text for details.

References

1. Bodian, D., A note on nodes of Ranvier in the central nervous system, *J. comp. Neurol.*, 94 (1951) 475–483.
2. Brown, A.G. and Fyffe, R.E.W., The morphology of group Ia afferent fiber collaterals in the spinal cord of the cat. *J. Physiol. (Lond.)*, 274 (1978) 111–127.
3. Brown, A.G., Rose, P.K. and Snow, P.J., The morphology of hair follicle afferent fibre collaterals in the spinal cord of the cat, *J. Physiol. (Lond.)*, 272 (1977) 779–797.
4. Hess, A. and Young, J.Z., The node of Ranvier, *Proc. roy. Soc. B*, 149 (1952) 301–320.
5. Hongo, T , Ishizuka, N., Mannen, H. and Sasaki, S., Axonal trajectory of single group Ia and Ib fibers in the cat spinal cord, *Neurosci. Lett.* (in press).
6. Iles, J.F., Central terminations of muscle afferents on motoneurones in the cat spinal cord. *J. Physiol. (Lond.)*, 262 (1976) 91–117.
7. Mannen, H., Reconstruction of axonal trajectory of individual neurons in the spinal cord using Golgi-stained serial sections, *J. comp. Neurol.*, 159 (1975) 357–374.
8. Robertson, J.D., Preliminary observations on the ultrastructure of nodes of Ranvier, *Z. Zellforsch.*, 50 (1959) 553–560.

Antagonist inhibition in sequential voluntary movements of ankle extension and flexion in man

REISAKU TANAKA

Department of Neurobiology, Tokyo Metropolitan Institute for Neurosciences, Fuchu, Tokyo 183, Japan

Hufschmidt and Hufschmidt reported that, when a human subject flexing his elbow strongly reacts to a sensory stimulus by extending the elbow, the voluntary EMG activity of the triceps brachii muscle is usually preceded by some 50 msec by disappearance of the tonic biceps activity[1]. The authors, describing this as *antagonist inhibition*, interpreted this reaction as a part of the voluntary reaction, but did not discuss its actual mechanism. The present investigation was primarily aimed at clarifying whether the phenomenon is caused by active inhibition of motoneurons or not. Ankle extensor (m. triceps surae) and flexor (m. tibialis ant.) muscles were chosen as the antagonistic pair for the test because the H-reflex can be used as an indicator of motoneuron excitability.

The subjects in this study were 4 healthy adults (ages, 21–26 years). The subject sat in a reclining chair. The foot was fixed to a pedal and contraction of the leg muscles was nearly isometric. The procedures for stimulation of the tibial and peroneal nerves and recording of EMG activities were the same as in the previous study[3]. An LED (light-emitting diode) which could indicate both green and red was placed in front of the subject for visual signals. The subject was requested to plantarflex his foot in response to a green signal and to keep it contracted while the green light was on. After 1 to 2 sec, the light turned red and the subject was then supposed to dorsiflex his foot quickly and phasically in response. The LED was turned off soon after the reaction and the subject relaxed and waited for the next signal. The signals were given at intervals of 6–10 sec. Thus, the motor paradigm was the same in principle as that of the Hufschmidts[1]. The nerve stimulation was applied with appropriate timing at the end of the triceps EMG or onset of the pretibial EMG.

In the present motor paradigm of ankle extension-flexion, the voluntary EMG activity of the pretibial muscles was almost always preceded by disappearance of the tonic triceps surae EMG, as was the case with elbow flexion-extension movement[1]. In an example illustrated in Fig. 1, the mean interval between the end of extensor EMG (GS off) and the onset of flexor EMG (TA on) was 40 msec ($n = 52$) and 80% of the trials were between 30 and 90 msec (horizontal bars with an open circle). The values in other subjects were similar.

Fig. 1 illustrates the excitability change of the triceps surae motor pool for GS off (A) or TA on (B). As shown in A, the H-reflex, which was facilitated during voluntary contraction, had larger amplitude than the control in the resting state even after GS off, but appeared to gradually decrease towards TA on. However, the time at which the facilitation turned into depression showed a fairly broad range and was not clear-cut. This is understandable, since the latency of TA on measured from GS off was variable and the antagonist inhibition might be more related to the agonist activity. It appears from plot B that some facilitation remained 10 msec prior to TA on but that depression started at or just after TA on. A clear-cut depression was observed after a few tens of milliseconds.

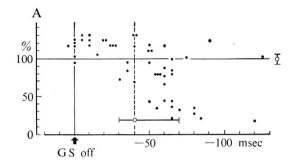

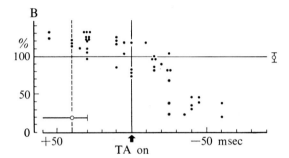

Fig. 1. Changes in the excitability of the triceps surae motor pool during ankle extension-flexion movements. The amplitude of the triceps H-reflexes (ordinates, expressed as a percentage of the control amplitude obtained in a resting state and indicated on the right-hand side with s.d.) are plotted against the intervals (abscissae) between the test H-reflexes and either GS off (A) or TA on (B). Further details are given in the text.

The results suggest that the *antagonist inhibition* of the Hufschmidts' motor paradigm is caused not by active inhibition of motoneurons but by disfacilitation due to withdrawal of descending excitatory signals. Active reciprocal inhibition occurs at or just after the onset of the agonist activity. Facilitation of the Ia inhibitory pathway to the triceps surae was observed between GS off and TA on (not illustrated), i.e., just prior to the pretibial activity, as was the case with simple dorsiflexion movement[3]. Reciprocal Ia inhibition may thus be related to the actual inhibition.

Thus, it seems that cessation of the motor command for the first contraction and initiation of the command to start the second contraction occur simultaneously in the brain. The first mover (later antagonist) ceases action immediately upon withdrawal of the excitatory command, while it takes some time to recruit the second mover and the Ia inhibitory pathway to the first mover, which should have been inhibited during the antagonist contraction[4]. This interpretation is in line with the view of Kots based on an H-reflex study with a slightly different motor paradigm from the present study[2].

REFERENCES

1. Hufschmidt, H.I. and Hufschmidt, T., Antagonist inhibition as the earliest sign of a sensrimotor reaction, *Nature (Lond.)*, 174 (1954) 607.
2. Kots, Ya. M., Supraspinal control of the segmental centres of muscle-antagonists in man. II. Reflex excitability of the motor neurones of muscle antagonists on organization of sequential activity, *Biophysics*, 14 (1969) 1146–1154.
3. Simoyama, M. and Tanaka, R., Reciprocal Ia inhibition at the onset of voluntary movements in man, *Brain Research*, 82 (1974) 334–337.
4. Tanaka, R., Reciprocal Ia inhibition during voluntary movements in man, *Exp. Brain Res.*, 21 (1974) 529–540.

Changes in monosynaptic EPSPs of quadriceps motoneurons in monkeys with the spinal cord chronically hemisected at the thoracic level

MAMORU AOKI and SHIGEMI MORI

Department of Physiology, Asahikawa Medical College,
Asahikawa, Hokkaido 078–11, Japan

Spinal cord hemisection at Th8 level in the rhesus monkey produces ipsilateral flaccid paralysis of the hind limb. However, the animal regains an ability to utilize the limb, seemingly free, several months after the infliction. In the course of such recovery, concurrent enhancement of knee-jerk and quadriceps monosynaptic reflex[1,2] was found to develop gradually on the hemisected side. This finding suggested that a change of synaptic efficacy may underlie the recovery of limb movement. Therefore, as an initial attempt to reveal the underlying neural mechanisms for recovery of the motor function, the time course of the monosynaptic excitatory postsynaptic potentials (EPSPs) at the unitary level was analyzed.

A series of experiments was carried out on 8 rhesus monkeys weighing 2.5–4.0 kg. The thoracic cord at Th 8–10 level was hemisected 3–6 months prior to the experiments and clear enhancement of knee-jerk was confirmed. Anesthesia was maintained with α-chloralose (50–70 mg/kg). The trachea was cannulated routinely and the animals were immobilized with gallamine triethiodide and artificially ventilated. Nerves to the quadriceps femoris muscles were dissected and indwelling bipolar electrodes (interpolar distance 8 mm) were fitted on both sides. Laminectomies were performed at L5–7 and cut L6 ventral roots were prepared for antidromic stimulation. GI afferent volleys were recorded monopolarly from the dorsal root entry zone with silver ball electrodes. Intracellular recordings from the quadriceps motoneurons were made with glass micropipettes filled with 3 M KCl in the usual manner. Conventional stimulating and recording apparatus was employed.

In 8 monkeys, a total of 48 quadriceps motoneurons were successfully penetrated, 19 on the control side and 29 on the hemisceted side. The resting membrane potentials were 65.2 ± 5.2 mV and 65.4 ± 3.0 mV, respectively, on the control and hemisected sides. However, it was noticed that GIa monosynaptic EPSPs had a shorter rise time on the hemisected side. Accordingly, the time to spike discharge was shorter on average by about 0.2 msec on the hemisceted side.

To compare the time courses of GIa EPSPs at the unitary level on both sides, GIa EPSPs were recorded with minimal stimulus intensity. The amplitudes of the unitary EPSPs ranged from 0.3 to 2.0 (mean 0.84) mV on the hemisected side and were slightly larger than 0.1–1.1 (mean 0.71) mV on the control side. As shown in Fig. 1, the rise times ranged from 0.7 to 1.4 (mean 1.10) msec and 0.5 to 1.2 (mean 0.85) msec, respectively, on the control and hemisceted sides. Thus, the rise times of unitary EPSPs on the hemisected side were shown to be 0.25 msec shorter than those on the control side. The half widths were 2.0–5.5 (mean 3.5) msec and 2.0–6.5 (mean 4.3) msec, respectively, on the control and hemisected sides. Thus, the unitary EPSPs on the hemisected side were found to have a faster rise time and slower decay time than those on the control side.

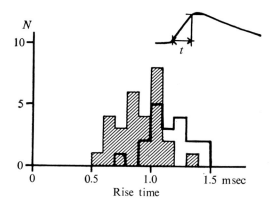

Fig. 1. Histograms of rise times (from 10 to 90% of the amplitude) of unitary GIa EPSPs. The shaded columns indicate the distribution on the hemisected side. Abscissa: rise time (t) in msec. Ordinate: no. of observations (N).

In keeping with our previous work[1,2], the present results provide further evidence for increased synaptic efficacy of monosynaptic transmission following spinal cord hemisection. The most straightforward interpretation of the changes in the time course of GIa EPSPs is to assume the occurrence of "collateral sprouting" from GIa fibers[4] and formation of new synaptic contacts at more proximal parts of the soma-dendritic membrane of motoneurons. Definite physiological evidence for such sprouting has recently been obtained in red nucleus neurons after destruction of the cerebellar nuclear input[5].

The relationship between increased synaptic efficacy and recovery of limb movement appears to be twofold. First, enhanced segmental reflex movements may function in part vicariously for the lost supraspinal control[3]. Second, some descending fibers through remaining spinal pathways may also form new functional connections with lumbosacral motoneurons on the hemisected side, thus contributing to the return of voluntary movements.

REFERENCES

1. Aoki, M., Mori, S. and Fujimori, B., Mechanisms of exaggerated knee-jerk in chronic spinal hemisected monkeys, *Proc. int. physiol. Sci.*, 11 (1974) 157.
2. Aoki, M., Mori. S. and Fujimori, B., Exaggeration of knee-jerk following spinal hemisection in monkeys, *Brain Research*, 107 (1976) 471–485.
3. Goldberger, M.E., Recovery of movement after CNS lesions in monkeys. In D.G. Stein *et al.* (Eds.), *Plasticity and Recovery of Function in the Central Nervous System*, Academic Press, New York, 1974.
4. McCouch, G.P., Austin, G.M., Liu, C.N. and Liu, G.Y., Sprouting as a cause of spasticity, *J. Neurophysiol.*, 21 (1958) 205–216.
5. Tsukahara, N., Hultborn, H., Murakami, F. and Fujito, Y., Electrophysiological study of formation of new synapses and collateral sprouting in red nucleus neurons after partial denervation, *J. Neurophysiol.*, 38 (1975) 1359–1372.

Statistical analysis of 'locked' motor unit spikes in the stretch reflex

SABURO HOMMA and YOSHIO NAKAJIMA

Department of Physiology, School of Medicine, Chiba University,
Inohana, Chiba 280, Japan

Vibratory stimulation of a muscle in man elicits its tonic contraction (tonic vibration reflex; TVR)[2]. Cross-correlograms between motor unit spike activity and vibratory stimuli in this reflex show that some motor unit spikes are well correlated with the vibration and some others are not [1,3]. These two groups of motor unit spikes were called 'phase-locked' spikes and 'phase-unlocked' spikes, respectively[3,4]. Since vibratory stimuli of a muscle activate spindle primary afferents in phase to the vibration, the 'locked' motor unit activities are supposed to be elicited monosynaptically by the excitatory post-synaptic potentials (EPSPs) from the primary afferent terminals[4]. In these cross-correlograms the 'locked' spike activity showed variable recurrence times (times from a stimulus to the resulting motor unit spike) and distributed widely, indicating relatively wide scattering of times of the primary afferent-motor neuron transmissions. The range of this time is called here the correlation time. In order to further confirm this phenomenon, intracellular motoneuron recordings were carried out on cats anesthetized with urethane and chloralose.

Fig. 1 shows one example of calculations for a motoneuron. Both the cross-correlogram between electric stimuli of the peripheral nerve and elicited motoneuron potentials (designated in Fig. 1 as PSTH) and averaged motoneuron EPSPs generated by the stimuli are illustrated on the same time scale (Fig. 1A). The abscissa represents recurrence time and the ordinate the probability of spike occurrence and EPSP magnitude. As shown, the primary correlation time of the correlation curve is almost the same as the time-to-peak values of the EPSP, i.e., 3.6 msec. Instead of electrical stimulation, the muscle was stretched triangularly at random intervals (10–100 msec) and the same analysis as in Fig. 1A was performed (Fig. 1B). Primary correlation time and time-to-peak value were 16.0 and 14.0 msec, respectively. These results of Fig. 1 indicate that the primary correlation time of the cross-correlogram corresponds to the time-to-peak of the average EPSPs.

Using a neuron model, Knox[6] showed in 1974 that the primary correlation time is related to the derivative of post-synaptic potentials. Our experimental results are in agreement with his theoretical point of view. In order to approximate the primary correlation time to the time-to-peak value of PSPs, it is considered prerequisite for motoneuron membrane potential to be depolarized near the firing level. As the vibratory stimulation of a muscle elicits both monosynaptic and polysynaptic EPSPs in motoneurons[5], the membrane is considered to be depolarized near the firing level. It is concluded from these considerations that the cross-correlogram of motor unit spikes with vibratory stimuli during TVR indicates the approximate time course of EPSP of the alpha-motoneuron.

The cross-correlogram between triangular waves of human Achilles tendon and motor unit spikes recorded from the soleus muscle is almost the same as those shown in Fig. 1. Mean values of the primary correlation time obtained from 55 soleus motor units was 8.33 ± 2.54 msec. This

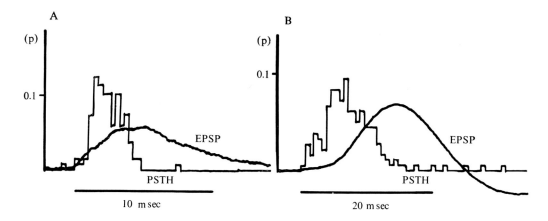

Fig. 1. Cross-correlograms and EPSPs during electrical stimulation of a peripheral nerve (A) and during triangular stretching of a muscle (B). See the text for details.

indicates that EPSP, whose time-to-peak value was around 8 msec, was elicited in the alpha-motoneuron by the triangular vibratory stimulation.

REFERENCES

1. Godaux, E., Desmedt, J.E. and Demaret, P., Vibration of human limb muscles: the alleged phase-locking of motor unit spikes, *Brain Research*, 100 (1975) 175–177.
2. Hagbarth, K.-E. and Eklund, G., Motor effects of vibratory muscle stimuli in man. In R. Granit (Ed.) *Nobel Symposium on Muscular Afferents and Motor Control*, Almqvist and Wiksell, Stockholm, 1966, pp. 177–186.
3. Hirayama, K., Homma, S., Mizote, M., Nakajima, Y. and Watanabe, S., Separation of the contributions of voluntary and vibratory activation of motor units in man by cross-correlograms, *Japan J. Physiol.*, 24 (1974) 293–304.
4. Homma, S. and Kanda, K., Impulse decoding process in stretch reflex, In A.A. Gydikov, N.T. Tankov and D.S. Kosarov (Eds.) *Motor Control*, Plenum Press, New York, 1973, pp. 45–64.
5. Kanda, K., Contribution of polysynaptic pathways to tonic vibration reflex, *Japan. J. Physiol.*, 22 (1972) 367–377.
6. Knox, C.K., Cross-correlation functions for a neuronal model, *Biophys. J.*, 14 (1974) 567–582.

Neuronal activity in cortical supplementary motor area responding to motor instructions

JUN TANJI

Department of Physiology, School of Medicine, Hokkaido University,
Kita-ku, Sapporo 060, Japan

An experiment was designed to determine whether the supplementary motor area (SMA) of the cerebral cortex is involved in performing motor tasks which require readiness for proper usage of somesthetic sensory inputs to start an intended movement. Evarts and Tanji[1,2] have reported that the response of motor cortex neurons to a somesthetic stimulus can be modified by a prior instruction telling the animal how to respond to the stimulus. This finding points to the existence of CNS structures responsible for adjusting the input-output relations of motor cortex in accord with requirements for performance of motor tasks triggered by somesthetic inputs. Experiments by Wiesendanger *et al.*[3] have demonstrated that electrical stimulation of the SMA modifies responses of neurons in the motor cortex to sensory inputs, raising the possibility that the SMA is involved in the system which modulates motor cortex responsiveness. In order to test this hypothesis, a monkey was trained to perform essentially the same task as in the report of Evarts and Tanji[1] and single-unit activity in the SMA was recorded.

A monkey was trained to grasp a handle and maintain it in a certain position which was signalled by a white lamp. In the course of training, the correct holding position was progressively narrowed until it limited the movement of the handle to within 0.5 cm. After correct holding of 1.5 to 3 sec, an instruction was given which told the monkey how he should respond to a perturbation of the handle which would occur subsequently. The instruction was a green or red light which appeared 2.5 to 5 sec prior to the onset of the handle perturbation. The red light informed the monkey that he should pull towards himself when the perturbation occurred, and the green light meant that he should push away from himself when the perturbation occurred. The perturbation, a sudden external load change, was produced by a torque motor. There were two different directions of perturbation, one being a movement of the handle towards the monkey and the other a movement of the handle away from the monkey. Thus, after the instruction, the monkey was required to keep holding the handle without any movement but to be prepared to push or pull the handle as instructed in response to the perturbation, regardless of the direction of the perturbation. It was previously shown that the motor cortex response differed greatly depending on the direction of the movement the animal intended to perform. According to the hypothesis that the SMA is responsible for this modification of the response, there should be activity changes in SMA neurons during a preparatory period when the monkey is instructed to push or pull the handle in response to a forthcoming perturbation.

A total of 276 neurons were recorded in the SMA contralateral to the arm performing the trained task. The recording site, examined histologically, extended from A 14 to A 26 of Horseley-Clarke's coordinates and from midline to L.6. Thirty-two neurons had neuronal activity which was reciprocally or differentially related with the direction of the intended movement. An example is shown in Fig. 1. This neuron increased its discharge when the monkey was instructed to pull but

174

A
Instruction : Pull

B
Instruction : Push

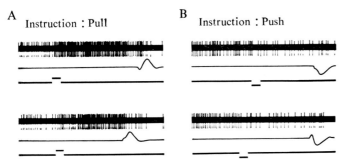

Fig. 1. Discharges of an SMA neuron the activity of which increased on instruction to pull but decreased on instruction to push the handle. In the four sets of traces, the top trace shows the discharges of an SMA neuron, the middle trace shows the position of the handle, and the bottom trace indicates the time of occurrence of the instruction signal. The duration of each display set is 4.8 sec.

decreased its discharge when he was instructed to push the handle. This evident response to the instruction appeared invariably over 64 trials. Discharges were then aligned in relation to the perturbation given to the handle and in relation to the onset of handle movement. Careful inspection of the display revealed no stable relation to the perturbation or to the movement. Thus the discharge of this neuron, like the other 31 instruction-related neurons, was not clearly related with the motor task *per se*, although at times it increased or decreased in various time relationships with the motor task. None of the 32 neurons was clearly driven by such natural sensory stimuli as tapping or stroking various body parts. The latency of the instruction-related neuronal response varied from 140 to 450 msec with a median value of 240 msec. Similar response to the instruction has been reported for motor cortex neurons[1]. It appeared that the latency of the response is shorter in the SMA.

The direction of the sensory triggering stimulus (perturbation of the handle), coming towards or away from the monkey, was usually randomized but in limited observations the direction was unchanged for 16 consecutive trials. In these trials, the monkey apparently anticipated the direction of perturbation as was evidenced by a gradual augmentation of short-latency muscle response. In parallel with the augmentation of the early muscle response, the activity changes of 6 SMA neurons during the anticipatory period appeared to be gradually augmented or suppressed in successive trials according to the direction of perturbation. Thus, the neuronal activity in the SMA was not only related to the direction of the intended movement but also differed greatly depending on whether the forthcoming perturbation was the one which aided or antagonized the intended movement.

In the present experiment the animal was highly trained to perform a motor task which required readiness to utilize the kinesthetic stimulus to start rapid movements. Thus, the instruction light required him to be prepared for a forthcoming movement in response to the perturbation to the handle. This preparatory "motor set" gave rise to activity changes of some neurons in the SMA as early as 140 msec after the onset of the instruction. During this preparatory period the monkey kept holding the handle in a narrow holding zone. He was specially trained not to make any movement of the handle or postural adjustments until the occurrence of the perturbation. As a result, EMG recordings from forelimb and trunk muscles revealed almost no activity changes in this period. On the other hand, in association with the monkey's repositioning of the handle after the performance of pushing or pulling, there was obvious EMG activity in the forelimb and trunk muscles. The activity of 32 neurons described in this report was not at all associated with this EMG activity. (Some neurons other than the 32 exhibited activity changes closely related to the repositioning movement; these will be described in a separate paper). Therefore, it is unlikely that their response to the instruction light is related to postural readjustments. In conclusion, it can be said that the neuronal response in the SMA described here substantiates the view that the SMA actually plays a part in modifying the input-output relation in the motor cortex, in a behavioral context where usage of the sensory input is essential for proficient performance of a motor task.

References

1. Evarts, E.V. and Tanji, J., Gating of motor cortex reflexes by prior instruction, *Brain Research*, 71 (1974) 479–494.
2. Evarts, E.V. and Tanji, J., Reflex and intended responses in motor cortex pyramidal tract neurons of monkey, *J. Neurophysiol.*, 39 (1976) 1069–1080.
3. Wiesendanger, M., Rüegg, D.G. and Lucier, G.E., Why transcortical reflexes?, *Canad. J. neurol. Sci.*, 2 (1975) 295–301.

Compensatory activities of pyramidal tract neurons after sudden target position shifts in awake monkeys

KEN'ICHI MATSUNAMI, SHINTARO FUNAHASHI AND KISOU KUBOTA

Department of Neurophysiology, Primate Research Institute, Kyoto University, Inuyama, Aichi 484, Japan

It has been found in movement control studies that the primate precentral neurons, including pyramidal tract neurons (PTNs), are involved in a movement mechanism compensating against an externally applied perturbation: precentral neurons responded with 20–40 msec latency to a sudden change of load applied to a muscle[1]. This load compensation appears to be accomplished by a transcortical long ascending reflex loop, because the timing relations support such a loop structure[1,7]. As for visually guided movement, it is not known how the motor cortex neurons behave if a preprogrammed visual target is changed. The present experiments were designed to determine in a visual tracking task how PTNs are concerned in compensatory mechanisms to a sudden change of a visually given target position after the start of the tracking movement.

Monkeys performed a single-step visual tracking task of zero order, moving a vertical handle with wrist extension or flexion. The task and manipulandum were described previously[6]. The monkey faced a panel with lamps (two-colored light-emitting diodes; LEDs) (Fig. 1A). The central portion of the range (64°) was divided equally into eight 8° zones, each corresponding to an appropriate lamp. Each of the lamps of the upper target row (T3-T6) indicated the target zone and lamps of the lower row (P1-P8) indicated angular displacement zones of the handle.

When the monkey moved the handle to the P1 or P8 zone (preparatory period), a green lamp was lighted in P1 or P8. After 1 sec, a green light was switched to red and simultaneously one of the target lights was turned on (GO signal). Then the monkey moved the handle to the target zone. If the handle was held there for 1 sec, he was rewarded (standard trial). In other trials, as soon as handle displacement started, the target lamp was changed, that is, an adjacent target lamp was lighted (for example, from T5, to T4 or to T6). Since the target zone was shifted randomly, and after movement had started, the monkey was unable to predict the final zone of the displacement. After the shift the monkey corrected the movement so that the handle was moved further (forward shift trial) or changed movement direction (backward shift trial). Reaction times for these corrections were, on the average, 200–250 msec and were not different from reaction times in standard trials.

Single PTN activity, recorded with a glass-coated Pt-Ir microelectrode (1–4 MΩ), was identified by invasion of the antidromic response by pontine stimulation (double pulses with 3 msec intervals, 0.1 msec duration). Intracortical microstimulation (300 Hz, 0.1 msec, 20 pulses) was routinely performed at a site at which the PTN activity had been recorded and contractions of finger or wrist muscles were evoked at an intensity of less than 50 μA. The cortical area of PTN recordings occupied 4×4 mm^2. In total, 54 PTNs were recorded from three monkeys. Of these, 32 increased their discharge rates during extension and 22 during flexion at the wrist joint.

Figure 1 shows a typical example of discharge pattern of a flexion-type PTN in standard

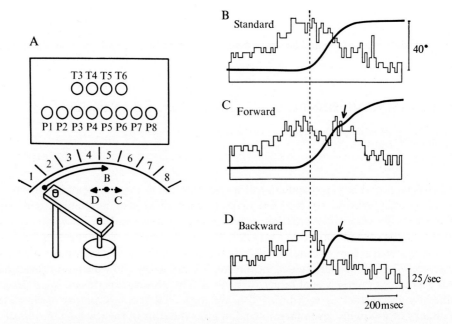

Fig. 1.   Schematic illustration of the task sequence.
       A: Lamp panel, manipulandum and temporal sequence. Above there is a panel with 12 LEDs and below is a vertical handle. The monkey gripped the handle with the left hand and moved it over a range of 110°. The middle portion is divided into 8 zones. When the handle is in one of the zones, the corresponding zone lamp (P1–P8) is on. Lamps in the upper row indicate target zones for trials (T3–T6).
       The sequence of the standard flexion task (40° range) illustrated in B is as follows. When the handle is in the P1 zone, the P1 lamp is turned on green. If it stays there for 1 sec, the color changes to red and simultaneously the T5 target lamp is turned on red. After this GO signal, the monkey moves the handle from the P1 to the P5 zone. Lamps P1–P5 are put on successively. If the T5 and P5 lamps are on for 1 sec, the monkey is rewarded. In position shift trials, the target lamp was changed from T5 to T4 (backward shift; D) or T6 (forward shift; C), as soon as the movement was started. It was detected by displacement change (threshold, 61°/s). On recognizing target change, the monkey further moved the handle to P6 or, changing the movement direction, returned the handle to the P4 zone. If the handle stayed there for 1 sec, he was rewarded. In B (standard trial), C (forward trial) and D (backward trial), 10 responses were averaged, taking the moment of target shift as zero axes in C and D and the timing of the handle entry into the P2 zone in B. Upper; PTN discharges and lower; displacement traces. Vertical broken lines: moments of target lamp shifts in C and D. From a PTN with 1.2 msec antidromic latency. Intracortical microstimulation, 50 μA with wrist flexion. Bin/25 ms.

(B), forward (C), and backward trials (D) of the flexion task. In standard trials the PTN activity gradually increased in firing rate during the preparatory period and after the GO signal it increased further, reaching a peak around the time of displacement onset. Then it started to decrease gradually, even before the handle reached the target zone (Fig. 1B). In forward shift trials the second displacement started 200 msec after the target shift, from the vertical line to the point indicated by an arrow. Corresponsding to this, another peak of activity was observed before the onset of the second displacement. This occurred about 150 msec after target shift. The discharge rate of the second peak was as high as that of the first one. In backward shift trials, the movement direction was changed about 200 msec after target shift. An abrupt decrease of the rate from an increased level occurred at about 150 msec after target shift. Thus, in the illustrated PTN a reciprocal discharge pattern related to sudden change of the target was seen before the compensatory movement of small amplitude.

In all examined PTNs, both flexion and extension type, a reciprocal pattern of the discharge rate was invariably observed. The peak rate at the second peak was slightly higher, lower or the same as that of the first peak. In these PTNs, onset timing of the rate change after the target shift was about 150 msec. Based on averaged responses, the onset of the second displacement of the handle occurred about 200 msec after target shift and was approximately equal to the reaction time values in standard trials. This latency value of PTNs was slightly longer than that reported in visually conditioned hand movement (the shortest latency was reported to be 80 msec[5] or 100 msec[2]). Therefore, although this difference requires explanation, a central program to elicit PTN discharges during standard tracking may be used in a compensatory tracking after target shift. A peripheral compensatory mechanism for load does not appear to contribute significantly to the visual compensatory mechanism, because its latency is too short to influence the 150 msec latency of visually triggered compensation of movement.

Thus, during a single-step visual tracking task at the wrist, target positions were changed slightly (backwards or forwards) after the tracking movement had started. Correction of the movement was detected about 200 msec after a sudden shift of the target. Thirty-two extension- and 22 flexion-related PTNs changed their firing rates in a reciprocal manner with a 150 msec latent period after target shift.

REFERENCES

1. Conrad, B., Meyer-Lohmann, J., Matsunami K. and Brooks, V.B., Precentral unit activity following torque pulse injections into elbow movements, *Brain Research*, 94 (1975) 215–236.
2. Evarts, E.V., Pyramidal tract activity associated with a conditioned hand movement in the monkey, *J. Neurophysiol.*, 29 (1966) 1011–1027.
3. Evarts, E.V. and Fromm, C., Sensory responses in motor cortex neurons during precise motor control, *Neurosci. Lett.*, 5 (1977) 267–272.
4. Fromm, C. and Evarts, E.V., Relation of motor cortex neurons to precisely controlled and ballistic movements, *Neurosci. Lett.*, 5 (1977) 256–265.
5. Hamada, I. and Kubota, K., Preparatory activity of monkey pyramidal tract neurons during visual tracking performance of single step, *J. physiol. Soc. Japan*, 39 (1977) 347.
6. Hamada, I. and Kubota, K., A mini-computer system (PDP-11/10) applied to analyze relations between single neuron activity and visual tracking performance. *Brain Theory News Lett.*, (1978) (in press).
7. Phillips, C.G., The Ferrier Lecture, 1968: Motor apparatus of the baboon's hand. *Proc. roy. Soc. B.*, 173 (1969) 141–174.

Corticospinal collateral actions on pontine nuclei of the cat

TOMOKAZU OSHIMA

Department of Neurobiology, Tokyo Metropolitan Institute for Neurosciences,
Fuchu, Tokyo 183, Japan

Many pontine nuclei (PN) cells receive an excitatory input from the collateral branches of pyramidal tract (PT) fibers[1]. This suggests that the "motor command" signal originating from the cerebral cortex is monitored to the cerebellum through PN. However, only the medullary pyramid (MP) was stimulated in our previous experiments[1] to test the action of PT collaterals. If the neural information carried by the corticofugal impulses be the "motor command", it should reach the motor apparatus in the spinal cord. This article describes an attempt to stimulate the fibers of the corticospinal tract (CST) at the C_2 level of the spinal cord in order to examine their collateral action on PN cells. A similar attempt has also been made on a relatively small sample of PN cells by Rüegg and Wiesendanger[2]. Employing a larger sample, the population of PN cells innervated by CST collaterals will be estimated below, together with measurements of the conduction velocity of CST fibers giving off these collaterals.

Cats were anesthetized with pentobarbital sodium (initial dose, 40 mg/kg i.p.), immobilized with gallamine triethiodide and artificially respirated. The experimental arrangement and procedure have been fully described in a previous paper[1]. As an additional technique the dorsolateral funiculus (DLF) of the cervical cord was stimulated with paired wire electrodes. A glass microelectrode filled with 2 M NaCl solution was inserted to record extracellular unit activities from a PN cell during stimulation of PT at the levels of the cerebral peduncle (CP), MP and DLF. The PN cell was antidromically identified as a projection neuron by stimulating the brachium pontis or regions near the interpositus and lateral nuclei.

A total of 92 PN cells was used. All were excited from CP. These cells were classified into three groups according to their response to stimulation of MP and DLF. Thirty-four cells (37%) could not be excited either from MP or DLF: these cells may be innervated only by the corticopontine fibers which terminate within the pons. Twenty cells (22%) received excitation only from MP: these cells are considered to represent the recipient of the collateral action of the PT fibers which terminate within the medulla and do not reach the spinal cord. The remaining 38 cells (41%) were excited from both MP and DLF: these cells would be capable of conveying the "motor command" to the spinal cord as well as to the cerebellum.

The excitatory connection from the CST to PN cells is proved to be monosynaptic. In Fig. 1, latency distribution histograms for stimulation to three different sites are presented according to distance (left scale; mm) along the course of corticofugal fibers. The upper histogram shows the distribution of the latency of excitation to CP stimulation. The scale for sample number is given on the right. The middle and lower histograms show the latencies from MP and DLF, respectively, employing the same scale. The base line of each histogram is positioned at the mean value of the distance (ordinate) from the recording site as origin (O) to the stimulated site. A minus sign on the ordinate indicates a position caudal to PN. Paired stimuli were used routinely to measure the

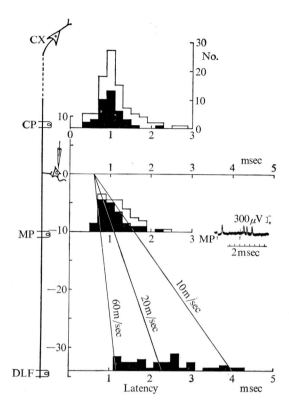

Fig. 1. Latency distribution histograms. For explanation, see text.

minimum value of the effective latency of unit firing (inset trace, *cf.* ref. 1). Filled columns in Fig. 1 show the population of PN cells excited from DLF, and open columns the other groups of cells. The latency varied considerably. Three straight lines are drawn to demonstrate the linear relationship between the latency and the conduction distance for representative fibers with fast (60 m/sec), intermediate (20 m/sec) and slow conduction velocities (10 m/sec). The wide range of these latencies thus indicates contribution of both fast and slow PT fibers to the collateral input on PN cells.

It is concluded that about 40% of PN cells receive a monosynaptic collateral input from fast and slow CST fibers.

REFERENCES

1. Allen, G.I., Korn, H., Oshima, T. and Toyama, K., The mode of synaptic linkage in the cerebro-ponto-cerebellar pathway of the cat. II. Responses of single cells in the pontine nuclei, *Exp. Brain Res.*, 24 (1975) 15–36.
2. Rüegg, D. and Wiesendanger, M., Corticofugal effects from sensorimotor area I and somatosensory area II on neurones of the pontine nuclei in the cat, *J. Physiol. (Lond.)*, 247 (1975) 745–757.

Automatic and reliable discrimination between simple and complex spikes of a cerebellar Purkinje cell

NORI-ICHI MANO AND KEN-ICHI YAMAMOTO*

Department of Neurophysiology, Tokyo Metropolitan Institute for Neurosciences, Fuchu, Tokyo 183, Japan

Automatic and reliable discrimination between simple and complex spikes generated by a cerebellar Purkinje cell (P-cell) is indispensable for analyses of P-cell activities using an electronic computer. Discrimination has been achieved in terms of the difference of amplitudes of the two sorts of spikes[1-3]. However, in many P-cells this method is often unreliable because of the small amplitude difference or the large fluctuation induced by background noise. We designed an improved discriminator based on the difference between the time courses of the two types of spikes[5].

Fig. 1 shows the principle (A), the block diagram (B) and the digital logic circuitry (C) of the discriminator. The logic circuitry was based on the K-series modules of DEC Inc. The procedure of the operation is as follows. 1) Trigger the oscilloscope sweep by a unitary spikes with a sweep speed fast enough (0.1–0.5 msec/div.) to catch all the simple and complex spikes. 2) The gain of the attenuator should be adjusted to make one division on the display of the oscilloscope exactly equal to one volt. Then a gain of 1.0 V/div. for reference voltages can always be used, regardless of AC input gain of the oscilloscope. This procedure is very convenient when the amplitude of the spikes gradually changes, because the only necessary operation is to adjust the AC input variable gain without readjustment of the two reference voltages (Ref. V. 1,2). 3) Find the largest difference of shape between the simple and complex spikes. Select a suitable delay (O.S. #1) and duration (O. S. #2) to open the AND GATE (1), so that the ref. volt. (1) is crossed while the GATE is open only by the complex spikes at the largest difference point, which is usually seen at the larger after-wave (Fig. 1A) or at the secondary spikes of the complex spike[4]. Thus, the output (1) gives a selectively transformed pulse of a complex spike. O.S. #3 and the counter (1) are not usually necessary, but are useful if one wants to select a complex spike with a certain number of secondary spikes. 4) The ref. volt. (2) should be set to slice all the simple spikes, but not the background noise level. A complex spike which crossed the ref. volt. (1) at the initial spike is blocked by the AND GATE 2 and only the simple spikes which cross ref. volt. (2) but not ref. volt. (1) can pass GATE 2. Thus, the output (2) gives a selectively transformed pulse of a simple spike. The counter (2) makes it possible to plot simple spikes of high frequency on a pen recorder of low frequency characteristics by dividing the frequency by two, four or eight. The delay of several milliseconds of simple spikes produced at O.S. #5 should be taken into consideration when data analyses are performed.

This discriminator is useful even when the amplitude difference between the two spikes is small or when the spike amplitudes fluctuate.

ACKNOWLEDGEMENTS: The basic idea for this type of discriminator was suggested by Dr. E.V. Evarts[5]. A part of this study was supported by a grant from the Ministry of Education of Japan.

* Present address: Division of Neurophysiology, Psychiatric Research Institute of Tokyo, 2–1–8, Kamikitazawa, Setagaya-ku, Tokyo 156, Japan

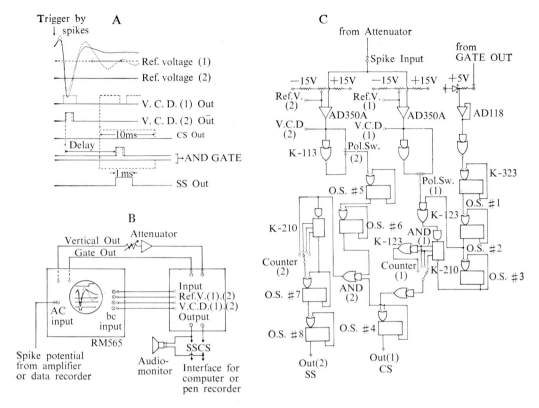

Fig. 1. The principle (A), the block diagram (B) and the digital logic circuitry (C) of the discriminator between simple and complex spikes of a P-cell. Two reference voltages and two outputs from the voltage crossing detector (V.C.D. 1,2) as well as the original spikes are monitored visually on the oscilloscope display. Final output pulses of simple and complex spikes are monitored with an audio-monitor.

REFERENCES

1. Ghelarducci, M.B., Ito, M. and Yagi, N., Impulse discharges from flocculus Purkinje cells of alert rabbits during visual stimulation combined with horizontal head rotation, *Brain Research*, 87 (1975) 66.
2. Gilbert, P.F.C. and Thach, W.T., Purkinje cell activity during motor learning, *Brain Research*, 128 (1977) 309.
3. Llinas, R. and Wolfe, J.W., Functional linkage between the electrical activity in the vermal cerebellar cortex and saccadic eye movements, *Exp. Brain Res.*, 29 (1977) 1.
4. Mano, N., Changes of simple and complex spike activity of cerebellar Purkinje cells with sleep and waking. *Science* 170 (1970) 1325.
5. Mano, N., Simple and complex spike activities of the cerebellar Purkinje cell in relation to selective alternate movement in intact monkey, *Brain Research*, 70, (1974) 381.

Cerebrocerebellar connections through the parvocellular part of the red nucleus

HIROSHI OKA AND KOHNOSUKE JINNAI

Department of Physiology, Institute for Brain Research, Faculty of Medicine, Kyoto University, Sakyo-ku, Kyoto 606, Japan

In our previous study[5], extracellular activities in the rostrolateral part of the red nucleus (RN) were explored in response to stimulation of the ipsilateral cerebral cortex, the contralateral cerebellar nucleus and the ipsilateral inferior olive in cats. Most of the neurons in this region were activated by stimulation of the parietal association cortex and the lateral cerebellar nucleus, but they hardly responded to stimulation of the frontal motor cortex and other cerebellar nuclei, fastigial and interpositus. Moreover, several of the neurons were identified as rubro-olivary ones with antidromically evoked response to inferior olive stimulation. On histological examination, these RN neurons were confirmed to be located in a fairly restricted area of the rostrolateral part of the nucleus. This area was mostly composed of relatively small-sized cells (cf. ref. 3). Based on their responsiveness to stimulation and their localization in the histological preparation, the neurons in the rostrolateral part of the RN could be identified as parvocellular RN neurons. In the present study, the effects of stimulus to or lesion of the parvocellular part of the RN were examined and analyzed in terms of cerebral-induced cerebellar responses.

The experiments were performed on eight cats under light anesthesia with sodium pentobarbital. Craniotomy was carried out to expose the cerebral hemisphere and the cerebellum. The superior colliculus was exposed after sucking out the overlying occipital lobe and the hippocampus. Bipolar stimulating electrodes were placed on the anterior sigmoid gyrus (frontal motor cortex) and the rostral portion of the middle suprasylvian gyrus (parietal association cortex). Concentric stimulating electrodes were introduced from the collicular surface to the rostrolateral part of the RN ipsilateral to the stimulated side of the cerebrum (see Fig. 1D) Through these electrodes brief pulse currents were delivered to the cerebral cortex or the parvocellular part of the RN. Recordings from the cerebellar cortex were made with gross surface electrodes using a silver ball. In other experiments, a thin cutting blade set in a frontal plane was advanced from the collicular surface to this RN part to form a lesion (see Fig. 1H), and the effects were observed upon the responses in the cerebellar cortex.

Stimulation of the rostrolateral part of the RN (R) as well as the parietal association (P) and frontal motor (F) cortices elicited markedly early mossy fiber (MF) and late climbing fiber (CF) responses in the contralateral paramedian lobule (Fig. 1A). The latency of R-evoked CF responses was about 12 msec, which is in accord with the results of Miller *et al.*[4] The latency of P-evoked CF responses was about 17 msec, about 3 msec longer than that of F-evoked CF responses. A similar difference in latencies was also seen in another experiment, shown in Fig. 1, E-F. Such a latency difference is consistent with the study of Sasaki *et al.*[6] As shown in Fig. 1B and C, P- or F-induced cerebellar responses were conditioned by R stimulation at various time intervals. The CF responses to P stimulation were almost completely suppressed by preceding R stimulation at an interval of about 57 msec, but those to F stimulation were only slightly affected (Fig. 1B).

184

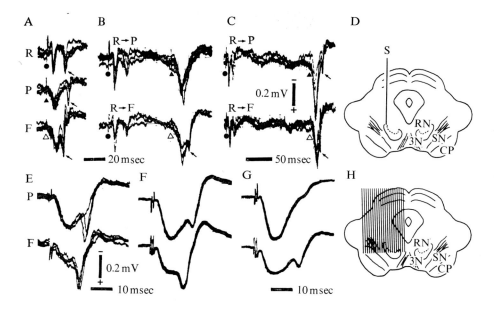

Fig. 1. Effects of stimulus (A–D) to and lesion (E–H) of the parvocellular part of the red nucleus upon cerebral-induced cerebellar responses. A: Sample and control records of cerebellar surface potentials upon stimulation of the rostrolateral part of the red nucleus (R), the parietal association (P) and frontal motor (F) cortices. B and C: Conditioning effects of R stimulation upon P- or F-induced cerebellar responses. Closed circles and closed and open triangles are placed below shock artifacts to R, P and F stimulations, respectively. Arrows indicate climbing fiber responses. For details see the text. 20 msec time scale for A and B, 50 msec for C. 0.2 mV calibration for all records. Three or four sweeps are superimposed in each frame. D: Location of a concentric stimulating electrode (S) in the midbrain presented schematically based on histological examination. E and F: Raw and averaged control records of cerebellar surface potentials on stimulation of the parietal (P) and frontal (F) cortices before lesion of the midbrain. G: Averaged records of the potentials after lesion. For further details, see the text. 10 msec time scale for all records and 0.2 mV calibration for E. 20 consecutive sweeps of cerebellar surface potentials are averaged in F and G. H: Location of a lesion in the midbrain indicated schematically by the shaded area with vertical lines, according to histological analysis. RN, red nucleus; SN, substantia nigra; CP, cerebral peduncle; 3N, oculomotor nerve.

Eoth CF responses recovered from the suppression to the control levels in about 152 msec (Fig. 1C). Such suppression occurred in most cases from about 20 msec to 130 msec after the preceding R stimulation. The suppressions are similar in nature to those in the inferior olive reported by Armstrong and Harvey[2]. The results mentioned above appear to indicate that the CF responses to P stimulation are relayed mostly through the rubro-olivary pathway originating in the rostrolateral part of the RN and that the CF responses to F stimulation are also conveyed partially through this pathway. When conditioned by R stimulation, MF responses to P or F stimulation were markedly enhanced for a long period (Fig. 1, B and C). These enhancements of MF responses should be investigated in detail, as frequency potentiation of the pontine nuclei potentials was reported by Allen *et al.*[1]

In order to clarify further the involvement of the rostrolateral part of the RN in cerebral-induced CF responses, the effects of lesion in this part were examined, as shown in Fig. 1, E-H. Fig. 1 E and F show, respectively, raw and averaged control records of cerebellar responses to parietal (P) and frontal (F) cortex stimulations before lesion of the midbrain. The recording site was in the contralateral paramedian lobule. The cutting blade was advanced to a depth of 10.5 mm from the collicular surface and then drawn up. Fig. 1 G shows averaged records of cerebellar responses after this procedure. The P-induced CF response almost disappeared, but the F-induced CF response was still well preserved. It should be noted here that the MF responses induced by both P and F stimulations were actually unchanged after lesion in this area. These findings support the view that the P-induced CF responses are conveyed mostly through the rubro-olivary pathway originating in and/or around the parvocellular part of the RN and that the F-induced CF responses are also transmitted to some extent through the pathway.

The present results suggest, in association with our previous results , that the parietal association area and the lateral cerebellar nucleus activate the rubro-olivary pathway at the parvocellular part of the RN. On the other hand, at the magnocellular part, the frontal motor area and the interpositus nucleus are predominant in acting on the rubro-spinal pathway.

References

1. Allen, G.I., Korn, H. and Oshima, T., The mode of synaptic linkage of the cerebro-ponto-cerebellar pathway of the cat. I. Responses in the brachium pontis, *Exp. Brain Res.*, 24 (1975) 1–14.
2. Armstrong, D.M. and Harvey, R.J., Responses in the inferior olive to stimulation of the cerebellar and cerebral cortices in the cat, *J. Physiol. (Lond.)*, 187 (1966) 553–574.
3. Berman, A.L., *The brain stem of the cat. A Cytoarchitectonic Atlas with Stereotaxic Coordinates*, University of Wisconsin Press, Madison, 1968, Plates 40 and 69.
4. Miller, S., Nezlina, N. and Oscarsson, O., Climbing fiber projection to cerebellar anterior lobe activated from structures in midbrain and from spinal cord, *Brain Research*, 14 (1969) 234–236.
5. Oka, H. and Jinnai, K., Electrophysiological study of parvocellular red nucleus neurons, *Brain Research*, 149 (1978) 239–246.
6. Sasaki, K., Oka, H., Matsuda, Y., Shimono, T. and Mizuno, N., Electrophysiological studies of the projection from the parietal association area to the cerebellar cortex, *Exp. Brain Res.*, 23 (1975) 91–102.

Neuronal circuits of cerebro-cerebellar interactions

KAZUO SASAKI, KOHNOSUKE JINNAI AND HISAE GEMBA

Department of Physiology, Institute for Brain Research, Faculty of Medicine, Kyoto University, Sakyo-ku, Kyoto 606, Japan

Electrophysiological studies on cerebro-cerebellar interconnections in cats have revealed that reciprocal innervations exist between the frontal motor cortex and the anterior lobe of the cerebellum and between the parietal association cortex and the posterior lobe of the cerebellum, respectively[5,6,7]. The cerebellar efferents originating from the lateral and interpositus nuclei project not only onto the motor cortex via the lateral ventral thalamic nucleus (as had been well known) but also onto the parietal association cortex (mainly area 5[3]) through the anterior ventral thalamic nucleus and its vicinities[5,6]. The parietal association area sends mossy fiber inputs back to the posterior lobe of the cerebellum via particular pontine nucleus neurons which are mostly different from those mediating mossy fiber volleys from the motor cortex to the anterior lobe of the cerebellum[4,7]. In the present study, cerebro-cerebellar interconnections were investigated electrophysiologically in monkeys as had been done in cats, since the posterior lobe of the cerebellum is far more developed in monkeys in connection with the motor and the association cortices than in cats.

Monkeys (*Macaca mulatta*, *M. iris* and *M. fuscata*) were first anesthetized with ketamin chloride and later with pentobarbital sodium which was administered intermittently during the experiments. In one group of experiments, the effects of stimulating various areas of the cerebral cortex were examined in the cerebellar cortex and shown to be due to mossy fiber and/or climbing fiber volleys by laminar field potential analysis with parallel fiber stimulation in the cerebellar cortex (see Eccles *et al.*[2]). In another group of experiments, stimulation of the medial, interpositus and lateral cerebellar nuclei was performed and the effects induced thereby were examined in different parts of the cerebral cortex. In some experiments, stimulating electrodes were also introduced in various thalamic nuclei in order to study the relay mechanism of the thalamic nuclei in the cerebello-cerebral projections. The sites of the stimulating electrodes in the cerebellar and thalamic nuclei were always checked histologically after the electrophysiological studies. The results are shown schematically in Fig. 1.

Stimulation of the motor cortex (area 4) and the parietal association area (area 5) induced mossy fiber and climbing fiber responses mainly in the anterior lobe of the cerebellum. Certain relationships were found between the somatotopical arrangement of the motor cortex and that of the anterior lobe of the cerebellum as reported previously[1,8], i.e., the medial part of the motor cortex (hindlimb area) projects predominantly on the rostral part of the anterior lobe and the lateral part (forelimb area) projects mainly to the caudal part of the anterior lobe, respectively. Besides the projection on the anterior lobe, the lateral part of the motor cortex (forelimb area) (4L) sends strong influences to the posterior lobe of the cerebellum (crus I, crus II and paramedian lobules) through mossy and climbing fiber systems (see upper diagram). The effects of stim-

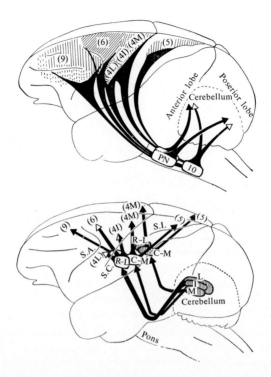

Fig. 1.   Schematical illustration of cerebro-cerebellar (upper diagram) and cerebello-cerebral (lower diagram) projections in monkeys. Numbers in the diagrams indicate cortical areas. In the upper diagram, the arrows in the cerebellum with filled and open triangles represent mossy and climbing fiber inputs, respectively. In the lower diagram, the arrows to the cerebral cortex with filled and open triangles represent deep (EPSP terminals in the deeper cortical layers) and superficial (EPSP terminals in the superficial cortical layer) thalamo-cortical projections, respectively. PN, Pontine nuclei; IO, inferior olive; L, I, and M, lateral, interpositus, and medial cerebellar nucleus; S.C., sulcus centralis; S.I., sulcus intraparietalis; S.A., sulcusarcuatus.

ulating the motor cortex were more marked on the contralateral than the ipsilateral cerebellar cortex.

Stimulation of the premotor cortex (area 6) induced mossy and climbing fiber responses not only in the anterior lobe but also in the posterior lobe, particularly in crus I. These responses were found more bilaterally than in the case of the motor cortex. Stimulation of the frontal association cortex (mainly area 9) elicited mossy and climbing fiber responses over even wider areas of the cerebellar cortex, especially in the posterior lobe. The main projection of the parietal association area (area 5) went to the anterior lobe and was similar to that of the medial and intermediate parts of the motor cortex.

The effects of stimulating the three cerebellar nuclei were explored in various areas of the cerebral cortex. They were examined by laminar field potential analysis in the cortex, as summarized in the lower diagram of Fig. 1. Stimulation of the medial nucleus (M) induced deep thalamo-cortical (T-C) responses in the medial part of the motor cortex (area 4) (4M) and the parietal association cortex (area 5) on both sides. Lateral nucleus stimulation evoked superficial T-C responses in the lateral part of the motor cortex (area 4) (mainly the forelimb area) (4L) and the premotor cortex (area 6) on the contralateral side. Interpositus nucleus stimulation evoked superficial T-C responses in the intermediate part of the motor cortex (area 4) (mainly the truncal area) (4I) and the premotor cortex (area 6) on the contralateral side. In addition to these effects on the motor and premotor cortices, stimulation of the lateral cerebellar nucleus was found to provoke deep T-C responses in the frontal association cortex (area 9) on the contralateral side.

The results of the present study reveal several interesting features in the cerebro-cerebellar interconnections of monkeys. The cerebellum sends influences back to both the motor cortex and the association cortex just as had been found in cats[5,6]. However, in monkeys, the cerebellum projects not only on the parietal association area but also on the frontal association area. The well developed premotor area in monkeys also receives cerebellar influences, particularly from the lateral part of the cerebellum, i.e., the neocerebellum. Furthermore, the lateral part of the motor cortex (mainly the forelimb area) in monkeys is intimately interconnected with the neocerebellum and is considered to have dual characteristics as motor and association cortices. This suggests that the enormously developed neocerebellum of primates plays an important role in controlling the forelimbs, especially the fine movements of the hands. On the other hand, the medial part of the cerebellum may be more closely related with control of the hindlimbs and the intermediate part of the cerebellum with that of the trunk.

The present study reveals a marked difference between monkeys and cats in the interconnections between the neocerebellum and the cerebral corex. The functional meaning of this difference will be exmined in future investigations.

REFERENCES

1. Adrian, E.D., Afferent areas in the cerebellum connected with the limbs, *Brain*, 66 (1943) 289–316.
2. Eccles, J.C., Sasaki, K. and Strata, P., Interpretation of the potential fields generated in the cerebellar cortex by a mossy fibre volley, *Exp. Brain Res.*, 3 (1967) 68–80.
3. Hassler, R. and Muhs-Clement, K., Architektonischer Aufbau des sensorimotorischen und parietalen Cortex der Katze, *J. Hirnforsch.*, 6 (1964) 377–420.
4. Oka, H., Sasaki, K., Matsuda, Y., Yasuda, T. and Mizuno, N., Responses of pontocerebellar neurones to stimulation of the parietal association and the frontal motor cortices, *Brain Research*, 93 (1975) 399–407.
5. Sasaki, K., Kawaguchi, S., Matsuda, Y. and Mizuno, N., Electrophysiological studies on cerebello-cerebral projections in the cat, *Exp. Brain Res.*, 16 (1972) 75–88.
6. Sasaki, K., Matsuda, Y., Kawaguchi, S. and Mizuno, N., On the cerebello-thalamo-cerebral pathways for the parietal cortex, *Exp. Brain Res.*, 16 (1972) 89–103.
7. Sasaki, K., Oka, H., Matsuda, Y., Shimono, T. and Mizuno, N., Electrophysiological studies of the projections from the parietal association area to the cerebellar cortex, *Exp. Brain Res.*, 23 (1975) 91–102.
8. Snider, R.S. and Eldred, E., Cerebro-cerebellar relationship in the monkey, *J. Neurophysiol.*, 15 (1952) 27–40.

The distribution of cerebellar projection neurons in the spinal cord of the cat, as studied by retrograde transport of horseradish peroxidase

MATSUO MATSUSHITA, YASUHIKO HOSOYA AND MICHIKO IKEDA*

Department of Anatomy, Institute of Basic Medical Sciences, University of Tsukuba,
Niihari-gun, Ibaraki 300–31, Japan, and
*Department of Anatomy, Kansai Medical School,
Moriguichi, Osaka 570, Japan

The ventral and the dorsal spinocerebellar tracts (VSCT and DSCT) are well known as pathways which transmit the proprioceptive as well as exteroceptive input from the periphery, especially from the hindlimb levels to the cerebellum (see refs. 7,8). Physiological studies have introduced the rostral spinocerebellar tract (RSCT) as the functional forelimb equivalent of the VSCT[7,8]. Although there are many reports of physiological studies on the function of the spinocerebellar tracts, a relatively few anatomical studies have appeared dealing with the cells of origin of these tracts[2,6,9,10,13].

In the present study we injected horseradish peroxidase (HRP) into the cerebellum, including the central nuclei and the surrounding white matter, in 30 cats, in order to identify all types of spinocerebellar tract neurons. Labeled neurons appeared bilaterally, and their distribution was mapped in the entire length of the spinal cord (Fig. 1). In 11 cases out of the total, the injections were preceded by hemisection at various cervical levels (C1, C2, C5, or C6) to find the ascending side of the axons within the spinal cord.

All the neurons of the central cervical nucleus (CCN) were labeled from the level of the spinomedullary junction to C4 (Fig. 1C1 and C3-CCN). Dorsal to the CCN, there was a group of labeled medium-sized neurons in the medial part of lamina VI from C2 to T1 (Fig. 1 thin arrows). In the cervical enlargement, three groups of labeled neurons appeared. The first, composed of neurons as large as motoneurons or medium-sized neurons, was located in the central to the lateral part of lamina VII from C6 to T1, being most developed at C7 to T1 (Fig. 1C7). The second group, which consisted of medium-sized neurons, was found in the lateral part of lamina V or the border region between laminae V and VI (Fig. 1C7 and T1). It was present throughout the thoracic cord and the first five lumbar segments. There were a few labeled neurons of medium-size in the medial part of lamina VII of C5 to T1 and scattered labeled neurons in lamina VIII of all cervical segments. In the thoracic cord both large and medium-sized neurons were labeled in Clarke's column and a very limited number of small neurons were also labeled. The great majority of the labeled neurons in lamina V were medium-sized, and a very few large ones were seen in the lower thoracic and lumbar segments (Fig. 1T4 and L3). Some were not confined to lamina V but were displaced ventral to lamina IV, or dorsal or lateral to the intermediolateral nucleus (ILN). From T10 to L6 neurons of the motoneuron type (spinal border cells) were labeled in the intermediate zone to the ventral horn and along the lateral or ventrolateral cord (Fig. 1SBC). Rostrally they were well localized to the lateral part (Fig. 1L3-SBC). They increased in number considerably in more caudal segments, and were distributed medially in the central to the lateral part of the inter-

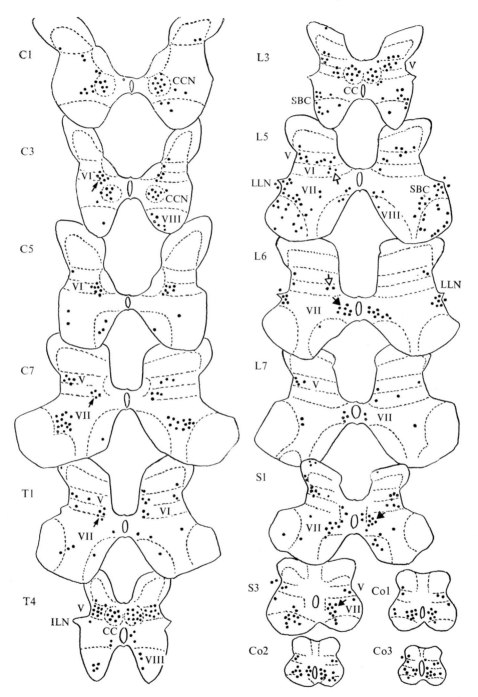

Fig. 1. Diagram showing the distribution of labeled neurons following injections of HRP into the cerebellum. CC, Clarke's column; CCN, central cervical nucleus; LLN, lateral lumbar nucleus; SBC, spinal border cells.

mediate zone and in the ventrolateral part of the ventral horn. In L5 and L6 there was a process of the gray matter which protruded into the lateral cord; the labeled neurons localized in this area, termed the "lateral lumbar nucleus" (Fig. 1L5 and L6-LLN) were smaller than the medially distributed ones. In the medial part of lamina VI at L5 and L6 a small number of large neurons were labeled (Fig. 1L5 and L6, open arrows), with a few displaced medially in lamina V. In L6 and L7 a group of labeled medium-sized or large neurons was consistently found lateral to the central canal, and others belonging to a similar category were encountered at the corresponding site in the sacral to coccygeal cord (Fig. 1L6 and S3, thick arrows). In the sacro-coccygeal cord labeled neurons were observed in three major locations; the lateral part of the base of the dorsal horn, which included medium-sized or giant multipolar neurons, the medial part of lamina VII (lateral to the central canal), and the ventral horn. The neurons of the latter were as large as motoneurons, and more frequent from S2 to the coccygeal cord.

The ascending side of the axons of these neurons was studied in cases with hemisections at the cervical levels. The CCN and scattered lamina VIII neurons were found to give rise to crossed axons while the medial lamina VI group of C2 to T1 (thin arrows) and the lamina VII group of the cervical enlargement gave rise to uncrossed axons. Axons of the lamina V neurons and Clarke neurons were exclusively uncrossed. Large neurons of the medial lamina VI of L5 and L6 (open arrows) also gave rise to uncrossed axons. The axons of the spinal border cells were completely crossed. However, no neurons were found in lamina V, with crossed axons projecting to the cerebellum in L5 and L6. The medial lamina VII neurons of L6 and those in more caudal segments, and other neurons in the sacro-coccygeal cord gave rise principally to crossed ascending axons.

In the present study the cells of origin of the spinocerebellar tracts were identified by means of retrograde axonal transport of HRP. They formed distinct groups and their occurrence was consistent. In addition to the CCN[2,6,9,13], two major groups were found in the cervical cord to project to the cerebellum; one was the group of the medial lamina VI, corresponding to Stilling's cervical nucleus in earlier descriptions[4,11,12] or to the centrobasilar nucleus[9,10]. Contrary to previous reports,[9,10] it existed from C2 to T1. Another group was that present in the central part of lamina VII of C7 to T1. Hirai et al.[3] found that this group consisted of two types of neurons, which were either excited or inhibited by the peripheral input. The RSCT has been considered to be a functional forelimb equivalent of the VSCT. However, the spinocerebellar tract arising from the cervical cord is never single, as demonstrated by the present study, and the cells of origin fulfilling the criteria of the RSCT seem to constitute only a proportion of the neuronal groups found in the cervical cord[3,5]. It is of particular interest that the neurons of the lateral lamina V of the thoracic and the lumbar cord project to the cerebellum via the ipsilateral ascending axons. Such projections have not been reported previously. Large to medium-sized neurons in the medial part of lamina VI of L5 and L6, which are distinct from the Clarke neurons, correspond to those identified physiologically[1]. Most of the labeled neurons in the lumbar cord gave rise to crossed ascending axons: these are the spinal border cells (the cells of origin of VSCT), the medial lamina VII neurons in the lumbosacral cord, which might be Stilling's lumbar and sacral nucleus[12], the neurons in the base of the dorsal horn and those in the ventral horn of the sacro-coccygeal cord.

The present study has shown that there are multiple groups of spinocerebellar tract neurons which have thus far not been reported and that they are present from the level of the spinomedullary junction to the coccygeal cord, projecting to the cerebellum through either crossed or uncrossed tracts. The relationship between the neurons and their projection areas in the cerebellum is now being studied.

REFERENCES

1. Aoyama, M., Hongo, T. and Kudo, N., An uncrossed ascending tract originating from below Clarke's column and conveying group I impulses from the hindlimb muscles in the cat, *Brain Research*, 62 (1973) 237–241.
2. Cummings, J.F. and Petras, J.M., The origin of spinocerebellar pathways. I. The nucleus cervicalis centralis of the cranial cervical spinal cord, *J. comp. Neurol.*, 173 (1977) 655–692.
3. Hirai, N., Hongo, T., Kudo, N. and Yamaguchi, T., Heterogeneous composition of the spinocerebellar tract originating from the cervical enlargement in the cat, *Brain Research*, 109 (1976) 387–391.
4. Jacobsohn, L., Ueber die Kerne des Rückenmarkes, *Neurol. Zentralblatt*, 27 (1908) 617–626.
5. MacKay, W.A. and Murphy, J.T., Responses of interpositus neurons to passive muscle stretch, *J. Neurophysiol.*, 37 (1974) 1410–1423.
6. Matsushita, M. and Ikeda, M., The central cervical nucleus as cell origin of a spinocerebellar tract arising from the cervical cord: a study in the cat using horseradish peroxidase, *Brain Research*, 100 (1975) 412–417.
7. Oscarsson, O., Functional organization of the spinocerebellar and cuneocerebellar tracts, *Physiol. Rev.*, 45 (1965) 495–522.
8. Oscarsson, O., Functional organization of spinocerebellar paths. In A. Iggo (Ed.) *Handbook of Sensory Physiology, Vol. 2, Somatosensory System*, Springer, Berlin, 1973, pp. 340–380.
9. Petras, J.M., Spinocerebellar neurons in the rhesus monkey, *Brain Research*, 130 (1977) 146–151.
10. Petras, J.M. and Cummings, J.F., The origin of spinocerebellar pathways. II. The nucleus centrobasalis of the cervical enlargement and the nucleus dorsalis of the thoracolumbar spinal cord, *J. comp. Neurol.*, 173 (1977) 693–716.
11. Reed, A.F., The nuclear masses in the cervical spinal cord of *Macaca mulatta*, *J. comp. Neurol.*, 72 (1940) 187–206.
12. Stilling, B., *Neue Untersuchungen über den Bau des Rückenmarks* (5 Vols), Hotop, Cassel, 1859, pp. 1192.
13. Wiksten, B., The central cervical nucleus—a source of spinocerebellar fibres, demonstrated by retrograde transport of horseradish peroxidase, *Neurosci. Lett.*, 1 (1975) 81–84.

Electrophysiological analysis of neuronal circuit in the cerebellar cortex of rolling mouse Nagoya

TADAO OHNO AND SHIGETO SASAKI

Department of Physiology, Institute of Basic Medical Sciences, The University of Tsukuba,
Niihari-gun, Ibaraki 300–31, Japan

Rolling mouse Nagoya (RMN) is a mutant mouse characterized by severe gait disturbance. This mouse was first found by Oda in the course of mating experiments between S III and C57 BL/6J Nga mice. Its condition is determined by an autosomal recessive gene[5]. Homozygotes (*rol/ rol*) are distinguishable from their littermates by 10 to 14 days after birth. When the mouse walks, its gait is usually interrupted every few steps by a lurching motion and it frequently falls over to one side or the other. The symptoms are more evident in the hindlimbs than in the forelimbs. We analyzed the locomotor movements of the hindlimb cinematographically, and found that stepping in RMN does not show any clear reproducible pattern and limb movement is not coordinated, whereas the step cycle of the normal mouse exhibits a regular pattern comprising a series of four phases (the F, E_1, E_2 and E_3 phases)[3]. For example, in RMN, just after one hindlimb leaves the ground, the ankle joint begins to flex excessively, while the knee and hip joints remain overextended. When the hindlimb is brought down, the ankle, instead of the toes, is the first to contact the ground. At rest, the limbs and trunk are slightly flaccid. Tremor is not observed.

Histological abnormalities have been found in the cerebellar anterior lobe of RMN, where the total number of granule cells, basket cells and stellate cells is reduced to about 60% of the normal value[4]. Furthermore, histofluorescence analysis has shown increases in the number and fluorescence intensity of noradrenaline nerve terminals in the cerebellum and in the entire cerebral cortex[1]. In the cerebellum, the increase is more distinct in the anterior lobe.

Since the symptoms of RMN are likely to be of cerebellar origin and histological abnormalities have been found in the cerebellum, we compared the functional connections in the mossy fiber-granule cell–Purkinje cell pathway and the effect of inhibitory neurons in RMN with those of the normal mouse.

Mice were anesthetized with Nembutal (25 mg/kg, intraperitoneally) and ventilated artificially. Field potentials were recorded from the cerebellar anterior lobe with glass micropipettes filled with 2 M NaCl. The white matter at the central part of the cerebellum was stimulated with a bipolar electrode (WM), and parallel fibers on the surface were stimulated with a concentric electrode (LOC) placed on the cortical surface several hundred microns apart from the point of microelectrode insertion (see Fig. 1A). Responses recorded in normal mice were regarded as the control. In the normal mouse (Fig. 1A), stimulation of WM evoked P_1–N_1 waves in the granular layer which are due to antidromic conduction of impulses along Purkinje cell axons and orthodromic conduction along afferent fibers[2]. P_1–N_1 waves were also recorded in the upper part of the molecular layer, indicating that the antidromic impulses in Purkinje cell axons can invade into the dendrites of Purkinje cells. Following the N_1 wave, N_2–P_2 waves were obtained in the granular layer, N_2 being generated by the current flow resulting from the excitatory synaptic action of mossy fibers onto granule and Golgi cells and P_2 being due to propagation of granule cell dis-

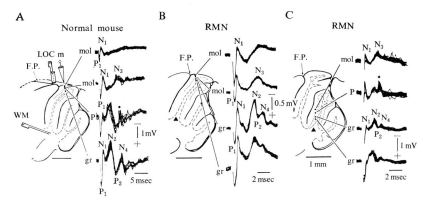

Fig. 1.   Field potentials evoked by stimulation of the white matter (WM) at the central part of the cerebellum. A, Records from a normal mouse. B and C, Records from different RMNs. ▲ in B and C indicate the positions of the tips of WM electrodes. Layers from which records were obtained (dots in the inset drawings) are indicated at the left side of the records. mol, Molecular layer. P, Purkinje cell layer. gr, Granular layer. ◆, Spike firings of a Purkinje cell. Calibrations and time scales are shown for each set of records. LOC, Concentric electrode placed on the surface of the anterior lobe. m, Glass microelectrode. F.P., Fissura prima.

charge into the molecular layer and the following excitation of Purkinje cells. In the molecular layer, N_3 wave was recorded as a sink for P_2[2]. When Purkinje cells fired, spike discharges were seen in the Purkinje cell layer and N_4 wave was recorded in the granular layer[2]. Thus, in the normal mouse, there are functional excitatory connections in the mossy fiber-granule cell-Purkinje cell pathway, just as in cat cerebellum[2]. Field potentials obtained from RMN (Fig. 1B and C) were composed of basically the same component waves as those observed in the normal mouse, indicating that the basic connections in the mossy fiber–granule cell–Purkinje cell pathway are present in RMN. Furthermore, both in RMN and in the normal mouse, the amplitude of N_1 and P_2 waves induced by WM stimulation was reduced by conditioning LOC stimulation. This result indicates that inhibition of Purkinje cells by basket cells and inhibition of granule cells by Golgi cells exist in RMN as well as in the normal mouse[2].

In summary, the basic excitatory connections in the mossy fiber–granule cell–Purkinje cell pathway and the inhibitory action of basket and Golgi cells exist in the cerebellum of RMN as they do in the normal mouse. A quantitative difference in these basic circuits or some involvement of other parts of the central nervous system may explain the motor disorders of RMN.

ACKNOWLEDGEMENTS: We wish to thank Dr. S. Oda for providing rolling mouse Nagoya and Miss M. Shibanuma for her technical assistance.

REFERENCES

1. Adachi, K., Sobue, I., Tohyama, M. and Shimizu, N., Changes in the cerebellar noradrenaline nerve terminals of the neurological murine mutant rolling mouse Nagoya: A histofluorescence analysis, *Neurobiol. Neurophysiol.*, 3 (1975) 329–330.
2. Eccles, J.C., Ito, M. and Szentágothai, J., *The Cerebellum as a Neuronal Machine*, Springer, Berlin-Heidelberg-New York, 1967, pp. 116–155.
3. Grillner, S., Locomotion in vertebrates: Central mechanisms and reflex interaction, *Physiol. Rev.*, 55 (1975) 247–304.
4. Nishimura, Y., The cerebellum of rolling mouse Nagoya, *Advanc. Neurol. Sci.* (*Japan*), 19 (1975) 58–60.
5. Oda, S., The observation of rolling mouse Nagoya (*rol*), a new neurological mutant, and its maintenance, *Exp. Anim.* (Japan), 22 (1973) 281–288.

Antidromic responses of thalamic VL neurons to cortical stimulation in cats

MASATAKE UNO, NOBUYUKI OZAWA AND KEN-ICHI YAMAMOTO

Psychiatric Research Institute of Tokyo,
Setagaya-ku, Tokyo 156, Japan

The ventrolateral nucleus of the thalamus (VL) is situated as a relay for both cerebellar and pallidal afferents destined for the motor cortex[1,3,5–8]. Physiological studies have shown that VL neurons receive excitatory afferents from cerebellar nuclei and send axons into the precruciate cortex in the cat[6,8]. On the other hand, the pallidothalamic pathway arising from the entopeduncular nucleus (ENT, the feline homolog of the medial segment of the globus pallidus) exerts an inhibitory influence monosynaptically on the neurons located in the rostromedial part of the VL-VA complex, but not on VL relay cells of the cerebello–thalamo–cortical pathway[9]. The present study was undertaken to determine whether these rostromedial VL neurons also terminate in the motor cortex.

Experiments were conducted on cats anesthetized with pentobarbital sodium (35 mg/kg). The ipsilateral ENT was stimulated with 6 tungsten electrodes insulated except for the very tip, and the contralateral brachium conjunctivum (BC) with 2 electrodes. Stimulation of the motor cortex was effected through an array of 6 tungsten electrodes, cemented together in a mediolateral plane at 1.5 mm intervals and placed inside the precruciate cortex at a depth of 1.5 mm. Stimulus pulses (0.08–0.1 msec, 50–400 μA) were applied with a constant current stimulator between two neighboring poles. For extracellular recordings, glass micropipettes filled with 2 M NaCl saturated with Fast Green FCF were inserted into the VL-VA region of the thalamus and the recording positions in the thalamus were identified in each animal by reference to spots of dye deposited electrophoretically from the electrode tip.

Stimulation of ENT evokes field potentials consisting of an initial positive-negative spike followed by a relatively slow positivity in the rostromedial portion of the VL-VA complex. These potentials are explicable, at least in part, by the sequential occurrence of impulses in the excited entopeduncular fibers and focal potentials of VL-VA neurons inhibited by the former[10]. Thirty–seven cells were recorded within the rostromedial VL region so determined and confirmed later by histological examination. They were identified as VL cells receiving pallidal afferents by suppression of spontaneous discharges for about 20 msec after ENT stimulation (Fig. 1A). In 28 of the cells, the antidromic response was obtained from one or two of the 6 electrodes in the precruciate gyrus with a stimulus strength less than 200 μA. Action potentials of negative or positive-negative polarity were considered to indicate antidromic activation of the cell if (1) they occurred at a constant latency with suprathreshold stimulus intensities and showed no more than 0.1 msec latency variation with the stimulus intensity straddling threshold, and (2) they followed each stimulus of double shocks delivered at intervals of less than 2.0 msec. Figs. 1B, C show action potentials excited antidromically with a latency of 3.5 msec from the precruciate cortex in the same cell as in Fig. 1A with threshold stimulus strength (1B) and suprathreshold double shock stimuli (1C). The antidromic latency in the 28 cells ranged from 1.2–4.1 msec (mean, 2.86 msec; S.D., 0.92 msec).

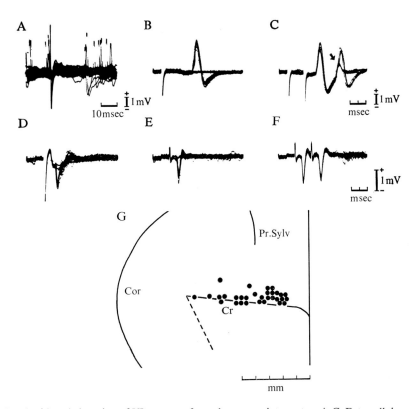

Fig. 1. Antidromic invasion of VL neurons from the precruciate cortex. A-C, Extracellular records from a rostromedial VL neuron. A, Spontaneous discharges were suppressed after ENT stimulation; B, action potentials evoked in an all-or-none manner by stimuli straddling the threshold to the precruciate cortex; C, a spike follows each of the suprathreshold double shocks at 2 msec intervals. The oblique arrow marks an inflection of the spike rising phase indicating a step conduction from the initial segment to the cell soma. D-F, Records from a caudodorsal VL relay cell. D, Action potentials evoked orthodromically by BC stimulation; E, F, antidromic responses to single (E) and double shock stimuli (F) to the cortex. G, Rostrodorsal aspect of the left pericruciate gyrus showing a projection area of rostromedial VL cells which received pallidal afferents. The plotted points represent the positions from which antidromic spikes were invaded with a threshold stimulus intensity of <200 μA. Cr, Cruciate sulcus; Cor, coronal sulcus; Pr. Sylv, presylvian sulcus.

As reported elsewhere[8,10], orthodromic excitation of action potentials by BC stimulation was observed in 69 cells located in the caudal VL. Of these, 52 cells responded to cortical stimulation. Figs. ID-F show spike potentials evoked with a latency of 1.4 msec after BC stimulation (1D) and those activated antidromically with a latency of 0.9 msec from the precruciate gyrus (1E,F). The antidromic latency in the 52 relay cells ranged from 0.8–2.9 msec (mean, 1.41 msec; S.D., 0.46 msec), which is significantly shorter than that obtained in the rostromedial VL neurons.

The site of termination of the thalamocortical projection from the rostromedial VL which receives pallidal afferents, was explored with the 6 needles implanted in the precruciate gyrus. Brief pulses of amplitude 50–400 μA were applied in turn between the two neighboring poles. The antidromic response was obtained from only one electrode in 25 cells and from two in 3 other cells with a stimulus strength of < 200 μA. Fig. 1G illustrates the frequency of occurrence of antidromic activation for these cells on the rostrodorsal aspect of the pericruciate gyrus. Clearly, the plotted points are scattered over the medial and middle parts of the precruciate gyrus, particularly the former. On the other hand, relay cells of the cerebello-thalamo-cortical pathway were activated rather from the lateral and middle parts of the gyrus (not illustrated).

The present study demonstrates that rostromedial VL neurons receive inhibitory afferents from ENT, the efferent neurons of basal ganglia, and send projections mainly to the medial precruciate gyrus. Physiological and anatomical studies on the representation of body parts on the surface of the cat motor cortex indicate that the axial part is represented within the region corresponding to area 6 on the medial part of the precruciate gyrus[2,7,11]. Certain clinical observations and experimental studies suggest that basal ganglia are particularly important in controlling postures[4]. The present results indicate therefore that separate functional zones exist in the VL for the control of postural adjustments and for movements of the extremities, as several authors have suggested[6,7], and that the rostromedial VL is mostly responsible for the former.

References

1. Cohen, D., Chambers, W.W. and Sprague, J.M., Experimental study of the efferent projections from the cerebellar nuclei to the brainstem of the cat, *J. comp. Neurol.*, 109 (1958) 233–259.
2. Hassler, R. und Muhs-Clement, K., Architektonischer Aufbau des sensomotorischen und parietalen Cortex der Katze, *J. Hirnforsch.*, 6 (1964) 377–420.
3. Kim, R., Nakano, K., Jayaraman, A. and Carpenter, M.B., Projections of the globus pallidus and adjacent structures: an autoradiographic study in the monkey, *J. comp. Neurol.*, 169 (1976) 263–289.
4. Martin, J.P., *The Basal Ganglia and Posture*, Pitman Medical, London, 1967, 149 pp.
5. Nauta, W.J.H. and Mehler, W.R., Projections of the lentiform nucleus in the monkey, *Brain Research*, 1 (1966) 3–42.
6. Rispal-Padel, L., Massion, J. and Grangetto, A., Relations between the ventrolateral thalamic nucleus and motor cortex and their possible role in the central organization of motor control, *Brain Research*, 60 (1973) 1–20.
7. Strick, P.L., Light microscopic analysis of the cortical projection of the thalamic ventrolateral nucleus in the cat, *Brain Research*, 55 (1973) 1–24.
8. Uno, M., Yoshida, M. and Hirota, I., The mode of cerebellothalamic relay transmission investigated with intracellular recording from cells of the ventrolateral nucleus of cat's thalamus, *Exp. Brain Res.*, 10 (1970) 121–139.
9. Uno, M. and Yoshida, M., Monosynaptic inhibition of thalamic neurons produced by stimulation of the pallidal nucleus in cats, *Brain Research*, 99 (1975) 377–380.
10. Uno, M., Ozawa, N. and Yoshida, M., The mode of pallido-thalamic transmission investigated with intracellular recording from cat thalamus, *Exp. Brain Res.*, (in press).
11. Woolsey, C.N., Organization of somatic sensory and motor areas of the cerebral cortex. In H.F. Harlow and C.N. Woolsey (Eds.), *Biological and Biochemical Bases of Behavior*, Univ. of Wisconsin Press, Madison, 1958, pp. 63–81.

Clinicophysiological studies of ocular movement in Parkinson's disease

HIROSHI SHIBASAKI AND SADATOSHI TSUJI

*Department of Neurology, Neurological Institute, Faculty of Medicine, Kyushu University,
Higashi-ku, Fukuoka 812, Japan*

Basal ganglia are believed to participate in the control of ocular movement, but the precise mechanism is poorly undertsood. Idiopathic Parkinson's disease is the most common degenerative disease of basal ganglia, involving primarily the dopaminergic nigro-striatal system. Although ocular motor abnormalities have been commonly found in Parkinson's disease[2], whether these abnormalities are directly related to the basal ganglia dysfunction has not yet been clarified. There is controversy as to whether bradykinesia and rigidity exist in the ocular movement or not. The present study was therefore undertaken to elucidate the relationship between the ocular motor abnormalities and the truncal and limb motor dysfunctions of patients with Parkinson's disease.

The subjects were 19 patients with idiopathic Parkinson's disease (8 males and 11 females). Their ages at the time of examination ranged from 49 to 69 yr. The control group consisted of 10 healthy males aged 42 to 58 yr.

Neuroophthalmologic investigations included, in addition to clinical observations, measurements of electrooculograms (EOG), reaction time (RT) and maximal saccadic velocity (MSV) of horizontal gaze. EOG, RT and MSV were studied in a sitting position, with the head fixed in a head-hold. Cup electrodes were placed on the outer and inner canthi for the horizontal movement, and above and below each eye for the vertical movement. The EOG was recorded on a 9–channel polygraph with a time constant of 1.5 sec for the original curve and 0.03 sec for the velocity curve. Target movement, saccadic and smooth pursuit, was produced with a Hamamatsu-TV oculomotor stimulator HTV-C 582, and projected onto a screen 1.5 m in front of the eyes.

The RT of horizontal gaze was determined using a Takei Whole Body Reaction Type II. The subject was made to respond as quickly as possible to a tone stimulus, presented from behind at random, by making a saccadic movement from a forward gaze position to fix on a target 26° lateral. The timer started with the beginning of the tone and stopped when the EOG had reached a certain level.

For obtaining MSV, the EOG at the time of RT examination was recorded on the polygraph at a paper speed of 6 cm/sec. A tangential line was drawn along the maximal gradient of the saccadic EOG and its angular velocity was measured. The test consisted of at least 2 blocks of 20 to 25 trials each.

As an index of akinesia, the RT of finger and truncal movements was determined on the same day. The subject was made to respond as quickly as possible to a tone stimulus either by pressing a button with one index finger or by stepping out of a mat from a standing position. The timer started with the tone and stopped when the button was depressed or when the subject had just stepped out of the mat.

EOG findings: On eye-tracking tests, the saccadic movement was abnormal in 16 of 18 patients for the horizontal movement, and in 13 of 18 for the vertical movement. The most fre-

Reaction time in Parkinson's disease

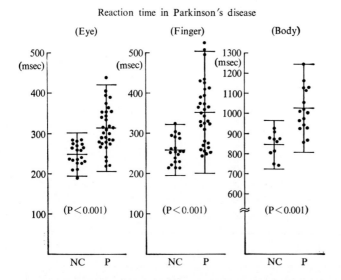

Fig. 1   Reaction time in 19 patients with Parkinson's disease (P) in comparison with the normal control group (NC). The mean TR in the patient group was 313 msec ($\sigma = 54$) for ocular, 352 msec ($\sigma = 76$) for finger, and 1026 msec ($\sigma = 109$) for truncal movement, whereas that in the control group was 248 msec ($\sigma = 27$) for ocular, 258 msec ($\sigma = 32$) for finger, and 843 msec ($\sigma = 61$) for truncal movement. The difference between the patient group and control was significant ($P < 0.001$, Mann-Whitney test) for each movement.

quent abnormality was of "hypometric or stepwise saccade". The smooth pursuit was abnormal in 6 of 18 patients for the horizontal movement, and in 12 of 18 for the vertical movement. The most frequent abnormality was of "saccadic pursuit". Saccadid movement in response to verbal command was found to be abnormal in 5 of 16 patients for the horizontal and also the vertical movement. The most frequent abnormality was "hypometric or stepwise saccade". Convergence was insufficient in 11 of 16 patients examined. Oculocephalic reflex was normal in all patients. Optokinetic nystagmus was insufficient in 1 of 18 patients for the horizontal movement, and in 4 of 18 for the vertical movement.

Reaction time (RT): RT was significantly longer in the patient group than in the control group for all movements: eyes, finger and trunk (Mann-Whitney test) (Fig. 1). The RT of ocullar movement was not significantly correlated with that of finger movement ($r = +0.29$, $0.1 < P < 0.2$, t test) or with that of truncal movement ($r = +0.44$, $0.05 < P < 0.1$, t test).

Maximal saccadic velocity (MSV): The mean MSV for the horizontal gaze was 337°/sec ($\sigma = 64$) in the patient group versus 392°/sec ($\sigma = 49$) in the control group ($p < 0.005$, t test). The MSV was not significantly correlated with the RT of horizontal gaze ($r = -0.33$, $0.05 < P < 0.1$, t test), but was significantly correlated with the RT of truncal movement ($r = -0.51$, $P < 0.05$, t test). The MSV was significantly correlated with the RT of finger movement when pressing the button with the finger ipsilateral to the direction of horizontal gaze ($r = -0.39$, $P < 0.05$, t test), but it was not so when pressing with the contralateral finger ($r = -0.28$, $0.1 < P < 0.2$, t test).

Hypometric saccade and saccadic pursuit are frequently encountered in Parkinson's disease[2,4,6]. These abnormalities have, however, been described in pathological involvements of the central nervous system other than of the basal ganglia[5]. The present study clearly demonstrated an increased RT of the horizontal gaze and a decreased MSV in Parkinson's disease. Similar findings have been reported previously[4,6]. Whether or not these abnormalities are directly related to the dysfunction of basal ganglia has not yet been elucidated.

In so far as limb movement is concerned, an increased RT in Parkinson's disease has been correlated with bradykinesia[1,3]. The present study demonstrated, for the first time to the authors' knowledge, a negative correlation between the MSV of horizontal gaze and RT of finger and truncal movements. It is particularly noteworthy that the MSV correlated with the RT of the finger ipsilateral to the direction of horizontal gaze, but not with that of the contralateral finger. These facts are interpreted to show the existence of ocular bradykinesia in Parkinson's disease.

ACKNOWLEDGEMENT: The authors are grateful to Prof. Yoshigoro Kuroiwa for his helpful advice and revision of this article.

REFERENCES

1. Brumlik, J. and Boshes, B., The mechanism of bradykinesia in parkinsonism, *Neurology,* 16 (1966) 337–344.
2. Corin, M.S., Elizan, T.S. and Bender, M.B., Oculomotor function in patients with Parkinson's disease, *J. Neurol. Sci.,* 15 (1972) 251- 265.
3. Heilman, K.M., Bowers, D., Watson, R.T. and Greer, M., Reaction times in Parkinson's disease, *Arch. Neurol.,* 33 (1976) 139–140.
4. Highstein, S., Cohen, B. and Mones, R., Changes in saccadic eye movements of patients with Parkinson's disease before and after L-Dopa, *Trans. Amer. neurol. Ass.,* 94 (1969) 277–279.
5. Hoyt, W.F. and Daroff, R.B., Supranuclear disorders of ocular control systems in man. Clinical, anatomical, and physiological correlations—1969, In P. Bach-y-Rita and C.C. Collins (Eds.), *The Control of Eye Movements,* Academic Press, New York, 1971, pp. 175–235.
6. Slatt, B., I oeffler, J.D. and Hoyt, W.F., Ocular motor disturbances in Parkinson's disease: Electromyographic observations, *Canad. J. Ophthal.,* 1 (1966) 267–273.

Cerebellar modification of involuntary movements

HIROTARO NARABAYASHI

Department of Neurology, Juntendo University, the Medical School, Bunkyo-ku, Tokyo 113, Japan

Cerebellar symptoms were well described by Thomas and Holmes more than fifty years ago. Although extensive microphysiological analyses of the cerebellum in animals have been reported, the role of the cerebellum in human patients with movement disorders is still not well understood. This paper proposes a simple method to analyze the role of the cerebellum in human patients in modifying the coexisting extrapyramidal manifestations.

Intention or postural tremor, one of the cerebellar signs, does not appear when the patient is completely at rest in a supine position. However, it does appear when some motor effort such as slow voluntary movement or slight postural change is performed. Psychological effort, such as counting of serial numbers in reverse order or simple arithmetic calculations, does not induce the tremorous movement. However, when tremor is already there due to slight muscle contraction, it is exaggerated by further addition of a psychological task.

It is known from the results of human stereotaxic surgery that either intention or postural tremor, like parkinsonian tremor, is almost completely relieved by making small surgical lesions in the ventralis intermedius nucleus (Vim) of the thalamus, but dysmetria is not modified. By using the microelectrode recording technique from this nucleus, rhythmic burst discharges, consisting of trains of several spike discharges, often synchronous in phase with peripheral tremor rhythm, are found. These rhythmic bursts have been interpreted as tremorogenic in nature, as well as reflecting the proprioceptive impulses produced by tremor movement, so the Vim has been considered as an important structure involved in the tremorogenic circuit. Stimulation of Vim immediately decreases increases tremor, and surgical lesion abolished the tremor.

In the case of parkinsonian tremor at rest, free from any cerebellar signs, similar features of neuron activities are found in the Vim. On the other hand, intention tremor is accompanied by cerebellar signs such as muscular hypotonia and dysmetria, in addition to the tremor mechanism focusing on the Vim. Thus, the clinical difference of intention or postural tremor from parkinsonian tremor at rest is assumed to be due to participation of cerebellar pathology.

Choreic movement of Huntington's disease is another example of involuntary movements, which has no pathology in cerebellar and its output structures. As shown in Fig. 1, choreic movement in Huntington's disease is present at rest (top), as well as in slight muscle contraction, such as touching the nose with the finger (middle). Choreic movement was markedly increased by psychological effort (bottom). Ordinary loads by standing or walking in routine neurological examinations, which are quite difficult balancing and coordination tasks for severely disabled patients, can be considered as a combination of both psychological and motor efforts.

As far as the cerebellar mechanisms are concerened, hemiballism, parkinsonian tremor, peroral dyskinesia, dopa-induced dyskinesia and dystonic posturings seem to belong to the same category as choreic movement. These are not modified by slight muscle contractions or posturings,

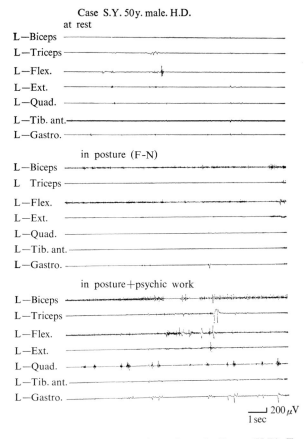

Case S.Y. 50y. male. H.D.

Fig. 1. Surface EMG recordings in a case of Huntington's disease (H.D.). Top: activities almost absent in the resting condition. EMGs were recorded from upper and lower muscles of the left side, as shown on the left. Middle: abnormal choreic movement does not increase upon slight posturing (touching the nose with the finger; F-N).
Bottom: EMG increased markedly by a psychological task (counting serial numbers backwards).

TABLE 1. Appearance of involuntary movement.

	Involuntary movements due to diencephalic pathophysioloigcal mechanism	Involuntary movements due to diencephalic mechanism plus cerebellar deficit	
Increase by slight posturing or slight contraction (motor effort)	−	+	
Increase by psychological task (psychological effort)	+	−	Psychological effort exaggerates the involuntary movements already existing under slight posturing.
Increase by difficult, complex performance (motor and psychological effort)	+	+	

but are very easily exaggerated by psychological effort of patients. On the other hand, postural or intention tremor was modified by these muscle changes.

The above clinical difference between the two groups, i.e., whether or not the involuntary movements are produced by simple introduction of slight voluntary movement and posturing, may corresdonp to whehert or not they are combined with cerebellar pathology. The cerebellar outflow to the cerebrum via the thalamus seems to exert a tonic facilitatory influence on the existing mechanism of involuntary movements in the diencephalon, inducing the involuntary movement exposed both at rest and at weak postural changes. When is it severely decreased, the involuntary movement appears only in movement or posturing (Table 1).

These distinctions may be of help in analyzing symptoms of multi-system degeneration such as dentato-rubro-pallido-Luysian atrophy and others. The most basic cerebellar feature in such a condition would be an interruption of tonic facilitatory influences on the mechanism of involuntary movements at the diencephalic level.

EMG study of human reflex blinking by air puff stimulation

MARI HIRAOKA AND MUNEO SHIMAMURA

Department of Neurophysiology, Tokyo Metropolitan Institute for Neurosciences, Fuchu, Tokyo 183, Japan

The blink reflex is a brief phasic contraction of the orbicularis oculi muscle evoked by stimuli such as a mechanical tap to the periorbital skin or an electrical current delivered to the branches of the trigeminal nerve. The evoked EMG presents two successive components: firstly, an early, brief and di– or triphasic reflex and secondly, a late, longer and multiphasic reflex. The former appears ipsilaterally and the latter bilaterally following a unilateral stimulus. We have designated the early component as the first response (R_1) and the late one as the second response (R_2) after Penders and Delwaide[3]. It has been established that both reflex components are exteroceptive in nature[3,5] and are mediated by the same group of afferent fibers.

Reflex blinks can also be evoked by stimuli such as a puff of air or light touch to the cornea[2,4]. Only one group of reflex response is elicited with longer and variable latency bilaterally. Due to the similarity of these features to the R_2 evoked by the electrical stimulus, we propose that the response can be termed R_2. However, it has been thought that the first response is not produced by these stimuli. We reported previously that both components appeared by tactile and electrical stimulation to the cornea of the cat and were exteroceptive in origin[1]. Further study of the human blink reflex was carried out to investigate the possibility of eliciting the exteroceptive first component by air puff stimulus.

Six healthy adult subjects were examined. Each was tested twice on different days. The subjects were asked to open their eyes naturally. An air puff stimulus controlled by an electromagnetic valve was applied to the cornea for several msec every 10 sec. Electrical stimulation was delivered via a pair of surface electrodes. The cathode was positioned near the point of emergence of the supraorbital nerve and the anode at a separation of 2 cm along the eyebrow. Stimuli were square waves of 0.3–0.5 msec duration and of supra-threshold intensity. A pair of surface electrodes with saline paste in them was fixed to each upper eyelid to record the response of the orbicularis oculi.

The air puff stimulus elicited a multiphasic response (R_2) bilaterally (Fig. 1 Aa). The latencies were 43.5 ± 5.4 (S.D.) msec on the side ipsilateral to the stimulus and 55.0 ± 8.1 on the opposite side. Fifty-times averaged EMG showed a diphasic spike wave with a latency of about 20 msec only on the ipsilateral side, but the maximum amplitude was about 1/10 that of R_2 (Fig. 1 Ab). We propose that this component represents R_1.

Next, the recovery curve of R_1 was obtained by delivering the air puff as a conditioning stimulus. The peak-to-peak amplitude of R_1 tested by the electrical stimulation was measured and plotted at various conditioning-testing intervals (Fig. 1B). The curve showed two supernormal phases: an early, short (10 msec) augmentation with a maximum (130%) at 15 msec and a late, long-lasting (35–100 msec) one with a maximum (270%) at 55 msec. The former can be augmented R_1 by the early component (R_1) of the conditioning stimulus and latter by the R_2.

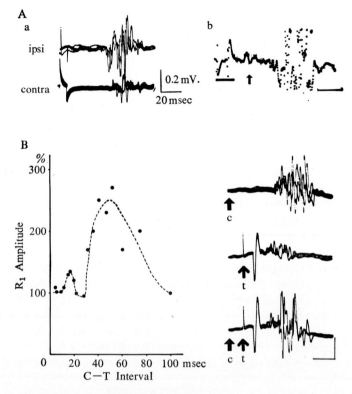

Fig. 1A.   a, Three-times superimposed reflex EMG responses of orbicularis oculi by air puff stimulation showing R₂ bilaterally. b, Fifty-times averaged EMG. The R₁ component (shown by an arrow) precedes R₂. The artefact of the stimulus is indicated by a black bar. The scale line represents 20 msec.

Fig. 1B.   R₁ recovery curve; the conditioning shock is an air puff and the test shock an electrical stimulation. An example is shown on the right (upper, response only by the conditioning stimulus; middle, response by the testing stimulus; lower, response by both stimuli). The vertical and horizontal scale lines represent 0.2 mV and 20 msec, respectively.

These observations support the idea that R₁ can be produced also by air puff stimulation. Since the afferent volleys would be dispersed compared to the electrical stimulus, the amplitude is lower and the latency is longer. On plain air puff stimulation, R₁ will be subliminal This contribution suggests the exteroceptive nature of the first component of reflex blinking.

REFERENCES

1. Hiraoka, M. and Shimamura, M., Neural mechanisms of the corneal blinking reflex in cats, *Brain Research*, 125 (1977) 265–275.
2. Magladery, J.W. and Teasdall, R.D., Corneal reflexes; An electromyographic study in man, *Arch. Neurol.*, 5 (1961) 51–56.
3. Penders, C.A. and Delwaide, P.J., Physiologic approach to the human blink reflex. In J.E. Desmedt (Ed.), *New Developments in Electromyography and Clinical Neurophysiology, Vol. 3*, Karger, Basel, 1973, pp. 649–657.
4. Rushworth, G., Observations on blink reflexes, *J. Neurol. Neurosurg. Psychiat.*, 25 (1962) 93–108.
5. Shahani, B., The human blink reflex, *J. Neurol. Neurosurg. Psychiat.*, 33 (1970) 792–800.

A brain stem mechanism responsible for cortical control of trigeminal motoneurons

YOSHIO NAKAMURA AND SHUICHI NOZAKI

Section of Physiology, Institute of Stomatognathic Science, Tokyo Medical and Dental University,
Bunkyo-ku, Tokyo 113, Japan

Single shocks applied to the orbital gyrus of cats have been reported to evoke a short-latency IPSP in masseteric motoneurons as well as a short-latency depression of the masseteric reflex in encéphale isolé preparations[2]. Previous studies in our laboratory have demonstrated (1) that the inhibitory effect was abolished by a circumscribed lesion in the medial reticular formation at the pontomedullary junction, i.e., just caudal to the trigeminal motor nucleus, and (2) that stimulation of the medial bulbar reticular formation induced an IPSP and EPSP, respectively, in masseteric and anterior digastric motoneurons with a latency of monosynatpic range (mean, *ca.* 0.8 msec)[5]. Based on these findings, it was assumed that inhibitory interneurons for masseteric motoneruons (I_M neurons) and excitatory interneurons for digastric motoneurons (E_D neurons), which were involved in the orbital cortical control of trigeminal motoneurons, were located in the medial bulbar reticular formation. The purposes of the present study were (1) to identify these interneurons and to determine their location in the bulbar reticular formation, and (2) to study their input and output modes.

Experiments were performed on cats anesthetized with α-chloralose. The orbito-frontal region of the cerebral cortex was exposed. Two pairs of silver ball electrodes were placed on the cortical surface, one on the orbital gyrus, of which stimulation exerted the maximum inhibitory effect on the masseteric reflex, and the other on another cortical area, from which no inhibitory effect was obtained on the masseteric reflex. The lingual nerve was sectioned peripherally and a bipolar collar-type electrode was attached to the central stump. Tungsten stimulating electrodes were inserted bilaterally into the dorsal and ventral reticulospinal tracts at C_2 level. Glass microelectrodes filled with 3 M KCl were used for intra- and extracellular recording from bulbar reticular neurons. Some glass electrodes were filled with 3 M KCl solution saturated with Fast green FCF, and the dye was deposited at the recording sites electrophoretically. Some reticular neurons were recorded intracellularly with electrodes filled with 3 M KCl solution containing 4% horseradish peroxidase (HRP), which was injected intracellularly at the conclusion of recording. These reticular neurons were located and identified histologically.

In order to identify I_M and E_D neurons from antidromic spike potentials evoked by selective stimulation of the masseteric and digastric motor nuclei, respectively, a tungsten electrode was inserted into each of the motor nuclei. These electrodes were fixed at the sites, from which the largest antidromic field potentials were recorded by stimulation of the masseteric and anterior digastric nerve, respectively. Electrical pulses of 0.1 msec duration at an intensity of less than 15 and 10 μA were applied respectively to the masseteric and digastric motor nuclei to localize the effect of stimulation within each motor nucleus.

In the medial bulbar reticular formation, neurons were found which responded with EPSPs and spike potentials selectively to stimulation of the orbital gyrus and with antidromic spike potentials to stimulation of either the masseteric or the digastric motor nucleus. For these identified I_M and E_D neurons, the following results were obtained.

(1) The latency of the antidromic spike potentials evoked in I_M and E_D neurons by stimulation of the masseteric and digastric motor nuclei were 0.2–0.5 msec (mean 0.38 msec) and 0.3–0.6 msec (mean 0.46 msec), respectively.

(2) Stimulation of the orbital gyrus evoked EPSPs in I_M and E_D neurons with a latency of 1.1–3.9 msec and 1.2–5.4 msec, respectively.

(3) Three of 10 I_M neurons (33 %) and 13 of 26 E_D neurons (50 %) responded antidromically to stimulation of the spinal cord at C_2 level with a latency of 0.5–0.8 msec (mean 0.59 msec).

(4) Only 1 of 10 I_M neurons (10 %) and 4 of 26 E_D neurons (18 %) responded with one or two spike potentials to stimulation of the lingual nerve.

(5) The sites of recording from I_M and E_D neurons which were marked by Fast green FCF were localized in the medial bulbar reticular formation bilaterally including the nucleus reticularis gigantocellularis. HRP-positive I_M and E_D neurons were found to be of medium size.

From these findings, the following conclusions were drawn.

(1) Judging from the latency of the orbital cortically induced EPSPs, I_M and E_D neurons would receive excitatory inputs monosynatpically from the orbital gyrus via the direct cortico-bulbar projection. Hence, the shortest pathway for orbital cortically induced inhibition of masseteric motoneurons and excitation of digastric motoneurons would be a disynatpic route. In addition, these reticular neurons would be activated polysynaptically from the orbital gyrus.

(2) Some I_M and E_D neurons possess bifurcating axons, the ascending and descending branches terminating in the trigeminal motor nucleus and the spinal cord, respectively.

(3) Few spikes were triggered in a small number of I_M and E_D neurons by lingual nerve volleys, although they were powerful inhibitory and excitatory inputs from the periphery to masseteric and digastric motoneurons, respectively[1,3]. It was also found previously that stimulation of the medial bulbar reticular formation did not activate supratrigeminal neurons[4], which are regarded as inhibitory neurons involved in lingually evoked inhibition of masseteric motoneurons[1]. Thus, the pathway for cortical control of trigeminal motoneurons via I_M and E_D neurons would be basically separate from the pathway responsible for peripheral control of trigeminal motoneurons.

REFERENCES

1. Goldberg, L.J. and Nakamura, Y., Lingually induced inhibition of masseteric motoneurons, *Experientia,* 24 (1968) 371–373.
2. Nakamura, Y., Goldberg, L.J. and Clemente, C.D., Nature of suppression of the masseteric monosynaptic reflex induced by stimulation of the orbital gyrus of the cat, *Brain Research*, 6 (1967) 184–198.
3. Nakamura, Y., Nagashima, H. and Mori, S., Bilateral effects of the afferent impulses from the masseteric muscle on the trigeminal motoneuron of the cat, *Brain Research*, 57 (1973) 15–17.
4. Nakamura, Y., Nozaki, S., Takatori, M. and Kikuchi, M., Possible inhibitory neurons in the bulbar reticular formation involved in the cortically evoked inhibition of the masseteric motoneuron of the cat, *Brain Research*, 115 (1976) 512–517.
5. Nakamura, Y., Takatori, M., Nozaki, S. and Kikuchi, M., Monosynaptic reciprocal control of trigeminal motoneurons from the medial bulbar reticular formation, *Brain Research*, 89 (1975) 144–148.

Lower brain-stem "locomotor region" in the mesencephalic cat

SHIGEMI MORI, HIROSHI NISHIMURA, CHIKAHARU KURAKAMI,
TAKEYASU YAMAMURA AND MAMORU AOKI

*Department of Physiology, Asahikawa Medical College,
Asahikawa, Hokkaido 078-11, Japan*

Stimulation of the mesencephalic locomotor region (MLR) induces "controlled locomotion" in the acute precollicular-postmamillary decerebrate cat. Stimulation of the pontine locomotor region (PLR) which extends ventrocaudally throughout the lateral pontine tegmentum, also induces controlled locomotion in the same preparation[2]. These studies indicate that the PLR mediates the effects of MLR stimulation through the bulbar structure to the spinal cord where the final stepping generator is presumed to exist.

To identify such a structure, microelectrodes were placed systematically at 0.5 mm intervals throughout the lateral bulbar tegmentum at levels ranging from P9 to P18 dorsoventrally (H-5 to H-10) and mediolaterally from L2 or R2 to L6 or R6. Through each electrode, rectangular pulses (less than 20 μA) of 0.5 msec duration at a frequency of 50 Hz were delivered to test their potential effects on locomotion in the acute precollicular-postmamillary decerebrate cat.

The experimental set-up was essentially the same as that described previously[2]. At the end of each experiment, electrolytic marks were made by passing a short current pulse of 2–3 mA through the stimulating electrodes. The locations of each electrode tip were determined and referred to histologically verified coordinates. The identified locations were then referred to the stereotaxic atlas of Berman[1] and plotted on appropriate schemas of the bulbar structure.

As with MLR and PLR stimulation, controlled locomotion could be evoked by ipsilateral stimulation of a discrete zone within the bulbar lateral tegmentum (hereafter termed the bulbar locomotor region, BLR). Such locomotion was, however, much more difficult to evoke than that evoked by either MLR or PLR stimulation. The mediolateral and dorsoventral dimensions of the locomotor strip were each less than 0.5 mm and were much more restricted than the PLR. To evoke controlled locomotion successfully without side effects, an adequate development of postural tonus after decerebration was necessary. When the postural tonus was not well developed, locomotion was not evoked even if an electrode was placed within the locomotor regions (PLR and BLR)[3]. The tip of the electrode should also be placed precisely within the locomotor region. In such a case, the stimulus intensity for evoking locomotion was less than 5 μA. If it was placed outside a zone, a stronger stimulus intensity was necessary and side effects such as respiratory arrest appeared.

The extent of the BLR was traced throughout the lateral bulbar tegmentum from P10 to P19. The most effective sites were 4 mm lateral to the midline and about 2 mm beneath the floor of the IVth ventricle as in the case of the PLR (i.e., H-6.5 at the P10 level, H-7 at P12, H-7 at P14, H-7.5 at P16, and H-8 at P18). Locomotion was elicited by the BLR stimulation except at the level of P18 which corresponds to the first cervical spinal segments, where only ipsilateral stepping of the hind-limb was elicited.

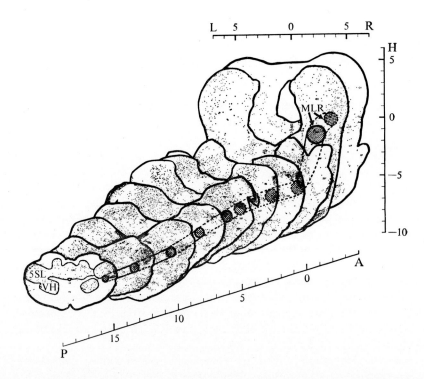

Fig. 1.   Representative locations of electrolytic lesions drawn on each corresponding drawing of frontal brain-stem sections along Horsley-Clarke coordinates. The assembled lesions constitute a pontobulbar locomotor strip originating from the cuneiform nucleus (MLR) through the lateral tegmentum to the dorsolateral funiculus of the C_1 spinal segment. The electrolytic lesions from P0.9 to P9.2 were redrawn from the previous study of Mori et al.[2] A, Anterior; P, posterior; L, left; R, right; H, dorsoventral depth, 5SL, laminal trigeminal nucleus; VH, ventral horn.

The representative electrolytic lesions were plotted in frontal sections as shown Fig. 1. Throughout the bulbar tegmentum, electrolytic lesions were located ventrally to the alaminal spinal trigeminal nucleus (5SP) and to the laminal trigeminal nucleus (5SL). At the level of P18.3, lesions were observed at the ventrolateral border of the most caudal laminal trigeminal nucleus which corresponds to the dorsolateral funiculus of the cervical spinal cord. Recently, Shik and Yagodnitsyn[5] also extended the MLR-PLR strip throughout the medulla to the level of the C_1 spinal segment (i.e., from P9 to P18). They found that the C_1 stepping point is located at the border of the spinal gray and the dorsolateral funiculus. Our stepping point agrees well with that of Shik and Yagodnitsyn[5] and appear to be the same site at which Sherrington[4] obtained stepping in decapitate cats.

The results of present study indicate that the BLR represents the functional continuity of the MLR and PLR strip. They also confirm the previous conclusion of Mori et al.[2] that the lateral reticular formation of the lower brain-stem contains a continuous strip whose activation results in controlled locomotion in the mesencephalic cat.

References

1. Berman, A.L., *The Brain Stem of the Cat. A Cytoarchitectonic Atlas With Stereotaxic Coordinates*, Univ. of Wisconsin Press, Madison, 1968.
2. Mori, S., Shik, M.L. and Yagodnitsyn, A.S., Role of pontine tegmentum for locomotor control in mesencephalic cat, *J. Neurophysiol.*, 40 (1977) 284–295.
3. Mori, S., Nishimura, H., Kurakami, C., Yamamura, T. and Aoki, M., Controlled locomotion in the mesencephalic cat: Distribution of facilitatory and inhibitory regions within the pontine tegmentum, *J. Neurophysiol.*, in press.
4. Sherrington, C.S., Flexion-reflex on the limb, crossed extension reflex, and reflex stepping and standing, *J. Physiol. (Lond.)*, 40 (1910) 28–121.
5. Shik, M.L. and Yagodnitsyn, A.S., Pontobulbar "locomotor strip", *Neurophysiology*, 9 (1977) 95–97 (in Russian).

Differential effects on locomotor movements of fore- and hindlimbs of the decerebrate cat induced by partial cooling of cerebellar intermediate and vermian cortices

MASAO UDO AND KANJI MATSUKAWA

Department of Biophysical Engineering, Faculty of Engineering Science, Osaka University, Toyonaka, Osaka 560, Japan

The stepping movements of decerebrate cats on a treadmill[3] have several advantages for investigations of cerebellar control of locomotion in that the effects of cerebellar lesions can be examined in acute experiments. By taking advantage of this procedure changes in brain stem neuronal activity could be reversibly induced by local cerebellar cooling[4]. Characteristic changes in locomotor movements have been reported in unrestrained walking cats with chronic cerebellar lesions, e.g., hyperflexion of limbs following cortical lesions in the intermediate part and stiff gait following those in the vermian part[1]. In the present work, we tested whether these changes in locomotor pattern in chronic cats also occur on partial cooling of different lobules of the cerebellar cortex in these so-called "stepping preparations".

Adult cats ($n = 25$) were decerebrated at the precollicular and premammillary level. After decerebration, stepping movements could be induced when the four limbs were driven by a treadmill at constant speeds of 34–59 cm/sec. Electrical stimulation of the brain stem locomotor region was not used to induce stepping. Vertebrae at the second cervical and first lumbar level and pelvis were rigidly fixed with clamps. In this preparation, vertical floor-to-foot forces (FFFs) were measured at each limb in every step by arranging four force plates beneath the treadmill belt. Under our experimental conditions, it was particularly important to choose preparations whose vertical FFFs were well developed to obtain consistent cooling effects. Thus, preparations developing more than 1000 g–weight at the forelimb and more than 800 g–weight at the hindlimb were chosen. The procedures of cooling of the cerebellar cortex and evaluation of the extent of its effectiveness were described previously[2,4]. Changes in a certain parameter of locomotor movements were taken as significant when the mean value for more than 10 succeeding steps during the cooling changed ($p < 0.05$) in comparison with the equivalent steps before and after cooling.

Cooling of Lobule V of the intermediate part induced mainly changes in the ipsilateral forelimb movements. As shown in Fig. 1A, the angular velocity of flexion movements of the elbow, shoulder and scapular joints increased in the swing phase (22% at the elbow, 29% at the shoulder, 11% at the scapular joint for peak velocity). The limb swung to a more rostral position (hyperflexion), as shown in the stick diagrams D and E. The duration of the swing phase became longer and more time was spent in placing down the limb, although in the late swing phase (E_1 phase) extension occurred with higher angular velocity. In contrast, the duration of the stance phase was shortened. There was virtually no change in the ipsilateral hindlimb movements.

Cooling of Lobule IV of the intermediate part was performed by placing the cooling probe on the cortical surface of Lobule IV after complete removal of the tentorium. However, during this cooling, the rostral part of Lobule V of the intermediate part was also cooled as judged by the changes of the cortical field potentials. Nevertheless, this cooling induced changes in the ipsilateral

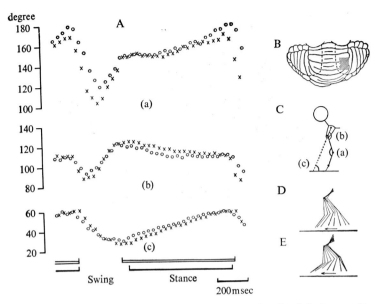

Fig. 1. Effects of partial cooling of the cerebellar cortex at Lobule V of the intermediate part upon the ipsilateral forelimb movements. The cooled cortical area is shown hatched in B. A, Time course of changes in joint angles of the forelimb: (a) for the elbow, (b) for the shoulder and (c) for the scapular joint. Angles of each joint were measured according to the scheme shown in C. Those before cooling are plotted as circles and those during cooling as crosses. Horizontal bars below indicate the stance phase before (double thin lines) and during (a thick line) cooling. D, E: Stick diagrams of the fore-limb in the first half of the swing phase before (D) and during (E) cooling. Horizontal lines indicate the surface of the treadmill belt.

hindlimb strikingly different from those induced by cooling of Lobule V. Angular velocities of joint flexion movements increased in the swing phase (34% at the hip, 13% at the knee and 35% at the ankle for peak velocity), and in the E_1 phase angular velocities of extension increased. The duration of the swing phase was shortened and the paw was placed at a more forward point. This resulted in the duration of the stance phase being somewhat prolonged. In the ipsilateral forelimb, changes similar to those shown in Fig. 1 occurred and this may be at least partly attributable to the concomitant cooling of Lobule V.

Cooling of Lobule V of the vermian part characteristically induced an enhancement of the am-plitudes of vertical FFFs at the ipsilateral fore- and hindlimb (30% for the fore- and 35% for the hindlimb for peak amplitudes). Changes in the limb movements differed from those observed on cooling of the intermediate part. In the ipsilateral hindlimb, there were changes in the relative an-gles at the hip, knee and ankle joints in the E_1 and stance phases. In the ipsilateral forelimb, there was an increase of angular velocity of extension mainly of the shoulder joint in the E_1 phase[4].

The present experiments demonstrate that by partial cooling of the cerebellar cortex of the "stepping preparation" hyperflexion or stiff gait occurred, as reported in unrestrained walking cats with chronic cerebellar cortical lesions[1]. Furthermore, these locomotor changes occurred in a different limb or limbs when each lobule of the cerebellar cortex was cooled. The present results, together with those for unrestrained walking cats, suggest that cerebellar efferent signals from each lobule contribute to adjust the timings of locomotor limb movements, or to adjust the amplitudes of vertical FFFs of a particular limb or limbs. Drastic changes might appear in locomotor patterns when the cooled area is extended to include several cerebellar areas ipsilaterally or bilaterally.

REFERENCES

1. Chambers, W.W. and Sprague, J.M., Functional localization in the cerebellum. II. Somatotopic organization in cortex and nuclei, *Arch. Neurol. Psychiat.*, 74 (1955) 653-680.
2. Eccles, J.C., Rosén, I., Scheid, P. and Táboříková, H., The differential effect of cooling on responses of cerebellar cortex, *J. Physiol. (Lond.)*, 249(1975) 119–138.
3. Shik, M.L. and Orlovsky, G.N., Neurophysiology of locomotor automatism, *Physiol. Rev.*, 56 (1976) 465–501.
4. Udo, M., Oda, Y., Tanaka, K. and Horikawa, J., Cerebellar control of locomotion: Discharges from Deiters neurones, EMG and limb movements during local cooling of cerebellar cortex. In S. Homma (Ed.) *Progress in Brain Research* Vol. 44, Elsevier, Amsterdam, 1976, pp. 544–559.

PART IV

CENTRAL NERVOUS SYSTEM CONTROL OF
CARDIOVASCULAR AND RESPIRATORY FUNCTIONS

HIROSHI IRISAWA

Department of Physiology, School of Medicine, Hiroshima University,
Kasumi, Hiroshima 734, Japan

Accurate and quantitative information on the circulatory and respiratory systems is usually obtained by analysis of the function of the individual organ and tissues under strictly controlled experimental conditions. For this purpose, an organ isolated from the rest of the body has often been used. However, normal integrated physiological function cannot be the result of an algebraic summation of the individual functions. This is particularly so when functions are controlled by the central nervous systems. Therefore, studies must be directed toward an understanding of the integrative mechanisms of the autonomic functions.

Non-invasive method for evaluation of the autonomic functions

Recordings of the input and output neural signals have mostly been done by the recording of impulses either at the peripheral or the central cut ends of the nerve fibers. In such an experimental procedure, one has to open the closed circuit. Recently, impulses from the intact sympathetic nerve have been recorded[7]. Since signals contain both afferent and efferent activities, a technique for the recording of afferent and efferent impulses separately from the intact nerve fibers without opening the circuits is of value. In addition to neural recording, many non-invasive techniques have been devised for monitoring the cardiovascular functions[3]. Simultaneous application of these techniques with neural recording is particularly valuable for analysis of the autonomic function in an intact, unanesthetized animal.

Rhythmic activities

Almost all autonomic functions show rhythmic activities. For example, various circadian and ultradian rhythms are known, but their origin and genesis have not been clarified. The rhythm formation in the multicellular sino-atrial node tissue in rabbit's heart has been studied extensively and possible ionic mechanisms have been suggested[4]. In the central nervous system, rhythmic discharges of the nerve impulses have also been frequently observed. However, it is not certain whether the origin of these rhythmic discharges is due to circus movement of the excitation or to intrinsic automaticity. Further information is required on the rhythmic impulse formation in the neuron pools of the brain.

Non-homogenous distribution of the sympathetic nerve activities

The baroceptor reflex originates from the major vascular wall and the impulses are integrated in the central nervous system. The resulting information is sent to various visceral organs via autonomic efferents. This well-known servomechanism has been studied since the middle of the last century, but recently there has been renewed interest in this area of research (Iriki and Simon, this section). A recent semiquantitative method has shown that impulses from the various efferent nerves exhibit regional inhomogeneity within the different sympathetic nerve activities. Efferent nerves to the stomach[8] and to the intestine[2,5] contain both quantitatively and qualitatively different neural activities from those to the kidney and the heart[5,6]. The latter two nerve activities are almost completely abolished by the baroceptor reflex, but only 20 to 30% of the activities of the former two nerves are abolished by the baroceptor reflex. Similarly the cutaneous sympathetic nerve fiber reacts in a different manner from those of the visceral sympathetic nerves. These observations are not compatible with the classical concept of the homogeneous distribution of the sympathetic efferent activities[11], and offer an area for exploration in the autonomic functions, particularly as regards the central nervous system.

Stereotyped responses in autonomic functions

Although the individual efferent nerve activities are not the same, many of the autonomic responses occur in a stereotyped fashion. It is now established that a region such as the hypothalamus contains a number of neuronpools from which specific and well-integrated autonomic response patterns are evoked. These responses are usually stereotyped and were mostly observed in combination with the motor and autonomic responses. For example an elevation of the carotid sinus pressure evoked a sleep-like state in an unanesthetized animal and stimulation of the hypothalamus elicited cardiovascular responses accompanied by a defense reaction[1] or by an exercise reaction.[12] The acts of standing, eating and exercise are all linked with increased heart rate, rate of rise of tension development, instantaneous aortic flow, stroke volume, peak power and stroke work as well as other cardiovascular responses[10]. Furthermore, the diving reflex occurred upon a mere threatening move towards a seal. These responses occur as if they were previously programmed within the central nervous system[9]. Accompanying these motor responses, an anticipatory cardiovascular response was always observed, indicating that there is participation of the higher central nervous system in these autonomic responses. Thus, the autonomic activities are more intimately connected with somatic functions, suggesting a need for further study on the correlation between these two major functions: autonomic and somatic.

REFERENCES

1. Folkow, B. and Neil, E., *Circulation*, Oxford University Press, New York, 1971.
2. Irisawa, H., Ninomiya, I. and Woolley, G., Efferent activity in renal and intestinal nerves during circulatory reflexes. *Japan. J. Physiol.*, 23 (1973) 657–666.
3. Irisawa, H. and Hirakawa, S., Evaluation of cardiac functions through noninvasive techniques – a symposium, *Japan. Circ. J.*, 41 (1977) 475–537.
4. Irisawa, H., Comparative physiology of the cardiac pacemaker mechanism *Physiol. Rev.*, 58 (1978) 461–498.
5. Ninomiya, I., Irisawa, H. and Woolley, G., Intestinal mechanoreceptor reflex effects on sympathetic never activity to intestine and kidney, *Amer. J. Physiol.*, 227 (1974) 684–691.
6. Ninomiya, I., Irisawa, A. and Nisimaru, N., Nonuniformity of sympathetic nerve activity to the skin and kidney, *Amer. J. Physiol.*, 224 (1973) 256–264.
7. Ninomiya, I., Yonezawa, Y. and Wilson, M.F., Implantable electrode for recording nerve signals in awake animals, *J. Appl. Physiol.*, 41 (1976) 111–114.
8. Nisimaru, N., Comparison of gastric and renal nerve activity. *Amer. J. Physiol.*, 220 (1971) 1303–1308.
9. Reis, D.J., Central neural mechanism governing the circulation with particular reference to the lower brainstem and cerebellum, In A. Zanchetti (Ed.) *Neural and Psychological Mechanism in Cardiovascular Diseases*, 11 Ponte, Milan, 1972, pp. 255–280.

10. Rushmer, R.F., *Cardiovascular Dynamics* (4th ed.), Saunders, Philadelphia, 1976.
11. Schaefer, H., Central control of cardiac function, *Physiol. Rev., Suppl. 4*, 40 (1960) 213–231.
12. Smith, O.A., Jabbur, S.J., Rushmer, R.F. and Lasher, E.P., Role of hypothalamic structures in cardiac control, *Physiol. Rev., Suppl. 4*, 40 (1960) 136–145.

Regional differentiation of sympathetic efferents

MASAMI IRIKI*[1] AND ECKERT SIMON*[2]

*[1] *Department of Physiology, Tokyo Metropolitan Institute of Gerontology,*
Itabashi-ku, Tokyo 173, Japan.
*[2] *Max-Planck-Institut für physiologische und klinische Forschung, W.G. Kerckhoff-Institut,*
Bad Nauheim, Germany

Introduction

The autonomic nervous system is involved in the maintenance of the homeostasis of the internal body status. One of the most important functions is its control of a major homeostatic effector system: the circulation. With respect to this control function, the roles of the two main components of the autonomic nervous system, the parasympathetic and sympathetic, have been considered to be different. The ability to induce regionally well defined changes of cardiovascular functions has been mainly ascribed to the parasympathetic system, while the sympathetic system was assumed to mediate "en masse" reactions[4]. This view, however, was derived only to a minor extent from analysis of circulatory control functions, and was largely based on general functional and morphological considerations. The assumption of a more or less diffuse mode of response appeared to correspond to the structure of the sympathetic nervous system, with its extensive branching. The fundamental work of Cannon[5] on the sympatho-adrenal system has been interpreted as supporting the view that the sympathetic cardiovascular innervation generally responds in a diffuse and generalized manner[49], although Cannon's concept had been derived from the endocrine-metabolic functions of the sympathetic system rather than from its cardiovascular control functions.

This study considers the concept of regional cardiovascular control by qualitative differentiation of the sympathetic outflow. This concept was put forward as a result of the combined hemodynamic and neurophysiological investigations of Kullmann, Schönung and Simon[39] and Walther, Iriki and Simon[58] on regional vasomotor control under conditions of apparently natural disturbance of thermal homeostasis. These and a number of subsequent investigations in this field have demonstrated regionally diverse changes of sympathetic activity as a mode of homeostatic control. Several other groups of studies were carried out on this theme following different lines of research, such as autonomic reflex analysis[34,48], evaluation of sympathetic efferents with specialized cardiovascular functions, e.g., active vasodilatation[1,16,56], and analysis of circulatory reflexes governed by the classical proprio- and chemoreceptors, as well as by newly discovered cardiovascular afferents[3,40-42].

Regional differentiation of cardiovascular functions – the law of Dastre and Morat

The present studies demonstrating the qualitative differentiation of the cardiovascular innervation are supported by a number of hemodynamic observations which conform to the so-called "law of Dastre and Morat". Referring to the work of these authors[8], this law expresses the finding that the direction of regional vascular responses may be diverse in different sections of the body. The validity of this "law" has been confirmed under a variety of natural and experimental conditions.

In general, a variety of mechanisms may account for regionally diverse adjustments of circulatory functions. Interaction of local metabolism with remote neural control may be common, particularly in metabolically active tissues. However, this explanation appears not to hold in many cases. Folkow et al.[10] suggested that regionally different adjustments of blood flow may result from a differential susceptibility to cardiovascular reflex inputs of the tonically active neuron pools controlling the sympathetic outflow to various sections of the circulation. Regionally different frequency-response characteristics of the nerve-effector connections could additionally contribute to hemodynamic differentiation. Interaction between dilator and constrictor innervation was discussed as early as 1887 by Dastre and Morat and was assumed to account for the characteristic blood flow distribution patterns in fight-flight conditions[56]. Many investigators, however, have felt for a long time that explanations of this kind might not suffice; e.g., "the thermoregulatory responses of the skin vessels are not consistent with the idea of a widespread diffuse action of the sympathetic system" (Barcroft, 1960)[2], or "many similarities with the organization of the complex control of somatomotor activity will be revealed by future work; this implies that the old concept that the sympathetic nervous system was largely diffuse in its activity, is far from correct" (Folkow, Heymans and Neil, 1965)[10]. The difficulty has been to confirm the regionally antagonistic innervations of functionally different cardiovascular sections suggested by the hemodynamic studies. Direct evidence was first presented by Walther, Iriki and Simon[53] and in a number of subsequent studies of the same group.

Regional differentiation of the sympathetic outflow

Cutaneo-visceral antagonism in thermoregulation:
The data reported on antagonistic differentiation of the sympathetic efferents are shown by Fig. 1. During selective spinal cord cooling, increased activity in the cutaneous sympathetic efferents was indicated by the recorded mass discharges as well as by the integrated activity. Rhythmic changes of activity synchronized with the respiratory cycles were observed during the pre- and post-cooling phases, but were more prominent during cooling. At the same time, the activity of the splanchnic sympathetic efferents was reduced. After the end of cooling the activities of both efferents changed towards their pre-stimulation levels.

Spinal cord cooling as a stimulus to alter regional sympathetic activity must be considered as a means to specifically alter the thermal input into the temperature regulation system. This follows from the presence of body temperature sensors in the spinal cord; they also exist in the hypothalamus and in the integument[53]. The evaluation of thermally induced sympathetic differentiation by stimulation of each of these thermosensitive sites was the aim of a first series of investigations[26,45,58]. The intention was to confirm that sympathetic differentiation was a specific autonomic control component in the thermoregulatory adjustments of heat loss from the body surface. At this state of evaluation it was important to demonstrate close correlations between the neurophysiological findings on regional sympathetic activity and the local hemodynamic reactions[39,44,50]; this established that the observed sympathetic antagonism was, indeed, of hemodynamic importance.

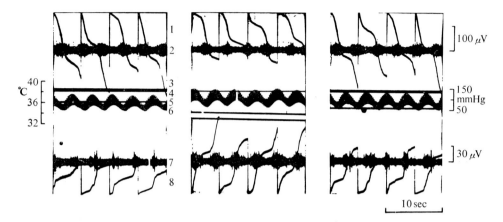

Fig. 1. Regional sympathetic activity in an anesthetized, paralyzed rabbit before (left), during (middle) and after (right) selective cooling of the spinal cord. Sections from original recordings: 1, integrated discharges of splanchnic sympathetic; 2, discharges of splanchnic sympathetic; 3, rectal temperature; 4, vertebral canal temperature; 5, skin temperature of right ear; 6, arterial pressure; 7, discharges of ear cutaneous sympathetic; 8, integrated discharges of ear cutaneous sympathetic[58]. (Source: ref. 58 Reproduced by kind permission of Springer Verlag, West Germany.)

Patterns of cutaneous, visceral and cardiac sympathetic differentiation:
(a) *Changes of blood gas composition.* Investigations of Iriki and associates (1971–1975) have incorporated changes of blood gas composition as a disturbance of homeostasis presumed to induce sympathetic differentiation[6,37]. These studies included the analysis of cardiac sympathetic efferents, the role of which appeared to be particularly important in the adjustment of heart functions during hypoxia and asphyxia[27]. Fig. 2 shows the time courses of cutaneous and splanchnic sympathetic activities (Fig. 2A) and of cardiac and splanchnic sympathetic activities (Fig. 2B), together with some other parameters during moderate arterial hypoxia. Rabbits were ventilated with 8% oxygen in nitrogen for 4–6 min. The changes of PaO_2, $PaCO_2$ and pH are indicated by columns. Thirty sec after the start of hypoxia, the discharge of the ear sympathetic nerves decreased and remained depressed throughout the hypoxic phase. A considerable rise of ear skin temperature, indicating increased skin blood flow, corresponded to the changes in local sympathetic activity. Cardiac sympathetic activity also decreased and remained depressed during hypoxic ventilation. The heart rate decreased in close correlation with cardiac sympathetic activity. In contrast to these two sympathetic branches, the activity of the splanchnic nerve began to increase within 30 sec after the start of hypoxia and was maintained in this state during hypoxia. After the end of hypoxic ventilation, regional sympathetic activities returned towards their pre-stimulation levels, as did the ear temperature and heart rate.

When the hypoxic stress became more severe, and PaO_2 fell below about 25 torr, the differentiated pattern of regional sympathetic activity changes turned into a general and strong activation[25,29]. This reaction may be considered as an emergency response corresponding to Cannon's concept of the sympatho-adrenal function, and contrasts with the apparently homeostatic adjustment induced by moderate hypoxia. The pattern of the latter appears to be species-dependent to some extent. For instance, depression of cutaneous sympathetic activity by arterial hypoxia was also found in cats[12], but a decrease of cardiac sympathetic activity could not be confirmed in this species[24]; cardiac sympathetic activity increased uniformly at all levels of arterial hypoxia.

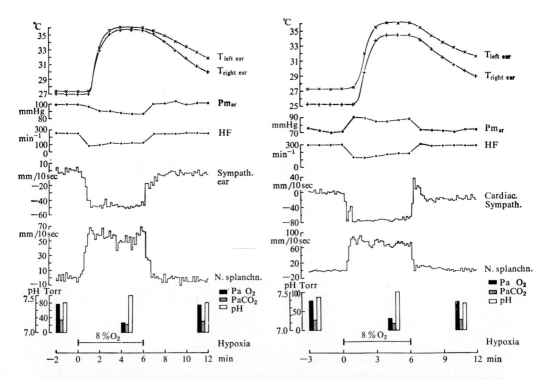

Fig. 2.   Differentiated responses of regional sympathetic efferents during hypoxia in the anesthetized, paralyzed rabbit. Regional cutaneous (sympath. ear), visceral (N. splanchn.) and cardiac (car diac sympath.) sympathetic activity. The courses of regional sympathetic activity are visualized by plotting the changes in amplitude of the integrator signals (in mm/10 sec); reference level: average integrator signal amplitude during the pre-stimulation period. Ear skin temperatures ($T_{left\ ear}$, $T_{right\ ear}$), arterial mean pressure (Pm_{ar}), heart rate (HF) and blood gas values (vertical bars)[28]. (Source: ref. 28 Reproduced by kind permission of Australian Journal of Experimental Biology and Medical Science.)

Hypercapnia induced the same pattern of regional sympathetic responses as those induced by hypoxia[55]. The qualitatively identical reactions of hypoxia and hypercapnia indicate the regulatory origin of the induced sympathetic response pattern, presumably by the same cardiorespiratory control system.

(b) *Thermal stimulation.* Inclusion of cardiac sympathetic efferents in the analysis of sympathetic differentiation has for the first time revealed differences between patterns of qualitative sympathetic differentiation corresponding to the underlying stimulus. The experimental period shown in Fig. 3A was selected to demonstrate the typical antagonism between splanchnic and cutaneous sympathetic activity in response to a central cold stimulus applied to the spinal cord. The close correlation between local cutaneous sympathetic activity and ear blood flow is again indicated by the fall of ear skin temperature. Fig. 3B shows the course of cardiac sympathetic activity under the same stimulus. The animal was vagotomized to ensure that the heart rate reflected changes in cardiac sympathetic innervation. A decrease of heart rate was found to accompany the reduction of cardiac sympathetic activity, indicating that the recorded discharges represented chronotropic control of the heart by sympathetic efferents.

The antagonism between cutaneous and cardiac sympathetic activity, in reversed states of

Spinal cord cooling

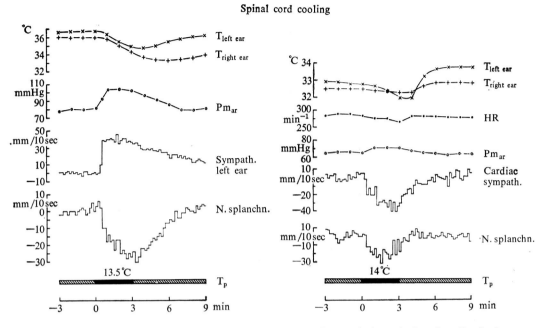

Fig. 3. Differentiated responses of regional sympathetic efferents during spinal cord cooling in the anesthetized, paralyzed rabbit[28]. Parameters are as in Fig. 2. (Source: ref. 28 Reproduced by kind permission of Australian Journal of Experimental Biology and Medical Science.)

activity, was also observed during spinal cord heating. However, this antagonism appeared to be less consistent as compared to the antagonism between cutaneous and splanchnic activity. As indicated by hemodynamic studies[11], hypothalamic cooling and heating did not consistently change cardiac sympathetic innervation in a direction opposite to that of cutaneous sympathetic activity, indicating that the specific thermoregulatory pattern of sympathetic differentiation may be partially modified by non-specific thermal effects on vasomotor neurons.

The conclusion to be drawn from the observations described above is that the patterns of sympathetic differentiation varied with the homeostatic system under evaluation. This implies that a multitude of patterns may be expected, depending on the kind of disturbance induced or stimulation applied. Table 1 summarizes our own (upper part) and other authors' (lower part) investigations which have demonstrated the existence of differentiated sympathetic responses. This table indicates clearly the different patterns of sympathetic differentiation under different conditions of stimulations.

Differentiation within the sympathetic outflow to single organs:

Regionally diverse changes of the sympathetic outflow, as revealed by recording mass discharges from nerve filaments, reflect the average changes of activity of a multitude of fibers which do not necessarily serve the same function. The only way to evaluate the significance of such average responses is to correlate them with local changes of function, e.g., by measuring regional blood flow and parameters of cardiac function. As emphasized in the preceding sections, this has been observed in the investigations which established the concept of qualitative sympa-

Table 1.   Summary of the results on regional differentiation of sympathetic efferents, investigated directly by recording of nerve discharges.

Experimental conditions	Sympathetic efferents					Literature
	Cutaneous	Splanchnic	Cardiac	Muscle	Renal	
Cold stimulation						
Cutaneous	+	−				45
Spinal cord	+	−	−			27, 58
Hypothalamus	+	−				26
Warm stimulation						
Cutaneous	−	+				45
Spinal cord	−	+	+			27, 58
Hypothalamus	−	+				26
Hypoxic stimulation						
Primary tissue	−	+	+			23
Mild arterial	−	+	−			25, 27, 29
Severe arterial	+	+	+			29
Hypercapnic stimulation	−	+	−			55
Chemoreceptor stimulation	−			+		20
Baroreceptor stimulation	∅	−	−	−	−	30, 41, 42, 43, 57
Atrial dilatation		∅	+	∅	−	33
Coronal occlusion	−	+				15, 38
Cutaneous stimulation						
Non-noxious	+ (−)			−		17
Noxious	− (+)			+		18
Mental arithmetic	+			−		9
Hyperventilation	+			−		9

+ : activation, − : inhibition, ∅ : no change.

thetic differentiation. If, as a consequence, it is taken for granted that the sympathetic nervous system is capable of a differential control of local functions, then it may be inferred that single fiber recording from the same filament will exhibit a diversity of response patterns on the basis of the presumption that different functions are fulfilled by different fibers. Evidence is accumulating that a considerable degree of differentiation of the sympathetic outflow occurs at the level of single unit activity. Several investigators have succeeded in identifying fibers on the basis of electrophysiological and functional properties and have suggested particular functions for the different fiber types.

(a) *Cutaneous sympathetic*. Jänig and co-workers[13,17,18,32] have identified four types of fibers in the sympathetic outflow to the skin of the cat which appear to have sudomotor, pilomotor, vasoconstrictor and possibly vasodilatator functions. Vasoconstrictor fibers exhibited the following properties: spontaneous activity, reflex inhibition by noxious and activation by mechanoreceptor stimulation, primary inhibition and subsequent activation by asphyxia, inhibition by heating and activation by cooling the spinal cord. Pilomotor fibers were not spontaneously active and were excited during terminal phases of asphyxia when visible piloerection occurred. Sudomotor fibers responded transiently to spinal heating, and their activity showed some coincidence with electrodermal reflex changes. Finally, fibers have been detected which are selectively activated by spinal cord heating and which may represent the cutaneous vasodilatator fibers whose involvement in thermoregulation had been demonstrated by Schönung et al.[51] Fig. 4 shows the inverse relationship of activities between these putative vasodilators and the vasoconstrictors in relation to spinal cord temperature. This antagonism between vasoconstrictor and dilator fibers confined to the same vascular region is particularly important as it confirms the differential control of different vasomotor mechanisms.

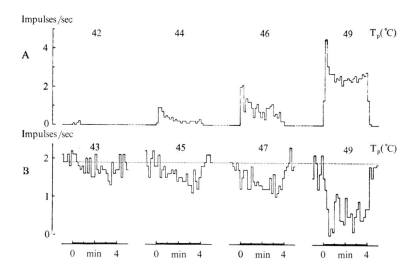

Fig. 4. Inverse relationship of activities of putative vasodilators (A) and vasoconstrictors (B) in relation to spinal cord temperature[13]. (A) Silent postganglionic neuron to the hairy skin. (B) Spontaneously active postganglionic neuron to the hairless skin. T_p, perfusion temperature of spinal cord thermode. (Source: ref. 13 Reproduced by kind permission of Springer Verlag, West Germany.)

(b) *Muscle sympathetic.* Two vasomotor fiber types could be discriminated by Horeysek *et al.*[19] in the cat. One spontaneously active fraction apparently represented vasoconstrictor fibers. A second group was not spontaneously active but could be activated by stimulations of hypothalamic structures known to elicit the complex pattern of the "defence reaction". Therefore, these fibers probably represent the muscle vasodilatators[16,56] accounting for the increase in muscle blood flow during the initial phase of this reaction. The observation is again important that a coordinated change of activity in muscle vasoconstrictor and dilatator fibers occurred at the onset of this reaction, so that initial activation of the vasodilatators partly coincided with a silent period in the vasoconstrictor discharges.

(c) *Cardiac sympathetic.* The first observation of a differentiation within the sympathetic supply of the heart under conditions of differentiated sympathetic activation was made by Simon and Riedel[55] when the activities of fine strands from the right cardioaccelerator nerve were simultaneously recorded. Single fiber preparations, particularly from the left cardioaccelerator nerve, have subsequently revealed a great diversity of response patterns under central thermal stimulation and changes of blood gas composition[46]. If it is presumed that these fibers serve functions in the control of cardiac performance, then a highly differentiated control of various components of cardiac function appears likely. The great technical difficulties in selectively evaluating the various parameters of cardiac function under conditions at which they may change independently of each other have, thus far, precluded detailed analysis of their nervous control. It could, however, be demonstrated that the activity of some cardiac sympathetic nerve fibers under various circumstances was always correlated with heart rate, while the activity of other fibers was not.

(d) *Renal sympathetic*. Differentiation at the level of single unit activity has also been demonstrated in the sympathetic supply to the rabbit kidney. Similar to the situation in the analysis of cardiac sympathetic innervation, the functions which particular fibers of the renal sympathetic system fulfil have remained obscure. In an attempt to evaluate functional differences between renal sympathetic fibers, Riedel and Peter[47] recently demonstrated two types of fibers responding differently to vasoactive substances. As shown in Fig. 5, one type was obviously reflexly inhibited by increases of blood pressure, due to intravenous application of noradrenaline or angiotensin II. Another type, however, was inhibited by noradrenaline but activated by angiotensin II. Although this observation does not clarify the functions of these two fiber populations, it suggests differences in their central control. This observation may offer a clue for further analysis of the mechanism of differentiation, because the same two different response types to the vasoactive substances have been observed in the sympathetic supply to all other organs investigated so far.

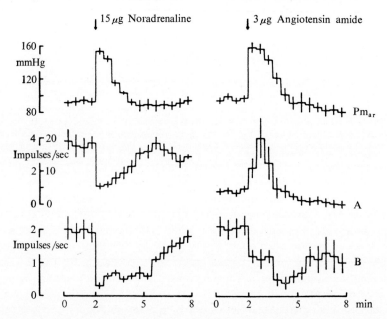

Fig. 5.   Response of renal sympathetic efferents (fiber types A and B) and of arterial mean blood pressure (Pm_{ar}) to i.v. injections of noradrenaline (15 μg) and angiotensin amide (3 μg). Mean values with standard deviations obtained from 9 animals. The right-hand scale of the ordinate for fiber type A refers to the effect of angiotensin amide[47]. (Source: ref. 47 Reproduced by kind permission of Birkhäuser Verlag, Swiss)

Some attempts to analyze the mechanism of regional sympathetic differentiation

As clearly shown in Table 1, the patterns of regional sympathetic differentiation differ from each other according to the modes, intensities and locations of stimulations and also to some extent with the species under investigation. The variability of the patterns strongly suggests that a considerable degree of functional independence must exist between the central vasomotor neuron pools controlling the various sections of the cardiovascular system. Functional separation between the neuronal networks of central vasomotor control of diverse regions may be established at different levels of integration. This is suggested by the different categories of stimuli which are able to induce regional sympathetic differentiation. Some of these stimuli, for instance those applied by Horeysek and Jänig[17,18], suggest interactions between spinal and supraspinal: reflex arcs as a mode of sympathetic differentiation. With respect to the viscerosympathetic reflex patterns[41,42] differentiation may be based on the differentiated connection of baro- and chemoreceptor inputs with the central tonic activities, as proposed by Korner[35]. However, no such explanation on the basis of reflex connection appears likely for the patterns of sympathetic differentiation observed in response to stimulation of temperature sensors in the skin and at sites of the body core as different as the hypothalamus and spinal cord. It may even be questioned whether the assumption of the reflex origin of differentiation holds for the patterns observed in response to changes of blood gas composition. The doubts arise from the fact that these stimuli naturally elicit complex homeostatic adjustments, including autonomic as well as somatomotor and behavioral activities. Patterns of sympathetic differentiation generated within the scope of these adjustments are, therefore, probably generated together with other activities at the highest levels of somatovisceral integration, i.e., at supramedullary levels, and require concepts of control rather than of reflex mechanisms for their analysis[36]. The following considerations regarding the central mechanisms of sympathetic differentiation have been guided by this view and are, therefore, restricted to response patterns with a presumed regulatory significance.

Role of baroreceptors in sympathetic differentiation:
(a) *Pattern generation.* According to the presumption that patterns of sympathetic differentiation in the course of homeostatic adjustment reactions are produced at high levels of central nervous integration, the main characteristics of particular differentiated responses are primary in nature. Nevertheless, interference of the descending signals of pattern generation with proprioceptive inputs at the medullary or lower levels may be critical for the final design of the differentiated response. Mechanisms of facilitation, inhibition and occlusion have to be taken into consideration as modifying mechanisms. The importance of interactions of this kind was first experimentally assessed by excluding the proprioceptive inputs from the circulation by sinoaortic denervation and vagotomy. In part of the experiments, the patterns of sympathetic differentiation induced by standard thermal stimuli or by changes of blood gas composition were analyzed directly by mass discharge recordings. In addition, or alternatively, indirect evaluation by hemodynamic analysis appeared more feasible in view of the great stresses imposed on the animals by opening the proprioceptive control loops.

Simon and Riedel[55] investigated the effect of sinoaortic denervation and vagotomy on the regional differentiation of sympathetic efferents in response to *central thermal stimulation* by mass discharge recordings. Fig. 6 summarizes the results obtained in two groups of experiments in which the spinal cord was selectively heated in rabbits with sinoaortic denervation and vagotomy. As in intact animals, cutaneous sympathetic activity was reduced by heating, while cardiac and intestinal sympathetic activities were simultaneously increased. Both rise of ear skin temperatures and cardiac acceleration corresponded to the local changes of cardiovascular innervation. Thus, the original pattern was preserved in qualitative respects, although circulatory homeostasis was lost. Hemodynamic studies in dogs have confirmed this preservation of the response pattern[7,54] as far as the response to heating is concerned. Quantitatively, sympathetic activation was more

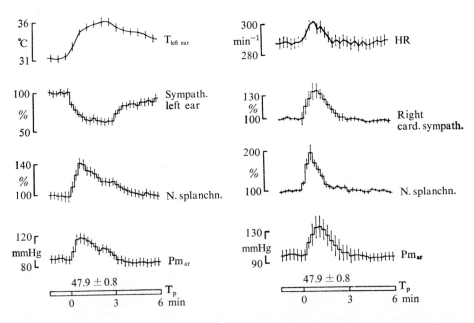

Fig. 6.   Responses of regional sympathetic efferents during selective spinal cord heating in anesthetized, paralyzed rabbits with sinoaortic denervation and vagotomy[55]. Mean value with standard error of 7 experiments. Parameters are as in Fig. 2.

pronounced after sinoaortic denervation and vagotomy with the result of considerable rises of blood pressure. The same preponderance of the activating components of the pattern of differentiation turned out to exist under conditions of spinal cord cooling, causing a qualitative deviation from the pattern of the intact animal. As shown by Simon and Riedel[55] and by Conradt *et al.*[7], spinal cord cooling after sinoaortic denervation and vagotomy caused a strong activation of splanchnic activity, contrasting to the inhibition of activity in intact animals, but cardiac and cutaneous sympathetic responses and the corresponding hemodynamic reactions were not qualitatively altered. The deviation of the response after denervation from that of the intact animal may, however, be ascribed to a unique, hitherto completely obscure effect of the spinal cord signal input on medullary vasomotor tone[52] and not to the loss *per se* of the baroreceptor input. This interpretation has been supported by recent hemodynamic investigations in which the changes of skin and intestinal blood flow and of cardiac functions during hypothalamic thermal stimulation were investigated comparatively in intact dogs and in those with sinoaortic denervation and vagotomy[11]. The typical response pattern of the intact animals was fully preserved after opening the proprioceptive control loop, indicating that the pattern of sympathetic differentiation in thermoregulation was generated completely independently of the baroreceptor control system[11].

With regard to the pattern of sympathetic differentiation induced by *changes of blood gas composition*, the role of the baroreceptor input could be observed only under conditions in which the pattern was presumably generated via central chemoreceptors, i.e., by hypercapnia, because the arterial chemoreceptors were excluded, together with the baroreceptor input, by sinoaortic denervation and vagotomy. As demonstrated by Simon and Riedel[55], rabbits with an interrupted proprioceptive control loop responded to strong hypercapnia with the same pattern of regional symphathetic differentiation as intact rabbits did according to Iriki et al.[27]. The conclusion may be drawn that interaction between the control information descending from supramedullary integrative centers to the medullary and/or spinal vasomotor neuron pools are not basically altered by the medullary or spinal reflex inputs. Thus, baroreceptor inputs do not form decisive components in the generation of those patterns of sympathetic differentiation which may be considered as the autonomic control components of complex homeostatic reactions.

(b) *Pattern modulation*. The modulating effect of the baroreflex on the various regional components of the sympathetic response pattern to arterial hypoxia have been experimentally assessed by Iriki, Dorward and Korner[21,22] with the additional aim of clarifying the interactions between baro- and chemoreceptor inputs in the generation of the sympathetic response. As shown in Fig. 7, arterial baroreceptor influences have been observed in renal, cardiac and splanchnic sympathetic efferents, but not in the cutaneous branches to the ear. Chemoreceptor influences exert excitatory effects (estimated from shifts of the upper plateau) on the renal efferents, but inhibitory effects on the cardiac and cutaneous efferents. Significant interactions (indicated by changes in the baroreflex curve parameters) occur in the renal sympathetic system, consisting of facilitatory interaction, i.e., more sympathetic activity at a given arterial pressure during hypoxia, and in the

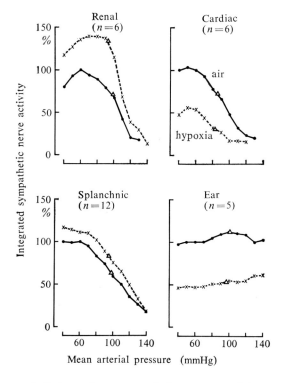

Fig. 7. Average sympathetic baroreflex curves, relating mean arterial pressure (mm Hg) to integrated sympathetic activity (%), during ventilation with room air (solid lines) and during arterial hypoxia (interrupted lines) in anesthetized, immobilized rabbits. Mean value of each experimental series. Triangles indicate the sympathetic activity at average resting mean arterial pressure[22].

cardiac sympathetic system, consisting of an inhibitory interaction. The corresponding moto-neuron pools involve elements that receive baroreceptor projections and elements under the control of chemoreceptor projections. However, the motoneuron pool of the cutaneous sympathetic system receives no substantial baroreceptor projections, while the splanchnic motoneuron pool receives little projection from chemoreceptor afferents. These results clearly indicate that differentiated changes of sympathetic efferent activity are basically primary responses and not secondary to reflex interferences with the baroreceptor inputs, and also that the pattern of interaction between baro- and chemoreceptor inputs is different in different pools of the sympathetic efferent system. The analysis allows a definition of the modulatory effects of the baroreceptor projections on the primary response.

The role of higher nervous centers:

As shown previously, the regional differentiation of sympathetic activity as a regulatory component in complex homeostatic adjustments must be considered as a primary response modulated to some extent by baroreflex interactions. Other, as yet undefined inputs may also interact, as suggested by some irregularities occasionally observed, e.g., different cardiac sympathetic responses to spinal and hypothalamic thermal stimulation in otherwise identical response patterns. Particularly for those inputs which evoke the response patterns, e.g., chemoreceptor and thermoreceptor inputs, their projections on the central vasomotor neuron pools presumably occur at different levels, including supramedullary structures. In order to evaluate the importance of the contributions of the various levels of projection to pattern generation, experiments were performed in animals with acute or chronic transections of the central nervous axis, mostly in decerebrated rabbits.

(a) *Thermal stimulation.* Fig. 8 shows the responses of regional sympathetic activities during spinal cord thermal stimulation in rabbits decerebrated at the midcollicular level. Spinal cord warming induced increases of splanchnic and simultaneous depression of cutaneous sympathetic activity. Cardiac sympathetic activity tended to increase, but this increase was not significant. However, in infracollicularly decerebrated animals the cardiac sympathetic response could be verified. Rectal temperature and arterial pressure did not change, while the heart rate rose, though insignificantly, and the ear temperature rose consistently in correlation with the local sympathetic inhibition. During spinal cord cooling the responses were inverse to those observed during warming. In midcollicularly decerebrated rabbits splanchnic activity decreased and cutaneous sympathetic activity increased. The decrease of cardiac sympathetic activity was again only significant after infracollicular decerebration.

The above results indicate that the same pattern of regional sympathetic differentiation as in intact animals can be produced by rabbits in which the classical thermoregulation center has been destroyed. Apparently, neural networks caudal to the midbrain level are capable of integrating the thermal input and produce the appropriate vasomotor adjustments. Upper midbrain structures appear, however, to exert some stabilizing influence on the lower cardiac sympathetic neuron pools, as indicated by the differences in cardiac sympathetic activity changes between animals with mid- and infracollicular decerebration.

Even integrative structures at the spinal level may acquire the ability to produce the essential features of the thermoregulatory differentiated sympathetic response. Fig. 9 shows the response to spinal cord cooling of a lightly anesthetized rabbit spinalized four days before at the C6 level. The integrated discharges from the splanchnic nerve show a considerable reduction of activity,

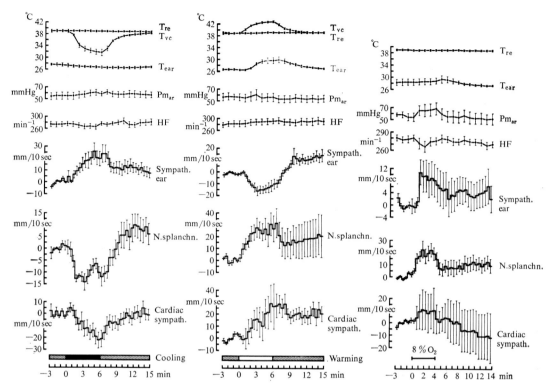

Fig. 8. Differentiated responses of regional sympathetic efferents during spinal cord cooling (left) and warming (middle) and during hypoxia (right) in anesthetized, immobilized rabbits after midcollicular decerebration. 24 Each value is the mean value with standard error of 8 experiments. Parameters are as in Fig. 2. (Source: ref. 24 Reproduced by kind permission of Spinger Verlag, West Germany.)

while the decline of ear skin temperature at a basically constant arterial pressure indicates an increased vasoconstrictor activity in this region. This state of opposite deviations of activity from the pre-stimulation conditions was maintained throughout the period of stimulation and gradually disappeared during the post-cooling control period.

The conclusion to be drawn from the transection experiments for the generation of the thermoregulatory patterns of sympathetic differentiation is that thermal inputs can be transformed into the appropriate regulatory signals to the autonomic effector systems at various levles along the central nervous axis. This does not indicate a simple reflex origin of this response, but is due to the multiple representation of thermoregulatory integrative networks in the central nervous system[53].

(b) *Arterial hypoxia.* During arterial hypoxia in rabbits decerebrated at the midcollicular level, splanchnic and cutaneous sympathetic activities were significantly increased. Cardiac sympathetic activity tended to increase, but this change could not be confirmed statistically. However, in infracollicularly decerebrated rabbits, activation of the cardiac sympathetic system during hypoxia could be demonstrated[24]. The summarized data are shown in the right-hand side of Fig. 8. The results demonstrate that suprabulbar integration is essential for the generation of the inhibitory components in the differential sympathetic response pattern during arterial hypoxia, which typi-

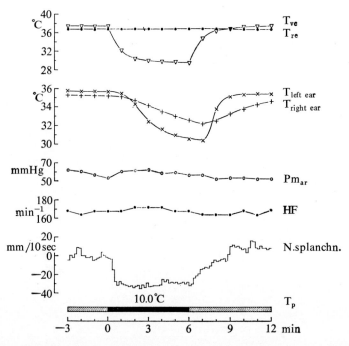

Fig. 9. Responses of ear skin temperatures and of visceral sympathetic activity during spinal cord cooling in a lightly anesthetized rabbit with spinal transection at C_6 four days before[59]. Parameters are as in Fig. 2. (Source: ref. 59 Reproduced by kind permission of Springer Verlag, West Germany.)

cally includes inhibition of cardiac and cutaneous sympathetic activity. In contrast to the thermo-regulatory sympathetic response pattern, interaction between different levels of integration appears to be necessary to generate the full regulatory autonomic component in the homeostatic reaction to a change of blood gas composition.

The results obtained in normal and decerebrated rabbits with several types of stimulation known to elicit differentiated sympathetic responses under normal conditions are summarized

TABLE 2. The pattern of regional sympathetic differentiation in normal and decerebrated animals

| | Sympathetic efferents | | | | | | | |
| | Normal | | | | Decerebrated | | | |
	Cutaneous	Splanchnic	Cardiac	Muscle	Cutaneous	Splanchnic	Cardiac	Muscle
Thermal stimulation								
Spinal cord warming	−	+	+		−	+	+	
Spinal cord cooling	+	−	−		+	−	−	
Hypoxic stimulation								
Primary tissue	−	+	+		+	+	+	
Arterial	−	+	−		+	+	+	
Cutaneous stimulation								
Non-noxious	+ (−)			−	∅			∅
Noxious	− (+)			+	+			+

$+$: activation, $—$: inhibition, $∅$: no change.

in Table 2, including the data of Jänig[31] on response patterns induced by cutaneous afferents. The effects of decerebration on the patterns generated by thermal stimulation, hypoxia and cutaneous stimulation show different contributions of bulbar and suprabulbar components to the response patterns. Not demonstrated are the responses of spinalized preparations in which further changes of the response to hypoxia and cutaneous stimulation were found. However, the thermal stimulus appears to be unique in that integrative networks appear to exist at all levels of the central organization of the sympathetic nervous system, which are able to produce the essential features of the specific pattern of regional sympathetic differentiation.

Conclusions

Recent progress in studies concerned with the concept of regional cardiovascular control by qualitative differentiation of the sympathetic outflow are summarized in the present report, centering around our own data. Qualitative differentiation has been proved directly by the recording of neuronal activities, not only in the sympathetic outflows to functionally different organs, but also of different neurons within the sympathetic outflow to single organs.

A variety of patterns of qualitative differentiation of sympathetic outflow is produced under various natural and experimental conditions. This means that the phenomenon of regional qualitative sympathetic differentiation is not the result of fixed autonomic reactions. The different patterns observed under different conditions may be regarded as specific autonomic regulatory responses, which are evoked in order to adjust cardiovascular function according to the special demands arising from the particular types of generalized stress. For instance, in temperature regulation the regional qualitative differentiation of the sympathetic vasoconstrictor outflow appears to be involved as a specific vasomotor response which permits regulation of heat transfer from the body core to the skin with the least possible alteration of general circulatory homeostasis. In arterial hypoxia, the blood flow away from certain vascular regions with higher need for oxygen, such as muscle and intestine, towards metabolically inert tissue such as the skin, may be considered as a reaction to save oxygen for mainly metabolically controlled vascular regions, such as the heart and brain, while, at the same time, avoiding excessive increases of systemic vascular resistance.

The differentiated changes of sympathetic outflow are basically primary responses and not secondary to reflex interferences with the reflexes concerned with circulatory homeostasis, such as the baroreflex. The mechanisms by which the central nervous system produces these responses are still obscure. It may be speculated that a complex system of a multitude of meshed reflex loops will ultimately emerge as the neuronal substrate by which a particular pattern of differentiation is brought about. However, in view of the apparent homeostatic character of at least some of the differentiated response patterns, the application of control theory for further analysis of these patterns should be a useful heuristic concept. The results obtained in decerebrated rabbits indicate that the effect of decerebration on the ability to produce differential sympathetic responses is quite different depending on the homeostatic system involved. This means that the interaction of anatomically separable integrative mechanisms at different levels of the brain stem is not a necessary precondition for the generation of a differential response. In other words, the influence of a brain stem lesion on a particular autonomic response pattern seems to depend on the degree to which special integrative (or control) functions have become concentrated in, or dispersed over, various parts of the central nervous system. This property of the mechanisms by which various patterns of differentiation are generated offers the possibility to investigate particular response components step by step, considering that the pattern of differentiation of the sympathetic outflow is not a fixed one but differs according to the mode and strength of the stimulus involved.

REFERENCES

1. Abrahams, V.C., Hilton, S.M. and Zbrozyna, A.W., The role of active muscle vasodilatation in the alerting stage of the defence reaction, *J. Physiol. (Lond.)*, 171 (1964) 189–202.
2. Barcroft, H., Sympathetic control of vessels in the hand and forearm skin, *Physiol. Rev.*, 40 Suppl. 4 (1960) 81–91.
3. Brown, A.M. and Malliani, A., Spinal sympathetic reflexes initiated by coronary receptors, *J. Physiol. (Lond.)*, 212 (1971) 685–705.
4. Burton, A.C., *Physiology and Biophysics of the Circulation*, Year Book Medical Publications, Chicago, 1965.
5. Cannon, W.B., *Bodily Changes in Pain, Hunger, Fear and Rage; An Account of Recent Researches into the Function of Emotional Excitement*, 2nd ed. (Reprint), Charles T. Branford Co., Boston, 1953.
6. Chalmers, J.P., Korner, P.I. and White, S.W., The control of the circulation in skeletal muscle during arterial hypoxia in the rabbit, *J. Physiol. (Lond.)*, 184 (1966) 698–716.
7. Conradt, M., Kullmann, R., Matsuzaki, T. and Simon, E., Arterial baroreceptor function in differential cardiovascular adjustments induced by central thermal stimulation, *Basic. Res. Cardio.*, 70 (1975) 10–28.
8. Dastre, A. and Morat, J.-P., Influence du sang asphyxique sur l'appareil nerveux de la circulation, *Arch. Physiol. norm. path.*, 16 (1884) 1–45.
9. Delius, W., Hagbarth, K.-E., Hongell, A. and Wallin, B.G., Manoeuvres affecting sympathetic outflow in human skin nerves, *Acta physiol. scand.*, 84 (1972) 177–186.
10. Folkow, B., Heymans, C. and Neil, E., *Integrated Aspects of Cardiovascular Regulation. In W.F. Hamilton (Ed.) Handbook of Physiol.*, Sect. 2, Vol. III, Amer. Physiol. Soc., Washington D.C., 1965, pp. 1787–1824.
11. Göbel, D., Martin, H. and Simon, E., Primary cardiac responses to stimulation of hypothalamic and spinal cord temperature sensors evaluated in anaesthetized paralyzed dogs, *J. thermal Biol.*, 2 (1977) 41–47.
12. Gregor, M. and Jänig, W., Effects of systemic hypoxia and hypercapnia on cutaneous and muscle vasoconstrictor neurones to the cat's hindlimb, *Pflügers Arch. ges. Physiol.*, 368 (1977) 71–81.
13. Gregor, M., Jänig, W. and Riedel, W., Response pattern of cutaneous postganglionic neurones to the hindlimb on spinal cord heating and cooling in the cat, *Pflügers Arch. ges. Physiol.*, 363 (1976) 135–140.
14. Grosse, M. and Jänig, W., Vasoconstrictor and pilomotor fibres in skin nerves to the cat's tail, *Pflügers Arch. ges. Physiol.*, 361 (1976) 221–229.
15. Handley, H.G., Costing, J.C. and Skinner Jr., N.S., Differential reflex adjustments in cutaneous and muscle vascular beds during experimental coronary artery occlusion, *Amer. J. Cardiol.*, 27 (1971) 513–521.
16. Hilton, S.M., Ways of viewing the central nervous control of circulation, old and new, *Brain Research*, 87 (1975) 213–219.
17. Horeyseck, G. and Jänig, W., Reflexes in postganglionic fibers within skin and muscle nerves after non-noxious mechanical stimulation of skin, *Exp. Brain Res.*, 20 (1974 a) 115-123.
18. Horeyseck, G. and Jänig, W., Reflexes in postganglionic fibers within skin and muscle nerves after noxious stimulation of skin, *Exp. Brain Res.*, 20 (1974 b) 125-134.
19. Horeyseck, G., Jänig, W., Kirchner, F. and Thämer, V., Activation and inhibition of muscle and cutaneous postganglionic neurones to hindlimb during hypothalamically induced vasoconstriction and atropine-sensitive vasodilation, *Pflügers Arch. ges. Physiol.*, 361 (1976) 231–240.
20. Horeyseck, G. and Mie, K., Chemoreceptor influence on sympathetic discharges to the skin and muscles, *Pflügers Arch. ges. Physiol.*, 339 (1973) R 36.
21. Iriki, M., Dorward, P. and Korner, P.I., Baroreflex "resetting" by arterial hypoxia in the renal and cardiac sympathetic nerves of the rabbit, *Pflügers Arch. ges. Physiol.* 370 (1977) 1–7.
22. Iriki, M., Kozawa, E., Korner, P.I. and Dorward, P., *Baroreflex "Resetting" in Various Regional Sympathetic Efferents during Arterial Hypoxia in Normal and Decerebrated Rabbits*, Proc. of XVIII International Congress of Neurovegetative Res., (1977) (in press).
23. Iriki, M. and Kozawa, E., Factors controlling the regional differentiation of sympathetic outflow – Influence of the chemoreceptor reflex, *Brain Research*, 87 (1975) 281–291.
24. Iriki, M. and Kozawa, E., Patterns of differentiation in various sympathetic efferents induced by hypoxic and by central thermal stimulation in decerebrated rabbits, *Pflügers Arch. ges. Physiol.*, 362 (1976) 101–108.
25. Iriki, M., Pleschka, K., Walther, O.-E. and Simon, E., Hypoxia and hypercapnia in asphyctic differentiation of regional sympathetic activity in the anesthetized rabbit, *Pflügers Arch. ges. Physiol.*, 328 (1971 a) 91–102.

26. Iriki, M., Riedel, W. and Simon, E., Regional differentiation of sympathetic activity during hypothalamic heating and cooling in anesthetized rabbits, *Pflügers Arch. ges. Physiol.*, 328 (1971 b) 320–331.
27. Iriki, M., Riedel, W. and Simon, E., Patterns of differentiation in various sympathetic efferents induced by changes of blood gas composition and by central thermal stimulation in anesthetized rabbits, *Japan. J. Physiol.*, 22 (1972) 585–602.
28. Iriki, M. and Simon, E., Differential autonomic control of regional circulatory reflexes evoked by thermal stimulation and by hypoxia, *AJEBAK*, 51 (1973) 283–293.
29. Iriki, M., Walther, O.-E., Pleschka, K. and Simon, E., Regional cutaneous and visceral sympathetic activity during asphyxia in the anesthetized rabbit, *Pflügers Arch. ges. Physiol.*, 322 (1971 c) 167–182.
30. Irisawa, H., Ninomiya, I. and Woolley, G., Efferent activity in renal and intestinal nerves during circulatory reflexes, *Japan. J. Physiol.*, 23 (1973) 657–666.
31. Jänig, W., Central organization of somatosympathetic reflexes in vasoconstrictor neurones, *Brain Research*, 87 (1975) 305–312.
32. Jänig, W. and Kümmel, H., Functional discrimination of postganglionic neurones to the cat's hindpaw with respect to the skin potentials recorded from hairless skin, *Pflügers Arch. ges. Physiol.*, 371 (1977) 217–225.
33. Karim, F., Kidd, C., Malpus, C.M. and Penna, P.E., The effects of stimulation of the left atrial receptors on sympathetic efferent nerve activity, *J. Physiol. (Lond.)*, 227 (1972) 243–260.
34. Koizumi, K. and Brooks, C. McC., The integration of autonomic reactions: a discussion of autonomic reflexes, their control and their association with somatic reactions, *Rev. Physiol. biochem. Pharmacol.*, 67 (1972) 1–68.
35. Korner, P.I., Integrative neural cardiovascular control. *Physiol. Rev.*, 51 (1971) 312–367.
36. Korner, P.I. and Simon, E., Regional organization of autonomic nervous system, *Brain Research*, 87 (1975) 339–340.
37. Korner, P.I., Uther, J.B. and White, S.W., Central nervous integration of the circulatory and respiratory responses to arterial hypoxemia in the rabbit, *Circul. Res.*, 24 (1969) 757–776.
38. Kullmann, R. and Junk, H.G., Differential sympathetic response during coronary occlusion, *Res. exp. Med.*, 160 (1973) 317–320.
39. Kullmann, R., Schönung, W. and Simon, E., Antagonistic changes of blood flow and sympathetic activity in different vascular beds following central thermal stimulation. I. Blood flow in skin, muscle and intestine during spinal cord heating and cooling in anesthetized dogs, *Pflügers Arch. ges. Physiol.*, 319 (1970) 146–161.
40. Malliani, A., Peterson, D.F., Bishop, V.S. and Brown, A.M., Spinal sympathetic cardiocardiac reflexes, *Circul. Res.*, 30 (1972) 158–166.
41. Ninomiya, I., Irisawa, H. and Nisimaru, N., Nonuniformity of sympathetic nerve activity to the skin and kidney, *Amer. J. Physiol.*, 224 (1973) 256–264.
42. Ninomiya, I., Nisimaru, N. and Irisawa, H., Sympathetic nerve activity to the splee, kidney, and heart in response to baroceptor input, *Amer. J. Physiol.*, 221 (1971) 1346–1351.
43. Nisimaru, N., Comparison of gastric and renal nerve activity, *Amer. J. Physiol.*, 220 (1971) 1303–1308.
44. Rein, H., Vasomotorische Regulationen, *Ergeb. physiol.*, 32 (1931) 28–72.
45. Riedel, W., Iriki, M. and Simon, E., Regional differentiation of sympathetic activity during peripheral heating and cooling in anesthetized rabbits, *Pflügers Arch. ges. Physiol.*, 332 (1972) 239–247.
46. Riedel, W. and Peter, W., Effect of thermal stimulation and of changes of blood gas composition on sympathetic nervous outflow, *Pflügers Arch. ges. Physiol.*, 365 Suppl. (1976) R 37.
47. Riedel, W. and Peter, W., Non-uniformity of regional vasomotor activity indicating the existence of 2 different systems in the sympathetic cardiovascular outflow, *Experientia (Basel)*, 33 (1977) 337–338.
48. Sato, A. and Schmidt, R.F., Somato-sympathetic reflexes: Afferent fibers, central pathways, discharge characteristics, *Physiol. Rev.*, 53 (1973) 916–947.
49. Schäfer, H., Central control of cardiac function, *Physiol. Rev.*, 40 Suppl. 4 (1960) 213–231.
50. Schönung, W., Jessen, C., Wagner, H. and Simon, E., Regional blood flow antagonism induced by central thermal stimulation in the conscious dog, *Experientia (Basel)*, 27 (1971) 1291–1292.
51. Schönung, W., Wagner, H. and Simon, E., Neurogenic vasodilatatory component in the thermoregulatory skin blood flow response of the dog, *Naunyn-Schmiedebergs Arch. Pharmacol.*, 273 (1972) 230–241.
52. Simon, E., Kreislaufwirkungen der spinalen Hypothermie, *J. Neuro-Vise. Re.*, 31 (1969) 223–259.
53. Simon, E., Temperature regulation—the spinal cord as a site of extrahypothalamic thermoregulatory functions, *Rev. Physiol. biochem. Pharmacol.*, 71 (1974) 1–76.
54. Simon, E., Iriki, M. and Riedel, W., Qualitative differentiation of regional sympathetic activity as regulatory response of autonomic control systems. In W. Umbach and H.P. Koepchen (Eds.) *Central Rhythmic and Regulation*, Hippokrates, Stuttgart, 1974, pp. 220–228.
55. Simon, E. and Riedel, W., Diversity of regional sympathetic outflow in integrative cardiovascular control; Patterns and mechanisms, *Brain Research*, 87 (1975) 323–333.
56. Uvnäs, B., Central cardiovascular control. In H.W. Magoun (Ed.) *Handbook of Physiology*, Sect. 1, Vol. II, Amer. Physiol. Soc., Washington D.C., 1960, pp. 1131–1162.

57. Wallin. B.G., Sundlöf, G. and Delius, W., The effect of carotid sinus nerve stimulation on muscle and skin nerve sympathetic activity in man, *Pflügers Arch. ges. Physiol.*, 358 (1975) 101–110.
58. Walther, O.-E., Iriki, M. and Simon, E., Antagonïstic changes of blood flow and sympathetic activity in different vascular beds following central thermal stimulation. II. Cutaneous and visceral sympathetic activity during spinal cord heating and cooling in anesthetized rabbits and cats, *Pflügers Arch. ges. Physiol.*, 319 (1970) 162–184.
59. Walther, O.-E., Riedel, W., Iriki, M. and Simon, E., Differentiation of sympathetic activity at the spinal level in response to central cold stimulation, *Pflügers Arch. ges. Physiol.*, 329 (1971) 220–230.

Effect of carotid sinus stimulation on the excitation of afferent cardiac sympathetic fibers during myocardial ischemia

YASUMI UCHIDA

Second Department of Internal Medicine, Faculty of Medicine, University of Tokyo, Bunkyo-ku, Tokyo 113, Japan.

It has been demonstrated that afferent fibers in the cardiac sympathetic nerves are excited during myocardial ischemia and their activity is influenced by sympathetic and vagal efferent fibers[1-3]. Stimulation of the carotid sinus baroreceptor is known to affect the activities of efferent cardiac sympathetic and vagal fibers by reflex. The present experiments were undertaken to examine the possibility that pressure stimulation of the carotid sinus might modulate the augmented activity evoked in the afferent cardiac sympathetic fibers by coronary constriction.

Nine mongrel dogs were anesthetized with pentobarbital sodium (35–40 mg/kg, i.v.). The trachea was intubated for positive pressure respiration with air. Action potentials were recorded from single afferent sympathetic fibers at the level of the upper thoracic communicating rami of the left side, and their receptive fields were identified to be in the apical area of the left ventricle by proving the ventricular surface. The proximal segment of the anterior descending coronary artery was constricted stepwise with a screw clamp to produce myocardial ischemia. A catheter was introduced in retrograde fashion into a small branch of the artery to measure the coronary blood pressure. A strain gauge was attached to the anterior wall of the left ventricle to measure the left ventricular tension. Another catheter was introduced into the right femoral artery to measure the systemic blood pressure. The right common carotid artery and right external carotid artery were cannulated. The internal carotid artery and other small arteries on the same side were ligated to reduce the sinus region to a blind sac. The carotid sinus pressure was elevated to 200 mm Hg by injection of warm saline through the cannula attached to the common carotid artery. This pressure level was maintained for about 20 sec and then the pressure was readjusted to the initial level by removing saline. The action potentials, left ventricular tension and systemic blood pressure were recorded simultaneously on moving films. At the same time, integrated curves of the action potentials, coronary blood pressure, left ventricular tension and carotid sinus pressure were recorded on a penoscillograph.

Action potentials were recorded from six A delta fibers and one C fiber. Before coronary constriction, the discharges of the fibers were sporadic in most preparations. An obvious increase in discharge frequency was observed in all preparations when the mean coronary blood pressure was lowered by constriction to below 50% of the control value.

Without coronary constriction, carotid sinus stimulation caused a slight decrease in discharge frequency. During partial constriction of the coronary artery, the same pressure stimulation of the carotid sinus produced a significant decrease in the augmented discharge frequency, while the magnitude of the decrease in heart rate and that of the fall in systemic blood pressure were not different from those of the control stimulation experiments (Figs. 1 and 2). During complete coronary constriction, the inhibition caused by carotid sinus stimulation was more significant than that caused during partial constriction. In addition, the decreased discharge frequency was maintained even after cessation of carotid sinus stimulation. During partial coronary constriction, cessation of carotid sinus stimulation induced a transient increase in discharge frequency as well as systolic bulge (passive stretching of the myocardium during systole). During complete coronary constriction, systolic bulge was reduced by stimulation and was augmented after cessation of stimulation. An augmented increase in discharge frequency was associated with the augmented systolic bulge.

The present results indicate that carotid sinus stimulation produces suppression of the excitation induced in afferent sympathetic fibers of left ventricular origin by coronary constriction. It is well known that activation of the carotid sinus nerves inhibits efferent sympathetic fiber activity and facilitates efferent vagal fiber activity, and as a consequence decreases heart rate and systemic blood pressure. It appears likely therefore that the decreases in heart rate and left ventricular after-load due to the lowered arterial pressure might have resulted in decreased oxygen consumption and, in turn, a reduction in ischemia level of the myocardium, and consequently the suppression of excitation of the afferent fibers might have occurred.

During partial constriction of the coronary artery, cessation of carotid sinus stimulation was followed by an augmented increase in discharge frequency and systolic bulge of the left ventricle. In a previous study[3], it has been shown that blood flow in partially constricted coronary artery remained reduced or was further reduced after cessation of stimulation of vagal efferents. Reflex excitation of efferent sympathetic fibers was also found to occur after cessation of carotid

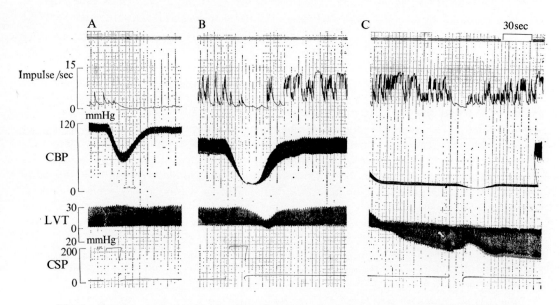

Fig. 1.   Sample records showing the effect of pressure stimulation on afferent neural activity of the cardiac nerve with and without coronary constriction. From top: integrated action potentials of an A delta fiber of left ventricular origin, coronary blood pressure, left ventricular tension, and carotid sinus pressure. A, Before coronary constriction; B, during partial coronary constriction; C, during complete coronary constriction.

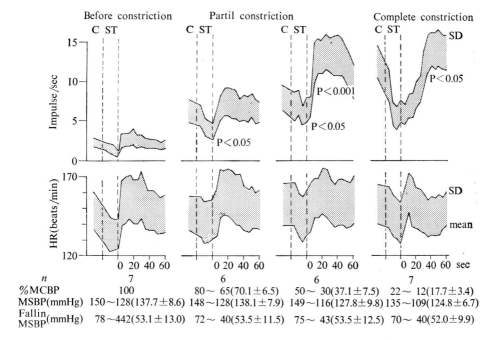

Fig. 2. Changes in discharge frequency of afferent fibers and heart rate induced by carotid sinus stimulation. The changes in mean systemic blood pressure induced by the stimulation are shown at the bottom. n = No. of fiber preparations. % MCBP = Mean coronary blood pressure expressed as percent of the control value. C = Discharge frequency before stimulation (average value of 30 sec). ST = Stimulation of carotid sinus. Abscissa indicates time (sec) from cessation of stimulation.

sinus stimulation. Accordingly, a decrease in coronary blood flow which would be enhanced by positive chronotropic and inotropic actions of efferent sympathetic fibers might have caused more severe myocardial ischemia, which would reasonably lead to augmented excitation of the afferent cardiac sympathetic fibers[1]. During complete coronary constriction, augmented excitation of the fibers occurred with a relatively long latency after cessation of carotid sinus stimulation (Fig. 2). Since no further decrease in blood flow could be produced, the possible explanation is that increased oxygen consumption due to reflex excitation of efferent sympathetic fibers might have occurred, and myocardial ischemia might accordingly have developed slowly, resulting in delayed excitation of the afferent fibers.

REFERENCES

1. Uchida, Y. and Murao, S., Excitation of afferent cardiac sympathetic nerve fibers during coronary occlusion, *Amer. J. Physiol.*, 226 (1974) 1094–1099.
2. Uchida, Y., Yoshimoto, N. and Murao, S., Excitation of afferent cardiac sympathetic nerve fibers induced by vagal stimulation, *Japan Heart J.*, 16 (1975) 548–563.
3. Uchida, Y. and Murao, S., Sustained decrease in coronary blood flow and excitation of cardiac sensory fibers following sympathetic stimulation, *Japan Heart J.*, 16 (1975) 265–278.

Depressor and pressor responses produced by muscular thin-fiber afferents

TAKAO KUMAZAWA, KAZUE MIZUMURA, EIKO TADAKI AND KIO KIM

Department of Physiology, School of Medicine, Nagoya University,
Showa-ku, Nagoya 466, Japan

Polymodal nociceptors have been found to exist in cutaneous tissue[1,2]. The majority of the thin afferent nerve fibers in the deep somatic and visceral organs, such as the gastrocnemius muscle and testis, have been shown to originate from the polymodal receptors in dogs[3-5]. Our previous study[6] has demonstrated that chemical stimulation of the muscle in dogs produced both an augmentation of ventilation and excitation of polymodal C fibers. The latency and relative magnitude of the latter response to various chemicals were similar to those of the respiratory response. The present experiments were designed to test whether electrical stimulation of polymodal afferent nerve fibers innervating the posterior limb muscle in the dog produced any changes in systemic arterial blood pressure and heart rate.

Dogs were anesthetized and paralyzed by continuous i.v. infusion of a mixture of chloralose, urethane and gallamine triethiodide and respirated artificially. The bilateral vagal nerves were transected at the cervical level. For recording arterial blood pressure a cannula connected to a pressure transducer was attached to the common carotid artery. When the afferent nerve fibers originating from the limb muscle were stimulated, either the remaining unobstructed common carotid artery was transiently ligated or the carotid sinus nerve on that side was previously transected to eliminate blood pressure changes due to the carotid sinus reflex which may be activated secondarily by the blood pressure response to stimulation of the muscle nerve. Each one of the nerves innervating the gastrocnemius-soleus, the biceps femoris and the semitendinosus muscles was isolated for stimulation and recording the evoked compound action potentials. The threshold intensity was determined for A-δ and for C fibers in each preparation from the corresponding responses in compound action potentials evoked by single pulses. Repetitive pulses of 2 and 8 or 16 Hz and 1 min duration were used for evoking responses in blood pressure. The end-tidal CO_2 and O_2 levels and body temperature were monitored throughout the experiment.

Stimulation of the muscle nerve at an intensity stronger than the threshold for A-δ fiber induced a decrease in blood pressure in most cases as shown in Fig. 1. As the stimulus intensity was increased up to a certain level, this depressor response was augmented. When the stimulus intensity was further increased, a response of increased blood pressure appeared, and became dominant as shown in Fig. 1. An increase and decrease in heart rate preceded the responses of increasing and decreasing blood pressure, respectively. High frequency stimulation exaggerated both responses in blood pressure (Fig. 1): this may be explained by temporal summation of neural transmission in the central nervous system. However, the response of increasing blood pressure was not always produced even by stimuli as strong as 5 times the threshold for C fiber.

When the respiratory tidal volume was increased to lower the end-tidal CO_2 level, depressor response was found to be far more dominant than response of increasing blood pressure at all stimulus levels when compared to the results obtained under normal acid-base balance (Fig. 1)

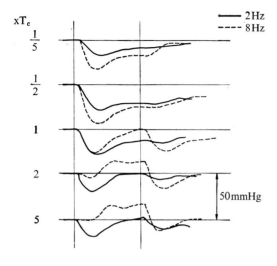

xT$_c$

$\frac{1}{5}$

$\frac{1}{2}$

1

2

5

—— 2 Hz
---- 8 Hz

50 mmHg

Fig. 1. Changes in blood pressure after electrical stimulation of the afferent fiber innervating the posterior limb muscle, the biceps femoris muscle, in the dog. The stimulus intensity used expressed as multiples of the threshold for activating C fibers T$_c$) is indicated on the left. Stimulus frequency, 2 Hz (——), 8 Hz (----); end-tidal CO$_2$, 4.2–4.4%; body temperature, 38.2°C.

at the same stimulus intensity and frequency. On the other hand, the response of increasing blood pressure was far more prominent than the depressor response when the end-tidal CO$_2$ level was increased by inhalation of air containing 2% CO$_2$.

Johanson[7] has demonstrated that somatic afferent A and C fibers mediate a decrease and an increase in blood pressure in response to stimulation of the muscle nerve, respectively. He proposed to call the A and C afferent fibers the depressor and pressor afferents, respectively. The present results obtained in dogs under normal acid-base balance appear to be consistent with Johanson's view. However, our results obtained under disturbed acid-base balance have demonstrated that the A and C afferent fibers in the muscle nerve do not always mediate the same responses in blood pressure under various physiological conditions such as those reported by Johanson. Most of the thin afferent fibers, including A-δ and C fibers, innervating the medial gastrocnemius muscle have been shown to originate from polymodal receptors in dogs[5]. It is likely therefore that the circulatory responses produced by stimulation of afferent fibers in the muscle nerve are due to activation of polymodal afferents.

REFERENCES

1. Bessou, P. and Perl, E.R., Response of cutaneous sensory units with unmyelinated fibers to noxious stimuli, *J. Neurophysiol.*, 32 (1969) 1025–1043.
2. Kumazawa, T. and Perl, E.R., Primate cutaneous sensory units with unmyelinated (C) afferent fibers, *J. Neurophysiol.*, 40 (1977) 1325–1338.
3. Kumazawa, T. and Mizumura, K., The polymodal C-fiber receptor in the muscle of the dog, *Brain Research*, 101 (1976) 589–593.
4. Kumazawa, T. and Mizumura, K., The polymodal receptors in the testis of dog, *Brain Research*, 136 (1977) 553–558.
5. Kumazawa, T. and Mizumura, K., Thin-fiber receptors responding to mechanical, chemical, and thermal stimulation in the skeletal muscle of the dog, *J. Physiol. (Lond.)*, 273 (1977) 179–194.
6. Mizumura, K. and Kumazawa, T., Reflex respiratory response induced by chemical stimulation of muscle afferents, *Brain Research*, 109 (1976) 402–406.
7. Johanson, B., Circulatory responses to stimulation of somatic afferents, *Acta physiol. scand.*, 57 (1962) Suppl. 198.

Origin of the cardio-inhibitory motoneurons in the medulla of the cat

MITSUHIKO MIURA AND TAKAMASA KITAMURA

Department of Physiology, School of Medicine, Gunma University,
Maebashi, Gumma 371, Japan

Recently, the site of origin of the preganglionic cardio-inhibitory motoneurons of cats has been identified electrophysiologically in the nucleus ambiguus (NA)[3]. However, anatomical evidence based on the horseradish peroxidase (HRP) method, has suggested as the sites the nucleus of the solitary tract (NTS) and the dorsal motor nucleus of the vagus (DMNV)[4]. Since this problem remains unsettled, the present experiments were undertaken to determine definitively by antidromic techniques the site of origin of cardio-inhibitory preganglionic fibers.

Forty-five cats (wt2–4kg) were anesthetized with a mixture of chloralose and urethane. The trachea was cannulated and the animal was artificially ventilated. The right chest was opened and the cranial and/or caudal branches of the cardiac vagus nerve (CN) were dissected free. The ipsilateral or bilateral carotid sinus nerves (CSN) were also dissected for stimulation. For recording the evoked field potentials glass micropipettes were filled with 2 M NaCl solution containing fast green dye for marking, and the resistance was 2 M .

While stimulating either cranial branch of the CN or CSN, the NTS and DMNV (163

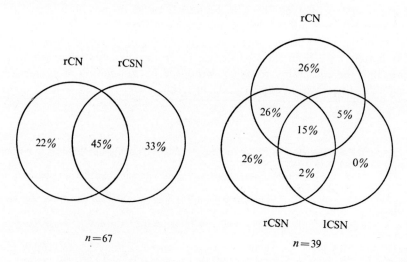

Fig. 1. Percentage distribution of evoked potentials elicited in the cat medulla oblongata by electrical stimulation of the cardiac nerve (CN) and/or the carotid sinus nerve (CSN). Overlapped compartments represent one and the same site at which the response was evoked by stimulation of either nerve. The left diagram indicates the results of stimulating the right CN and the right CSN. The right diagram shows the results of stimulating the right CN, the right CSN and the left CSN in each recording site.

tracks) and the NA and dorsal lateral tegmental field (dFTL) (169 tracks) were explored. Evoked potentials elicited by 50 repetitive stimuli applied to the CN were averaged. For each site of recording, either ipsilateral CSN or bilateral CSN were also tested for evoking response. The percent distribution of evoked responses to stimulation of the different nerves is summarized in Fig. 1. Over 40% of the evoked potentials were elicited by stimulation of the CSN in addition to the CN.

Since the cardiac branch of the vagus nerve contains both afferent and efferent fibers, the evoked potentials elicited by stimulation of the CN can be attributed to either orthodromically or antidromically evoked responses. As efferent fibers of the CN have been classified as B fibers[1,2], and the approximate distance between the stimulating site of the CN and the medulla oblongata was about 150 mm, the latency of the antidromic response evoked and conducted along B fibers must be longer than 10 msec. We attempted to classify the responses to CN stimulation into two groups according to whether their peak latency was longer or shorter than 10 msec.

Fig. 2 illustrates the percent distribution of the responses to CN stimulation according to the recording sites and peak latencies. When the testing stimulus was given 20 msec after a conditioning stimulus in the paired pulse experiments, the threshold for the testing stimulus to evoke the

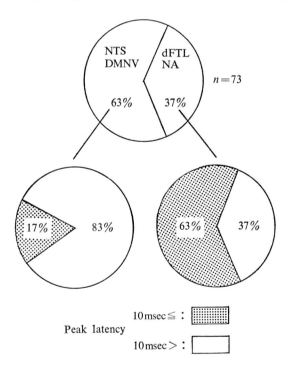

Fig. 2. Percentage distribution of latency of the field potentials elicited in the cat medulla oblongata by electrical stimulation of the cardiac branch of the vagus nerve. The upper diagram represents the percentage compartments of the site of recording responses. The lower left diagram shows the percentage distribution of latency of the responses recorded in the NTS and the DMNV, and the lower right diagram shows the percentage distribution of the responses recorded in the dFTL and the NA. DMNV, Dorsal motor nucleus of the vagus; dFTL, dorsal lateral tegmental field; NA, nucleus ambiguus; NTS, nucleus of the solitary tract.

long latency response was found to be higher than that for the conditioning stimulus. This result appears to suggest that the nerve fibers producing the long latency responses are B fibers. The sum of the peak latency of the responses recorded at the same single site to stimulation of the CN and the CSN was longer than 20 msec, which is comparable to the reflex time as estimated by stimulating the CSN and recording the evoked response from the CN.

The results in Figs. 1 and 2 lead us to conclude the following. (1) Both the NTS and NA are possible sites of origin of the vagal efferent motoneurons innervating the heart; and the NA appears to contain the majority of them. (2) The bilateral CSN's converge onto both the NTS and the NA from which vagal efferent fibers arise.

References

1. Grundfest, H., The properties of mammalian B fibers, *Amer. J. Physiol.*, 127 (1939) 252–262.
2. Kunze, D.L., Reflex discharge patterns of cardiac vagal efferent fibers, *J. Physiol. (Lond.)*, 222 (1972) 1–15.
3. McAllen, R.M. and Spyer, K.M., The location of cardiac vagal preganglionic motoneurons in the medulla of the cat, *J. Physiol. (Lond.)*, 258 (1976) 187–204.
4. Todo, K. Yamamoto, T., Satomi, H., Ise, H., Takatama, H. and Takahashi, K., Origin of vagal preganglionic fibers to the sino-atrial and atrio-ventricular node regions in the cat heart as studied by the horseradish peroxidase method, *Brain Research*, 130 (1977) 545–550.

Effects of cord section on blood pressure in different experimental hypertensive rats

JURO IRIUCHIJIMA AND YOSHINOBU NUMAO

Department of Physiology, School of Medicine, University of Tokyo,
Bunkyo-ku, Tokyo 113, Japan

Comparison of blood pressure between hypertensive and normotensive rats after spinal cord section is considered to provide information on the participation of the cardiovascular centers in hypertension. By suitably selecting the level of cord section, blood pressure can be observed in rats breathing spontaneously with the connection between the medulla and the thoracolumbar spinal segments interrupted. If cord section is performed under ether anesthesia and the ether is withdrawn immediately after section, it is possible to observe blood pressure free from the effects of anesthetic within a few hours. This is a great advantage in the study of hypertension, since some anesthetics exert a profound, direct influence on peripheral hypertensive mechanisms also[2]. The purpose of the present study was to examine the role played by the cardiovascular centers in different kinds of experimental hypertension in the conscious state.

In a previous study[3] the above experiment was performed on spontaneously hypertensive rats (SHR; Okamoto and Aoki[4]). SHR and normotensive control rats (NCR) were anesthetized with ether. The femoral artery was cannulated for measurement of the arterial pressure. The spinal cord was transected between vertebrae C7 and Th 1. In both SHR and NCR, the arterial pressure first dropped steeply to a minimum value of about 50–60 mm Hg in 1–2 min and then recovered gradually. For the first several minutes, the arterial pressures of both groups were similar but they gradually diverged. From 30 min after transection, the arterial pressure of SHR was significantly higher than that of NCR. Two hr after cord section, the mean arterial pressure $\pm$ S.D. for SHR was 124 $\pm$ 13.6 mm Hg, while that for NCR was 98.2 $\pm$ 12.7 (each $n = 10$). This difference was significant by the t-test ($P < 0.001$).

The above result indicates that the hypertensive factors of SHR are not confined to the supraspinal centers. The blood pressure was also significantly higher in SHR than in NCR even after pithing the spinal cord below the vertebra of Th 1. Therefore, the activity in the spinal sympathetic centers is not indispensable for the higher pressure in SHR than in NCR following cord section. After cord section or cord pithing, subsequent pentobarbital sodium anesthesia abolished the significant difference in pressure between the two groups of rats. The blood pressure after either cord section or pithing tended to increase with age in SHR but not in NCR. These findings indicate the presence of certain age-dependent peripheral hypertensive factors which are susceptible to pentobarbital and probably myogenic in nature, considering the direct inhibitory effects which this anesthetic exerts on cardiac and vascular smooth muscles[1].

The same cord section experiment was performed in chronic neurogenic hypertensive rats (NHR) prepared by sino-aortic denervation according to the procedure of Krieger[5]. The mean arterial pressure $\pm$ S.D. from 6 NHRs is plotted against the time elapsed after cord section in Fig. 1 (crosses). In contrast to SHR, the blood pressure in NHR did not exceed that of NCR (circles) after cord section. This finding may be interpreted to indicate that the neurogenic hypertension is

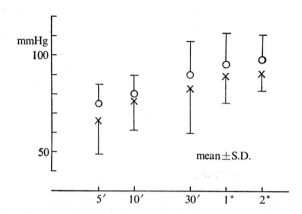

Fig. 1. Time course of change in arterial pressure after cord section. Crosses are for neurogenic hypertensive rats and circles for normotensive control rats. Each value is given as mean ± S.D. from 6 rats (neurogenic hypertensive rats) or 10 rats (controls). The neurogenic hypertensive rats were 23 ± 7-week-old and 7.8 ± 3.1 weeks after sino-aortic denervation. The controls were 25 ± 7-week-old. Prior to the experiment, in the conscious state, the mean tail blood pressure ± S.D. of the hypertensive rats was 179 ± 11.1 mm Hg.

maintained almost exclusively by an elevated sympathetic tone due to descending impulses to the thoracolumbar centers. The non-neural hypertensive factor as assumed in adult SHR was not observed in NHR.

DOCA salt hypertension was produced in male rats by unilateral nephrectomy at 10–11 weeks of age and thereafter by injecting deoxycorticosterone acetate subcutaneously at a dose of 20 mg/kg per week and giving 1% sodium chloride in the drinking water. Cord section was performed 1–7 weeks after nephrectomy, when the tail blood pressure was over 170 mm Hg in the conscious state. The arterial pressure 2 hr after cord section ranged widely from 75 to 140 mm Hg, the mean ± S.D. being 99.6 ± 20.3 mm Hg ($n = 13$). The pressure was not significantly related to the duration of DOCA and salt administration, the correlation coefficient being 0.222 ($n = 13$).

Since the variance was large, the above result does not necessarily indicate a paramount importance for the medullary cardiovascular centers in maintaining the DOCA salt hypertension. The fact that the pressure after cord section was unusually high in a few rats suggests the presence of some extremely unstable non-neural hypertensive factors, which become manifest only in a minority of DOCA salt hypertensive rats after cord section.

Although cord section was not performed on renovascular hypertensive rats, cord pithing was carried out in 2 one-kidney renovascular hypertensive rats. The blood pressure values 2 hr after cord pithing were 149 and 112 mm Hg. These values were considerably high compared to the corresponding values of spontaneously hypertensive rats.

Of the several experimental hypertensive rats tested in this study, only the one produced by sino-aortic denervation met the condition for being purely neurogenic. Its hypertensive state was thought to be maintained by an incessant barrage of impulses from the medullary cardiovascular centers to the thoracolumbar spinal segments.

REFERENCES

1. Altura, B.T. and Altura, B.M., Pentobarbital and contraction of vascular smooth muscle, *Amer. J. Physiol.*, 229 (1975) 1635–1640.
2. Iriuchijima, J. and Numao, Y., Hypotensive effects of pentobarbital and diuretics on sympathectomized spontaneously hypertensive rats, *Arch. int. Pharmacodyn. Ther.*, 226 (1977) 149–155.
3. Iriuchijima, J. and Numao, Y., Effects of cord section and pithing on spontaneously hypertensive rats, *Jap. J. Physiol.*, 27 (1977) 801–809.
4. Okamoto, K. and Aoki, K., Development of a strain of spontaneously hypertensive rats, *Jap. Circulat. J.*, 27 (1963) 282–293.
5. Krieger, E.M., Neurogenic hypertension in the rat, *Circulat. Res.*, 15 (1964) 511–521.

Inhibition of renal sympathetic discharge during trigeminal depressor response

NAOHITO TERUI*[1], MAMORU KUMADA*[1] AND DONALD J. REIS*[2]

*[1] *Institute of Basic Medical Sciences, The University of Tsukuba, Niihari-gun, Ibaraki 300–31, Japan*
*[2] *Laboratory of Neurobiology, Department of Neurology, Cornell University Medical College, New York 10021, U.S.A.*

Stimulation of the spinal trigeminal tract and its nucleus (i.e., the spinal trigeminal complex) evokes a profound fall in arterial pressure and bradycardia—the trigeminal depressor response (TDR)[3,4]. We have suggested that the fall in arterial pressure is due to inhibition of the discharge of sympathetic vasoconstrictor nerves, since the hypotension of TDR persists after blockade of the bradycardia by vagotomy and α-adrenergic block. In the present study, we attempted to investigate the inhibitory influence of TDR on sympathetic nervous activity, which reflects almost exclusively vasoconstrictor activity[1,2], during elicitation of TDR.

Adult New Zealand rabbits were anesthetized, paralyzed and artificially ventilated. The procedures for preparation of the animals, exposure of the brainstem and stereotaxic placement of the stimulating electrodes in the spinal trigeminal complex have been described in detail elsewhere[3,4]. The electrical stimulus consisted of isolated square wave pulses of 0.5 msec duration delivered at a frequency of 5 Hz with variable stimulus currents and pulse trains.

To record renal sympathetic discharges, the left renal nerve was approached dorsally through a flank incision, and was prepared near the renal artery. The central cut-end of the nerve was placed on a pair of bipolar Ag-AgCl electrodes connected to an amplifier (Grass P 15B) and an oscillosocope (Tektronix 5113). The lower and higher cut-off frequencies of the recording system were 30 and 1 kHz, respectively. Evoked sympathetic discharges were rectified, passed through a low-pass filter (time constant 20 msec), averaged during 32 to 64 successive sweeps with a data processing computer (ATAC-350, NIHON KOHDEN), and displayed on an X–Y recorder (Watanabe 4401).

A single pulse delivered to the spinal trigeminal complex resulted in inhibition of renal sympathetic discharge as illustrated by the recording from a single oscilloscopic sweep (Fig. 1A) or as the averaged evoked responses (Fig. 1B). Inhibition, lasting more than 500 msec after a single pulse, could be elicited by stimulation of the ipsi- or contralateral spinal trigeminal complex, and was not usually preceded by sympathetic excitation. The threshold current for sympathetic inhibition by stimulation of the spinal trigeminal tract was 5 to 40 μA. Stimulus currents 2 to 3 times the threshold for sympathetic inhibition elicited a period of complete disappearance of renal sympathetic discharge, i.e., a silent period. The duration of this silent period was prolonged as the stimulus current was further increased up to 5–7 times the threshold. Inhibition of sympathetic vasoconstrictor discharges thus occurs during TDR.

An attempt was next made to determine whether the trigeminal stimulation also inhibited reflexly elicited discharges in sympathetic nerves. An inhibitory curve for the effect of TDR on reflex sympathetic excitation was obtained by stimulating the brainstem with a pair of pulses having varying time intervals between them, i.e., conditioning and test stimuli. The test stimulus

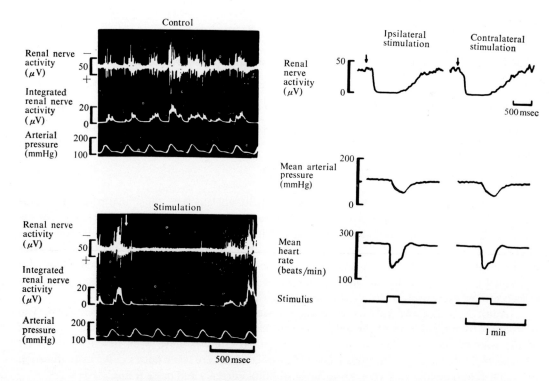

Fig. 1.   Renal sympathetic activity recorded from the left renal nerve, and its inhibition by stimulation of the spinal trigeminal complex. Left drawings (A) comprise a single sweep record of spontaneous renal sympathetic discharges (upper drawing) and their inhibition by a single pulse (100 μA, 0.5 msec) applied to the left spinal trigeminal complex at the time indicated by the arrow (lower drawing). In the top tracings in B, renal sympathetic discharges are rectified, integrated and averaged for 64 successive sweeps repeated at a rate of once every 3 sec. The responses of renal nerve discharges to stimulation of the ipsi- (left) or contralateral (right) spinal trigeminal complex are shown. The coordinates of the stimulus sites were 2 mm posterior to the obex, 2.5 mm lateral to the mid-saggital plane and 0.5 mm below the surface of the brain. At these sites, stimulation by a 12-sec train of pulses (100 μA, 0.5 msec) at a frequency of 5 Hz elicited comparable changes in arterial pressure or heart rate as shown in the lower tracings.

was delivered through an electrode placed in the medullary pressor area, specifically within the nucleus parvocellularis reticularis. Stimulation of this area elicited a powerful sympathetic excitation as shown in Fig. 2. The conditioning stimulus was delivered to the spinal trigeminal tract 50 to 1000 msec prior to the test stimulus, and diminished the sympathetic excitation evoked by the test stimulus. The maximum inhibition, which diminished the evoked response to less than 15% of the control value, occurred with an interval of 300 msec (Fig. 2). Complete recovery of the sympathetic excitation occurred at about 1 sec after the conditioning stimulus.

In summary, therefore, a single shock stimulus of the spinal trigeminal complex suppresses tonic sympathetic vasoconstrictor discharges for more than 500 msec. During this silent period, sympathetic discharges evoked by stimulation of the medullary reticular pressor area are also inhibited. The results indicate therefore that the hypotension in TDR is a result of inhibition of both tonic and evoked sympathetic vasoconstrictor discharges.

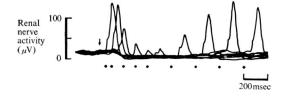

Renal
nerve
activity
(μV)

100

0

200 msec

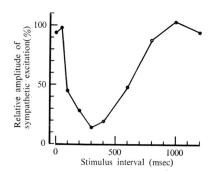

Relative amplitude of sympathetic excitation(%)

100

50

0

0   500   1000
Stimulus interval (msec)

Fig. 2. Inhibitory curve of the trigeminal depressor response. A single pulse (100 μA, 0.5 msec) was given to the spinal trigeminal complex as conditioning stimulus. The test stimulus consisted of two pulses (200 μA, 0.5 msec, separated by an interval of 5 msec) applied to the medullary pressor area within the nucleus parvocellularis reticularis at 6 mm anterior to the obex. The interval between the conditioning and test stimuli was varied up to 1200 msec. The upper drawing consists of superimposed tracings of renal nerve activity elicited by the test stimuli given at the intervals indicated by small dots. In the lower drawing, the decrease in renal nerve activity is plotted as a function of time interval.

ACKNOWLEDGEMENT: This work was supported by a grant from the Ministry of Education of Japan to M. Kumada and grants from NIH and NASA to D.J. Reis.

REFERENCES

1. Christensen, K., Lewis, E. and Kuntz, A., Innervation of the renal blood vessels in the cat, *J. comp. Neurol.*, 95 (1951) 373–385.
2. Concha, J.M. and Norris, B., Studies on renal vasomotion, *Brit. J. Pharmacol.*, 34 (1968) 277–290.
3. Kumada, M., Dampney, R.A.L. and Reis, D.J., The trigeminal depressor response: a cardiovascular reflex originating from the trigeminal system, *Brain Research*, 92 (1975) 485–489.
4. Kumada, M., Dampney, R.A.L. and Reis, D.J., The trigeminal depressor response: A novel vasodepressor response orginating from the trigeminal system, *Brain Research*, 119 (1977) 305–326.

Role of the central monoaminergic system in the control of arterial blood pressure in the rat

MASAYORI OZAKI, KAZUNOBU SUGAWARA, YUHZO FUJITA AND NAOKO TAKAMI

2nd Department of Pharmacology and Department of Neurosurgery, School of Medicine, Nagasaki University, Sakamoto, Nagasaki 852, Japan

Accumulating evidences have so far suggested that the central monoaminergic system may play an important role in the control of arterial blood pressure. The present experiments aimed to investigate the effects of blocking drugs of the central monoamine system on both monoamine contents in various parts of the brain and arterial blood pressure in normotensive and spontaneously hypertensive rats.

Male rats of normotensive Wistar and spontaneously hypertensive strains weighing 250–400g were used. Techniques for local administration of the blocking drugs, estimating monoamine contents in various parts of the brain and recording arterial blood pressure have been reported elsewhere[2].

Normotensive rats: 6-Hydroxydopamine (6-OHDA) which is known to degenerate nor-adrenaline (NA)-containing neurons specifically was injected bilaterally into the nucleus locus coeruleus (LC) at a dose of 6–12 μg in a 3–6 μl of solution containing 0.9 % NaCl and 0.1 % ascorbic acid. After the injection the blood pressure and heart rate increased significantly; the mean values were 172 ± 12 mm Hg and 460 ± 10 beats/min, respectively. The hypertensive state lasted for about 12 days and then the blood pressure was restored to the level before the drug. The magnitude of the induced hypertension was well related to the decrease in NA content in the cerebral cortex ($r = 0.74$, $P < 0.02$, $n = 10$). Previous injection of either 6-OHDA or desipramine, an inhibitor of NA uptake by NA-releasing axon terminals, blocked the development of hypertension after 6-OHDA injection into the LC. Fluoromicroscopic observations depicted degeneration of perikarya of NA-containing cells in the LC and of NA-containing axons around the nucleus. These results suggest that NA-containing neurons in the LC may be continuously activating the neural mechanism which depresses blood pressure and after lesions of these NA systems some other neural mechanisms may compensatorily take over the function in about 2 weeks.

Two weeks after the bilateral injection of 6-OHDA into the LC, the contents of both serotonin (5-HT) in the spinal cord and of 5-hydroxyindole acetic acid in the spinal cord and cerebral cortex increased significantly. The turnover rate of 5-HT was also found to be increased in the cerebral cortex (+314%) and spinal cord (+204%) as estimated from the decrease in 5-hydroxyindole acetic acid content. Intraperitoneally administered *p*-chlorophenylalamine elevated the blood pressure. 5,6-Dihydroxytryptamine injected into the spinal cord at the C4 level induced a small but significant increase in blood pressure. These results seem to suggest that 5-HT-containing neurons may be involved in the neural mechanism which depresses blood pressure.

Spontaneously hypertensive rats (SHR): Seven SHR fetuses were injected subcutaneously with 6-hydroxydopa (6-OHDOPA) at a dose of 50 mg/kg for each injection on the 19th and 21st days of gestation. Seven control SHR fetuses received the same amount of the vehicle (0.9 % NaCl containing 1 mg/ml ascorbic acid). The systolic blood pressure of conscious SHR was measured at intervals of a week by the tail cuff biophysiographic method between the ages of 6 and 12 weeks. Control SHR became hypertensive at 6–8 weeks of age. 6-OHDOPA delayed the onset of the hypertensive state in SHR. Namely, the systolic blood pressure of SHR injected with 6-OHDOPA was significantly lower than that of control SHR ($P < 0.05$), progressively rose thereafter and reached the same hypertensive level (176 ± 4 mm Hg) as that of control SHR (179 ± 6 mm Hg).

The NA content of the lower brain stem including the pons and the medulla oblongata as estimated at 12 weeks of age was significantly higher in the 6-OHDOPA-treated SHR (1530 ± 238 ng/g wet tissue, $n = 6$ than in the control SHR (732 ± 67 ng/g, $n = 6$). On the other hand NA contents of the remaining part of the brain (343 ± 18 ng/g) and the spinal cord (56 ± 10 ng/g) in the six 6-OHDOPA-treated SHR were markedly lower than those of the remaining brain (535 ± 36 ng/g) and the spinal cord (463 ± 41 ng/g) in six control SHR. The NA contents of the heart and the kidney were not significantly different between 6-OHDOPA-treated and control groups.

α-Methyl dopa (α-MD) was injected intraperitoneally into the control and 6-OHDOPA-treated SHR at 50–60 weeks of age at a dose of 300 mg/kg. α-MD lowered the blood pressure in both groups of SHR. However, the magnitude of the depressive response to α-MD was significantly smaller in 6-OHDOPA-treated SHR than in the control SHR.

Contents of NA and α-methyl noradrenaline (α-MeNA) in various parts of the brain and the spinal cord were determined 4 hr after α-MD injection by gas-liquid chromatography utilizing electron capture detection[1]. The content of α-MeNA in the spinal cord was significantly lower in the 6-OHDOPA-treated SHR, in which the depressive action of α-MD was partially antagonized. In addition, when 6-OHDA was injected into the spinal cord at the C_4 level, the contents of both NA and α-MeNA in the spinal cord caudal to the injection site were much lower than those in an uninjected animal 2 weeks after the injection. These results appear to suggest that NA-containing neurons are involved in the control of blood pressure at the level of the spinal cord as well as the lower brain stem.

REFERENCES

1. Kawano, T., Niwa, M., Fujita, Y., Ozaki, M. and Mori, K., An improved method for analysis of catecholamines—Gas-liquid chromatography (GLC) equipped with electron-capture detector, *Japan. J. Pharmacol.*, 28 (1978) 168–171.
2. Ogawa, M., Fujita, Y., Niwa, M., Takami, N. and Ozaki, M., Role on blood pressure regulation of noradrenergic neurons originating from the Locus coeruleus in the Kyoto-Wistar rat, *Japan. Heart J.*, 18 (1977) 586–587.

Bulbar neural mechanisms originating intrinsic respiratory rhythms in the central respiratory mechanisms

TAKEHIKO HUKUHARA, SIGERU KAGEYAMA, YURIKO KIGUCHI, KAZUTOSHI GOTO, YOSHINOBU NISHIKAWA AND KAZUO TAKANO

Department of Pharmacology II, Jikei University School of Medicine, Minato-ku, Tokyo 105, Japan

Neural mechanisms generating respiratory rhythms have been shown to exist in the brain stem including the pontine and medullary reticular formation[6]. The purpose of this experiment was to determine the precise localization of the primary neural network generating the intrinsic rhythmic neural activitity responsible for the eupneic breathing pattern. Therefore, the mainten-

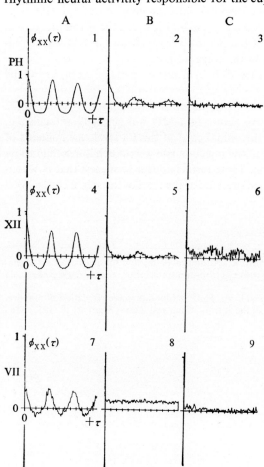

Fig. 1. Autocorrelation analysis of spontaneous activities recorded simultaneously in the phrenic (PH), hypoglossal (XII) and facial (VII) nerves. The autocorrelograms in A (1,4,7) were obtained after sectioning the vagosympathetic trunks and the carotid sinus nerves. Those in B (2,5,8) represent results obtained during 6.50% CO_2 in O_2 inhalation after transection of the brain stem at the ponto-bulbar junction. Note the persistent rhythm in both the phrenic and hypoglossal nerve activities. C (3,6,9) represents results obtained during 4.10% CO_2 in O_2 inhalation after brain stem transection at the ponto-bulbar junction and additional transection at the bulbo-spinal junction. Note that periodicity is maintained in the hypoglossal nerve activity. The ordinates indicate relative units and one division on the axis of the abscissae represents 900 msec.

254

ance of spontaneous periodic burst activity of bulbar respiratory neurons, hypoglossal, facial, trigeminal and phrenic nerves after brain stem transection at the level of the ponto-bulbar and bulbo-spinal junctions was examined.

Cats were vagotomized and paralyzed with d-tubocurarine or gallamine triethiodide, and respirated artificially under local anesthesia. The carotid sinus nerve was cut bilaterally. The end-tidal O_2 and CO_2 levels, Po_2 of the arterial blood and the medullary tissue, and systemic arterial blood pressure were all monitored continuously.

Efferent nerve activity was recorded simultaneously from the trigeminal, facial, hypoglossal and phrenic nerves. All of these nerves showed periodic burst discharges in the inspiratory phase. Autocorrelograms and crosscorrelograms indicated that the period of the burst in the efferent nerve activities of these cranial nerves was synchronous with that of the phrenic nerve, which contains inspiratory motor nerve fibers, as shown in Fig. 1. The duration and period of the burst were found to be fairly constant in the phrenic nerve, while varying rather widely in the trigeminal and facial nerves, as measured by the coefficient of variation of both burst parameters. The power

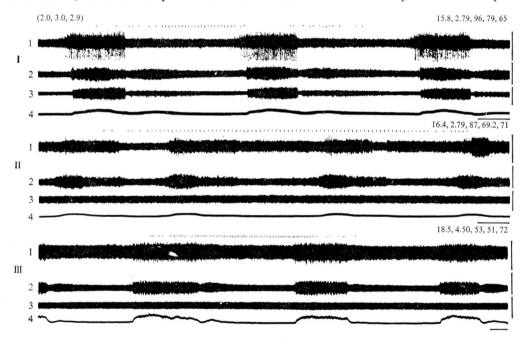

Fig. 2. Changes in discharge patterns recorded from the phrenic nerve, the hypoglossal nerve and a bulbar inspiratory unit, caused by transection of the brain stem at the ponto-bulbar junction and additional transection at the bulbo-spinal junction. 1: Discharges of a bulbar inspiratory unit recorded in the lateral area of the medullary reticular formation; 2: hypoglossal nerve activity; 3: phrenic nerve activity; 4: integrated neurogram of the hypoglossal nerve activity. I: After sectioning the vagosympathetic nerve trunks and the carotid sinus nerves and after transection of the brain stem at the ponto-bulbar junction; II: after additional transection at the bulbo-spinal junction (note the persistent respiratory rhythm in both the inspiratory unitary discharges and hypoglossal nerve activity); III: 9 min after commencing 4.10% CO_2 in O_2 inhalation. The horizontal scale lines indicate 1 sec. The vertical scale lines indicate 100 μV. The end-tidal O_2 and CO_2 levels and arterial blood pressure were 15.8%, 2.79% and 65 mm Hg in I, 16.4%, 2.79% and 71 mm Hg in II, and 18.5%, 4.50%, and 72 mm Hg in III, respectively.

spectrum of the phrenic nerve activity showed a prominent peak in the range of 60–120 Hz, while no peak was found in the power spectra of the cranial nerves.

When the brain stem was transected at the level of the ponto-bulbar junction, the periodic burst discharges disappeared completely in the trigeminal and facial nerves. The periodicity was not recovered, even under a hypercapnic condition induced by inhalation of 6.50% CO_2 in O_2 as shown in Fig. 1. (B, 8). However, periodic burst discharges were maintained after pontobulbar transection of the brain stem in the inspiratory and expiratory units recorded from the medullary reticular formation and the hypoglossal nerve, as well as the phrenic nerve. They showed neither an apneustic breathing pattern nor a gasping pattern (Fig. 2) as long as the arterial and the medullary tissue Po_2 levels were within a certain normal range.

In cats whose ponto-bulbar junction had been previously transected, and additional bulbo-spinal transection of the neuroaxis completely abolished the periodic burst discharges in the phrenic nerve. Even under a hypercapnic state elicited by inhalation of 4.10% CO_2 in O_2, the rhythmic activity did not reappear. However, the bulbar inspiratory units and the hypoglossal nerve were found to maintain their periodic burst activities and inhalation of 4.10% CO_2 in O_2 remarkably enhanced these periodic burst activities (Fig. 2).

The present results clearly demonstrate that the neural mechanisms in the medulla oblongata can generate an intrinsic and spontaneous periodic activity of eupneic rhythms independently of the neural inputs mediated by the afferent vagal pathways, from the pontine respiratory mechanisms, and the respiratory mechanisms in the spinal cord. The respiratory motor nerve activity in the trigeminal, facial and phrenic nerves is dependent on the medullary neural mechanisms. The present results thus support our previous view[3,4] that the periodic activity originating in the medullary neural mechanisms is dominant with respect to the spontaneity over other rhythmic activities. This has been observed in other neural mechanisms in the central nervous system, such as the pneumotaxic mechanisms in the pons[1], the pneumotaxic-apneustic center complex[2,6] and the respiratory neural mechanisms in the spinal cord[5].

References

1. Bertrand, F., Hugelin, A. and Vibert, J.F., A stereologic model of pneumotaxic oscillator based on spatial and temporal distributions of neuronal bursts, *J. Neurophysiol.*, 37 (1974) 91–107.
2. Cohen, M.I., Piercey, M.F., Gootman, P.M. and Wolotsky, P., Respiratory rhythmicity in the cat, *Fed. Proc.*, 35 (1976) 1967–74.
3. Hukuhara, T., Jr., Neuronal organization of the central respiratory mechanisms in the brain stem of the cat, *Acta neurobiol. exp.*, 33 (1973) 219–244.
4. Hukuhara, T., Jr., Functional organization of brain stem respiratory neurons and rhythmogenesis. In W. Umbach and H.P. Koepchen (Eds.), *Central Rhythmic and Regulation*, Hippokrates-Verlag, Stuttgart, 1974, pp. 35–49.
5. Sears, T.A., The respiratory motoneuron and apneusis, *Fed. Proc.*, 36 (1977) 2412–20.
6. Wyss, O.A.M., Die nervöse Steuerung der Atmung, *Ergebn. Physiol.*, 54 (1964) 1–479.

Effects of picrotoxin on vagal respiratory inhibition in the rabbit

KYUHACHIRO SHIMADA, YASUYUKI KITADA AND YOSHIAKI YAMADA

Department of Physiology, School of Dentistry, Niigata University,
Gakko-cho, Niigata 951, Japan

It has been reported that picrotoxin augments the increase of inspiratory volume in response to direct electrical stimulation of the inspiratory center in cats[2]. However, there is very little direct evidence as to the site of action of picrotoxin. In the present investigation the vagal inhibitory effect on the inspiratory and expiratory activity was studied in rabbits intravenously injected with picrotoxin.

Experiments were carried out in rabbits anesthetized with urethane (1.0 g/kg). After tracheotomy, venous cannulation and bilateral vagotomy, the anesthetized animal was paralyzed with gallamine triethiodide and artificially ventilated.

As shown in Fig. 1, picrotoxin increased the frequency of respiration up to about 80/min. The phrenic nerve activity in each inspiratory phase was also augmented. Shortening of the expiratory phase was very marked (Fig. 1B). With an increased dose of picrotoxin, the augmented burst activity of the phrenic nerve was changed to short burst activities. Since division of each augmented burst activity did not occur simultaneously, the rhythm of the phrenic activity became irregular. When all augmented burst activities had changed into short burst activities, the rhythm of the activity became regular again (Fig. 1C). The maximum frequency of the activity was 8/sec. With further application of picrotoxin the phrenic activity became irregular, and the rhythmicity of respiration disappeared. The phrenic nerve discharges persisted though the magnitude of the discharge fluctuated irregularly (Fig. 1D).

In some animals short burst activity was not observed, and the pattern of respiration changed directly to that shown in Fig. 1D.

Slight increases in the discharge frequency of single phrenic nerve fibers were observed during application of picrotoxin. The effect of picrotoxin on the respiratory activity was characterized by a change in the duration of the respiratory phase rather than in discharge frequency.

In order to examine the vagal respiratory inhibition during application of picrotoxin, the following experiments were preliminarily performed. Stimulation of the vagus nerve of the control animal shortened the inspiratory phase of the respiratory movement. As the stimulus frequency was increased, the inspiratory phase shortened further (Fig. 2A). The expiratory phase was also shortened by the stimulation, but the maximum shortening of the expiratory phase was observed at a relatively low stimulus frequency (Fig. 2B). The effect of vagal stimulation on the discharge frequency of single phrenic nerve fibers was similar to that in the inspiratory phase.

In a rabbit injected with picrotoxin the shortening effect of vagal stimulation on the inspiratory phase was clearly reduced, as shown in Fig. 2A. Expiratory arrest did not occur on high frequency vagal stimulation (100–200 Hz), and short burst activity of the phrenic nerve was observed. The expiratory phase was also slightly shortened. The inhibitory effect of low frequency stimulation on the expiratory phase decreased slightly. The disinhibitory effect of picrotoxin on the va-

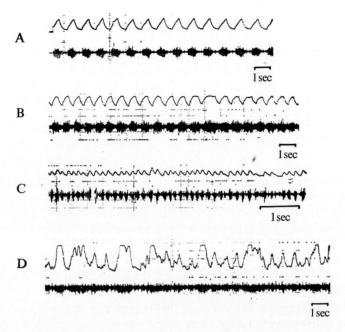

Fig. 1.   Effect of picrotoxin on respiration. In each record the upper trace is the integrated phrenic activity and the bottom trace is the phrenic activity. Picrotoxin (3 mg/ml, 20 ml) was intravenously applied. A, control; B, picrotoxin 9 mg/kg; C, 15 mg/kg; D, 20 mg/kg.

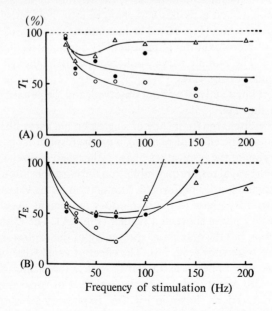

Fig. 2.   Disinhibitory effect of picrotoxin on vagal inhibition of the inspiratory (A) or expiratory (B) activity. Shortening of the inspiratory or expiratory phase indicates an inhibition of the inspiratory or expiratory activity, respectively. T_I, duration of the inspiratory phase; T_E, duration of the expiratory phase;—○—, control; —●—, picrotoxin 4.3 mg/kg; —△—, 5.1 mg/kg.

gal inhibition of the expiratory activity appears to be smaller than that on the inspiratory activity (Fig. 2A and B). When the phrenic activity became irregular and the respiratory rhythmicity disappeared after picrotoxin administration, as shown in Fig. 1, vagal stimulation did not produce any change in phrenic activity. Reduction or disappearance of the inhibitory effect of vagal stimulation on respiratory activity after picrotoxin administration may be due to a possible disinhibition of neuronal activity in the respiratory reflex center, since picrotoxin is known to block inhibitory synaptic transmission by GABA-releasing neurons. Irregular phrenic activity or disappearance of rhythmicity may also be caused by a disinhibition of both inspiratory and expiratory neurons in the respiratory center, since these are considered to have reciprocal inhibitory neural circuits[1].

REFERENCES

1. Baumgarten, V.R. and Nakayama, S., Spontane und reizbedingte Änderungen der antidromen Erregbarkeit von bulbaren respiratorischen Nervenzellen der Katze, *Pflüg. Arch. ges. Physiol.*, 281 (1964) 245–258.
2. Wells, J.A., Fox, C.A., Rambach, W.A., Dragstedt, C.A. and Windle, W.F., Effect of picrotoxin on electrical excitability of the respiratory center, *Proc. Soc. exp. Biol. Med.*, 56 (1944) 176–178.

A quantitative evaluation of hypoxic drive in ventilation from the peripheral chemoreceptors

YOSHIYUKI HONDA, NAMIYO HATA, YOSHIKAZU SAKAKIBARA AND
SETSUKO AKIYAMA

*Department of Physiology, Chiba University School of Medicine,
Inohana, Chiba 280, Japan*

The observation of breath-by-breath ventilation for a period of 5 to 20 sec after a sudden change of oxygen content in the inspired air is known to be a measure for determining the isolated activity of the peripheral chemoreceptors. This is because within such a limited period no blood altered in oxygen content would have reached the central nervous structures, so that no secondary effect will distort the real peripheral chemosensitivities. Since Dejours[1] first advocated this procedure, a number of modifications have been developed. Among these, the withdrawal test, in which hypoxic and/or hypercapnic stimulation to the peripheral chemoreceptors were withdrawn by one or two breaths of 100% O_2, was suggested to be most reliable by Miller *et al.* Their reasoning was as follows. 1) Respiration is augmented by hypoxia and/or hypercapnia, so the magnitude of ventilation tends to be uniform. 2) When end-tidal P_{O_2} is elevated above 200 mm Hg by 1–2 breaths of O_2 (withdrawal procedure), peripheral chemoreceptor activities will be suppressed practically to zero, irrespective of the level of alveolar-arterial P_{CO_2}. 3) Because the results of the test are evaluated by depression of ventilation, the subject can easily tolerate the procedure and usually realizes when the test effect is terminated. Thus, disturbance due to subjective feeling is not of great importance.

In the present study, the method used by Miller *et al.*[3]. was improved in two respects. 1) Instead of administering gas mixtures with given O_2 or CO_2 content for chemical stimulation, the breath-by-breath alveolar carbon dioxide (P_{ACO_2}) and oxygen pressure (P_{AO_2}) were continuously observed and monitored. 2) Withdrawal effects were determined at three different hypoxia levels. Thus, the ventilatory responses were evaluated as a continuous function of P_{O_2}, rather than evaluating at one particular hypoxia level as was done by Miller *et al.*

Ten healthy subjects were tested twice on different days. The experimental setup and the method of withdrawal testing have been described elsewhere[2]. Withdrawal procedures were conducted at P_{AO_2} levels of 75, 65 and 55 mm Hg with P_{ACO_2} 5 mm Hg higher than the control level. The difference in ventilation between pre- and post-O_2 breaths was determined and designated as $\Delta \dot{V}$. In order to eliminate differences in ventilation due to different body sizes, all the ventilatory data were normalized by multiplying by the allometric coefficient,[5] (70/body weight in kg)[75].

Fig. 1 shows three series of withdrawal tests on subject I. H. Upon breathing O_2 twice, ventilation was clearly depressed and alveolar P_{O_2} increased. It was also seen that the stronger the degree of hypoxia before O_2 breathing, the greater the effect of withdrawal.

The depression of ventilation as determined by the withdrawal test ($\Delta \dot{V}$) was found to be a linear function of alveolar as well as arterial P_{O_2} when $\Delta \dot{V}$ was plotted on a logarithmic scale. Therefore, the relationship was analyzed as in $\Delta \dot{V} = \alpha(P_{O_2} - \beta)$, where α is the regression slope and β is the intercept with the abscissa. Using this qeuation, we calculated $\Delta \dot{V}_{50}$ (defined as $\Delta \dot{V}$

at $P_{O_2} = 50$ mm Hg). From plots of P_{AO_2} vs. in $\Delta \dot{V}$, the mean slope and $\Delta \dot{V}_{50}$ were found to be -0.048 ± 0.042 and 9.04 ± 6.87 1/min, respectively (mean $\pm$ S.D.). On the other hand, plots of arterial P_{O_2} (P_{AO_2}) vs. in $\Delta \dot{V}$ gave a mean slope and $\Delta \dot{V}_{50}$ of -0.048 ± 0.043 and 9.18 ± 7.51 1/min, respectively. Thus, there was fairly good agreement in both parameters.

As suggested by Rebuck and Campbell[4], arterial oxygen saturation (Sao_2) was found to be linearly related to $\Delta \dot{V}$ in this experiment. The slope of the Sao_2 vs. $\Delta \dot{V}$ curve and $\Delta \dot{V}$ at Sao_2 of 85% (defined as $\Delta \dot{V}_{85\%}$) were -0.67 ± 0.67 1 min/Sao_2 and 8.5 ± 7.61 1/min, respectively (mean $\pm$ S.D.). The mean $\Delta \dot{V}_{85\%}$ was nearly the same as the mean $\Delta \dot{V}_{50}$.

The magnitude of $\Delta \dot{V}_{50}$ or $\Delta \dot{V}_{85\%}$ was found to be smaller than that obtained from the steady-state response, i.e., the increments in ventilation from hyperoxia to P_{AO_2} or P_{AO_2} 50 mm Hg or Sao_2 85% with P_{ACO_2} control + 5 mm Hg before withdrawal (termed $\Delta \dot{V}_{50\ (s)}$ or $\Delta \dot{V}_{85\%}$ (s)] exceeded the $\Delta \dot{V}_{50}$ or $\Delta \dot{V}_{85\%}$ values. $\Delta \dot{V}_{50}$'s obtained from plots of P_{AO_2} vs. in $\Delta \dot{V}$ and Pao_2 vs. in $\Delta \dot{V}$ were 66 ± 34 and $68 \pm 35\%$ of $\Delta \dot{V}_{50(s)}$, respecively. $\Delta \dot{V}_{85\%}$ obtained from Sao_2 vs. $\Delta \dot{V}$ analysis was $60 \pm 32\%$ of $\Delta \dot{V}_{85\%\ (s)}$. Even if maximal depression in breath-by-breath ventilation during 5–20 sec after withdrawal was obtained (termed $\Delta \dot{V}_{50(max)}$, or $\Delta \dot{V}_{85\%(max)}$), $\Delta \dot{V}_{50(max)}$ as determined by P_{AO_2} vs. in $\Delta \dot{V}$ analysis and $\Delta \dot{V}_{85\%(max)}$ as determined by Sao_2 vs. $\Delta \dot{V}$ analysis were 83 ± 37, 82 ± 36, and $78 \pm 38\%$ of $\Delta \dot{V}_{50(s)}$, and $\Delta \dot{V}_{85\%(s)}$, respectively. These results suggest the existence of central modification of the peripheral chemoreceptor input.

Subj. I. H.

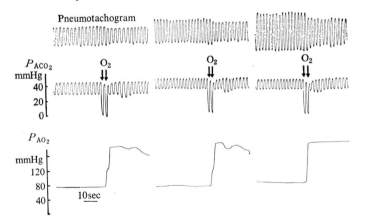

Fig. 1. An example of the withdrawal test with subject I.H. From left to right, P_{AO_2} was kept at 75, 65 and 55 mm Hg, respectively, with P_{ACO_2} 5 mm Hg higher than the control level. Then two breaths of 100% O_2 were given with spontaneous respiration. Upon O_2 breathing, P_{AO_2} promptly increased and ventilation decreased. Inspiration was downward in the pneumotachogram. It was noted that the stronger the preliminary hypoxic stimulation, the more pronounced the withdrawal effect.

The distribution of the breath sequence as related to the maximal depression on withdrawal further supported the possibility of central modification as described above. This was mainly observed at about 15 sec after O_2 administration. Since the circulation time from the lung to the carotid body is 5–6 sec, the remaining 10 sec or so is necessary to elicit maximal depression from the carotid body desensitization to respiratory movement. The conduction times from the peripheral chemoreceptor, peripheral nerve pathways to the neuromuscular junctions of the respiratory muscles total less than a few seconds. Therefore, at least several seconds should be available for the central respiratory mechanism to elicit maximal depression and modification.

References

1. Dejours, P., Labrousse, Y., Raynaud, J. and Teillac, A., Stimulus oxygène chémoréflexe de la ventilation à basse altitude (50 m) chez l'homme. I. Au repos, *J. Physiol. (Paris)*, 49 (1957) 115–124.
2. Honda, Y., Watanabe, S., Hasegawa, S., Mjojo, S., Takizawa, H., Sugita, T., Kimura, K., Hasegawa, T., Kuriyama, T., Saito Y., Katsuki, H. and Severinghaus, J.W., Breathing without carotid chemoreceptors in man. In H.H. Loeschcke (Ed.) *Acid-base Homeostasis of the Brain Extracellular Fluid and the Respiratory Control System*, Georg Thieme Verlag, Stuttgart, 1976, pp. 88–94.
3. Miller, J.P., Cunningham, D.J.C., Lloyd, B.B. and Young, J.M., The transient respiratory effects in man of sudden changes in alveolar CO_2 in hypoxia and in high oxygen, *Respir. Physiol.*, 20 (1974) 17–31.
4. Rebuck, A.S. and Campbell E.J.M., A clinical method for assessing the ventilatory response to hypoxia, *Amer. Rev. Respir. Dis.*, 109 (1973) 345–350.
5. Severinghaus, J.W., Ozanne, G. and Massuda, Y., Measurement of the ventilatory response to hypoxia, *Chest*, 70 (1976) 121–124, Suppl.

PART V

NEURAL CONTROL OF THE DIGESTIVE SYSTEM

YUTAKA MATSUO

The 3rd Department of Internal Medicine, Faculty of Medicine, University of Tokyo, Bunkyo-ku, Tokyo 113, Japan

As is well-known, control of the digestive system, especially the gastrointestinal tract, involves the enteric plexus for neural regulation and the gastrointestinal hormones for humoral regulation. Recently it has been proved that these two regulatory systems work conjointly under control by the brain. There are many interesting questions as to how the integrative control functions of the brain are represented in the digestive system. Since stress stimulus through the central nervous system causes peptic ulcers and many other digestive disorders, studies in this field should be valuable in elucidating pathological states of digestive diseases and in developing new diagnostic methods and treatments.

The present group study has been conducted along the following four lines; 1) movement of the gastrointestinal tract; 2) secretion of the digestive juice; 3) metabolic regulation in the pancreas and liver; 4) structure and function of paraneurons. The term "paraneurons" was proposed by Fujita (1975)[2] to describe those cells which in general have not been considered as neurons, but which in regard to their origin, structure, function and metabolism have many features in common with neurons. They are in fact recepto-secretory cells, including endocrine cells (APUD cells as described by Pearse[3]) and also various sensory cells. The concept of the "paraneuron" originated from studies of the gastrointestinal and pancreatic systems, and can be regarded as characteristic of the digestive system.

Gastrointestinal hormones releasing cells are scattered in the mucosa of the gatrointestinal tract, and their release is triggered by constituents of the ingested food and the digestive juices. These hormones are of two kinds; one is the so-called endocrine hormone, which is released into the blood, and the other is the paracrine hormone[1] which acts directly on the neighboring cells without being mediated by the blood. D cells of islets of the pancrease were found to release somatostatin[5], which directly affects the proximate A and B cells. This mode of paracrine action also applies to D cells in the mucosa of the gastrointestimal tract. For this reason and because many of the gastrointestinal hormones are also found in the brain, it has become more difficult to place a clear-cut boundary between endocrine hormones and neural transmitters. The relationship of the enteric plexus to the gastrointestinal hormones now appears to be very similar to the relationship of nervous pathways to neurochemical transmitters in the brain. The gastrointestinal system thus may act as a "small brain" in which the integrative control functions of the brain are represented in a simplified, condensed manner.

REFERENCES

1. Feyrter F., *Uber die peripheren Endokrine (Paracrinen) Drüsendes Menschen*, Wilhelm Mandrich, Wien, 1953.
2. Fujita, T., The gastro-enteric endocrine cell and its paraneuronic nature. In R.E. Coupland and T. Fujita (Eds.) *Chromaffin, Enterochromaffin and Related Cells*, Elsevier, Amsterdam, 1976, pp. 191–208.

3. Pearse, A.G.E. and Polak, J.M., Neural crest origin of the endocrine polypeptide (APUD) cells of the gastrointestinal tract and pancreas, *Gut*, 12 (1971) 783–788.
4. Pearse, A.G.E., Peptides in brain and intestine, *Nature* (Lond.), 262 (1976) 92–94.
5. Polak, J.M., A.G. Pearse, L. Grimelius, *et al.*, Growth hormone release inhibiting hormone in gastrointestinal and pancreatic D cells, *Lancet* (1) (1975) 1220–1222.

Central nervous regulation of motility of alimentary canals in the dog

TAKEHIKO SEMBA AND KAZUMOTO FUJII

*Department of Physiology, School of Medicine, University of Hiroshima,
Kasumi, Hiroshima 734, Japan*

Summary

This study is concerned with the mechanisms of the neural reflex which involves in extrinsic nerves and controls movements of the gastrointestinal tract in the dog.

Intestinal inhibitory reflex, i.e., a reflex producing an inhibition of movement of a part of the gastrointestinal tract by afferent impulses originating from some other part of the tract, was found to be functioning in an animal in which the spinal cord was transected at the level between the cervical and the thoracic cord, and the splanchnic nerves were left intact. Either lesions of the thoracic and lumbar cord or bilateral transection of the splanchnic nerve abolished the inhibition of movements due to the reflex. During the inhibition, the rates of efferent impulses of the splanchnic nerve increased.

In addition to the sacral cord with the pelvic nerve, the thoracolumbar spinal cord with the splanchnic nerve was shown under certain conditions to mediate the effects of the gastrointestinal excitatory reflex, i.e., the reflex producing a facilitation of gastrointestinal tract movements.

Stimulation of ventral parts of the lateral and the medial muclei of the thoracic and the lumbar cord, both of which were isolated by dual transection, produced an inhibition of gastrointestinal motility, while stimulation of dorsal parts of the nuclei evoked a facilitation of movement. In the sacral cord which had been isolated from the lumbar part by transection, facilitation of colonic motility was observed following stimulation of the intermedial substance of the sacral gray matter. In the cervical cord stimulation of ventral and dorsal parts of the intermedial substance of the gray matter produced an inhibition and a facilitation of gastrointestinal movements, respectively, through an excitation of efferent fibers in the splanchnic nerve.

Units recorded in the lateral intermedial nucleus of the isolated thoracic spinal cord showed excitation during the evoked inhibitory reflex and inhibition during the evoked excitatory reflex. On the other hand, unit activity recorded in the dorsal nucleus of the isolated thoracic cord was augmented during the excitatory reflex and reduced during the inhibitory reflex.

In the medulla oblongata stimulation of the dorsomedial nucleus of n. vagi, the nucleus of the tractus solitarius and the dorsal region of the medullary reticular formation produced a facilitation of gastric motility in some cases and an inhibition in others. Gastric excitatory points and inhibitory points were found in the dorsomedial nucleus of the n. vagi, in which an increase in the rates of unit firings was observed during the facilitation and inhibition of gastric motility, respectively.

The activities of both units, recorded in the excitatory and inhibitory points of the thoracic cord, were depressed immediately after transection of the cervical cord and recovered to the previous level within 42 min after the transection. In the intact dog, stimulation of the excitatory and inhibitory points in the dorsomedial nucleus of the n. vagi excited the units recorded in the excitatory and inhibitory points of the thoracic cord. During the gastric inhibitory reflex, which involves an activation of neurons in the medullary inhibitory points, the firing rates of the units in the gastric inhibitory point of the thoracic cord increased.

Introduction

Many authors have suggested that the extrinsic nerves (vagal and splanchnic nerves) which innervate alimentary canals have both excitatory and inhibitory effects on the gut[23]. In order to study both effects of extrinsic nerves, we investigated whether the vagal nerve is the efferent pathway of the intestinal inhibitory reflex[24] and also whether the splanchnic nerve is the efferent pathway of the intestinal excitatory reflex[23]. A spinal autonomic processes in the term of sympathetic reflex paths have been suggested by Réthelyi[19], but he considered only the inhibitory motor center. We sought the location of the excitatory motor center as well as the inhibitory motor center in the spinal cord[27].

It was demonstrated by Kōsaka and Yagita[12] that the origin of the vagal nerve for excitation of gastric motility was the dorsal nucleus of n. vagi. However, a number of physiological and histological findings have indicated that the stimulation of this nucleus and its vicinity produces many sympathetic responses, such as inhibition of gastric motility[15]. We attempted to demonstrate the location of the inhibitory reflex center as well as the excitatory reflex center in the medulla oblongata.

Harding and Leek[9] induced electrical activities from the dorsal nucleus of n. vagi and its vicinity and classified the gastric preganglionic motoneurons, interneurons and afferent-like neurons from the patterns of spike discharge during vago-vagal gastric reflex. To study the mechanisms of alimentary motility, an attempt was made to determine the influence of the intestinal reflex on electrical activities of excitatory and inhibitory motor centers in the medulla oblongata and spinal cord.

Methods and materials

Dogs were used under anesthesia with sodium pentobarbital (Nembutal, Abbott, 25 mg/ kg body weight i.v.). The movement of the stomach (antral portion), small intestine (6 cm loop of the ileum) and distal colon were recorded by means of a balloon pressure transducer (Nihon Kohden MPU-0.5), an electronic manometer (Nihon Kohden MP-3A) and an ink-chart oscillograph (Nihon Kohden WI-180). For stimulation, a square wave stimulator (Nihon Kohden MSE-3R) was used which generated impulses having an intensity of 1–7 V, a pulse width of 0.1–1.0 msec and a frequency of 10–50 Hz. The stimulating period was varied from 30 to 120 sec. A monopolar or bipolar electrode was employed for stimulation of the extrinsic nerve. To stimulate the spinal cord or medulla oblongata, a monopolar electrode with a diameter of 25 μ and a bare tip was used. After changes in the motility of the gut on stimulation had been recorded, the position of the tip of electrode was determined histologically.

Changes in the electrical activities of one of the gastric branches of the splanchnic nerve or the gastric antral branch of the vagal nerve during intestinal reflex were recorded by means of a bipolar electrode.

To record electrical activities from the thoracic cord or medulla oblongata, dogs in which the nerve connection between the stomach and central nervous system was maintained either via the major splanchnic nerve or the vagal nerve were used. A coaxial needle electrode having a diameter of less than 5 μ was employed for recording electrical activities. The indifferent electrode was fixed on the surface of the spinal cord or medulla oblongata. The electrical activities were observed with an oscilloscope (Nihon Kohden VC-6) and recorded with a continuous recording camera (Nihon Kohden PC-IB). After recording the discharge electrical stimulation was applied without moving the position of the electrode, with the center of the coaxial electrode being negative and the mantle electrode being positive. According to the gastric response produced by stimulation, the site of the electrode tip was determined to be located in either the inhibitory point or excitatory point. The site of the electrode tip was then examined histologically.

To produce the vestibulo-gastric excitatory reflex[11], afferent stimulation was applied to the central cut end of the vestibular nerve. To produce the ileo-gastric inhibitory reflex[30], the intraluminal pressure of a loop of the ileum 6 cm in length was elevated to 60–100 mm Hg for 30 sec with Ringer's solution.

Results

Spinal cord as an intestinal reflex center:

(a) *Intestinal inhibitory reflex.* Intestinal inhibitory reflex was observed in an animal in which the bilateral vagosympathetic nerve trunks were severed and also in an animal in which the spinal cord was transected between the cervical and thoracic cord. Bilateral section of the major, minor and lumbar splanchnic nerves abolished the inhibitory reflex. Destruction of the thoracic and lumbar cord also abolished the inhibitory reflex. These observations demonstrate that the inhibitory reflex centers are located in the thoracic and lumbar cord, and afferent and efferent paths are in the splanchnic nerve.

In Fig. 1 A, the nerve connection between the thoracic cord and stomach was maintained only by the major splanchnic nerve. When the intraluminal pressure of a loop of the ileum was elevated rapidly to 100 mm Hg, gastric motility was depressed. The efferent discharge of impulses of the gastric branch of the splanchnic nerve increased markedly during inhibitory reflex[8].

(b) *Intestinal excitatory reflex.* Excitatory reflexes related to the spinal cord have been confined to the sacral cord and pelvic nerve[20], but it has recently been reported that the major, minor and lumbar splanchnic nerves, which are the efferent nerve pathways of inhibitory reflexes, also serve as an efferent nerve pathway for excitatory reflexes. In a dog with transection of the brain stem at the level between the superior and inferior colliculus and with severed bilateral vagosympathetic nerve trunks in the cervical region, the stomach and central nervous system have nerve connections only with the major splanchnic nerve. Afferent stimulation of the vestibular nerve produced a gastric excitatory response. The frequency of discharges of the gastric branch of the major splanchnic nerve increased during the vestibulo-gastric excitatory reflex, as shown in Fig. 1 B[8].

Efferent stimulation of the major splanchnic nerve of the dog produced an inhibitory response of the gastric and ileal motilities. However, when the celiac ganglion was painted with nicotine, stimulation of the same nerve under the same conditions reversed the response of the gastric and ileal motilities, i.e., excitatory responses were produced[23]. A similar response was demonstrated in the motility of the distal colon of the dog on stimulating the lumbar splanchnic nerve. When nicotine was applied to the inferior mesenteric ganglion, the inhibitory response of the

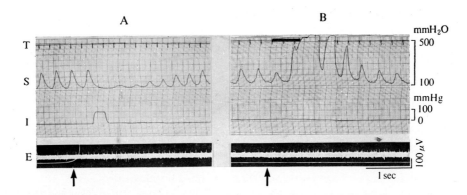

Fig. 1. Simultaneous recordings of the discharge of impulses of the gastric branch of the major splanchnic nerve and gastric response. The nerve connection was maintained only by the major splanchnic nerve between the stomach, ileum and central nervous system. A, Ileo-gastric inhibitory reflex; B, vestibulo-gastric excitatory reflex.
Symbols: T, time marks in 10 sec. At signal afferent stimulation was applied to the vestibular nerve; S, gastric motility; I, intraluminal pressure of the ileum; E, efferent discharge of the major splanchnic nerve; ↑, onset of gastric reflexes.

distal colon reversed to an excitatory response[22]. Responses reversed by the application of nicotine to the ganglia were also observed in various intestinal reflexes, such as the vesico-gastric, colon-gastric, ileo-ileal, vesico-colonic and ileo-colonic reflexes[21]. In these cases, the major, minor and lumbar splanchnic nerves, which are the efferent pathways of inhibitory reflexes, act as an efferent pathway of excitatory reflexes. The observation of these phenomena in the spinalized animal shows that the excitatory reflex center may be located in the thoracic and lumbar cord.

Localization of reflex centers in the spinal cord:

(a) *Thoracic cord.* The thoracic cord of the dog was transected at the upper level and at the lower level. A monopolar electrode was inserted into the thoracic cord from the dorsal surface. When the position of the electrode tip was relatively far from the dorsal surface (1.5–2.0 mm in depth from the surface), inhibitory response of the stomach was readily obtained by stimulation. When the tip of the electrode was located more superficially (0.5–1.0 mm in depth from the surface), excitatory response of the stomach was readily obtained by stimulation. The positions of the electrode tip required to produce inhibitory or excitatory response were examined histological-ly, and the distribution of these points is shown in Fig. 2. Both of these points were found in the lateral and medial intermedial nuclei. The dorsal region of these nuclei corresponds to the excitatory points, while the ventral region corresponds to the inhibitory points[27].

(b) *Lumbar cord.* Similar results were obtained for the distribution of inhibitory and excitatory points to colonic motility in the lumbar cord. The excitatory points were found mostly in the dorsal region of the intermedial substance and the inhibitory points were located mostly in the ventral region of the intermedial substance[18].

(c) *Sacral cord.* The sacral cord was stimulated in an animal transected between the lumbar and sacral cord. Histologically, the excitatory points which produced excitation of colonic motility were found to be located in the intermedial substance of the sacral gray matter,

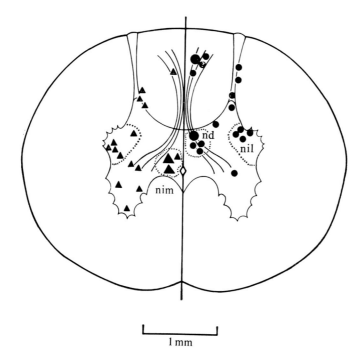

Fig. 2. Distribution of the inhibitory and excitatory points of gastric motility in the thoracic cord; cross section at level T-9 of a dog. nd, nucleus dorsalis; nil, nucleus intermedio lat.; nim, nucleus intermedio med.; ▲, inhibitory point; ●, excitatory point (large one, 3 examples; small one, 1 example). Inhibitory and excitatory points are illustrated on the left and right sides, respectively.

i.e., they were found in the parasympathetic gray and medial myoleioticus nucleus, and others were located in the dorsal column[29].

(d) *Cervical cord.* Extrinsic nerves were not supplied to the gut from the cervical cord. However, both inhibitory and excitatory responses of the gut to stimulation of the cervical cord were obtained via the splanchnic nerve. The inhibitory points were found to be located in the ventral region of the intermedial substance of the gray matter, while the excitatory points were located in the dorsal region of the gray matter. Both points were distributed continuously to the medulla oblongata[16].

Electrical activities of the inhibitory and excitatory points for gastric motility in the spinal cord:

(a) *Gastric inhibitory point.* The brain stem was transected at the level between the superior and inferior colliculus and at the level between the thoracic and lumbar cord. The bilateral vagosympathetic nerve trunks were severed in the cervical region. Thus the stomach and small intestine had nerve connection only via the splanchnic nerve to the central nervous system. Ileo-gastric inhibitory reflex was induced by distension of the ileac wall. The frequency of discharges of the inhibitory point in the T-9 segment of the thoracic cord increased remarkably during inhibitory reflex (Fig. 3 A and C,a). On the other hand, the frequency of discharges of the same inhibitory point was reduced during vestibulo-gastric excitatory reflex (Fig. 3 B and C,b)[4].

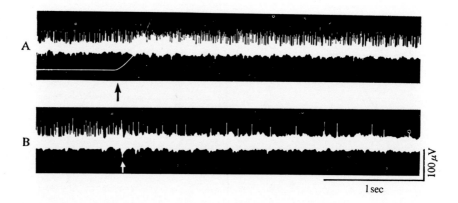

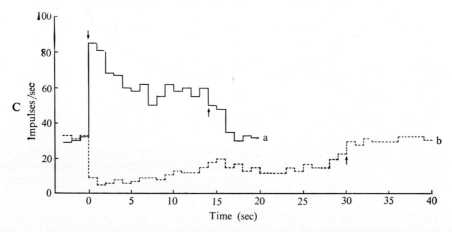

Fig. 3.   Changes in the frequency of discharges of the Type 1 gastric inhibitory point in the thoracic cord during gastric reflexes. Discharge of impulses was induced from the nucleus intermedio lát. of T-9 segment. The splanchnic nerve was the only nerve connection between the stomach, ileum and central nervous system.

A, Ileo-gastric inhibitory reflex; B, vestibulo-gastric excitatory reflex; ↑, onset of gastric reflexes; C, changes in the frequency of discharges; a, inhibitory reflex; b, excitatory reflex; ↕, onset and suspension of gastric reflexes.

Histologically, this inhibitory point was found to be located in the lateral intermedial nucleus. The point where increase of the frequency of discharges of the inhibitory point during inhibitory reflex was followed by a decrease of the frequency of discharges during excitatory reflex is called the Type 1 point, and is distinguished from the others[7].

(b) *Gastric excitatory point.*   The spinal cord was transected between the thoracic and lumbar cord and the bilateral vagosympathetic nerve trunks were severed. During vestibulo-gastric excitatory reflex the frequency of discharges of the T-9 segment of the gastric excitatory point increased (Fig. 4b) and the frequency of discharges of this point fell during ileo-gastric inhibitory reflex (Fig. 4a)[4]. This point is a Type 1 point (see preceding section). Histological examination showed this point to be the dorsal nucleus[7].

Medulla oblongata as an intestinal reflex center:

(a) *Intestinal excitatory reflex.*   The brain stem was transected at the level between the

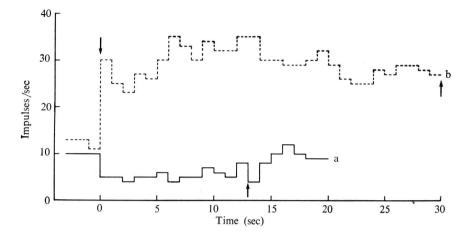

Fig. 4.   Changes in the frequency of discharges of Type 1 gastric excitatory point in the thoracic cord during gastric reflexes. The splanchnic nerve was the only nerve connection between the stomach, ileum and central nervous system. Discharge of impulses was induced from nucleus dorsalis of the T-9 segment.

a, Ileo-gastric inhibitory reflex; b, vestibulo-gastric excitatory reflex; ⇕, onset and suspension of gastric reflexes.

superior and inferior colliculus and the bilateral vagosympathetic nerve trunks were severed. The alae cinerea of the medulla oblongata and the upper region of the cervical cord were stimulated by inserting a monopolar electrode from the dorsal surface. The excitation of gastric motility was produced through the splanchnic nerve. The excitatory points were confined to the oral region of the obex at the upper level and were distributed continuously caudally to the cervical cord. On the other hand, in a spinalized dog in which the spinal cord was transected at the level between the cervical and thoracic cord and in which the vagal nerves were intact, stimulation of the alae cinerea in the medulla oblongata also produced gastric excitatory responses through the vagal nerve. The distribution of the excitatory points obtained from this experiment ranged from the oral region of the alae cinerea at the upper level to the caudal region of the obex at the lower level[25]. This shows that the excitatory responses of the stomach on stimulation of the medulla oblongata were produced through two pathways, i.e., the vagal nerve, and the splanchnic nerve via the spinal cord. It is also clear that the efferent nerve was the vagal nerve in the excitatory reflex, and further that the major and minor splanchnic nerves might have acted as an excitatory efferent pathway. It was observed that the frequency of discharges of the vagal nerve increased during the vestibulo-gastric excitatory reflex, as shown in Fig. 5A[5]. These experiments indicated that one of the gastric reflex centers might be located in the medulla oblongata. Excitatory responses through the vagal or splanchnic nerves were demonstrated in the gastro-gastric, ileo-gastric, colon-gastric and labyrintho-gastric excitatory reflexes.

(b) *Intestinal inhibitory reflex.*   Inhibitory pathways from the medulla oblongata to the gut were obtained in two pathways. One of the pathways of these inhibitory reflexes was through the medulla oblongata via the spinal cord to the splanchnic nerve (see Fig. 1A) and another was observed through the vagal nerve. Stimulation of the small intestine, colon, bladder and labyrinth, and afferent stimulation of the vagal nerve produced inhibitory responses of the stomach. Efferent and afferent pathways of the gastro-gastric inhibitory reflex through the vagal nerve were

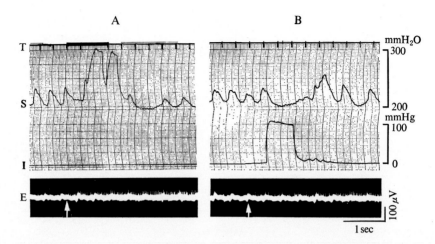

Fig. 5. Simultaneous recordings of the discharge of impulses of the gastric branch of the vagal nerve and gastric response. The vagal nerve was the only nerve connection between the stomach, ileum and medulla oblongata. A, Vestibulo-gastric excitatory reflex; B, ileo-gastric inhibitory reflex.
Symbols: T, time marks in 10 sec. At signal the vestibular nerve was stimulated afferently; S, gastric motility; I, intraluminal pressure of the ileum; E, efferent discharge of the vagal nerve; ↑, onset of gastric reflexes.

also observed. Discharge of impulses of the gastric branch of the vagal nerve during ileo-gastric inhibitory reflex was demonstrated, as shown in Fig. 5B[6].

Localization of reflex centers in the medulla oblongata:

The dorsomedial nucleus of n. vagi is responsible for the excitation of the gastric motility. But the inhibitory points, as well as the excitatory points, were found in this nucleus. The points which influence gastric motility are located not only in the dorsal nucleus of n. vagi, but also in the gray matter of the medulla oblongata. When a monopolar electrode was inserted into this nucleus and its vicinity from the dorsal surface and stimulated, many excitatory and inhibitory responses of gastric motility were observed. The distribution of these points which produced excitatory and inhibitory responses was determined histologically and is shown in Fig. 6. Both points were concentrated especially in the dorsal nucleus of n. vagi, the solitary tract and its nucleus and the dorsal regions of the reticular formation. Stimulation of the above regions produced not only excitation or inhibition of gastric motility but also changes in the motility of the small intestine and colon[26].

Electrical activities of the excitatory and inhibitory points of gastric motility in the medulla oblongata:

(a) *Gastric excitatory points.* Transection of the brain stem was done at the level between the superior and inferior colliculus and also between the C-1 and C-2 segments of the spinal cord, and the bilateral major and minor splanchnic nerves were severed. Thus, the vagal nerve was the only nerve connection between the medulla oblongata and the gut. It was demonstrated that the frequency of discharges of the excitatory points increased during the vestibulo-gastric excitatory reflex (Fig. 7b), but fell during the ileo-gastric inhibitory reflex (Fig. 7a)[3]. This point was found to be located in the dorsomedial nucleus of n. vagi by histological examination[6]. The point where increase in the frequency of discharges of the excitatory points during the excitatory reflex was followed by a decrease during the inhibitory reflex is called Type 1 point.

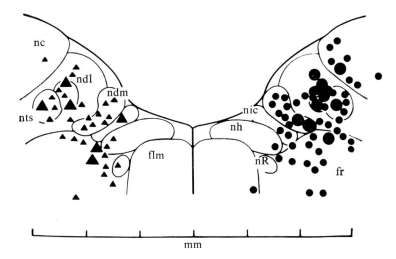

Fig. 6. Distribution of inhibitory and excitatory points of gastric motility in the medulla oblongata of the dog; middle of the alae cinerea, frontal section. The inhibitory points are placed on the left and excitatory points on the right.

▲, Inhibitory point; ●, excitatory point (large one, 3 examples; small one, 1 example); flm, fasciculus longitudinalis med.; fr, formatio reticularis; nc, nucleus cuneiformis; ndl, nucleus dorsolateralis n. vagi; ndm, nucleus dorsomedialis n. vagi; nh, nucleus hypoglossi; nic, nucleus intercalatus; nR, nucleus Rolleri; nts, nucleus tractus solitarii.

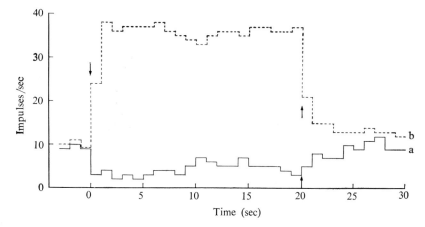

Fig. 7. Changes in the frequency of discharges of the Type 1 excitatory point in the medulla oblongata during gastric reflexes. The vagal nerve was the only nerve connection between the stomach, ileum and medulla oblongata. Discharge of impulses was induced from the dorsomedial nucleus of n. vagi.

a, Ileo-gastric inhibitory reflex; b, vestibulo-gastric excitatory reflex; ⇵, onset and suspension of gastric reflexes.

(b) *Gastric inhibitory points.* In an animal whose only nerve connection between the medulla oblongata and the gut was the vagal nerve, the inhibitory point in which an increase in the frequency of discharges was recorded during the ileo-gastric inhibitory reflex (Fig. 8a)[3] showed a decrease in the frequency of discharges during the vestibulo-gastric excitatory reflex (Fig. 8b)[3]. This point is a Type 1 point, as shown in the preceding experiments. The inhibitory point was found to be located in the dorsomedial nucleus of n. vagi by histological examination[6].

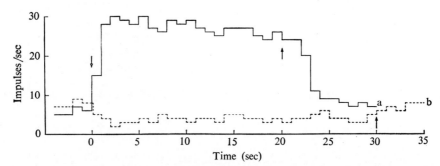

Fig. 8. Changes in the frequency of discharges of the Type 1 inhibitory point in the medulla oblongata during gastric reflexes. The vagal nerve was the only nerve connection between the stomach, ileum and medulla oblongata. Discharge of impulses was induced from the dorsomedial nucleus of n. vagi.
a, Ileo-gastric inhibitory reflex; b, vestibulo-gastric excitatory reflex; ↓↑, onset and suspension of gastric reflexes.

Positive and negative relationship between the medulla oblongata and spinal cord:

Fig. 9 shows the electrical activities recorded continuously from the inhibitory point of the thoracic cord. The frequency of discharges was temporarily increased immediately after transection of the cervical cord at the level between the C-1 and C-2 segments and thereafter the frequency of discharges fell rapidly and disappeared within 6 min. Electrical activities recovered to the pretransection level within 42 min after transection of the spinal cord (Fig. 9a). A similar phenomenon was also observed in the excitatory point of the thoracic cord (Fig. 9b). These observations demonstrate that the inhibitory and excitatory points in the thoracic cord not only receive tonic influence from the medulla oblongata but also are able to act spontaneously, independently of the medulla oblongata[8].

In an animal with an intact spinal cord, electrical stimulation of the inhibitory point of the medulla oblongata produced an increase in the frequency of discharges in the Type 1 inhibitory point in the thoracic cord. Stimulation of the excitatory point in the medulla oblongata also produced an increase in the frequency of discharges in the Type 1 excitatory point in the thoracic cord[4].

Similar responses were observed during the gastro-gastric inhibitory reflex. That is, the stomach was functionally divided into two portions. Distension of a portion of the gastric body produced tonic inhibition of the gastric antrum. This gastro-gastric inhibitory reflex arc consisted of the gastric body, vagal nerve, medulla oblongata, thoracic cord, major splanchnic nerve and gastric antrum. Thus, excitation of the inhibitory point in the medulla oblongata which was induced by the vagal afferent impulses due to the distension of the gastric body, produced an increase in the frequency of discharges of the inhibitory point (lateral intermedial nucleus) in the thoracic cord. During this period, discharge of impulses of the excitatory point in the thoracic cord decreased. A similar response was observed in the vestibulo-gastric excitatory reflex. Afferent stimulation of the vestibular nerve excited the excitatory point in the medulla oblongata and an

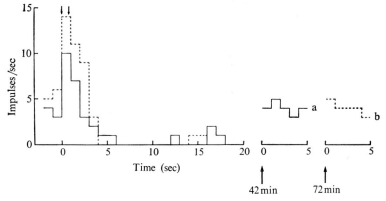

Fig. 9. Changes in the frequency of discharges of the Type 1 inhibitory and excitatory point in the thoracic cord due to transection of the spinal cord at the level between the C-1 and C-2 segments (↓↓). a, Discharge of impulses of the inhibitory point; b, discharge of impulses of the excitatory point. The abscissa shows time lapse at 20 sec immediately after transection of the spinal cord, and after 42 min and 72 min. The ordinate shows the frequency of dishcarges per sec.

increase in the frequency of discharges of the excitatory point in the thoracic cord, as shown in Fig. 4b.

Discussion

The frequency of discharges of the gastric branch of the major splanchnic nerve increased during the inhibitory reflex (Fig. 1A), but the frequency of discharges of this nerve also increased during the excitatory reflex, as shown in Fig. 1B. This shows that the splanchnic nerve has both inhibitory and excitatory efferent pathways of intestinal reflexes. Kuré et al.[13] suggested in their theory of the spinal parasympathetic nervous sytem the existence of an excitatory response of the gut by nerve stimulation from the thoracic and lumbar cord. Semba[23], one of the present authors, observed that excitatory responses of gastric and ileal motility were produced by a relatively weak stimulation of the splanchnic nerve and inhibitory responses by a relatively strong stimulation. Conditions required to produce excitation of the gut have been examined by many investigators[2,10]. After the celiac ganglion had been painted with nicotine, stimulation of the major splanchnic nerve consistently produced an excitatory response of the gut. This suggests that both inhibitory and excitatory nerve fibers are admixed in the splanchnic nerve, and that inhibitory nerves have synaptic connections in the celiac ganglion, while excitatory nerve fibers do not. The same phenomenon was observed in the synaptic connections involved in the inferior mesenteric ganglion and lumbar splanchnic nerve. The excitatory response is obtained by stimulation of the thoracic cord[27] and lumbar cord[18]. Excitatory points are found in the dorsal region of the intermedial substance, though an inhibitory point is found in the ventral region of the intermedial substance of the gray matter. An excitatory response is obtained by stimulation of the cervical cord and also the medulla oblongata through the splanchnic nerve. Thus, the splanchnic nerve plays a role as an excitatory efferent pathway (see Fig. 1 B).

The intestinal excitatory reflex involving the medulla oblongata was observed via the vagal nerve. The experiments shown in Fig. 5 A and B show that the vagal nerves have efferent pathways of both excitatory and inhibitory reflexes. The possibility that the vagal nerve may have an inhibitory response has been known since the study of Langley[14]. Abrahamsson[1] reported that the efferent pathway was the vagal nerve in the receptive relaxation mechanism of gastric motility. The origin of the vagal nerve which is responsible for gastric excitation is located in the dorsal nucleus of n. vagi[12]. However, a number of physiological findings have been presented indicating that the stimulation of this nucleus produces many sympathetic responses, such as inhibition of gastric motility[15]. Stimulation of the dorsomedial nucleus of n. vagi produced not only excitation of gastric motility but also gastric inhibition.

The excitatory and inhibitory points in the medulla oblongata were concentrated in the dorsal nucleus of n. vagi, the solitary tract and its nucleus and the dorsal region of the reticular formation, as illustrated in Fig. 6[26]. These points produced not only excitation and inhibition of gastric motility but also changes in the motility of the small intestine and colon[18]. At the present stage of studies, these regions may be assumed to be the regulatory motor centers of the alimentary canals[25]. These regulatory motor centers respond to afferent stimulation from various regions; one of the efferent pathways of the excitatory system is the vagal nerve and others are the major, minor and lumbar splanchnic nerves and also the pelvic nerve. The efferent fiber is cholinergic and also non-cholinergic[29]. As for the inhibitory system to the gut, one of the efferent pathways is the vagus nerve, which is non-adrenergic[17], and another descends via the spinal cord. The efferent nerves are the major, minor and lumbar splanchnic nerves, which are adrenergic and non-adrenergic. Thus, it has been demonstrated that the extrinsic nerves except for the pelvic nerve have both inhibitory and excitatory activities to the gut.

The experiments shown in Figs. 3 and 4 for the spinal cord or Figs. 7 and 8 for the medulla oblongata demonstrated that changes of discharge of impulses of Type 1 points were in inverse relation during inhibitory and excitatory reflexes. Thus, an increase in the discharge of impulses of the Type 1 inhibitory point during the inhibitory reflex was followed by a decrease of impulses in the Type 1 excitatory point, as shown in Figs. 3 and 8. This suggests that inhibitory interneurons of the excitatory preganglionic motoneurons may exist. The postulated neuron connection during the inhibitory reflex may be illustrated as shown in Fig. 10 A. It should be noted that the proposed inhibitory interneurons are located before the excitatory preganglionic motoneurons. A similar phenomenon was obtained in the Type 1 excitatory point during the excitatory reflex. The increase of discharge of impulses of the Type 1 excitatory point was followed by a decrease of discharge of impulses in the Type 1 inhibitory point, as shown in Figs. 4 and 7. Inhibitory interneurons of the inhibitory preganglionic motoneurons may thus be assumed to exist. The postulated neuron connection of the preganglionic motoneurons and inhibitory interneurons during excitatory reflex is shown in Fig. 10 B. The inhibitory interneurons may be located before the inhibitory preganglionic motoneurons. Thus, the Type 1 inhibitory and excitatory points which are responsible for gastric motility in the thoracic cord may have an inverse relation during intestinal reflex, like the inhibitory and excitatory points in the medulla oblongata[6].

On the other hand, the relation between the medulla oblongata and spinal cord is demonstrated in the experiments shown in Fig. 9. The preceding results may be summarized as showing that the Type 1 inhibitory or excitatory points in the medulla oblongata have a close positive relation to the Type 1 inhibitory or excitatory points in the spinal cord during intestinal reflexes, respectively. However, a negative relation is observed between the Type 1 inhibitory or excitatory points in the medulla oblongata and the Type 1 excitatory or inhibitory points in the spinal cord, respectively, and both points show a negative relation in the medulla oblongata or in the spinal cord. Thus, the existence of inhibitory interneurons may be assumed. Thus, the excitatory re-

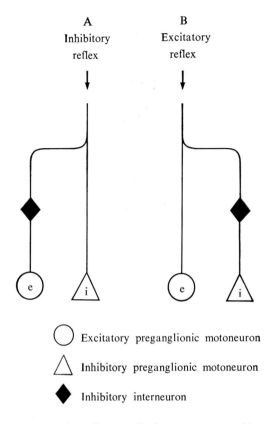

Fig. 10. The postulated neuron connections of preganglionic motoneurons and interneurons. A, inhibitory reflex; B, excitatory reflex.

sponse of motility of the alimentary canals depends not only on an increase of activities of the excitatory motoneurons but also on a decrease of activities of the inhibitory motoneurons. The inhibitory response of the gut is due to an increase of activities of the inhibitory motoneurons on the one hand and also to a decrease of activities of the excitatory motoneurons on the other hand[28].

ACKNOWLEDGEMENTS: We wish to express our gratitude to Dr. T. Mizonishi for technical assistance and to Mr. T. Kobayashi for his assistance in preparing the illustrations and photographs.

REFERENCES

1. Abrahamsson, H., Studies on the inhibitory nervous control of gastric motility, *Acta physiol. scand.*, 88, Suppl., 390 (1973) 1–38.
2. Brown, G.L. and McSwiney, B.A., The sympathetic innervation of the stomach. IV, Reversal of sympathetic action by luminal, *J. Physiol. (Lond.)*, 74 (1932) 179–194.
3. Fujii, K., Mizonishi, T. and Mizonishi, Y., Electrical activities of the gastric motor centers in the dog's medulla oblongata, *The autonomic nervous system*, 10 (1973) 133–139 (in Japanese).
4. Fujii, K., Mizonishi, T. and Mizonishi, Y., Electrical activities of the gastric motor centers in the thoracic cord, *The autonomic nervous system*, 11 (1974) 113–116 (in Japanese).

5. Fujii, K. and Mizonishi, T., Electrical activities of the gastric motor centers during the vestibulo-gastric excitatory reflex, *Japan. J. Smooth Muscle Res.*, 10 (1974) 202–203 (in Japanese).
6. Fujii, K. and Mizonishi, T., The central neural mechanism of the gastric motility in the dog's medulla oblongata on the vagal inhibitory and excitatory reflexes, *Japan. J. Smooth Muscle Res.*, 12 (1976) 77–85 (in Japanese).
7. Fujii, K., Mizonishi, T. and Nagao, Y., The central mechanisms of the gastric inhibitory and excitatory reflexes via the splanchnic nerves, *Brain and nerve*, 28 (1976) 345–352 (in Japanese).
8. Fujii, K., The central mechanisms of the gastric inhibitory and excitatory reflexes, *Clin. Physiol.*, 6 (1976–77) 299–306 (in Japanese).
9. Harding, R. and Leek, B.F., The locations and activities of medullary neurones associated with ruminant forestomach motility, *J. Physiol.* (Lond.), 219 (1971) 587–610.
10. Hukuhara, T., Is the small intestine innervated by the so-called spinal parasympathetic nervous system?, *Quart. J. exp. Physiol.*, 24 (1935) 37–44.
11. Kimura, N., On the labyrintho-gastric reflex, *Med. J. Hiroshima Univ.*, 14 (1966) 575–582 (in Japanese).
12. Kōsaka, K. and Yagita, K., Experimentelle Untersuchungen über den Ursprung des N. Vagus und die centrale Endigung der dem Plexus nodosus entstammenden sensiblen Vagusfasern, sowie über den Verlauf ihrer sekundären Bahn, *Mitt. Med. Ges. Okayama*, 17 (1905) 1–15.
13. Kuré, K., Ichiko, K. and Ishikawa, K., On the spinal parasympathetic. Physiological significance of the spinal parasympathetic system in relation to the digestive tract, *Quart. J. exp. Physiol.*, 21 (1931) 1–19.
14. Langley, J.N., On inhibitory fibres in the vagus for the end of oesophagus and stomach, *J. Physiol.* (Lond.), 23 (1898–99) 407–414.
15. Laughton, N.B., The effects on the stomach of stimulation of the dorsal vagus nuclei, *Amer. J. Physiol.*, 89 (1929) 18–23.
16. Noda, H., Motor response of dog's stomach caused by the stimulation of the spinal cord, *J. Hiroshima Med. Ass.*, 11, Orig. Ser., 11 (1958) 1537–1539 (in Japanese).
17. Ohga, A., Nakazato, Y. and Saito, K., Considerations of the efferent nervous mechanism of the vago-vagal reflex relaxation of the stomach in the dog, *Japan. J. Pharmacol.*, 20 (1970) 116–130
18 Ohya, S , Central neural regulation of the colonic motility of dogs, *Med. J. Hiroshima Univ.*, 17 (1969) 561–571 (in Japanese)
19 Réthelyi, M , Spinal transmission of autonomic processes. *J. Neural Transmission*, Suppl., 11 (1974) 195–212.
20. Semba, T., Mishima, H., Date, T. and Hiraoka, T., Reflex pathways of the pelvic nerves in the spinal cord., *J. Hiroshima Med. Ass.*, 8, Orig. Ser., 3 (1955) 942–943 (in Japanese).
21. Semba, T., The motor response of the stomach and small intestine to the stimulation of the urinary bladder, *Japan. J. Physiol.*, 6 (1956) 294–299.
22. Semba, T., Motor effect of the distal colon caused by stimulating the dorsal roots of the dog's lumbar nerves, *Japan. J. Physiol.*, 6 (1956) 321–326.
23. Semba, T. and Hiraoka, T., Motor response of the stomach and small intestine caused by stimulation of the peripheral end of the splanchnic nerve, thoracic sympathetic trunk and spinal roots, *Japan. J. Physiol.*, 7 (1957) 64–71.
24. Semba, T., Fujii, K. and Kimura, N., The vagal inhibitory responses of the stomach to stimulation of the dog's medulla oblongata, *Japan. J. Physiol.*, 14 (1964) 319–327.
25. Semba, T., On the gastric motor centers, *Japan. J. Smooth Muscle Res.*, 2 (1966) 67–84 (in Japanese).
26. Semba, T., Kimura, N. and Fujii, K., Bulbar influence on gastric motility, *Japan. J. Physiol.*, 19 (1969) 521–533.
27. Semba, T., Fujii, K. and Fujii, Y., The responses of gastric motility and their location by stimulating the thoracic cord of the dog, *Hiroshima J. Med. Sci.*, 19 (1970) 73–85.
28. Semba, T., The central neural regulation of the motility of the gastro-intestinal tracts, *J. Hiroshima Med. Ass.*, 27 (1974) 775–782 (in Japanese).
29. Semba, T. and Mizonishi, T., Atropine-resistant excitation of motility of the dog stomach and colon induced by stimulation of the extrinsic nerves and their centers, *Japan. J. Physiol.* 28 (1978) 239–248.
30. Youmans, W.B., *Nervous and Neurohumoral Regulation of Intestinal Motility*, Interscience, New York 1949, pp. 46–63.

Rhythmic fluctuations of postsynaptic potentials recorded in masseteric neurons during mastication

TADAAKI SUMI

Department of Physiology, Fujita-Gakuen University, School of Medicine,
Toyoake, Aichi 470–11, Japan

It is well known that mechanical stimulation of sensory receptors in the oral and dental structures or electrical stimulation of the frontal cerebral cortex has been found to evoke rhythmic jaw movements which resemble mastication in man[4] and in rabbit[6]. A "chewing center" has been shown to exist in the lower brain-stem[2,3]. In previous work, the hypoglossal motoneurons were shown to receive neural inputs from the cerebral cortex and to produce rhythmic neural activity which in turn evoked chewing movements[7]. It has also been demonstrated that stimulation of the proprioceptor in the masseteric muscle evokes reflex contraction in the muscle. In order to obtain further information on the neural mechanisms controlling mastication, the present experiments were undertaken to record both membrane potentials of the masseteric motoneurons intracellularly and the monosynaptically evoked efferent neural activity of the masseteric nerve, and to investigate the relationship between these neural activities and the cortically evoked rhythmic jaw movements.

Twenty-two lightly anesthetized adult rabbits were used. For recording the membrane potentials intracellularly, glass pipette microelectrodes filled with 3 M KCl were used. Monosynaptically evoked efferent neural activity was recorded from the proximal cut end of the masseteric nerve with a bipolar platinum electrode following stimulation of the mesencephalic nucleus of the trigeminal nerve with a concentric needle electrode[1]. Cortical stimulation was effected with repetitive pulses of 30–50 Hz (0.2 msec, 5–7 V). Electromyograms were simultaneously recorded from the digastric muscle.

At each phase of jaw-closing during the rhythmic jaw movements, the membrane potentials of the masseteric motoneurons showed a slow depolarization superimposed with bursting spikes (Fig. 1). Each spike occurred only when the membrane depolarization crossed beyond a certain critical level, and the frequency of bursting discharges was thus influenced by the slow depolarization. When the jaw began to open, the membrane turned to repolarize and showed no spike discharge as illustrated in Fig. 1. These rhythmic fluctuations of membrane potential in the masseteric motoneurons still remained after the animal was paralyzed with gallamine triethiodide (3 mg/kg, i.v.).

Stimulation of the proprioceptors in the masseteric muscle has been shown to produce a reflex contraction of the muscle. Accordingly, the neural activity monosynaptically evoked in the masseteric motor nerve by stimulation of the mesencephalic nucleus of the trigeminal nerve was facilitated during the period of jaw-closing and inhibited during the period of jaw-opening. The phases of facilitation and inhibition of the monosynaptic reflex activity were being locked to those of jaw-closing and jaw-opening, respectively. Paralysis of the animal enhanced the facilita-

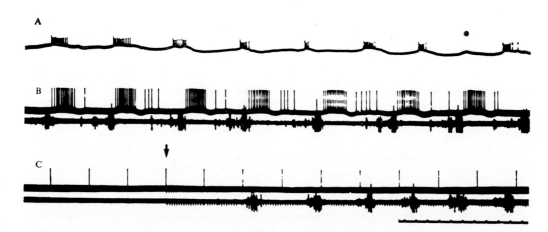

Fig. 1.   Membrane potentials recorded in three masseteric motoneurons during rhythmic jaw movements. Mylohyoid EMGs are shown in the lower trace of B and C. In A, the slow depolarizing potential marked by a dot was abortive in initiating spike action potentials. The spike potentials at regular intervals in C represent antidromically conducted action potentials. The arrow in C indicates the beginning of repetitive cortical stimulation. Time marks indicate 0.1 sec.

tion and inhibition of the monosynaptic reflex. These results suggest that afferent impulses elicited by masticatory movements may normally depress the facilitatory and inhibitory effects on the monosynaptic reflex control of the masseteric motoneurons.

A difference in characteristics has been shown to exist between the alpha and gamma motoneurons in the masseteric motor nucleus[5]. However, the physiological significance of these motoneurons and those exhibiting activity with no relation to rhythmic mastication as shown in Fig. 1C, remains to be studied. In addition, the motoneurons producing jaw-opening have not yet been characterized.

References

1. Hugelin, A. et Bonvallet, M., Étude électrophysiologique d'un réflexe monosynaptique trigéminal, *C. r. Soc. Biol.* (*Paris*), 150 (1956) 2067–2071.
2. Kawamura, Y., Neurogenesis of mastication. In Y. Kawamura (Ed.), *Frontiers of Oral Physiology, Vol. 1,* Karger, Basel, 1974, pp. 77–120.
3. Magoun, H.W., Ranson, S.W. and Fisher, C., Corticifugal pathways for mastication, lapping and other motor functions in the cat, *Arch. Neurol. Pyschiat.*, 30 (1933) 292–308.
4. Penfield, W. and Boldrey, E., Somatic motor and sensory representation in the cerebral cortex of man as studied by electrical stimulation, *Brain*, 60 (1937) 389–443.
5. Sessle, B.J., Identification of alpha and gamma trigeminal motoneurons and effects of stimulation of amygdala, cerebellum, and cerebral cortex, *Exp. Neurol.*, 54 (1977) 303–322.
6. Sumi, T., Some properties of cortically-evoked swallowing and chewing in rabbits, *Brain Research*, 15 (1969) 107–120.
7. Sumi, T., Activity in single hypoglossal fibers during cortically induced swallowing and chewing in rabbits, *Pflügers Arch.*, 314 (1970) 329–346.

Role of the myenteric plexus in the control of defecation in the guinea pig

SOSOGU NAKAYAMA, TERUHIRO YAMASATO, MASATOSHI MIZUTANI,
TOSHIAKI NEYA AND MIYAKO TAKAKI

Department of Physiology, Okayama University Medical School,
Shikata-cho, Okayama 700, Japan

In the guinea pig, defecation is still possible after either transection of the middle lumbar segment or pithing the spinal cord below the lower lumbar segment. The possibility thus arises that the myenteric neural plexus may control defecation in the guinea pig. The present experiments were designed to elucidate the possible role of the myenteric plexus in the control of defecation in the guinea pig.

Rectal motility was recorded by means of the balloon-pressure transducer method. Several days after transection or pithing of the spinal cord, the animals showed rhythmic rectal contractions at a rate of 8 to $10/min^{-1}$ which is similar to the frequency observed in the intact guinea pig.

In the intact animal, distension of the rectum by a balloon induced an increase in basal pressure and intermittently occurring phasic contractions as shown in Fig. 1. The frequency and

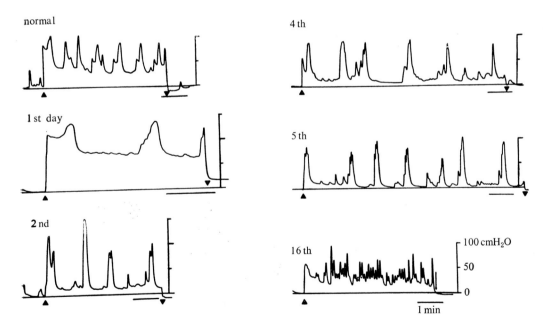

Fig. 1. Effect of distension of the rectum by inflating a balloon on its motility in pithed guinea pig.
(▲ ▼): Duration of distention of the rectum. ↓ : Evacuation of the balloon.

283

duration of the contractions were 1 to 2 min^{-1} and about 30 sec, respectively. One day after pithing, rectal distension elicited a marked increase in basal pressure and phasic contractions of low frequency. Two days later, the frequency and amplitude increased slightly, while the basal pressure decreased. From the 4th day onwards, the pattern of contraction elicited by rectal distension was similar to that of the normal intact animal as shown in Fig. 1. Administration of pentobarbital sodium at a large dose or atropine abolished the contractions.

For *in vitro* experiments, the rectum and distal colon (5 cm long) were isolated from the anesthetized guinea pig and immersed in a bath warmed at 37° C. For recording the spike potentials of the rectal muscle, Ag-AgCl wire of 100 μm diameter enclosed in a thin glass tube 25 mm long was used. When a plastic bolus of the same size and form as guinea-pig feces was inserted into the lumen of the isolated rectal loop from the oral end, a tonic contraction wave was initiated in the vicinity of the oral side of the bolus which gradually moved the bolus to the anal end. At the same time spike potentials were recorded during transportation of the bolus to the anal end. Immediately after insertion of the bolus, previously occurring spike potentials in the area just anal to the bolus disappeared. Both atropine (10^{-6} g/ml) and nicotine (10^{-5} g/ml) completely abolished the contraction wave evoked by the bolus. On the other hand, hexamethonium bromide did not completely inhibit the rectal contraction *in vitro*. These results suggest that the cholinergic neurons in the myenteric plexus play an important role in the control of defecation by guinea pig rectum.

In the guinea pig, the rectum is usually filled with feces, while in carnivores such as the dog and cat it is kept empty except at the time of defecation. This suggests that there is a difference between the defecation mechanisms of these two types of animals. In the carnivora, there is a different mechanism for transportation of feces in the colon and in the rectum, whereas in the guinea-pig rectum, the feces are transported by the same mechanism in both the colon than the rectum. It is supposed that defecation in higher animals such as man, dog and cat is mainly controlled by the higher nervous system, while in lower animals such as the guinea pig, the lower nervous system, i.e., Auerbach's plexus is most important.

Reflex facilitation and inhibition of gastric motility from various skin areas in rats

HIDEKI KAMETANI, AKIO SATO, YUKO SATO AND KIKUKO UEKI

*The 2nd Department of Physiology, Tokyo Metropolitan Institute of Gerontology,
Itabashi-ku, Tokyo 173, Japan*

It has been shown that stimulation of the somatic afferent nerves can influence the functions of the gastrointestinal tract. This response is a somato-autonomic reflex[1-5]. In a previous study[5], we systematically investigated the effect on gastric motility of pinching various skin areas along the mamillary lines of the trunk in rats. It was found that pinching the abdominal skin increased the reflex activity of the gastric sympathetic nerves and inhibited gastric motility. Similar inhibition of jejunal motility was produced by pinching the abdominal skin, while excitation of jejunal motility was elicited by pinching the paws (Koizumi *et al.*, *unpublished*). However, it has not yet been determined whether paw pinching produces any reflex effect on gastric motility.

The present experiment was undertaken to examine systematically the effects on gastric motility which can be produced by pinching various skin areas. Five rats were anesthetized with chloralose and urethane (50 mg/kg and 500 mg/kg, i.p., respectively). The trachea was always cannulated. The animals were usually permitted to breathe spontaneously, but when they were immobilized with gallamine triethiodide (10–20 mg/kg) during the experiment, respiration was maintained with an artificial respirator. All other experimental techniques, including measurement of the gastric motility with a balloon in the pyloric antrum and stimulation of the skin (area about 5×5 mm²) by pinching with forceps (about 2 kg force), were as described previously[5].

When the balloon pressure was increased from 0 to about 100–130 mm H_2O by expanding the volume of the balloon with water, rhythmic contraction waves of 5–6 min⁻¹ corresponding to peristaltic movements were observed and continuously recorded. Fig. 1A–F shows specimen records of gastric motility reflex responses elicited by pinching the various skin areas indicated in G. The responses in A,B,E and F represent reflex excitation; those in C and D represent reflex inhibition. The criteria for reflex excitation were an increase in the amplitude of gastric contraction and/or an increase in basic gastric tone; those for reflex inhibition were a decrease in the amplitude of gastric contraction and/or a decrease in basic gastric tone. All pinching was of 20 sec duration. Both reflex excitation and inhibition of gastric motility began 1–5 sec after the onset of pinching and reached a maximum within 10–30 sec. The responses returned to normal within an additional 20–60 sec. The response patterns for reflex inhibition with and without gallamine were identical, but the reflex excitation responses with gallamine were generally slower than those without.

Fig. 1G,H illustrate the results of pinching the different skin areas in 5 rats. In all rats, each area was pinched for 20 sec every 2–3 min (a minimum of 3 times), and the mean response was calculated. The magnitude of each response was measured as indicated in J. In each rat, all mean responses were expressed as percent of the maximum mean response elicited at one site. The various response magnitudes are indicated by different circle sizes (K), where open circles indicate reflex excitation and filled circles indicate inhibition. Clearly, pinching of the abdominal skin

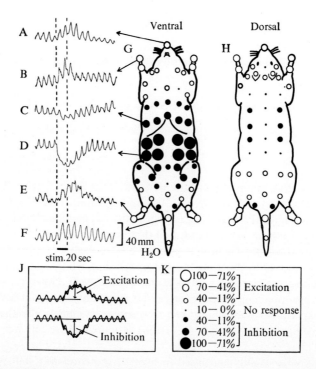

Fig. 1.   Effect on gastric motility of pinching various skin areas in rats. A–F, Specimen records of gastric motility. Pinching of 20 sec duration is shown by the bar and vertical dotted lines. The upward direction indicates gastric contraction; the downward direction indicates gastric relaxation. G and H, Schematic diagrams relating skin areas pinched to reflex changes in gastric motility. J, Model illustrating the method of estimating the magnitude of the reflex response. A mid-line for each wave was drawn and the maximum shift of this line from the pre-stimulus level gave the magnitude of the reflex response. The largest mean absolute value in each rat was taken as 100%, and all other mean reflex responses in the same rat were expressed as percent of this value. K, Open circles indicate excitation; filled circles indicate inhibition; circle size indicates magnitude.

produced strong inhibition: the maximum value was 50 mm H_2O, and the average following 37 trials in the 5 rats was 20.9 ± 12.9 mm H_2O. Pinching of the middle and caudal ventral, and the dorsal thorax produced moderate or weak inhibition. On the other hand, pinching of the paws produced excitation: the maximum value was 50 mm H_2O, and the average following 67 trials in the 5 rats was 14.2 ± 11.9 mm H_2O. Pinching of the nose, forearms, and tail produced a similar excitation, and pinching of the face, ears, neck, legs, and sacral area produced weak excitation.

It is noteworthy that the effect on gastric motility of pinching various skin areas appeared to have a relation to spinal segmental arrangement. When spinal inputs entering the mid- and caudal thoracic spinal levels were stimulated, inhibition was observed. Gastric sympathetic nerves emanate from the mid- and caudal thoracic spinal cord. Thus, it can be suggested that the spinal inputs of these cutaneous nerves increase the gastric sympathetic efferent nerve activity resulting in gastric inhibition. This is consistent with the results of Sato et al.[5]. On the other hand, pinching of the nose, face, ears, neck, arms, legs, paws, sacral area, and tail produced gastric excitation. This suggests that stimulation of cutaneous afferent nerves which enter the central nervous system far from the mid- and caudal thoracic spinal levels may produce either a reflex increase in gastric vagal efferent excitatory activity or a decrease in gastric sympathetic efferent inhibitory activity, each of which is well known to produce gastric excitation. The reflex excitation of jejunal motility produced by paw pinching was due to decreased intestinal sympathetic efferent activity (Koizumi *et al.*, *unpublished*). However, in the present experiment, it was shown that increase in gastric vagal efferent activity was responsible for such gastric excitation (detailed data to be published elsewhere).

In summary, pinching of skin areas of the abdomen, the middle and caudal ventral, and the dorsal thorax was found to inhibit gastric motility and/or reduce muscle tonus in the stomach, while pinching of the skin of nose, face, ears, neck, arms, legs, paws, sacral area, and tail excited gastric motility and/or increased muscle tonus. The inhibition of gastric motility was produced by an increase in gastric sympathetic efferent activity, while the excitation of gastric motility was possibly due to an increase in gastric vagal efferent activity.

REFERENCES

1. Babkin, B.P. and Kite, W.C., Jr., Central and reflex regulation of motility of pyloric antrum, *J. Neurophysiol.*, 13 (1950) 321–334.
2. Jansson, G., Effect of reflexes of somatic afferent of the adrenergic outflow to the stomach in the cat, *Acta physiol. scand.*, 77 (1969) 17–22.
3. Kuntz, A., Anatomic and physiologic properties of cutaneo-visceral vasomotor reflexes, *J. Neurophysiol.*, 8 (1946) 421–429.
4. Lehman, A.V., Studien über reflektorische Darmbewegungen beim Hunde, *Pflügers Arch. ges. Physiol.*, 149 (1913) 413–433.
5. Sato, A., Sato, Y., Shimada, F. and Torigata, Y., Changes in gastric motility produced by nociceptive stimulation of the skin in rats, *Brain Research*, 87 (1975) 151–159.

Interdigestive motor activity and gut polypeptides

ZEN ITOH, SHINJIN TAKEUCHI AND ISAMU AIZAWA

Department of Surgery, School of Medicine, Gunma University,
Maebashi, Gunma 371, Japan

The control mechanism of interdigestive gastrointestinal motor activity by gut hormones was studied in 10 conscious dogs and 20 healthy volunteers.

Gastrointestinal motor activities from the lower esophageal sphincter (LES) to the terminal ileum were continuously recorded on a polygraph by means of chronically implanted force transducers[3] in 10 conscious dogs. Human gastric motor activity was also measured by a balloon method in 20 healthy volunteers. Plasma gastrin and motilin were measured by radioimmunoassay. Synthetic motilin (Yanaihara), pentagastrin (I.C.I.) and pure natural secretin (Karolinska Institute) were used in the present study. These hormonal preparations were dissolved in normal saline and continuously infused intravenously via a chronically implanted silastic tube into the jugular vein.

It was found that the 24-hr gastrointestinal motor activity consisted of two major patterns; the digestive and interdigestive patterns[2]. The interdigestive motor activity was characterized by a cyclically recurring, caudally migrating band of strong contractions interrupted by a long-lasting motor quiescence. When one band of strong contractions reached the distal ileum, another developed again in the LES, stomach and duodenum simultaneously and propagated in a caudal direction. Such recycling episodes repeatedly occurred until the next meal. After the ingestion of food, gastrointestinal motor activity was quickly shifted to the digestive pattern. Synthetic motilin (0.3–0.9 μg/kg-hr) was continuously infused i.v. in both states. In the digestive state, an i.v. infusion of motilin in a dose up to 8.0 μg/kg-hr had no effect upon the gut motor activity. On the other hand, when motilin was infused during the interdigestive state 10 min after the termination of the natural contractions, it induced a pattern precisely similar to the naturally occurring contractions in the LES, stomach and duodenum simultaneously, and the motilin-induced contractions migrated caudally in a similar fashion to the natural interdigestive contractions. The naturally occurring interdigestive contractions and motilin-induced contractions were similarly inhibited by the ingestion of food or an i.v. infusion of pentagastrin (1.0 μg/kg-hr) for 10 min. On the other hand, secretin (8.0 cu/kg-hr) did not have any significant effect on the natural or motilin-induced contractions.

When plasma motilin concentration was measured by radioimmunoassay at one-hr intervals for 24 hr together with a continuous record of the gut motor activity, it was found that plasma motilin level was very low and could not be detected during the digestive state. However, when the gut motor activity shifted to the interdigestive pattern, plasma motilin level was increased. During the interdigestive state, plasma motilin concentration fluctuated in complete association with the interdigestive contractions in the LES, stomach and duodenum. When the gastric motor activity was in motor quiescence, the plasma motilin level was very low and could not be measured. However, when the gastric motor activity increased, plasma motilin level was also increased.

Immediately after a meal, it was observed that plasma motilin was increased, but at 60 min after the ingestion of food, motilin concentration in plasma was always below the detectable range in all measurements. Changes in gastrin concentration in plasma were opposite to those of motilin; the gastrin level was high during the digestive state and low during the interdigestive state.

When a duodenal cannula was left open to drain out duodenal contents during the interdigestive state, it was found that interdigestive contractions did not occur regularly due to the absence of any increase of motilin in the plasma. Direct infusion of food or nutrients into the duodenum strongly inhibited the occurrence of the interdigestive contractions due to a decrease in motilin concentration in the plasma.

In the human study, it was found that during the interdigestive state, plasma motilin concentration also fluctuated with an increase in gastric motor activity.

Bloom *et al*[1]. developed a radioimmunoassay technique for motilin and measured its plasma concentration in humans. It was found that the plasma motilin concentration in 100 fasting healthy subjects was from 5 to 300 pmol/l. This wide variation of plasma motilin level can be reasonably explained by fluctuations of motilin level associated with gut motor activity, as shown in the present experiments. On the other hand, Lee *et al*. measured plasma motilin level in dogs with duodenal motor activity monitored by means of implanted electrodes. They found that cyclic elevation of motilin concentration in plasma was accompanied by an concomitant increase in motor activity during the interdigestive state[4].

In conclusion, the interdigestive gut motor activity may be controlled by the polypeptide motilin. Motilin is an interdigestive hormone whose release, in contrast to all other known gut hormones, is induced by lack of food.

REFERENCES

1. Bloom, S.R., Mitznegg, P. and Bryant, M.G., Measurement of human plasma motilin, *Scand. J. Gastroent.* 11, Suppl. 39 (1976) 47–52.
2. Itoh, Z., Aizawa, I., Takeuchi, S. and Takayanagi, R., Diurnal changes in gastric motor activity in conscious dogs, *Amer. J. Dig. Dis.*, 22 (1977) 117–124.
3. Itoh, Z., Honda, R., Takeuchi, S., Aizawa, I. and Takayanagi, R., An extraluminal force transducer for recording contractile activity of the gastrointestinal smooth muscle in the conscious dogs: Its construction and implantation, *Gastroent. Jap.*, 12 (1977) 275–283.
4. Lee, K.Y., Chey, W.Y., Tai, H.H., Wagner, D. and Yajima, HI, Cyclic changes in plasma motilin levels and interdigestive myoelectric activity of canine antrum and duodenum, *Gastroenterology*, 72 (1977) 1162 (abstract).

Central noradrenergic neuron system: its relation to gastric mucosal blood flow and acid secretion in rats

YOSHITSUGU OSUMI, YASUNORI NAGASAKA AND MOTOHATSU FUJIWARA

Department of Pharmacology, Faculty of Medicine, Kyoto University,
Sakyo-ku, Kyoto 606, Japan

Gastric physiological functions are controlled by the autonomic nervous system and gastrointestinal hormones. There is a lack of information, however, regarding the central regulatory mechanism of gastric functions, particularly regulation as related to the central noradrenergic neuron system. In studies on urethane anesthetized rats[5], intraventricularly applied noradrenaline (NA) (10 μg/rat) decreased the basal gastric mucosal blood flow (MBF) and acid output. It also inhibited increases in these gastric parameters induced by electrical stimulation of the lateral hypothalamic area. The same dose of dopamine or acetylcholine did not affect the basal levels of these gastric parameters. As increases in MBF and acid output induced by stimulation of the lateral hypothalamic area were also blocked by intravenous administration of atropine, such effects may be mediated by activation of the pathway from the lateral hypothalamic area to the brain-stem vagal nuclei. It would appear that a central noradrenergic inhibitory mechanism is involved in the regulation of gastric function.

We undertook further experiments to determine the role of the central noradrenergic nervous system. Male Wistar rats weighing 220–250 g were deprived of food for 16 hr, and anesthetized with urethane. A single carotid artery and femoral vein were cannulated and a round-tipped cannula was inserted into the stomach via an incision in the duodenum. Two ml of prepared gastric solution prewarmed to 38°C was placed in the stomach at the beginning of each 15–min collection period to determine the MBF. The composition of the gastric solution was a 1/5 (v/v) mixture of glycine and mannitol, adjusted to 300 mosm and pH 3.5. MBF was measured by the aminopyrine clearance technique developed by Jacobson *et al.*[2]. The experimental procedures have been described in our previous report[5]. The animal was placed in a steroetaxic instrument. Following stabilization of acid output, the locus coeruleus was unilaterally stimulated, using a stainless-steel bipolar electrode, for 10 min with 0.5 mA, 2 msec pulses at 10 cycles/sec. At the end of the experiments, a small electrolytic lesion was made to identify the position of the electrode tip. The brain was then removed for histological observation.

Electrical stimulation of the locus coeruleus decreased both the gastric MBF and acid output in rats No. 1, 2, and 4, as shown in Fig. 1. In the case of rat No. 3, the electrode tip was in the region just medial to the locus coeruleus; acid output was decreased by the stimulation but no corresponding decrease in MBF was observed. In another 4 animals, in which the electrode tip had been placed in an area other than the locus coeruleus, both MBF and acid output were increased by the stimulation (data not included in Fig. 1). Thus, activation of the NA neuron system originating in the locus coeruleus does apparently exert an inhibitory effect on the gastric MBF and acid secretion. According to recent histochemical observations, both the brain-stem vagal nuclei and the lateral hypothalamic area have a large number of noradrenergic nerve terminals[1,3,4,6]. The former region receives noradrenergic nerve terminals originating from the locus coeruleus, but not from any other noradrenergic cell body in the medulla oblongata[7], while the latter region is probably not innervated by the locus coeruleus. Thus, the intraventricularly applied NA, and stimulation of the locus coeruleus do inhibit vagal activity, most probably at the level of the brain-stem vagal nuclei.

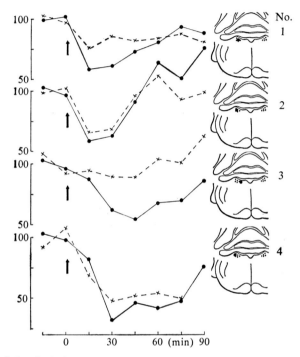

Fig. 1. Effects of electrical stimulation of the locus coeruleus on the gastric mucosal blood flow (MBF) and acid output. Results are expressed as percent changes from the respective basal value (mean of two values preceding treatment). X, MBF; ●, acid output. Upward arrows indicate electrical stimulation. In the diagrams on the right, large closed circles indicate the site of stimulation, and scattered small closed circles the location of the locus coeruleus.

REFERENCES

1. Fuxe, K., Evidence for the existence of monoamine neurons in the central nervous system, *Acta physiol. Scand.* *64 Suppl.* 247 (1965) 39–85.
2. Jacobson, E.D., Rinford, R.H. and Grossman, M.I., Gastric secretion in relation to mucosal blood flow studied by a clearance technic, *J. clin. Invest.*, 45 (1966) 1–12.
3. Loizou, L.A., Projection of the nucleus locus coeruleus in the albino rat, *Brain Research*, 15 (1969) 563–566.
4. Olson, L. and Fuxe, K., Further mapping out of central noradrenaline neuron system: Projections of the 'sub-coeruleus' area, *Brain Research*, 43 (1972) 289–295.
5. Osumi, Y., Aibara, S., Sakae, K. and Fujiwara, M., Central noradrenergic inhibition of gastric muocsal blood flow and acid secretion in rats, *Life Sci.*, 20 (1977) 1407–1416.
6. Swanson, L.W. and Hartman, B.K., The central adrenergic system. An immunofluorescence study of the location of cell bodies and their efferent connections in the rat utilizing dopamine-β-hydroxylase as a marker, *J. comp. Neurol.*, 163 (1975) 467–487.
7. Takahashi, Y., Satoh, K., Sakumoto T., Yamamoto, K., Kimoto, Y., Tohyama, M., Kamei, I. and Shimizu, N., Noradrenaline innervation of the ala cinerea, *Acta histochem. cytochem.*, 11 (1978) 120.

Secretory responses to stimulation of the vagus nerve and to acetylcholine in rat pancreas perfused *in situ*

TOMIO KANNO, ATSUSHI SAITO AND YOSHIAKI HABARA

Department of Physiology, Faculty of Veterinary Medicine, Hokkaido University, Kita-ku, Sapporo 060, Japan

In mammals, the control of pancreatic secretion has been divided into cephalic, gastric and intestinal phases by Thomas[9]. The cephalic phase of pancreatic secretion has been clearly demonstrated in the dog[6] and man[5,7], but was not found[1] or was of only minor importance in the rat[8]. In some rats, sham feeding increased both volume flow and amylase output, but it failed to do so in animals whose gastric juice was drained. It is possible that the pancreatic responses to sham feeding might not have been a true cephalic phase but rather, secondary to the small amounts of acid produced during the cephalic phase of gastric secretion[4]. It is also possible that the pancreatic responses might have been secondary to dilatation of the blood vessels supplying the pancreas[2].

The present experiments were undertaken to test the possibility that the vagus nerve may play some role in controlling secretion of the exocrine pancreas in rats. Wistar strain male rats weighing about 250 g were fasted for 24 hr before the experiments but were allowed water. Cannulation was performed under ether anesthesia: the inlets for vascular perfusion were the superior mesenteric and coeliac arteries, and the outlet was the portal vein. Modified Krebs-Henseleit solution[3] preheated at 37° C was then perfused, the rate of vascular flow being maintained at 2 ml/min with the aid of a roller pump. The hepatic end of the duct was ligated and pancreatic juice was collected from the duodenal end through a stainless steel cannula. Blood supply to the liver and spleen was halted by ligation of the arteries.

The pancreas, duodenum and mesentery were not isolated from the body, and their innervation was left intact. The ventral vagus nerve was cut in the thorax, and its peripheral end was stimulated electrically with a suction electrode. The stimulation, a train of square pulses of 10 msec duration at a frequency of 10 Hz, was continued for 5 min.

Pancreatic juice flow and amylase output into the common duct were estimated during the course of electrical stimulation of the vagus nerve applied regularly at 10-min intervals. The amylase output induced by the vagal stimulation initially increased by about 8 times the resting level and this was followed by a rapid diminution in the subsequent response. Fig. 1A gives an example of the results. The rapid decline in the secretory response may not be due to tachyphylaxis of the pancreatic acinar cells to acetylcholine (ACh), since application of ACh revived the secretory response in the same pancreas even when the response to the nerve stimulation had declined (Fig. 1A). Simultaneous increase and decrease in pancreatic juice flow and amylase output were observed (Fig. 1A). The rapid decline in the responses to successive stimulations of the vagus nerve was little affected by simultaneous application of 0.5 mU cholecystokinin-pancreozymin (CCK-PZ)/ml (Fig. 1B).

Lack of tachyphylaxis of the pancreatic acinar cells to ACh was confirmed. The amylase

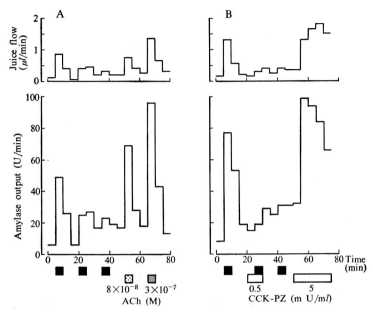

Fig. 1. Pancreatic juice flow and amylase output of rat pancreas perfused *in situ* during the course of intermittent stimulation of the vagus nerve or by acetylcholine (ACh) with (B) or without (A) cholecystokinin-pancreozymin (CCK-PZ).

output induced by intermittent stimulations with the same concentration of ACh (1×10^{-6} M or 3×10^{-6} M) showed a slight tendency to decline.

The present experiments indicate that only the first of the intermittent stimulations of the vagus nerve was effective in evoking secretory responses of the exocrine pancreas of the rat, and suggest that the rapid decline in the subsequent stimulations may be due to a rapid decrease in the ACh output from the endings of the vagus nerve. This is consistent with the view that the cephalic phase of secretion of the exocrine pancreas of the rat is only active, if at all, at the beginning of lasting secretion mediated mainly by endogenous secretion of CCK-PZ and secretin.

REFERENCES

1. Alphin, R.S. and Lin, T.M., Effect of feeding and sham feeding on pancreatic secretion of the rat, *Amer. J. Physiol.*, 197 (1959) 260–262.
2. Harper, A.A., Progress report. The control of pancreatic secretion, *Gut*, 13 (1972) 308–317.
3. Kanno, T., Suga, T. and Yamamoto, M., Effects of oxygen supply on electrical and secretory responses of humorally stimulated acinar cells in isolated rat pancreas, *Jap. J. Physiol.*, 26 (1976) 101–115.
4. Lin, T.M. and Alphin, R.S., Cephalic phase of gastric secretion in the rat, *Amer. J. Physiol.*, 192 (1958) 23–26.
5. Novis, B.H., Bank, S. and Marks, I.N., The cephalic phase of pancreatic secretion in man, *Scand. J. Gastroenterol.*, 6 (1971) 417–422.
6. Preshaw, R.M., Cooke, A.R. and Grossman, M.I., Sham feeding and pancreatic secretion in the dog, *Gastroenterology*, 50 (1966) 171–178.
7. Sarles, H., Dani, R., Prezelin, G., Souville, C. and Figarella, C., Cephalic phase of pancreatic secretion in man, *Gut*, 9 (1968) 214–221.
8. Shaw, H.M. and Heath, T.J., The phases of pancreatic secretion in rats, *Quart. J. exp. Physiol.*, 58 (1973) 229–237.
9. Thomas, J.E., *The External Secretion of the Pancreas*, Thomas, Springfield, Ill, 1950.

Inhibition of gastric acid secretion of somatostatin, secretin and CCK-PZ

YUTAKA MATSUO AND ATSUKO SEKI

The 3rd Department of Internal Medicine, Faculty of Medicine, University of Tokyo,
Bunkyo-ku, Tokyo 113, Japan

The inhibitory actions of somatostatin, a paracrine type[1] of gastrointestinal hormone, and of secretin and CCK-PZ on gastric acid secretion were studied. Gastric acid secretion and serum gastrin release were estimated in Schild's rats, Heidenhain pouch dogs and gastric fistula dogs.

A study was made of the effect of intravenous administration of 35–44 μg/kg/hr of somatostatin, 10 μg/kg/hr of secretin, and 6 μg/kg/hr of CCK-PZ on the gastric juice induced by administration of 1 mg/kg of tetragastrin intravenously, 40 μg/kg of histamine subcutaneously, 2 μg/kg of carbachol intravenously, and 25% meat extract orally.

Somatostatin markedly inhibited the gastric juice secretion induced by tetragastrin, carbachol (Fig. 1) and histamine (Fig. 2). In the Heidenhain pouch dogs, both the gastric juice secretion and serum gastrin release induced by food were inhibited by somatostatin. However, on discontinuance of somatostatin administration, the serum gastrin increased and gastric acid secretion was observed (Fig. 3).

In the gastric fistula dogs, secretin showed a marked inhibitory effect on the gastric acid secretion induced by oral administration of meat extract. However, it did not show any inhibitory effect on the gastric acid secretion induced by histamine and carbachol. The inhibitory effect of CCK-PZ on gastric acid secretion was similar to that of secretin.

Somatostatin, in contrast to secretin and CCK-PZ, inhibited the gastric acid secretion induced by carbachol and histamine; it can be said that this action resembled that of gastric inhibitory polypeptide (GIP)[3]. The inhibition of the gastric acid secretion induced by histamine has been found to be due to the characteristic action of enterogastrone, discovered by Kosaka and

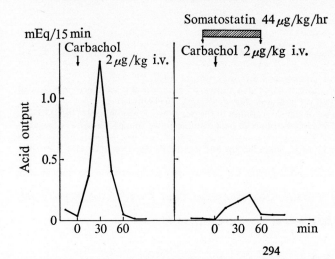

Fig. 1. Effect of intravenous infusion of somatostatin on carbachol-induced gastric acid output in gastric fistula dogs (mean ± SEM of 3 experiments).

Lim[2]. The present results indicate that somatostatin as well as GIP may exert an enterogastrone-like action.

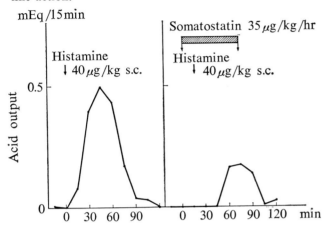

Fig. 2. Effect of intravenous infusion of somatostatin on histamine-induced gastric acid output in gastric fistula dogs (mean ± SEM of 3 experiments).

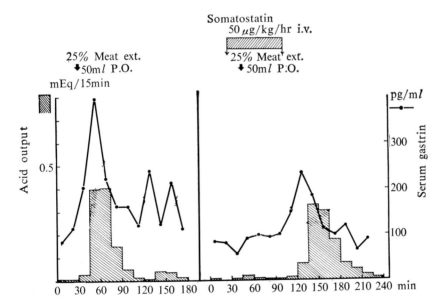

Fig. 3. Effect of intravenous infusion of somatostatin on the gastric acid induced by oral administration of 25% meat extract in Heidenhain pouch dogs (mean ± SEM of 3 experiments).

REFERENCES

1. Feyrter, F., *Über die peripheren Endokrine (paracrinen) Drüsen des Menschen*, Wilhelm Mandrid, Wien, 1953.
2. Kosaka, T. and Lim, R.K.S., Demonstration of the humoral agent in fat inhibition of gastric secretion, *Proc. Soc. Exp. Biol. Med.*, 27 (1930) 890–891.
3. Pederson R.A., and Brown, J.C., Inhibition of histamine-, pentagastrin-, and insulin-stimulated canine gastric secretion by pure "gastric inhibitory polypeptide", *Gastroenterology*, 62 (1972) 393–400.

Effect of intraluminally administered lidocaine upon the pancreozymin-producing endocrine cells of the canine duodenum

TSUNEO FUJITA, YOKO MATSUNARI, SUSUMU MURAKI, KAZUNORI SATO AND KOKI SHIMOJI

Departments of Anatomy and Anesthesiology, Niigata University School of Medicine, Asahi-machi, Niigata 951, Japan

It is now widely accepted that different intestinal hormones are produced by different types of mucosal endocrine cells, and that the cells release their hormones in response to chemical stimuli in the gut lumen perceived by the microvillous cell apex[3]. The present paper reports preliminary results showing that the hormone-releasing response to luminal stimuli of the gut endocrine cells may be inhibited by luminally administered local anesthetics. The effect of lidocaine on the pancreozymin-producing cells of the canine duodenum was examined.

Dogs of either sex, weighing 8–10 kg, were anesthetized by neuroleptoanalgesia and the abdomen was opened. A duodenal loop, 20–25 cm in length immediately anal to the pylorus, was made. The bile duct and the main pancreatic duct were cannulated. Outputs of bile and pancreatic juice were measured every 5 min in terms of their length in the tubes, while the protein contents of the pancreatic juice were measured every 15 min by spectrophotometry at 280 nm.

First, the loop was washed with 40 ml of warm saline and 3 min later, 40 ml of warm saline containing 50 mM/l tryptophan and 50 mM/l phenylalanine was perfused into the loop; 10 min later, the loop was washed with 100 ml of warm saline. A few minutes after administration of the amino acid solution, the pancreatic juice was markedly increased in both volume and protein content, reaching a peak at 15 min and returning to the base level in 45 min. The bile output was markedly but not consistently increased, apparently by contraction of the gallbladder. These reactions of the pancreas and gallbladder suggest a release of pancreozymin from the duodenal mucosa stimulated by the amino acids.

The second experimental procedure was initiated 1 hr after the first stimulation. The loop was infused with 40 ml of warm saline containing 0.25, 0.5, 1, or 5% lidocaine; 3 min later, saline having the same content of amino acids as in the first step but containing lidocaine at the concentration previously used was introduced into the loop; the loop was washed 10 min later. The reactions of the pancreas and gallbladder evoked by the first procedure did not occur in the presence of 1% and 5% lidocaine. Lidocaine at 0.5% suppressed the reactions strongly but not completely. The inhibition by 0.25% lidocaine was only slight.

The third procedure, 1 hr after the second perfusion with amino acids, was a repetition of the first procedure. Conspicuous reactions of the pancreas, often even larger than the first ones, and inconsistent contraction of the gallbladder were reproduced, suggesting that the pancreozymin-releasing ability of the duodenum was retained.

Fig. 1 shows the changes in protein content of the pancreatic juice through the three experimental procedures, showing the clear inhibitory effect of 0.5% and 1% lidocaine.

It seems reasonable to consider that the pancreozymin-producing cells themselves were

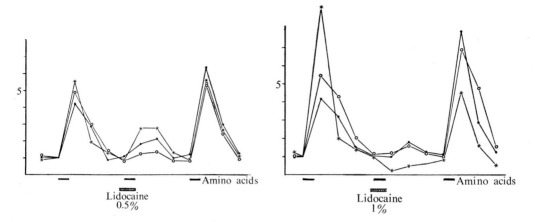

Fig. 1. Protein outputs every 15 min after stimulation with amino acids with and without infusion of lidocaine into the gut of dogs. Three different experiments are shown, using 0.5% (left) and 1% (right) lidocaine.

made either insensitive to amino acids or incapable of releasing hormones by lidocaine, the former possibility being more likely as the anesthetic directly attacks the receptor portion of the cell. Although lidocaine in the gut was partly absorbed into the circulation, it could be proved by providing pancreozymin exogenously that the pancreas remained quite sensitive to this hormone during the second procedure of the present experiment.

Inhibition of pancreozymin release[4,6] and secretin release[5,6] in response to acid stimulus has been reported upon application of local anesthetics to the duodenal mucosa. These findings have been thought to support the "nervous mechanism" of gut hormone release[1,4,5,6]. Recent results, however, show that gut hormones are released by their source cells quite independently of nervous control. According to our recent view, the gut endocrine cells are paraneuronal elements comparable in structure and function to sensory cells and neurons[2,3]. The probable direct effect of lidocaine on the gut endocrine cells shown in the present study, therefore, seems to support the view that the cells are neuron-like also in their response to anesthetics.

REFERENCES

1. Berry, H. and Flower, R.J., The assay of endogenous cholecystokinin and factors influencing its release in the dog and cat, *Gastroenterology*, 60 (1971) 409–420.
2. Fujita, T., The gastro-enteric endocrine cell and its paraneuronic nature. In R.E. Coupland and T. Fujita (Eds.), *Chromaffin, Enterochromaffin and Related Cells*, Elsevier, Amsterdam, 1976, 191–208.
3. Fujita, T. and Kobayashi, S., The cells and hormones of the GEP endocrine system. The current of studies. In T. Fujita (Ed.), *Gastro-Entero-Pancreatic Endocrine System—A Cell-Biological Approach*, Igaku Shoin Ltd., Tokyo, 1973, 1–16.
4. Hong, S.S. and Magee, D.F., Pharmacological studies on the regulation of pancreatic secretion in pigs, *Ann. Surg.*, 172 (1970) 41–48.
5. Schapiro, H. and Woodward, E.R., Inhibition of the secretin mechanism by local anesthetics, *Amer. Surg.* 31 (1965) 139–141.
6. Slayback, J.B., Swena, E.M., Thomas, J.E. and Smith, L.L., The pancreatic secretory response to topical anesthetic block of the small bowel, *Surgery*, 61 (1967) 591–595.

The effects of glucose, mannose and 2-deoxyglucose on the efferent discharge rate of the hepatic nerve in the rabbit

AKIRA NIIJIMA

Department of Physiology, Niigata University School of Medicine,
Asahi-machi, Niigata 951, Japan

It has been reported that hyperglycemic response and the depletion of glycogen reserves in the liver occur following stimulation of the peripheral cut end of the splanchnic nerve in calves and other animal species with both adrenal glands removed[2-4]. It was observed in the isolated liver of toad that a remarkable increase in glucose concentration in the perfusate of the liver occurred in response to stimulation of the hepatic branch of the splanchnic nerve[6].

Anand[1], Oomura and other workers[8,9] have demonstrated the existence of glucose-sensitive nerve cells in the hypothalamic region by means of the electrophysiological technique. It may be that these glucose-sensitive nerve cells send signals to the liver through the splanchnic pathway.

Experiments were conducted to study the effects of *d*-glucose, *l*-glucose, *d*-mannose and 2-deoxy-*d*-glucose on the efferent discharge rate of the hepatic nerve. Adult rabbits of both sexes were used. The animals were anesthetized by i.v. injection of pentobarbitone (35 mg/kg). Glucose and other test solutions were injected through a catheter placed in the cranial side of the left carotid artery or cardiac side of the left jugular vein. Before the intraarterial injection, both sides of the depressor nerves were cut and the sinus nerves on both sides were pinched with a pair of forceps to eliminate the effect of baroreceptor reflex following injection. Samples of arterial blood were withdrawn from a catheter inserted into the cardiac side of the carotid artery for the estimation of glucose content.

Efferent discharges were recorded from fine filaments dissected from nerve branches innervating the liver along the portal vein. Discharges were amplified by a condenser-coupled amplifier and stored on magnetic tape. Nervous activity was analyzed after conversion of spikes to standard pulses through a window discriminator. The standard pulses were then fed to a rate meter for analysis. On-line analysis of discharges was also carried out.

An injection of *d*-glucose (200 mg/kg, 2 ml) into the carotid artery caused a remarkable decrease in the efferent discharge rate of the hepatic nerve which lasted about 3 min. An intraarterial injection of *l*-glucose and *d*-mannose (200 mg/kg, 2 ml each) showed no decrease in firing rate. An i.v. injection of the same amount of *d*-glucose showed a smaller effect on firing rates.

It has been reported that the administration of 2-deoxy-*d*-glucose increases the firing rate of the adrenal nerve[7] in response to decreased glucose utilization[10], which in turn increases catecholamine release from the adrenal medulla[5]. As shown in the lower trace of Fig. 1, an i.v. injection of 2-deoxy-*d*-glucose caused a remarkable increase in firing rates, which lasted longer than 3 hr. Bilateral vagotomy, indicated by an arrow, did not change the firing rate, indicating that the nerve signals are not mediated by the vagus nerve but through the splanchnic nerve.

In the next experiments, the relationship between glucose content in the arterial blood and efferent discharge rate in the hepatic nerve was studied. A gradual decrease in blood glucose concentration from 130 mg/dl to 110 mg/dl following i.v. injection of regular insulin (Novo, 40 U/kg) caused a gradual increase in discharge rate (Fig. 2).

These results show that the increase in glucose levels in the carotid arterial blood cuases the decrease, and the decrease in glucose levels results in an increase in efferent discharge rate in the hepatic branch of the splanchnic nerve. The existence of a nervous pathway from glucose-sensitive nerve cells in the hypothalamus to the hepatic branch of the splanchnic nerve is suggested.

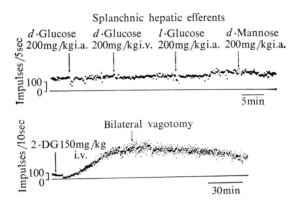

Fig. 1. The effects of *d*-glucose, *d*-mannose, *l*-glucose and 2-deoxy-*d*-glucose on the efferent discharge rate of the hepatic nerve.

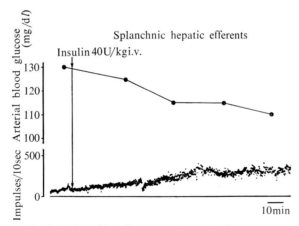

Fig. 2. The effects of i.v. injection of insulin on the efferent discharge rate and blood glucose level. Upper trace, time course of blood glucose content. Lower trace, time course of discharge rate.

REFERENCES

1. Anand, B.K., Chhina, G.S., Sharma, K.N., Dua, S., and Singh, B., Activity of single neurons in the hypothalamic feeding centers: effect of glucose, *Amer. J. Physiol.*, 207 (1964) 1146–1154.
2. Edwards, A.V. and Silver, M., The glycogenolytic response to stimulation of the splanchnic nerves in adrenalectomized calves, *J. Physiol. (Lond.)*, 211 (1970) 109–124.
3. Edwards, A.V., The glycogenolytic response to stimulation of the splanchnic nerves in adrenalectomized calves, sheep, dogs, cats and pigs, *J. Physiol. (Lond.)*, 213 (1971) 741–759.

4. Edwards, A.V., The hyperglycaemic response to stimulation of the hepatic sympathetic innervation in adrenalectomized cats and dogs, *J. Physiol. (Lond.)*, 220 (1972) 697–710.

5. Hokfelt, B., and Bydgeman, S., Increased adrenaline production following administration of 2-deoxy-d-glucose in the rat, *Proc. Soc. exp. Biol. (N.Y.)*, 106 (1961) 537–539.

6. Niijima, A. and Fukuda, A., Release of glucose from perfused liver preparation in response to stimulation of the splanchnic nerves in the toad, *Japan. J. Physiol.*, 23 (1973) 497–508.

7. Niijima, A., The effect of 2-deoxy-*d*-glucose and *d*-glucose on the efferent discharge rate of sympathetic nerves, *J. Physiol. (Lond.)*, 251 (1975) 231—243.

8. Oomura, Y., Kimura, K., Ooyama, H., Maeno, T., Iki, M., and Kuniyoshi, M., Reciprocal activites of the ventromedial and lateral hypothalamic areas of cats, *Science*, 143 (1964) 484–485.

9. Oomura, Y., Ooyama, H., Yamamoto, T., Ono, T. and Kobayashi, N., Behavior of hypothalamic unit activity during electrophoretic application of drugs, *Ann. N. Y. Acad. Sci.*, 157 (1969).

10. Smith, G.P. and Epstein, A.N., Increased feeding in response to decreased glucose utilization in the rat and monkey, *Amer. J. Physiol.*, 217 (1969) 1083–1087.

Central cholinergic regulation of hepatic enzymes

TAKASHI SHIMAZU, MASAKO OZAWA, KOICHI ISHIKAWA AND HIROSHI MATSUSHITA

Division of Neurochemistry, Psychiatric Research Institute of Tokyo,
Setagaya-ku, Tokyo 156, Japan

Electrical stimulation of the lateral hypothalamic nucleus (LH) in rats and rabbits results in enhanced glycogenesis[10,12], reduced gluconeogenesis[13], and increased activities of tryptophan pyrrolase[7] and tyrosine aminotransferase in the liver. Evidence was also obtained recently[9,11] that cholinergic stimulation of the LH by focal application of acetylcholine or carbachol caused activation of hepatic glycogen synthetase, an enzyme catalyzing the rate-limiting step of glycogenesis. Further studies have now shown that acetylcholine-sensitive neurons in the LH are specifically concerned with this enzyme regulation, and that the mode of transmission of the impulse from these neurons is through a cholinergic neural pathway that directly influences the hepatic enzyme, rather than through modification of pancreatic hormone secretion. Similarly, acetylcholine-sensitive neurons of the LH are also implicated in the regulation of another hepatic enzyme, tyrosine aminotransferase, but probably through glucocorticoid mediation. These results are reported in this communication.

Male Wistar rats, weighing 250–300 g, were used. Double-walled cannulas with inner and outer diameters of 0.30 mm and 0.65 mm were stereotaxically implanted into the LH of rats under pentobarbital anesthesia, as described previously[11,13]. Two weeks after the implantation, intrahypothalamic microinjections of different neurotransmitters were given, each in a single dose (5×10^{-8} mol in 1 μl of 0.9% saline) through the inner cannula. To minimize the effects of circadian variations of glycogen synthetase and tyrosine aminotransferase activities in the liver, all the experiments were started at 1100 hr and the animals were not fed for 3 hr before and during the experiments. One hr (for glycogen synthetase assay) and 4 hr (for tyrosine aminotransferase assay) after intrahypothalamic microinjection of transmitters, the animals were anesthetized by intraperitoneal injection of sodium pentobarbital (50 mg/kg), the abdominal wall was cut open, and a portion of the liver was quickly removed and immersed in liquid nitrogen. The activities of glycogen synthetase[11] and tyrosine aminotransferase[4] were then assayed.

As shown in Table 1, cholinergic stimulation of the LH neurons by focal application of acetylcholine greatly increased the activities of glycogen synthetase-*I* (active form) and tyrosine aminotransferase in the liver, as compared with the control group similarly treated with saline. Noradrenergic, dopaminergic, serotonergic and GABA-ergic stimulations of the LH neurons, on the other hand, did not affect the activity of either enzyme.

The time courses of the increases in enzyme activities after cholinergic stimulation indicated that the response of glycogen synthetase was faster than that of tyrosine aminotransferase. Nearly maximum increases of glycogen synthetase and tyrosine aminotransferase were obtained at 1 hr and 4 hr, respectively, after intrahypothalamic microinjection of acetylcholine. This difference in the responses of the two enzymes may reflect the difference in their regulatory mechanisms. The increase of glycogen synthetase-*I* activity was shown to be due to activation of the enzyme[9,11],

TABLE 1.   Effects of microinjections of various neurotransmitters into the lateral hypothalamic nucleus (LH) on the activities of glycogen synthetase and tyrosine aminotransferase in rat liver.
For glycogen synthetase, animals were killed 1 hr after the neurotransmitters had been administered. For tyrosine aminotransferase, the animals were killed 4 hr after. The doses of neurotransmitters were 5×10^{-8} mol, and the injection volume was 1 μl. One unit of glycogen synthetase-I was defined as the amount which catalyzes the incorporation of 1 μmol of glucose from UDP-[U-^{14}C]glucose into glycogen per min, and one unit of tyrosine aminotransferase was defined as the amount catalyzing the formation of 1 μmol of p-hydroxyphenylpyruvate from tyrosine in 1 min. Results are means $\pm$ SE of 4–8 determinations. *Significantly different from the saline group at $P < 0.05$.

Neurotransmitter	Enzyme activities (munits/mg protein)	
	Glycogen synthetase-I	Tyrosine aminotransferase
Saline (control)	0.96 ± 0.11	10.3 ± 0.9
Acetylcholine	2.05 ± 0.33*	36.3 ± 2.3*
Serotonin	0.94 ± 0.16	11.7 ± 1.0
Norepinephrine	1.30 ± 0.23	9.9 ± 0.2
Dopamine	0.97 ± 0.12	9.9 ± 0.7
γ-Aminobutyric acid	0.81 ± 0.10	12.3 ± 0.8

that is, conversion of the inactive synthetase (D form) to active synthetase (I form), whereas the increase of tyrosine aminotransferase activity was probably due to induction of the enzyme, $i.e.$, enhanced synthesis of the enzyme protein.

To examine whether acetylcholine injected into the LH acts through cholinergic transmission in the LH, a cholinolytic agent (atropine) was injected into the LH 10 min before local application of acetylcholine (Table 2, Exp. 1). Pretreatment of LH neurons with atropine resulted in almost complete blockage of the increases in glycogen synthetase and tyrosine aminotransferase in response to cholinergic stimulation of the LH. These results suggest that acetylcholine-sensitive neurons in the LH are particularly involved in the regulation of glycogen synthetase and tyrosine aminotransferase activities in the liver.

TABLE 2.   Effect of cholinergic blocking agents on the responses of liver glycogen synthetase and tyrosine aminotransferase to cholinergic stimulation of the LH.
In Exp. 1, atropine (1×10^{-7} mol in 1 μl saline) was applied to the LH, 10 min before intrahypothalamic application of acetylcholine (5×10^{-8} mol in 1 μl saline). In Exp. 2, N-methylatropine (10 mg/kg in 0.5 ml saline) was given intraperitoneally 30 min before intrahypothalamic microinjection of acetylcholine (Ach). Other exeprimental conditions were the same as in Table 1. *Significantly different from the saline group at $P < 0.05$.

Pretreatment	Stimulation of LH with	Glycogen synthetase-I	Tyrosine aminotransferase
		(munits/mg protein)	
Exp. 1 (intrahypothalamic)			
Saline	Saline	0.65 ± 0.12	10.5 ± 0.9
Saline	ACh	1.69 ± 0.33*	35.4 ± 2.1*
Atropine	ACh	0.73 ± 0.13	12.2 ± 1.7
Exp. 2 (intraperitoneal)			
Saline	Saline	0.76 ± 0.04	10.3 ± 0.7
Saline	ACh	1.38 ± 0.02*	35.9 ± 1.8*
N-methylatropine	ACh	0.73 ± 0.11	26.4 ± 3.5*

It is known that the vagal cholinergic nerves exert direct neural regulation on glycogen synthetase[8] and tyrosine aminotransferase[2] of the liver. To see whether the effects of cholinergic stimulation of the LH on the liver enzymes are mediated by this neural pathway, a cholinolytic agent was also administered peripherally. As shown in Exp. 2 of Table 2, activation of glycogen synthetase after cholinergic stimulation of the LH was completely blocked by a previous intraperitoneal injection of *N*-methylatropine, an anticholinergic agent that does not readily penetrate the blood-brain barrier. This may be explained by assuming that the effect of cholinergic stimulation of the LH is mediated by the peripheral cholinergic system. It has already been shown that the LH-vagal pathway is an important neural component for controlling glycogen synthesis in the liver[8,12]. In addition, it is known that acetylcholine can stimulate glycogen synthetase in isolated, perfused rat liver[6] and in isolated hepatocytes[1]. Therefore, the neural regulation of liver glycogen synthetase appears to be mediated by the cholinergic system centrally as well as peripherally, via the LH-vagal pathway.

Induction of tyrosine aminotransferase after cholinergic stimulation of the LH, on the other hand, was partially blocked by *N*-methylatropine administered peripherally. This result, different from that observed for glycogen synthetase, is consistent with the view that the hypothalamic cholinergic influence on this enzyme may be through some hormonal mediation, rather than through cholinergic neural pathways. Glucocorticoid is a possible mediator hormone, since this hormone is known to induce tyrosine aminotransferase and cholinergic stimulation of the hypothalamus reportedly causes glucocorticoid secretion[5]. This possibility was tested by injecting acetylcholine into the LH of adrenalectomized rats. The results showed that the levels of hepatic tyrosine aminotransferase 4 hr after cholinergic stimulation of the LH in adrenalectomized rats (13.3 ± 1.9 munits/mg protein) were not significantly different from the levels in adrenalectomized controls (11.8 ± 0.7 munits/mg protein). Hence, the response of tyrosine aminotransferase to cholinergic stimulation is mainly mediated by adrenal corticosteroids.

Presumably the acetylcholine-sensitive neurons of the hypothalamus comprise the origin of the hypothalamico-vagal neural pathways, which participate in the regulation of hepatic glycogenesis, and also act as a regulator for the hypothalamico hypophysial-adrenal axis, which controls hepatic tyrosine aminotransferase. In contrast, it has recently been shown that norepinephrine-sensitive neurons of the hypothalamus are concerned with the regulation of hepatic glycogenolysis[9] and of pancreatic hormone secretion[3].

REFERENCES

1. Akapan, J.O., Gardner, R. and Wagle, S.R., Studies on the effects of insulin and acetylcholine on activation of glycogen synthase and glycogenesis in hepatocytes isolated from normal fed rats, *Biochem. Biophys. Res. Commun.*, 61 (1974) 222–229.
2. Black, I.B. and Reis, D.J., Cholinergic regulation of hepatic tyrosine transaminase activity, *J. Physiol.*, 213 (1971) 421–433.
3. De Jong, A., Strubbe, J.H. and Steffens, A.B., Hypothalamic influence on insulin and glucagon release in the rat, *Amer. J. Physiol.*, 233 (1977) E380–E388.
4. Granner, D.K. and Tomkins, G.M., Tyrosine aminotransferase (rat liver). In H. Tabor and C.W. Tabor (Eds.) *Methods in Enzymology, Vol. XVIIA,* Academic Press, New York, 1970, pp. 633–637.
5. Krieger, H.P. and Krieger, D.T., Chemical stimulation of the brain: effect on adrenal corticoid release, *Amer. J. Physiol.*, 218 (1970) 1632–1641.
6. Ottolenghi, C., Caniato, A. and Barnabei, O., Effect of acetylcholine on glycogen formation and the activity of glycogen synthetase in isolated perfused rat liver, *Nature (Lond.),* 229 (1971) 420–422.
7. Shimazu, T., Role of the hypothalamus in the induction of tryptophan pyrrolase activity in rabbit liver, *J. Biochem.*, 55 (1964) 163–171.
8. Shimazu, T., Regulation of glycogen metabolism in liver by the autonomic nervous system: V. Activation of glycogen synthetase by vagal stimulation, *Biochim. Biophys. Acta*, 252 (1971) 28–38.

9. Shimazu, T., Reciprocal functions of the ventromedial and lateral hypothalamic nuclei in regulating carbohydrate metabolism in liver, and their relevance to food intake control. In Y. Katsuki, M. Sato, S. Takagi and Y. Oomura (Eds.) *Food Intake and Chemical Senses*, University of Tokyo Press, Tokyo, 1977, pp. 575–585.
10. Shimazu, T., Fukuda, A. and Ban, T., Reciprocal influences of the ventromedial and lateral hypothalamic nuclei on blood glucose level and liver glycogen content, *Nature (Lond.)*, 210 (1966) 1178–1179.
11. Shimazu, T., Matsushita, H. and Ishikawa, K., Cholinergic stimulation of the rat hypothalamus: Effects on liver glycogen synthesis, *Science*, 194 (1976) 535–536.
12. Shimazu, T., Matsushita, H. and Ishikawa, K., Hypothalamic control of liver glycogen metabolism in adult and aged rats, *Brain Research*, 144 (1978) 343–352.
13. Shimazu, T. and Ogasawara, S., Effects of hypothalamic stimulation on gluconeogenesis and glycolysis in rat liver, *Amer. J. Physiol.*, 228 (1975) 1787–1793.

PART VI

NEUROENDOCRINE CONTROL MECHANISMS

KINJI YAGI

Department of Physiology, Jichi Medical School,
Kawachi-gun, Tochigi 329–04, Japan

For more than a hundred years various physiological and pathological observations which appeared to reflect normal and abnormal neuroendocrine control mechanisms have been described, and since early this century, when the concept of the hormone as a chemical messenger was first introduced by British physiologists, many endocrinologists have studied the endocrine control mechanisms experimentally. These approaches involved specific stimulations and lesions of a particular endocrine system or, in other words, determinations of input-output relationships in the endocrine system. Many endocrinologists came to support the existence of integrative control mechanisms involving both the central nervous system and the endocrine glands, but in my view the concept of neuroendocrine control was not placed on a firm footing until 1955, when the famous book *Neural Control of the Pituitary Gland* by Professor G. W. Harris[1] was published.

The presently available information suggests that each of the neuroendocrine control systems is comprised of one or two of the three elementary mechanisms, the open loop neuroendocrine reflex, the modulating (parametric) control of endocrine reflex and the feedback control mechanism, as illustrated diagramatically in Fig. 1. As an example of the neuroendocrine reflexes, it is well known that environmental stresses stimulate adrenocorticotrophin secretion by the anterior pituitary gland and, in turn, glucocorticoid secretion. As another example, one can point out that both distension of the uterine cervix and touch stimuli of the nipple trigger oxytocin secretion by posterior pituitary gland. Modulating control of endocrine reflexes has been demonstrated in autonomic nervous control of insulin secretion by B cells of the endocrine pancreas and of renin secretion by the juxtaglomerular cells of the kidney. Either a negative or positive feedback mechanism, or both mechanisms in some cases are associated with a particular neuroendocrine reflex. For example, information on plasma osmolarity is passed back in a negative feedback fashion to the hypothalamo-neurohypophysial system controlling vasopressin secretion to keep the body fluid osmolarity constant. As another example, in female rats the plasma estrogen level influences gonadotrophin secretion by negative feedback control of the medial basal hypothalamus on the one hand and on the other hand by positive feedback control of the medial preoptic area in triggering the preovulatory surge of gonadotrophin.

Recently most neuroendocrine control systems have been shown to produce a periodic or episodic secretion of hormone. The period varies widely from a few hours to 28 days in the case of the ovulatory surge of luteinizing hormone in the woman. In my opinion the biological clock system which appears to exist in the brain and generates the circadian rhythm of endocrine activity seems to play an important role in producing such periodic secretions of hormone, in addition to the brain functions receiving inputs of physicochemical parameters from the external and internal environment and producing neuroendocrine outputs. However, the mechanisms of these integrative neural functions of the central nervous system are largely unknown at present. The integrative functions have been thought to involve the hypothalamus and related diencephalic

A   Neuroendocrine reflexes

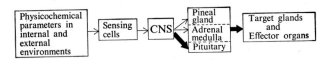

B   Modulating control of endocrine reflex

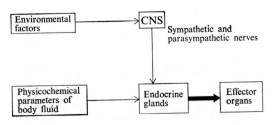

C   Feedback mechanism

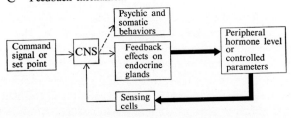

Fig. 1.   Neuroendocrine control mechanisms. Either a negative or a positive feedback mechanism is involved in most neuroendocrine reflexes, and in each of them the whole system functions as a closed loop control system under physiological conditions. CNS: the central nervous system. Thin arrows indicate the flow of neural impulses and thick arrows represent the flow of hormonal signals. A dashed line indicates functions other than feedback control.

structures as a central information processing unit of the neural machine in association with the pineal gland, the limbic brain and the lower brain stem.

This section presents a review and progress reports of a study group involving 13 outstanding Japanese neuroendocrinologists. The aim of this study group is to delineate from the following three standpoints the neuroendocrine control mechanisms of the brain which produce periodic activities of the hypothalamo-hypophysial system and the pineal system. First, to identify morphologically and functionally the neural circuit which is specific to each of the neuroendocrine functions. Second, to describe the chain of events in terms of molecular biology or biophysics from hormone binding to the feedback receptor to hormone secretion by the pituitary and the pineal glands, including hormone metabolism. Third, to elucidate the modulating control mechanism, especially the modulating control of hypothalamic neuroendocrine reflexes by the limbic brain, including the hippocampal formation and the amygdala. Experimental techniques which are suitable for analyzing and elucidating the functional "black boxes" of the brain have been developed rapidly during the past 20 years. Among others one can cite the techniques for analyzing specific neural circuitry by the use of axonal transport of horseradish peroxidase or radioisotope-labelled substances, immunohistochemistry and electrophysiological methods; neurochemical and neuropharmacological techniques applicable to very restricted parts of the brain; radioimmunoassay techniques which can now detect and quantitatively determine almost all kinds of hormones within the body fluid; the technique of recording the electrical activity of single neurons for long periods of time even in a conscious and freely moving mammal.

The results of experiments being conducted under the present research strategy, I believe, will identify the specific neural circuits for each particular neuroendocrine control mechanism and explain its functions at the molecular level, and as a consequence will elucidate the neural mechanism producing periodicity in the neuroendocrine control system of higher mammals, including man.

REFERENCES

1. Harris, G.W., *Neural Control of the Pituitary Gland*, Arnold London, 1955.

Membrane electrical properties of anterior pituitary cells and their relation to hormone secretion

SEIJI OZAWA

Department of Physiology, Jichi Medical School,
Kawachi-gun, Tochigi, 329–04, Japan

Secretion of anterior pituitary hormones is regulated by neurohormones produced in the hypothalamus and transported to their adenohypophysial targets by the hypophysial portal system. Among these hypophysiotropic hormones, TRH (thyrotropin releasing hormone)[3,7], LH–RH (luteinizing hormone releasing hormone)[6,26] and somatostatin[5] have been chemically identified. However, the exact mechanism by which the neurohormones facilitate or inhibit secretion of adenohypophysial hormones remains to be elucidated. Cyclic AMP has frequently been claimed to mediate the action of the hypophysiotropic hormones as an intracellular messenger. However, several experimental results are clearly incompatible with this hypothesis. Eto and Fleischer[12] have shown that TRH has no detectable effect on the adenylate cyclase level of TSH-producing mouse pituitary tumor cells, although the neurohormone enhances TSH release from these cells. They have further shown that prostaglandin E_1 stimulates adenylate cyclase activity and elevates cyclic AMP levels without enhancing TSH release. Hinkle and Tashjian[18] failed to observe any significant effect of TRH on the activities of both adenylate cyclase and cyclic nucleotide phosphodiesterase in rat tumor cells which increased prolactin secretion by the application of TRH. These results suggest that the effect of hypophysiotropic hormones must be mediated by mechanisms other than the cyclic AMP system.

Recently, there has been accumulating evidence that several kinds of endocrine cells are electrically excitable[1,2,4,8–10,20,27,30–32,36]. Pancreatic islet B cells and adrenal chromaffin cells have been shown to produce electrical activities which are dependent on Ca ions in the extracellular fluid[4,10]. Since hormone secretion is believed to be triggered by Ca-entry from the extracellular to the intracellular space in most endocrine cells[11], these Ca-dependent electrical activities may be involved in stimulus-secretion coupling. Concerning anterior pituitary cells, Kidokoro[20] has demonstrated that the clonal cell line GH_3 of rat anterior pituitary tumor cells which secretes growth hormone and prolactin, generates Ca-dependent action potentials and that the frequency of Ca spike increases when the external saline contains 30 nM thyrotropin releasing hormone (TRH) which is known to increase prolactin secretion in these cells. Biales et al.[2] have shown that the action potential of GH_3 cells is dependent on extracellular Na^+ as well as Ca^{2+}. Our previous experiments have also indicated that both GH_3 cells and pituitary cells of normal rats generate Na– and Ca–dependent action potentials[30,31].

This article summarizes our data on the membrane electrical properties of anterior pituitary cells, both clonal cell line GH_3 of rat anterior pituitary tumor and normal rat pituitary cells. The possibility that these electrical activities may play a significant role in the control of hormone secretion by anterior pituitary cells is discussed.

Membrane electrical properties of clonal cell line GH₃

Clonal cell line GH₃ was established by Tashijian *et al.*[35], and shown to secrete both prolactin and growth hormone continuously[19]. The present author commercially obtained GH₃ cells prepared and characterized by the American Type Culture Collection (Rockville, Maryland) through Dainihon Seiyaku (Osaka, Japan). The cells were grown as monolayers in plastic dishes (35 × 10 mm) (Falcon) containing 2.5 ml of Ham's F–10 medium supplemented with 15% horse serum and 2.5% fetal bovine serum in a humidified atmosphere of 95% air and 5% CO_2. Experiments were conducted at room temperature (23–25° C). The normal saline used had the following composition (mM): NaCl 150, KCl 5, $CaCl_2$ 2.4, $MgCl_2$ 1.3, glucose 10, and either Tris–HCl or Hepes–NaOH buffer 5 at pH 7.4. Glass micropipettes for recording the intracellular membrane potentials were filled with 4 M K-acetate and the resistance ranged from 70 to 100 MΩ.

Action potentials: The resting membrane potential of the GH₃ cells was between −40 and −60 mV in normal saline. Immediately after penetration, the resting potential was usually less negative than this value, but reached a more negative stable level within 10–20 seconds. Action potentials could be generated in an all–or–none fashion by current pulses injected through the recording electrode. The critical membrane potential for initiation of the action potentials ranged from −40 to −50 mV in most cases. When the resting potential was less ngeative than −50 mV, the action potential was evoked at termination of the hyperpolarizing current pulses (Fig. 1A). It was evoked by a depolarizing current pulse when the resting potential was more negative than −50 mV (Fig. 1B). The maximum rate of rise in the action potential under good

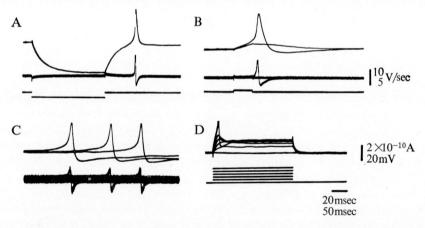

Fig. 1.   Intracellular recordings of action potentials of GH₃ cells in normal saline. A, An action potential evoked at termination of a hyperpolarizing current pulse. The resting potential was –47 mV. B, An all-or-none action potential elicited by a short depolarizing current pulse. C, Action potentials which occurred spontaneously in normal saline. Three traces are superimposed. D, Example of graded responses to depolarizing current pulses of increasing intensity. The resting potential was –55 mV. Five traces were superimposed by using a storage oscilloscope. The middle traces in A and B, and the lower trace in C represent the first order derivatives of the potential changes. The calibration of 10 V/sec is applicable to A and B, and of 5 V/sec to C. The time calibration of 20 msec applies only to record B.

conditions was 15 V/sec. Action potentials occurred spontaneously in a small number of cells (Fig. 1C).

Several cells failed to generate action potentials in an all–or–none fashion, as shown in Fig. 1D and the inset of Fig. 2. Both the amplitude and rate of rise of the spike response in these cells gradually increased with increasing intensity of depolarizing current pulses. The action potentials of all–or–none type became abortive probably due to reduction in the inward ionic current through the membrane by rapidly developing outward-going rectification as demonstrated in the next section.

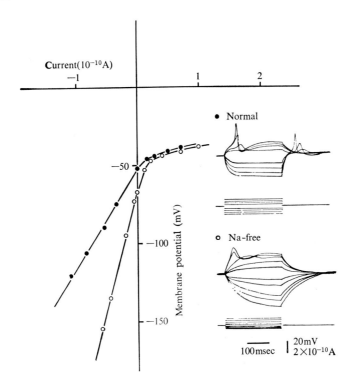

Fig. 2. Steady-state current voltage relations of GH₃ cells in normal saline (filled circles) and Na-free solution (open circles). Na-free solution was prepared by replacement of Na^+ with choline. The membrane potential changes measured at the end of 250 msec current pulses were plotted. Insets: sample records showing the time course of potential changes. The potential difference across the recording electrode was completely cancelled by using a bridge circuit.

Current-voltage relationship: A steady-state relation between the applied current and resultant voltage deviation was obtained at the end of a 250 msec current pulse in normal saline and Na–free solution (Fig. 2). The relation was linear when the membrane potential was more negative than −60 mV. The mean input resistance estimated from the linear portion in normal saline was 457 ± 35.9 MΩ (mean $\pm$ S.E., $n = 17$). A remarkable outward-going rectification was always observed in the membrane potential range more positive than −50 mV. In Na–free solution the resting membrane potential was more negative, and the input resistance averaged 992 ± 77.6 MΩ (mean $\pm$ S.E., $n = 13$). This result indicates that the GH₃ cell membrane has significant permeability to Na ions in the resting state. Outward-going rectification was also found in Na–free solution.

Na and Ca components of action potentials: Action potential of all–or–none type could not be evoked in Na–free solution, but graded responses were induced instead by depolarizing current pulses of increasing intensity (Fig. 3A). The presence of this graded response suggests that a potential-dependent increase in the membrane permeability to Ca^{2+} could have occurred in the GH₃ cells. This possibility was tested by the following experiments. When the Ca^{2+} concentration was increased 10–fold to 24 mM, an all–or–none action potential could be evoked in Na–free solution (Fig. 3B). In excitable cells which generate Ca spikes, Sr^{2+} and Ba^{2+} are known to be replaceable by Ca^{2+} as the inward current carrier[14]. Replacement of 24 mM Ca^{2+} with iso-molar Sr^{2+} was therefore carried out, and in this medium a depolarizing current pulse elicited an all–or–none action potential (Figs. 3C,D). In Na–free solution containing 24 mM Ba^{2+}, the GH₃ cells showed a resting potential less negative than -35 mV, and a prolonged regenerative response was generated at termination of the hyperpolarizing current pulse. A sample record is given in Fig. 3E. This cell had a resting potential of -5 mV and showed an inflection which indicated the onset of a Ba-dependent action potential after cessation of the current pulse. An all–or–none long-lasting action potential was evoked when the membrane potential was maintained at a more

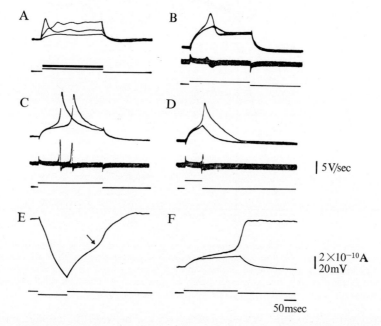

Fig. 3.   Regenerative responses in Na-free solution. A, Depolarizing responses in Na-free solution containing 2.4 mM Ca^{2+}. The amplitude of graded responses increased with increasing current pulses. B, An all–or–none action potential in Na-free, 24 mM Ca^{2+} solution. C, D, Action potentials in Na-free, 24 mM Sr^{2+} solution. The duration of the falling phase tended to be prolonged in Sr^{2+} solution. E, F, Prolonged action potentials in Na-free, 24 mM Ba^{2+} solution. The resting potential was -5 mV in E and a prolonged anode break excitation occurred at termination of the hyperpolarizing current pulse. The arrow indicates the inflection which reflects the critical membrane potential for initiation of the action potential. After the membrane potential was maintained at -65 mV by a DC hyper-polarizing current, a depolarizing pulse elicited an all–or–none prolonged action potential in F. The middle traces in B, C, and D represent the first order derivatives of the potential changes.

negative level than -60 mV by a DC hyperpolarizing current (Fig. 3F). The prolonged action potential is probably due to a suppressive effect by Ba ions on the development of delayed rectification, as has been demonstrated in other excitable tissues[16].

These results indicate that one of the inward current carriers producing action potential in GH_3 cells is Ca^{2+} in normal saline. Further, the fact that the rate of rise in the action potential decreased remarkably in Na–free solution suggests that the contribution of Na ions is also important in the generation of action potential in GH_3 cells. This notion is supported by the present observation that a significant spike response could be evoked in Ca-free solution containing a high concentration of Mg^{2+} (13 mM). It appears reasonable to conclude therefore that the GH_3 cell is capable of generating action potentials which are dependent on both Ca^{2+} and Na^+ as inward current carriers.

Prolactin secretion by GH_3 cells

Incubation of the anterior pituitary gland in a high concentration of potassium ions enhances the secretion of adrenocorticotropic hormone (ACTH)[22], luteinizing hormone[39], thyrotropin (TSH)[38], prolactin and growth hormone[25,33]. An attempt was therefore made to determine the effect of a high K^+ concentration in the medium on prolactin release from GH_3 cells under the same experimental conditions as for the electrophysiological study. The rate of prolactin relase increased from 13.0 ± 1.0 (mean $\pm$ S.E., $n = 4$) to 32.6 ± 2.8 ng/hr/mg cell protein (mean $\pm$ S.E., $n = 6$) when the K^+ concentration in the medium was raised 10–fold to 50 mM (Fig. 4). The increase in prolactin secretion by high K^+ was completely abolished in Ca–free solution. Gautvik and Tashjian have obtained similar results, although they reduced the extracellular Ca^{2+} in Ham's F–10 medium by adding 1 mM Na–EGTA[15]. The effect of high K^+ can be explained as follows. The membrane permeability of GH_3 cells to Ca ions increases when the membrene potential is depolarized. Hence, the membrane depolarization caused by high K^+ augments Ca^{2+} influx. The resultant increase in the intracellular Ca^{2+} concentration may, in turn, activate the exocytotic process. The potential-dependent increase in membrane permeability to Ca^{2+} in GH_3 cells was demonstrated by the electrophysiological method described in the previous section.

Effects of thyrotropin releasing hormone (TRH) and 4-aminopyridine (4-AP) on electrical activities in GH_3 cells

Effect of TRH: Thyrotropin releasing hormone (TRH) has been shown to cause an increase in prolactin secretion by GH_3 cells in a dose-dependent manner within the range up to 30 nM.[19] Kidokoro[20] has recorded the action potentials of GH_3 cells extracellularly using a suction electrode. He demonstrated that the frequency of spontaneous firing in GH_3 cells increased to 1.75 times that of the control after the addition of TRH at a concentration 30 nM, and suggested that this increase in spike frequency could cause an increase in prolactin secretion following the application of TRH. We have undertaken further studies on the effects of TRH on the membrane electrical properties of GH_3 cells by recording intracellular potentials.

TRH caused an increase in the number of cells which showed spontaneously occurring action potentials. Spontaneous discharges were found in 13 of 26 cells impaled in the medium containing TRH (100–200 nM) (Fig. 5A), but in only two of 22 cells in the control solution. The frequency of the spontaneous firings ranged from 0.5 to 2 Hz. This result indicates that TRH induces spontaneous firing in silent GH_3 cells. However, Kidokoro[20] has observed spontaneous firings in almost all cells tested in normal saline by the microsuction technique. At present, no

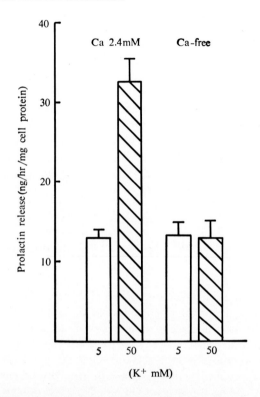

Fig. 4.   Effects of a high concentration of potassium (50 mM) on the release of prolactin from **GH₃** cells. The blank columns represent the mean values $\pm$ S.E. of prolactin secreted into the media containing 5 mM K⁺ in 1 hr, and the shaded columns those into the media containing 50 mM K⁺. The two columns on the left give results for solutions containing 2.4 mM Ca^{2+}, and the columns on the right those for Ca-free solutions. The sample numbers for each case were 4, 6, 3, and 3, respectively (from left to right). The experimental procedures were as follows: 2.5 ml aliquots of cell suspension at a concentration of 3.3×10^4 cells/ml were placed in 35×10 mm Falcon dishes. The experiment was carried out 10–14 days after plating, since it has been shown that the intracellular hormone content is larger at this subculture age than in the earlier phase[17]. In the experiment, the media were removed and the cells were washed three times with normal saline. New test solutions were added and the cells were incubated for 1 hr at room temperature. Ca-free solution was prepared by replacement of $CaCl_2$ with isotonic $MgCl_2$, without adding EGTA. The high potassium solution was prepared by substitution of K⁺ for Na⁺. The amount of prolactin released into the test solution in 1 hr was determined by radioimmunoassay. The data are expressed as ng rat prolactin (NIAMDD-rat prolactin RP-1)/hr/mg cell protein. The cell protein was measured by the method of Lowry et al.[24].

reasonable explanation can be suggested for this discrepancy. The present observations, however, agree with the data of Kidokoro in that TRH tended to increase the occurrence of spontaneous firings in GH₃ cells.

As illustrated in three successive traces in Fig. 5A, spontaneously occurring action potentials recorded in the TRH medium had a prolonged duration and occasionally showed two peaks (*cf.* the record in normal solution in Fig. 1C). An action potential with prolonged duration was also evoked by the application of current pulses in 7 of the 13 cells which showed spontaneous discharges in TRH solution (Fig. 5B, C). One possible explanation for the prolonged action potential

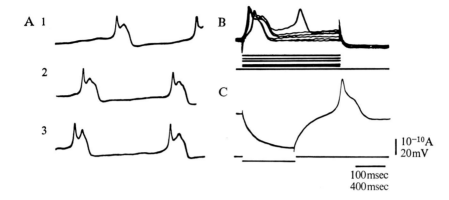

Fig. 5. Prolonged action potentials observed in the saline containing 200 nM TRH. A, Three successive traces of action potentials which occurred spontaneously. The time calibration of 400 msec applies only to these records. B, C, Prolonged action potentials evoked by depolarizing and hyperpolarizing current pulses, respectively (Ozawa, Miyazaki and Sand[31]). (Source ref. (31): By kind permission of John Wiley & Sons, Inc.)

is that the delayed rectification may be partially blocked by TRH. This notion is supported by the observation that the outward-going rectification was less prominent in the I-V curves in these cells than those in the control solution[31].

Increase in the frequency of spontaneous firings and prolonged duration of each action potential may lead to an increase in Ca influx into the cell, since the action potential has a Ca component as demonstrated above. This would in turn lead to an enhancement of prolactin secretion.

Fig. 6A shows a high gain amplitude oscilloscope display of the spontaneous action potentials of a GH_3 cell in TRH solution. Small potential fluctuations are seen to occur randomly, and action potentials appear to be initiated from the peak of these potentials. The amplitude of the potential fluctuations decreased as the membrane was hyperpolarized increasingly by a DC inward current. In Fig. 6A, the mean resting potential level was -51 mV without current injection. The potential fluctuations were becoming smaller when the membrane was hyperpolarized to -59 mV (B), -64 mV (C), and -69 mV (D). In general, these potentials were almost completely abolished at a membrane potential level of around -70 mV. When the membrane was further hyperpolarized beyond -70 mV in a few cells, the amplitude of the potential fluctuations again increased. Potential fluctuations of moderate amplitude were also found in Na–free solution. These results suggest that the fluctuations of the membrane potential are due to spontaneously occurring changes in K^+ permeability of the cell membrane. Assuming that the action potential is initiated when these small potential fluctuations exceed the critical membrane potential level in GH_3 cells, the spike initiation would have to be hindered by the outward–going rectification which was shown in the previous section to develop prominently around the membrane potential level of -50 mV. This level coincides with the critical membrane potential for spike initiation in these cells. The possibility must arise therefore that TRH may reduce the outward–going rectification and so facilitate an initiation of all–or–none action potential from these small potential fluctuations. In order to test this possibility, the effect of 4-aminopyridine (4–AP) was studied.

Effect of 4–AP: It has been demonstrated that 4–AP selectively blocks the potassium channels in giant axons of the cockroach[34] and the squid[40], when applied either from the internal or

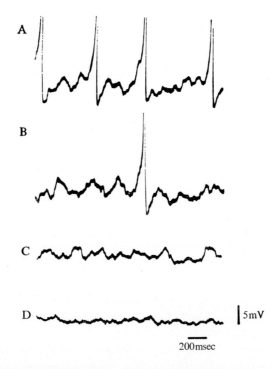

Fig. 6.   Spontaneous potential fluctuations of a GH₃ cell in the saline containing 200 nM TRH. The resting potential was –51 mV (A), from which it was shifted to –59 mV (B), –64 mV (C) and –69 mV (D) by increasing DC hyperpolarizing current (Ozawa, Miyazaki and Sand[31]). (Source ref. 31 : By kind permission of John Wiley & Sons, Inc.)

external surfaces of the membrane. The duration of the action potential is prolonged by 4–AP, but this effect is not so marked as that produced by intracellular application of tetraethylammonium, since the blocking effect of 4–AP on the K⁺ channels is relieved as the membrane depolarizes[40]. In the medium containing 4–AP at a concentration of 1–2 mM, 18 of 22 GH₃ cells tested showed spontaneously occurring action potentials (Fig. 7C). The spike frequency ranged between 0.5 and 5 Hz. When the action potential was evoked by current pulses injected via the recording electrode, the falling phase was prolonged and a hump was seen during the falling phase (Fig. 7B). The second action potential was occasionally initiated from this hump. Although the lowest effective concentration of 4–AP was not determined, these effects were clearly seen at a concentration of as low as 0.2 mM. Iontophoretically applied 4–AP was also found to be effective, as shown in Fig. 7A. 4–AP delivered by an outward current of 50–200 nA intensity from a micropipette containing 100 mM 4–AP abolished the after-hyperpolarization of the action potential and induced a hump at the termination of the falling phase as shown in Fig. 7A1 and 2. The first derivative of the potential change recorded in the middle traces clearly indicates that 4–AP lowered the maximum rate of fall. On the other hand, 4–AP occasionally increased the maximum rate of rise. This latter effect can be explained by assuming that 4–AP suppressed the increase in K⁺ conductance which might otherwise have occurred during the rising phase of the action

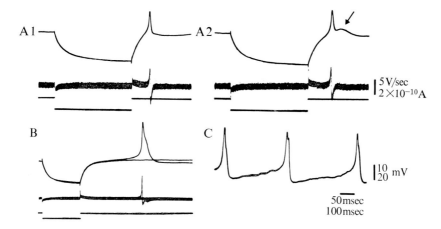

Fig. 7. Effects of 4-aminopyridine (4-AP) on the electrical activities of GH₃ cells. A, Effect of iontophoretically applied 4-AP. A double-barrelled glass micropipette was used for this experiment. One
barrel was filled with normal saline to which 4-AP and HCl were added so as to give a final 4-AP concentration of 100 mM and pH 7.4. The other barrel was used for the control and filled with normal
saline. The double-barrelled micropipette was located about 10 μm over the cell from which the intracellular potential was recorded. A1, An action potential evoked at termination of the hyperpolarizing current (control). A2, Change induced by iontophoretically applied 4-AP by an outward current
of 200 nA in intensity. The resting potential of this cell was –43 mV and did not change with the iontophoretic application of 4-AP. The middle traces of A1, A2 and B represent the first order derivatives
of the potential changes. B, An all-or-none action potential evoked by a current pulse in the solution
containing 1.5 mM 4-AP. C, Action potentials which occurred spontaneously in 1.5 mM 4-AP solution.
The spike was initiated from the membrane potential level of –42 mV. The time scale of 100 msec is
applicable to records B and C, and the voltage calibration of 10 mV only to record C.

potential. The effects of 4–AP on pituitary hormone secretion have not yet been investigated.
There have been several reports that application of 4–AP at a low concentration (4 μM–2 mM)
augments release of the neurotransmitters[21,23,29].

Action potentials of normal anterior pituitary cells

Since the GH₃ cells are tumor cells in culture, it could be argued that the electrical properties
of the GH₃ cells described above may have derived from unphysiological factors. In order to test
this possibility, electrophysiological experiments were carried out using the anterior pituitary
gland of normal rats[30,31]. Slices of 300–500 μm thickness prepared from the anterior pituitary
gland of female rats were superfused with oxygen-saturated saline, the temperature of which was
maintained at 37 ± 1°C.

The resting potential of the anterior pituitary cells ranged from −20 to −60 mV. Relatively
low values of resting potential were apparently due to cell injury caused by electrode penetration.
Sixteen of 51 cells tested generated action potentials at termination of the hyperpolarizing current pulse injected through the recording electrode (Fig. 8A). Repetitive firing was also observed
in several cells (Fig. 8B). In three other cells the resting potential was more negative than −55
mV, and action potentials were elicited by depolarizing current pulses in an all–or–none fashion
(Figs. 8C,D). The maximum rate of rise in the action potential ranged from 11 to 45 V/sec. In the

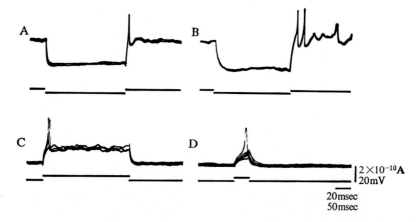

Fig. 8.   Intracellular recordings of action potentials of normal anterior pituitary cells. A, B, Action potentials elicited at the termination of hyperpolarizing current pulses. C, D, Action potentials evoked by depolarizing current pulses. The time scale of 20 msec is applicable to record D (Ozawa, Miyazaki and Sand[31]). (Source ref. 31 : By kind permission of John Wiley & Sons, Inc.)

remaining 32 cells, smaller and more slowly rising graded regenerative responses were evoked by current injection.

A steady-state relation between injected current and induced voltage deviation was obtained at the end of a current pulse of 200–300 msec duration in the cells which showed action potentials. The relationship was linear in the range of membrane potential more negative than -60 mV. The slope resistance decreased when the membrane potential shifted to the range less negative than -40 mV. This feature of the I-V relation resembles that of GH_3 cells. The mean input resistance estimated from the linear portion of the I-V relation was 274 ± 48.6 MΩ (mean $\pm$ S.E., $n = 19$).

The main component of the inward action current in normal pituitary cells is carried by Na^+, since all–or–none action potentials were never observed several minutes after the medium superfusing the slice had been switched to Na–free solution. Significant graded depolarizing responses, however, almost always occurred at termination of the hyperpolarizing current pulse or during the depolarizing pulse. This suggests that a potential-dependent increase in membrane permeability to Ca^{2+} may also occur in normal pituitary cells. The increase in membrane permeability to Ca ions could not result in an all–or–none potential change, probably because it would be too small to overcome the increase in K^+ permeability induced by the membrane depolarization. In order to examine the possible involvement of Ca^{2+} in the generation of the spike response evoked in Na–free medium, the Ca^{2+} concentration of the medium was increased 10–fold to 24 mM. In this high Ca^{2+}, Na–free solution, it was found that there was an increase in regenerative responses (Fig. 9A) and that all–or–none action potentials could be elicited by a depolarizing current pulse when the membrane potential was held to a level more negative than -70 mV by a DC hyperpolarizing current (Fig. 9B). Both Sr^{2+} and Ba^{2+} could replace Ca^{2+} as inward current carriers in normal pituitary cells (Fig. 9C, D). In Na–free solution containing Ba^{2+}, the resting potential of the cells was less negative than in the normal solution, and several cells even displayed positive values. In this solution prolonged action potentials were observed. Fig. 9E shows action potentials which occurred spontaneously in Na–free solution containing 24 mM Sr^{2+}. Small

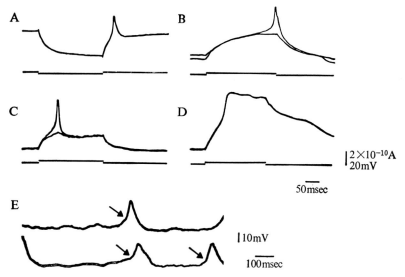

Fig. 9.   Action potentials of normal anterior pituitary cells in Na-free saline containing a high concentration of Ca^{2+}, Sr^{2+}, or Ba^{2+}. A, An anode break response in Na-free, 24 mM Ca^{2+} solution. The resting potential was –44 mV. B, An all-or-none action potential evoked by a depolarizing current pulse after the membrane potential had been shifted to become more negative than –70 mV by a DC hyperpolarizing current. C, An action potential evoked by a depolarizing current pulse in Na-free, 24 mM Sr^{2+} solution. The membrane was preliminarily hyperpolarized to –75 mV by a DC hyperpolarizing current. D, A prolonged action potential in Na-free, 24 mM Ba^{2+} solution under similar conditions to B and C. E, Two successive traces of spontaneous action potentials in Na-free, 24 mM Sr^{2+} solution. The action potentials were initiated by small fluctuations of the membrane potential. Arrows indicate the transition between these fluctuating potentials and the action potentials. The resting potential was –35 mV (Ozawa, Miyazaki and Sand[31]). (Source ref. 31 : By kind permission of John Wiley & Sons, Inc.)

potential fluctuations of less than 5 mV in amplitude were seen, and action potentials were occasionally initiated from the peak of these potential fluctuations.

These results indicate that the membrane electrical properties of normal anterior pituitary cells are essentially similar to those of GH_3 cells. It is concluded therefore that the membrane properties of GH_3 cells reflect physiological events in such pituitary cells.

Discussion and conclusion

Investigations of electrical activities and their relation to hormone secretion have been carried out mainly in pancreatic islet B cells and adrenal chromaffin cells. Meissner and Schmelz[27] were able to induce membrane depolarizations with superimposed spike activities in pancreatic B cells of mice by increasing the glucose concentration of the superfusing solution to more than 5.5 mM. They plotted the relative duration of these burst discharges against glucose concentration and found a dose-response relationship similar to that between insulin release and glucose concentration. These electrical activities, like insulin release, were dependent on the presence of Ca ions in the medium. Pace *et al.*[32] have recently demonstrated that somatostatin (2.5 nM) hyperpolarizes the membrane of cultured rat islet cells (mainly B cells) and abolishes their electrical activities irrespective of the presence of glucose (16.6 mM) in the medium. They have also shown that the insulin release induced by glucose (16.6 mM) is completely inhibited by 2.5 nM somato-statin. These observations strongly suggest a direct relation between the electrical activity and insulin secretion by glucose.

In cultured adrenal chromaffin cells, it has been reported that action potentials can be evoked either by electric current pulses injected through the recording electrode or by iontophore-tic application of acetylcholine (ACh)[1,4]. Calcium ions have been shown to contribute significant-ly to the generation of action potential in chromaffin cells, although Na ions carry a major frac-tion of the action current. It has been suggested that this Ca-influx during action potentials may play an important role in controlling the release of catecholamine under normal physiological conditions, since the dose-response relation between increase in spike frequency and ACh con-centration in the medium agrees well with that between catecholamine secretion and ACh con-centration[4].

The present results clearly demonstrate that both neoplastic GH_3 cells and normal anterior pituitary cells are capable of generating action potentials which are partially dependent on Ca^{2+}. It seems most probable that this potential-dependent increase in membrane permeability to Ca^{2+} is related to an increase in hormone secretion. A high concentration of K^+ in the medium has been shown to stimulate hormone release in a variety of endocrine glands. In the present experi-ments, high K^+ increased prolactin release from GH_3 cells, and this effect of high K^+ was Ca-dependent. Although such a Ca-dependency exists in the hormone release evoked by high K^+ as well as the generation of action potentials in the pituitary cells, it is still questionable whether the effect of high K^+ actually reflects physiological processes. The most important problem to be solved at present is whether the action potential due partly to an increase in membrane permea-bility to Ca^{2+} is involved in the control of hormone secretion effected by physiological secreta-gogues. The electrophysiological evidence so far available appears to suggest an affirmative answer to this question for the pituitary cells, since an increase in frequency of spontaneous action potentials in GH_3 cells was induced by TRH, a physiological secretagogue for prolactin.

Several studies have demonstrated that the increase in pituitary hormone secretion induced by hypothalamic releasing factors is inhibited in Ca–free medium[12,37]. Milligan and Kraicer[28], however, have shown in experiments using $^{45}Ca^{2+}$ that the hormone release induced by high K^+ is associated with an influx of Ca^{2+}, whereas that induced by a crude extract of hypothalamic-stalk-median eminence is not. Eto et al.[13] further demonstrated that the release of TSH by TRH, and those of GH and ACTH by crude hypothalamic extract were not inhibited by verapamil which is known to block the potential-dependent Ca^{2+} influx. Furthermore, they failed to observe a signi-ficant increase in intracellular $^{45}Ca^{2+}$ accumulation in the anterior pituitary after application of these physiological secretagogues. The above observations appear to suggest that hypothalamic releasing factors do not exert their effects on pituitary cells by augmenting potential-dependent Ca^{2+} influx. In order to establish the physiological significance of the electrical activities of pituitary cells, further information is obviously needed, especially with regard to (1) the effects of physiological secretagogues on the membrane electrical properties of pituitary cells, and (2) the effects of agents which modify the electrical activities of these cells (for instance 4–AP) on hormone secretion. Experiments along these lines are currently in progress in our laboratory.

Acknowledgements: The author wishes to thank Drs. K. Yagi and S. Miyazaki for their critical reading of the manuscript. He is also indebted to the NIAMDD Rat Pituitary Hormone Program for supply of the Rat Prolactin RIA Kit.

REFERENCES

1. Biales, B., Dichter, M.A. and Tischler, A., Electrical excitability of cultured adrenal chromaffin cells, *J. Physiol. (Lond.)*, 262 (1976) 743–753.
2. Biales, B., Dichter, M.A. and Tischler, A., Sodium and calcium action potential in pituitary cells, *Nature (Lond.)*, 267 (1977) 172–174.
3. Boler, J., Enzman, F., Folkers, K., Bowers, C.Y. and Schally, A.V., The identity of chemical and hormonal properties of the thyrotropin releasing hormone and pyroglutamyl-histidyl-proline amide, *Biochem. biophys. Res. Commun.*, 37 (1969) 705–710.
4. Brandt, B.L., Hagiwara, S., Kidokoro, Y. and Miyazaki, S., Action potentials in the rat chromaffin cell and effects of acetylcholine, *J. Physiol. (Lond.)*, 263 (1976) 417–439.
5. Brazeau, P., Vale, W., Burgus, R., Ling, V., Butcher, M., Rivier, J. and Guillemin, R., Hypothalamic polypeptide that inhibits the secretion of immunoreactive pituitary growth hormone, *Science*, 179 (1973) 77–79.
6. Burgus, R., Butcher, M., Ling, N., Monahan, M., Rivier, J., Fellows, R., Amoss, M., Blackwell, R., Vale, W. et Guillemin, R., Structure moléculaire du facteur hypothalamique (LRF) d'origine ovine contrôlant la sécrétion de l'hormone gonadotrope hypophysaire de lutéinisation (LH), *C. r. Acad. Sci. (Paris)*, 273 (1971) 1611–1613.
7. Burgus, R., Dunn, T.F., Desiderio, D., Ward, D.N., Vale, W. and Gillemin, R., Characterization of ovine hypothalamic hypophysiotropic TSH-releasing factor, *Nature (Lond.)*, 226 (1970) 321–325.
8. Davis, M. and Hadley, M., Spontaneous electrical potentials and pituitary hormone (MSH) secretion, *Nature (Lond.)*, 261 (1976) 422–423.
9. Dean, P.M. and Matthews, E.K., Glucose-induced electrical activity in pancreatic islet cells, *J. Physiol. (Lond.)*, 210 (1970) 255–264.
10. Dean, P.M. and Matthews, E.K., Electrical activity in pancreatic islet cells: Effect of ions, *J. Physiol. (Lond.)*, 210 (1970) 265–275.
11. Douglas, W.W., Stimulus-secretion coupling: The concept and clues from chromaffin and other cells, *Brit. J. Pharmacol.*, 34 (1968) 451–474.
12. Eto, S. and Fleischer, N., Regulation of thyrotropin (TSH) release and production in monolayer cultures of transplantable TSH-producing mouse tumors, *Endocrinology*, 98 (1976) 114–122.
13. Eto, S., Wood, J.M., Hutchins, M. and Fleischer, N., Pituitary $^{45}Ca^{2+}$ uptake and release of ACTH, GH, and TSH: Effect of verapamil, *Amer. J. Physiol.*, 226 (1974) 1315–1320.
14. Fatt, P. and Ginsborg, B.L., The ionic requirements for the production of action potentials in crustacean muscle fibres, *J. Physiol. (Lond.)*, 142 (1958) 516–543.
15. Gautvik, K.M. and Tashjian, A.H.Jr., Effects of cations and colchicine on the release of prolactin and growth hormone by functional pituitary tumor cells in culture, *Endocrinology*, 93 (1973) 793–799.
16. Hagiwara, S. and Naka, K., The initiation of spike potential in barnacle muscle fibres under low intracellular Ca^{2+}, *J. gen. Physiol.*, 48 (1964) 141–162.
17. Haug, E., Tjernshaugen, H. and Gautvik, K.M., Variations in prolactin and growth hormone production during cellular growth in clonal strains of rat pituitary cells, *J. cell. Physiol.*, 91 (1977) 15–30.
18. Hinkle, P.M. and Tashjian, A.H.Jr., Adenylyl cylacse and cyclic nucleotide phosphodiesterases in GH-strains of rat pituitary cells, *Endocrinology*, 100 (1977) 934–944.
19. Hinkle, P.M. and Tashjian, A.H.Jr., Interaction of thyrotropin-releasing hormone with pituitary cells in culture. In K.W. McKerns (Ed.), *Hormone and Cancer*, Academic Press, New York, 1974, pp. 203–227.
20. Kidokoro, Y., Spontaneous calcium action potentials in a clonal pituitary cell line and their relationship to prolactin secretion, *Nature (Lond.)*, 258 (1975) 741–742.
21. Kirpekar, M., Kirpekar, S.M. and Part, J.C., Effect of 4-aminopyridine on release of noradrenaline from the perfused cat spleen by nerve stimulation, *J. Physiol. (Lond.)*, 272 (1977) 517–528.
22. Kraicer, J., Milligan, J.V., Gosbee, J.L. and Conrad, R.G., *In vitro* release of ACTH: Effects of potassium, calcium and corticosterone, *Endocrinology*, 85 (1969) 1144–1153.
23. Llinas, R., Walton, K. and Bohr, V., Synaptic transmission in squid giant synapse after potassium conductance blockade with external 3- and 4-aminopyridine, *Biophys. J.*, 16 (1976) 83–86.
24. Lowry, O.H., Rosenbrough, N.J., Farr, A.L. and Randall, R.J., Protein measurement with the Folin phenol reagent, *J. biol. Chem.*, 193 (1951) 265–275.
25. MacLeod, R.M. and Fontham, E.H., Influence of ionic environment on the *in vitro* synthesis and release of pituitary hormones, *Endocrinology*, 86 (1970) 863–869.
26. Matsuo, H., Baba, Y., Nair, R.M.G., Arimura, A. and Schally, A.V., Structure of the porcine LH- and FSH releasing hormone. I. The proposed amino acid sequence, *Biochem. biophys. Res. Commun.*, 43 (1971) 1334–1339.
27. Meissner, H.P. and Schmelz, H., Membrane potentials of beta-cells in pancreatic islets, *Pflügers Arch.*, 351 (1974) 195–206.

28. Milligan, J.V. and Kraicer, J., ^{45}Ca uptake during the *in vitro* release of hormones from the rat adenohypophysis, *Endocrinology*, 89 (1971) 766–773.
29. Molgo, J., Lemeignan, M. and Lechat, P., Effects of 4-aminopyridine at the frog neuromuscular junction, *J. Pharmacol. exp. Ther.*, 203 (1977) 653–663.
30. Ozawa, S. and Sand, O., Electrical activity of rat anterior pituitary cells *in vitro*, *Acta physiol. scand.*, 102 (1978) 330–341.
31. Ozawa, S., Miyazaki, S. and Sand, O., Electrical activity of anterior pituitary cells and its functional implication, In M. Otsuka and Z.W. Hall (Eds), *Neurobiology of Chemical Transmission*, John Wiley, New York, in press.
32. Pace, C.S., Murphy, M., Conant, S. and Lacy, P.E., Somatostatin inhibition of glucose-induced electrical activity in cultured rat islet cells, *Amer. J. Physiol.*, 233 (1977) C164–C171.
33. Parsons, J.A., Effects of cations on prolactin and growth hormone secretion by rat adenohypophyses *in vitro*, *J. Physiol. (Lond.)*, (1970) 973–987.
34. Pelhate, M. and Pichon, Y., Selective inhibition of potassium current in the giant axon of the cockroach, *J. Physiol. (Lond.)*, 242 (1974) 90p–91p.
35. Tashijian, A.H.Jr., Yasumura, Y., Levine, L., Sato, G.H. and Parker, M.L., Establishment of clonal strains of rat pituitary tumor cells that secrete growth hormone, *Endocrinology*, 82 (1968) 342–352.
36. Tischler, A., Dichter, M.A., Biales, B., Delellis, R. and Wolf, H., Neural properties of cultured human endocrine tumors of proposed neural crest origin, *Science*, 192 (1976) 902–904.
37. Vale, W., Burgus, R. and Guillemin, R., Presence of calcium ions as a requisite for the *in vitro* stimulation of TSH-release by hypothalamic TRF, *Experientia (Basel)*, 23 (1967) 853–855.
38. Vale, W., Burgus, R. and Guillemin, R., Potassium-induced stimulation of thyrotropin release *in vitro*. Requirement for presence of calcium and inhibition by thyroxine, *Experientia (Basel)*, 23 (1967) 855–857.
39. Wakabayashi, K., Kamberi, I.A. and McCann, S.M., *In vitro* response of the rat pituitary to gonadotropin-releasing factors and to ions, *Endocrinology*, 85 (1969) 1046–1056.
40. Yeh, J.Z., Oxford, G.S., Wu, C.H. and Narahashi, T., Dynamics of aminopyridine block of potassium channels in squid axon membrane, *J. gen. Physiol.*, 68 (1976) 519–535.

Ultrastructural changes of stellate cells in rabbit anterior pituitary gland under various endocrine conditions

TADAYASU BAN AND YAHE SHIOTANI

Department of Anatomy, Osaka University Medical School,
Kita-ku, Osaka 530, Japan

The presence of agranular cells in the anterior pituitary gland of rabbits has been reported by some authors[2-4]. These cells were called stellate cells and were thought to correspond to the follicular cells in rats[1], although their functional significance remained unknown.

In the present study, the ultrastructure of the stellate cells of rabbits was observed under normal and experimental conditions. All rabbits were perfused with 4% glutaraldehyde solution under Nembutal anesthesia. Their pituitary glands were cut into small pieces, post-fixed in 2% OsO_4 solution, dehydrated, and embedded in Epon 812. Ultrathin sections were stained with uranyl acetate and lead hydroxide, and observed with a Hitachi electron microscope HU-12.

Stellate cells in normal rabbits were found to have scanty cytoplasm around the nucleus and some slender processes extended between the secretory cells. The nucleus was irregular in shape and the chromatin evenly distributed. The nucleolus was usually unclear. In the perikaryon or processes, a number of microfilaments were found to run in various directions. Besides them, mitochondria, Golgi apparatus, rough- and smooth-surfaced endoplasmic reticulum were present in the cytoplasm, although their development was rather poor. Secretory granules were never observed. The processes of the stellate cells were linked to each other by desmosomes, forming a meshwork as a whole, but some processes ended freely around the pericapillary space.

In the anterior pituitary gland of the lactating rabbit, in which mammotrophs and gonadotrophs showed enhanced secretory activity, the stellate cells were also found to be hypertrophied. In the cytoplasm, their Golgi apparatus and rough-surfaced endoplasmic reticulum were strongly developed, and small vacuoles were increased. Lysosomes and lipid droplets were frequently encountered, and a very large secondary lysosome was sometimes observed (Fig. 1). Between adjacent stellate cell processes, intercellular canals were very well developed and a number of microvilli were noticed.

In the anterior pituitary gland of the adrenalectomized rabbit after 7 days, the stellate cells became larger, and development of the cell organella was prominent, suggesting stimulated functions. In the anterior pituitary gland of the thyroidectomized rabbit after 7 days, in addition to the appearance of thyroidectomy cells, hypertrophied stellate cells were observed which contained well-developed Golgi apparatus and lipid droplets. In the anterior pituitary gland of the orchidectomized rabbit after 98 days, in which castration cells were prominent, the stellate cells had well-developed Golgi apparatus in the processes as well as in the perikaryon. In the anterior pituitary gland of rabbits subjected to repeated injection of LH–RH, the stellate cells also contained well-developed Golgi apparatus and lipid droplets.

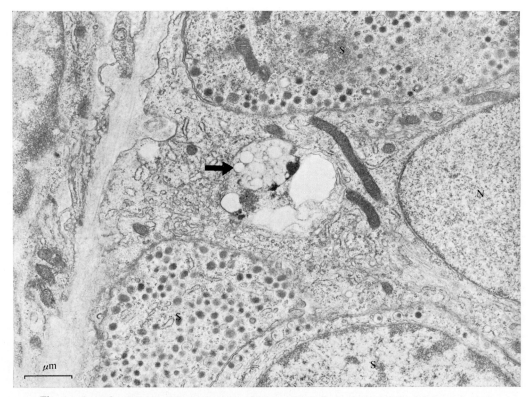

Fig. 1.   Part of a stellate cell in the anterior pituitary gland of a lactating rabbit. A large secondary lysosome (arrow) is present in the cytoplasm. N, Nucleus of the stellate cell; S, secretory cells.

Based on the above data, it becomes clear that stellate cells show morphological signs of stimulated function, whenever the secretory activity of the anterior pituitary gland is enhanced. It is therefore suggested that stellate cells may not only be supporting or sustentacular elements, but may play important roles such as in the supply of materials to secretory cells, or the disposal of waste products.

References

1. Rinehart, J.F. and Farquhar, M.C., The fine vascular organization of the anterior pituitary gland. An electron microscopic study with histochemical correlations, *Anat. Rec.*, 121 (1955) 207–240.
2. Salazar, H., The pars distalis of the female rabbit hypophysis: An electron microscopic study, *Anat. Rec.*, 147 (1963) 469–497.
3. Schechter, J., The ultrastructure of the stellate cell in the rabbit pars distalis, *Amer. J. Anat.*, 126 (1969) 477–488.
4. Young, B.A., Foster, C.L. and Cameron, E., Some observations on the ultrastructure of the adenohypophysis of the rabbit, *J. Endocrinol.*, 31 (1965) 279–287.

Effect of sex steroid hormones on rat anterior pituitary LH-RH receptor

MICHIYOSHI TAGA, HIROSHI MINAGUCHI, TOMONORI KIGAWA AND
SHOICHI SAKAMOTO

*Department of Obstetrics and Gynecology, School of Medicine, University of Tokyo,
Bunkyo-ku, Tokyo 113, Japan.*

Recent research has indicated that luteinizing hormone releasing hormone (LH-RH) acts initially by binding with receptor of the anterior pituitary plasma membrane[2]. We investigated the mechanism of action of LH-RH by analyzing rat anterior pituitary LH-RH receptor and changes in it caused by sex steroid hormones.

[3]H-LH-RH *binding assay*[1]: Homogenized rat anterior pituitaries were incubated with ^{3}H-LH-RH (specific activity 30 Ci/mmol) in the presence or absence of a 100-fold amount of cold LH-RH for 80 min at 0°C. The reaction was terminated by the addition of buffer and the binding part was separated with a Millipore filter (pore size 0.2 μm).

Responsiveness of rat anterior pituitary to LH-RH: Blood samples were collected from the jugular vein before and 20 min after i.v. injection of 0.4 μg LH-RH. The serum concentration of LH was measured with an NIAMDD radioimmunoassay kit.

The buffer solution for incubation required Mg^{2+} and K^+ for binding assay and the LH-RH binding saturated in 30 min at 0°C. A kinetic study showed that the dissociation constant of LH-RH receptor of castrated adult female rat and number of binding sites were 2.08×10^{-8} M and 27.6 fmol/mg protein, respectively (Fig. 1).

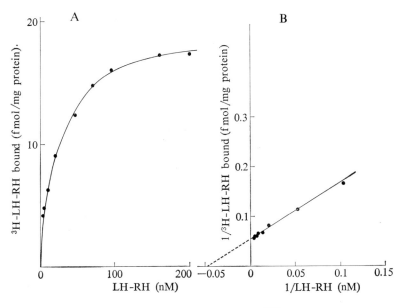

Fig. 1. Kinetic study of LH-RH receptor interaction. A, Binding of ^{3}H-LH-RH to anterior pituitary homogenate. B, Double-reciprocal (Lineweaver-Burk) plot of the same data. Dissociation constant, 2.08×10^{-8} M; no. of binding sites, 27.8 fmol/mg protein.

Concerning the effect of sex steroid hormones, daily subcutaneous injection of 20 μg 17β-estradiol or 20 μg estradiol with 2 mg progesterone to castrated adult female rats for 10 days, decreased the number of LH-RH receptor binding sites significantly ($p < 0.01$), but progesterone alone did not change the number significantly (Fig. 2). Daily injection of 20 μg estradiol for 2 and 4 days significantly increased the number of LH-RH receptor binding sites, but that for 6–10 days decreased them. On the other hand, the serum concentrations of LH after i.v. injection of LH-RH increased after daily administration of 20 μg estradiol. Thus, estradiol exhibited stimulatory effect on LH secretion at the level of the anterior pituitary.

We have clarified that rat anterior pituitary had a specific LH-RH receptor (dissociation constant 2.08×10^{-8} M) and that estradiol exerted an effect on both the level of rat anterior pituitary LH-RH receptor and the responsiveness of the anterior pituitary to LH-RH. The changes in LH-RH receptor levels coincided with the responsiveness of the anterior pituitary to LH-RH in rats injected daily with 20 μg estradiol for 2 and 4 days. These data indicate that estradiol regulates gonadotropin secretion by acting directly at the pituitary level and modulating the responsiveness of the anterior pituitary to LH-RH by changing the LH-RH receptor levels.

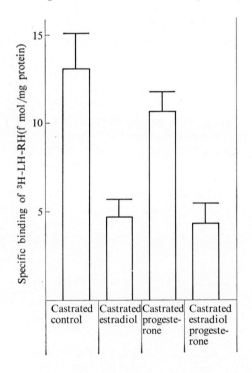

Fig. 2.   Effect of subcutaneous injections of 17β-estradiol, progesterone, or a combination of both for 10 days on anterior pituitary ³H-LH-RH binding in castrated adult female rats. Estradiol or estradiol with progesterone significantly decreased the number of LH-RH receptor binding sites but progesterone alone did not.

References

1. De Léan, A., Ferland, L., Drouin, J., Kelly, P.A. and Labrie, F., Modulation of pituitary releasing hormone receptor levels by estrogens and thyroid hormones, *Endocrinology*, 100 (1977) 1496–1504.
2. Spona, J., Hypothalamic hormone receptors. In A.L. Charro, R. Fornandez-Durango and J.G. Lopez del Campo (Eds.), *Basic Application and Clinical Uses of Hypothalamic Hormones*, Excerpta Medica, Amsterdam-Oxford, American Elsevier Pub. Co. Inc., New York, 1976, pp. 87–99.

Function of tanycytes in the hypothalamic median eminence

HIDESHI KOBAYASHI, MASUMI NOZAKI AND HARUKO UEMURA

*Misaki Marine Biological Station, Faculty of Science, University of Tokyo,
Miura, Kanagawa 238–02, Japan*

The tanycytes of the median eminence in mammals and birds have been suggested to absorb some hormones in the cerebrospinal fluid, transport them to the hypophysial portal vessels, and so contribute to the regulation of the adenohypophysial function[1,3]. Recently, however, we demonstrated that electrical destruction of the tanycytes of the median eminence did not lead to any significant disturbance of the estrous cycle of the rat or the photostimulated testicular growth of the Japanese quail[5]. This paper presents data which indicate that the tanycytes of the median eminence may not be involved in the regulation of the adenohypophysial function.

Absorption of peroxidase by tanycytes of the median eminence fixed in glutaraldehyde: Eight rats were killed by decapitation and a small piece of hypothalamic tissue including the median eminence was removed within 2 min of decapitation and immersed in Ringer's solution maintained at 37°C. The tissue was sliced transversely with a razor blade into several pieces (thickness 1–2 mm) in Ringer's solution within 10 min. They were then fixed in 5% glutaraldehyde solution for 30 min at 4°C. After washing in cold 0.1 M Tris buffer (pH 7.6), the slices were incubated in peroxidase solution (10 mg/1 ml saline) for 10 min at room temperature, and then post-fixed in 5% glutaraldehyde solution for 5 hr at 4°C. They were next washed in 0.1 M Tris buffer (pH 7.6) and cut to a thickness of 40 μm with a freezing microtome. Control slices were not pretreated with glutaraldehyde. The method of Karnovsky (1967) was used for the demonstration of peroxidase. It was found that the tanycytes fixed with glutaraldehyde, as well as the tanycytes of the control slices, showed the peroxidase reaction in their perikarya and processes.

Previously, we demonstrated that the tanycytes of the median eminence absorb intraventricularly injected peroxidase and transport it to the portal vessels through their processes, and therefore suggested that the tanycytes may perhaps be involved in the regulation of the adenohypophysial function[2,4]. However, it is apparent from the present study that the peroxidase reaction in the tanycytes is not due to physiological absorption, since the peroxidase reaction took place in tanycytes fixed with glutaraldehyde *in vitro*. It is too early to conclude from the previous peroxidase experiments[2,4] that tanycytes play a role in the regulation of the hypophysial function.

Serum LH level after electrical cautery of tanycytes: Thirty-one rats were subjected to electrical cautery and 10 rats received a sham operation. For complete destruction of the tanycytes in the median eminence, cautery was stereotaxically performed at the anterior and posterior portions of the median eminence in the same rat. An anodal electrode was inserted into the third ventricle just above the ventricular surface of the median eminence. To guide the needle tip into the desired position, two roentgenographs, which were taken from the lateral and frontal sides of the brain, were consulted. A cathodal electrode was inserted under the skin of one leg. A direct current of 1 mA was allowed to flow for 7 sec. Until 10 days after electrical cautery, 0.3 ml of blood was withdrawn by heart puncture under light ether anesthesia in the morning (10:30–11:30) on

329

every other day. Histological examinations showed that complete destruction of the tanycytes of the median eminence was successful in 8 rats (Fig. 1). The serum LH level of these 8 rats showed no significant change (Table 1). The weights of the adenohypophysis, throyids, adrenals and testes of the rats subjected to electrical cautery were not significantly different from those in sham-operated rats. The above results suggest that the tanycytes are not involved in the gonadotropic activity of the adenohypophysis. The lack of change in weight of the thyroids, adrenals and testes following tanycyte destruction also suggests that the tanycytes play no role in other adenohypophysial activities. Thus, it appears that the tanycytes of the median eminence may not participate in the mechanisms controlling adenohypophysial function.

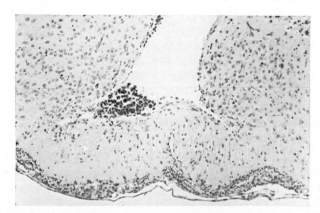

Fig. 1. Median eminence of the rat with lesioned ependymal linings 10 days after the operation.

TABLE 1.   Serum LH level after electrical cautery of tanycytes of the median eminence of the rat

Days after cautery	Controls ($n = 8$)	Rats with lesioned tanycytes ($n = 8$)
0	1.29 ± 0.17†	1.44 ± 0.16
2	1.13 ± 0.18	1.28 ± 0.17
4	1.14 ± 0.18	1.34 ± 0.12
6	1.18 ± 0.20	1.12 ± 0.19
8	1.37 ± 0.21	1.15 ± 0.12
10	1.39 ± 0.22	1.16 ± 0.11

†Value is expressed in terms of NIH-LH-SI. Mean ± SE

References

1. Knigge, K.M., Joseph, S.A., Sladek, J.R., Notter, M.F., Morris, M., Sundberg, D.K., Holzwarth, M.A., Hoffman, G.E. and O'Brien, L., Uptake and transport activity of the median eminence of the hypothalamus, *Int. Rev. Cytol.*, 45 (1976) 383–408.
2. Kobayashi, H., Wada, M., Uemura, H. and Ueck, M., Uptake of peroxidase from the third ventricle by ependymal cells of the median eminence, *Z. Zellforsch.*, 127 (1972) 545–551.
3. Kobayashi, H., Absorption of cerebrospinal fluid by ependymal cells of the median eminence. In K.M. Knigge, D.E. Scott, H. Kobayashi and S. Ishii (Eds.) *Brain-Endocrine Interaction, Vol. II, The Ventricular System*, Karger, Basel, 1975, pp. 109–122.
4. Nozaki, M., Absorption of intraventricularly injected peroxidase by tanycytes of the median eminence of the neonatal rat, *Zbl. vet. Med. C. Anat. Hist. Embryol.*, 6 (1977) 351–354.
5. Uemura, H. and Kobayashi, H., Effects on gonadal function by lesioning tanycytes in the median eminence of the rat and Japanese quail, *Cell Tissue Res.*, 178 (1977) 143–153.

Constant illumination blocks the effects of infundibulo-preoptic pathways in female rats

YUKIKO SAWAKI AND KINJI YAGI

Department of Physiology, Jichi Medical School,
Kawachi-gun, Tochigi 329–04, Japan

Our previous study has shown in rats that axon collaterals of tubero-infundibular (TI) neurosecretory neurons project to the medial preoptic nucleus (MPO) and mediate inhibition and excitation in MPO neurons[6]. Since the MPO is known to be the neural structure which triggers the surge of luteinizing hormone during the pre-ovulatory period as a consequence of an activation of TI neurons, the possibility arises that this 'infundibulo-preoptic' projection may be involved in the control of ovulation in rats. In order to test this possibility we investigated whether there is a sex difference in the frequency of occurrence of the MPO neurons which receive the infundibulo-preoptic projection and whether constant illumination, which is known to block spontaneous ovulation in rats[1], influenced the effects of this neural projection.

The tip of a concentric bipolar electrode (0.6 mm, o.d.) was placed on the surface of the median eminence of rats (Wistar strain) anesthetized with urethane (1.5 g/kg, s.c.) and either a single pulse (0.2 msec and 0.5 mA) or 5 pulses of 100 Hz were used to stimulate tubero-infundibular axons in the external layer of the median eminence[4,6]. The percentages of spontaneously firing MPO neurons that responded to the stimulation were not significantly different in the two sexes (Table 1).

In order to investigate the influence of environmental illumination on the ovulatory cycles and the effects of infundibulo-preoptic pathways, two groups of rats (an intact rat group for examining the estrous cycle by vaginal smears and an ovariectomized rat group for unit recording) were kept in an animal room under continuous light for 3 to 5 weeks and another two groups were kept in continuous darkness. The age of the rats was 5–9 months old at the unit recording. Intact rats exhibited a persistent estrous state after 3 weeks of constant illumination, while those kept in the dark were cyclic. The percentage of MPO units receiving the infundibulo-preoptic projection was significantly lower in ovariectomized rats kept in the light than in those kept in the dark (Table 1).

Since continuous lighting is known to induce polycystic ovaries in anovulatory rats[1], we conducted similar experiments in ovariectomized rats treated with estrogen at high doses. The ovariectomized rats received an intramuscular injection of 50 μg of 17 β-estradiol dipropionate each week during 3 to 5 weeks in either continuous light or continuous darkness. None of the MPO units recorded in the ovariectomized and estrogen-injected rats kept in continuous light responded to stimulation of the median eminence, while some of the MPO units sampled in animals kept in the dark responded (Table 1). Although the results cannot be statistically tested, they suggest a tendency for continuous light to block neural transmission through the infundibulo-preoptic pathway. Based on the results obtained from rats with and without estrogen injection, it appears that estrogen suppresses the effects of the infundibulo-preoptic projection.

It is also well known that young rats are resistant to the blocking action of continuous light-

TABLE 1.   Inhibition and excitation evoked in medial preoptic nucleus neurons by stimulation of the median eminence

| Conditions | Number of units | | | χ^2-test |
	Inhibited (%)	Excited (%)	Unresponsive (%)	
Sex				
Female	6 (11)	13 (24)	35 (65)	
Male	5 (19)	5 (19)	17 (62)	n.s.
Ovariectomized rats (5–9 months old)				
Light	6 (8)	3 (4)	66 (88)	
Dark	11 (26)	6 (14)	25 (60)	$P < 0.01$
Ovariectomized and estrogen-injected rats (5–9 months old)				
Light	0 (0)	0 (0)	49 (100)	
Dark	3 (4)	5 (7)	67 (89)	
Ovariectomized rats (3–4 months old)				
Light	4 (11)	5 (14)	27 (75)	
Dark	12 (16)	8 (11)	53 (73)	n.s.

ing on ovulation[1]. We therefore conducted similar experiments in young rats. Their age was 3 to 4 months old at the unit recording. The intact rats showed a rather regular ovulatory cycle even after 3 weeks of constant illumination. The percentages of MPO neurons that were inhibited and excited by stimulation of the median eminence were not significantly different between ovariectomized rats kept in continuous light and continuous darkness (Table 1).

The present results clearly demonstrate that the infundibulo-preoptic projection is not directly influenced by light stimulus *per se* but is related to the blocking of ovulation control. The results are, therefore, consistent with the view that the infundibulo-preoptic pathway may be involved in the control of ovulation. Both excitatory and inhibitory visual inputs have been observed in suprachiasmatic nucleus neurons in female rats[3]. Since this hypothalamic nucleus has been suggested to be involved in the biological clock mechanism producing circadian rhythm[2], the inhibitory actions of continuous light on both ovulation and neural transmission through the infundibulo-preoptic pathway may be dependent on the biological clock mechanism. In relation to the neural control of ovulation, we have proposed a reverberating neural circuit model involving the infundibulo-preoptic projection[7] to explain the recurrent excitation of tubero-infundibular neurosecretory neurons[4,5].

REFERENCES

1. Everett, J.W., Central neural control of reproductive functions of the adenohypophysis, *Physiol. Rev.*, 44 (1964) 373–431.
2. Moore, R.Y. and Klein, D.C., Visual pathways and the central neural control of a circadian rhythm in pineal serotonin *N*-acetyltransferase activity, *Brain Research*, 71 (1974) 17–33.
3. Sawaki, Y., Retinohypothalamic projection: electrophysiological evidence for the existence in female rats, *Brain Research*, 120 (1977) 336–341.
4. Sawaki, Y. and Yagi, K., Inhibition and facilitation of antidromically identified tubero-infundibular neurones following stimulation of the median eminence in the rat, *J. Physiol. (Lond.)*, 260 (1976) 447–460.
5. Yagi, K. and Sawaki, Y., Recurrent inhibition and facilitation: demonstration in the tubero-infundibular system and effects of strychnine and picrotoxin, *Brain Research*, 84 (1975) 155–159.
6. Yagi, K. and Sawaki, Y., Medial preoptic nucleus neurons: inhibition and facilitation of spontaneous activity following stimulation of the median eminence in female rats, *Brain Research*, 120 (1977) 342–346.
7. Yagi, K. and Sawaki, Y., Electrophysiological characteristics of identified tubero-infundibular neurons, *Neuroendocrinology*, 26 (1978) 50–64

Projection from the arcuate nucleus to the preoptic area revealed by retrograde transport of horseradish peroxidase

YASUHIKO IBATA, HARUO KINOSHITA, HIROSHI KIMURA*, KENJI WATANABE, YOSHIAKI NOJYO AND HAJIME FUJISAWA

*Department of Anatomy, Kyoto Prefectural University of Medicine,
Kamigyo-ku, Kyoto 602, Japan*
**Department of Anatomy, Shiga University of Medical Science,
Otsu, Shiga 520–21, Japan*

The preoptic area receives most of its neuronal input from the limbic system such as the amygdala and hippocampal formation via the stria terminalis and the fornix[6,8,9]. Efferent fibers from the preoptic area to the limbic system, midbrain and hypothalamic nuclei have also been identified[2], and more recently direct efferent fibers from the preoptic area to the median eminence have been reported[3,7]. On the other hand, the preoptic area has been shown by immunohistochemistry to contain LH-RH synthesizing neurons[1].

Our present work, which was designed to investigate the origin of an afferent pathway to the preoptic area using the method of retrograde transport of horseradish peroxidase (HRP), has yielded evidence of the existence of an afferent pathway from the arcuate nucleus to the preoptic area. Male adult Sprague-Dawley rats were used in the present study. Under Nembutal anesthesia, 0.1 to 0.5 μl of 50% HRP solution was injected stereotaxically into the medial preoptic area. After a survival period of 48 hr, the animals were perfused with saline followed by a mixture of 1% glutaraldehyde and 1% paraformaldehyde adjusted to pH 7.4 with phosphate buffer. After removal of the brain, additional fixation was carried out with the same fixative and blocks of brain tissue were transferred to 20% sucrose solution. Frontal serial sections of thickness 20 μm including the hypothalamus were cut in a cryostat and each section was floated on 0.1 M phosphate buffer. To determine the histochemical reaction to HRP, sections were incubated in 0.02 M 3, 3'-diaminobenzidine in Tris buffer with 0.03% H_2O_2 for 15 min, and then transferred to 0.1 M phosphate buffer. After mounting the sections on slides coated with gelatin, they were stained with cresylecht violet and examined by dark field and ordinary light microscopy. Dark field preparations showed a relatively large number of nerve cells in the arcuate nucleus with a positive HRP reaction (Fig. 1a). HRP granules were also observed in the perikarya of nerve cells. The nuclei appeared to be devoid of HRP granules by ordinary light microscopy (Fig. 1b). Ependymal cells of the third ventricle also failed to show HRP granules. A projection from medial basal hypothalamic neurons, including nerve cells in the arcuate nucleus, to the preoptic area has been identified electrophysiologically[5]. The influence of axon collaterals of the tuberoinfundibular neurons on inhibition and facilitation of the activity of medial preoptic nucleus neurons has also been reported using antidromic stimulation of the median eminence[10]. Our present study demonstrates morphologically an afferent pathway from the arcuate nucleus to the preoptic area and so supports the electrophysiological observations. The possibility of a neuronal circuit producing a reciprocal influence between these two areas could be postulated, since they both accept afferent inputs from each other. This system may play a significant role in the releasing/inhibiting hormonal regulation

333

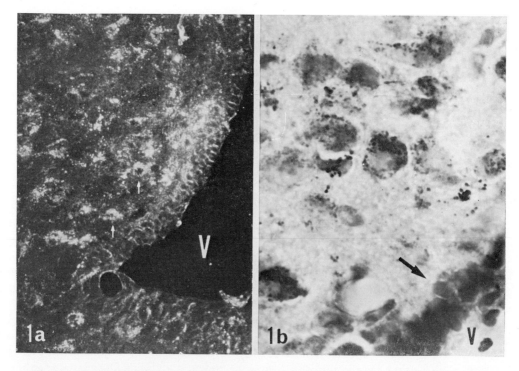

Fig. 1a.   Dark field micrograph of the arcuate nucleus ($\times$ 180). Many nerve cells with HRP granules are present (arrows). V, Third ventricle.

Fig. 1b.   High magnification micrograph of nerve cells in the arcuate nucleus ($\times$ 600). HRP granular deposits are observed in the perikarya, but appear to be absent from the nuclei. HRP granules are not apparent in the ependymal cells (arrow). V, Third ventricle.

of the anterior pituitary. It is generally accepted that a large proportion of the neurons in the arcuate nucleus contain dopamine and project into the external layer of the median eminence[4]. It is still uncertain, however, whether the neurons with an axonal projection to the preoptic area belong to the dopamine system. Also, it has not been possible to exclude the existence of neurons in the arcuate nucleus which have afferent connections with the preoptic area but lack an axonal projection to the median eminence. These points will be assessed in further investigations.

REFERENCES

1. Barry, J., Dubois, M.P. and Poulain, P., LRF producing cells of the mammalian hypothalamus. A fluorescent antibody study, *Z. Zellforsch.*, 146 (1973) 351–366.
2. Conrad, L.C.A. and Pfaff, D.W., Axonal projections of medial preoptic and anterior hypothalamic neurons, *Science*, 190 (1975) 1112–1114.
3. Daikoku, S., Matsumura, H. and Shinohara, Y., Efferent projection of the nucleus preopticus medialis to the median eminence in rats, *Neuroendocrinology*, 21 (1976) 130–138.
4. Fuxe, K., Cellular localization of monoamines in the median eminence and the infundibular stem of some mammals, *Z. Zellforsch.*, 61, (1974) 710–724.
5. Harris, M.C. and Sanghera, M., Projection of medial basal hypothalamic neurons to the preoptic anterior hypothalamic areas and the paraventricular nucleus in the rat, *Brain Research*, 81 (1974) 401–411.

6. Heimer, L. and Nauta, W.J.H., Hypothalamic distribution of the stria terminalis in the rat, *Brain Research,* 13 (1969) 284–297.
7. Ibata, Y., Nojyo, Y., Mizukawa, K. and Sano, Y., Direct projection from the medial preoptic area to the median eminence of the cat, *Endocrinol. japon.*, 24 (1977) 497–502.
8. Nauta, W.J.H., Hippocampal projections and related neuronal pathways to the midbrain in the rat, *Brain*, 81 (1958) 319–340.
9. Raisman, G. and Field, P.M., Sexual dimorphism in the preoptic area of the rat, *Science*, 173 (1971) 731–733.
10. Yagi, K. and Sawaki, Y., Medial preoptic nucleus neurons: inhibition and facilitation of spontaneous activity following stimulation of the median eminence in female rats, *Brain Research*, 120 (1977) 342–346.

Vasopressin release from guinea-pig hypothalamo-neurohypophysial system in organ culture

SHO YOSHIDA, SAN-E ISHIKAWA AND TOSHIKAZU SAITO

Department of Endocrinology and Metabolism, Jichi Medical School,
Kawachi-gun, Tochigi 329–04, Japan

In order to study the mechanism of secretion of vasopressin from the neurohypophysis, an organ cultured system of guinea-pig hypothalamo-neurohypophysial complex (HNC) has been developed. Activities of Na-K dependent ATPase and ability of DNA synthesis were maintained in the explant after 5 days culture *in vitro*. Vasopressin was released from the cultured HNC by 56 mM K Locke's solution. As shown by previous investigators[1-3], the organ cultured system of HNC can be used as a tool for *in vitro* studies of the mechanism of vasopressin secretion.

A block of tissue was taken from male guinea-pigs weighing 170–250 g. The blocks included an area about 2 mm rostral to the optic chiasma, 3 mm lateral to either side of the central medial line, and 2 mm caudal to the median eminence. The block was undercut at a depth of 1–2 mm. The anterior pituitary was removed and discarded. The posterior pituitary was retained intact. The explants were cultured in a culture-well containing 1.5 ml of Delbecco's Modified Eagle Medium fortified with 10% fetal calf serum, 100 μ/ml penicillin G and 0.1 mg/ml streptomycin. The culture dish was maintained in a humidified incubator at 37°C under 95% oxygen and 5% CO_2.

The rate of incorporation of [^{3}H]-thymidine into DNA was measured by incubation of the explants with [^{3}H]-thymidine (10 μc/dish) for 3 hr. The Na-K ATPase activites were measured as liberated inorganic phosphate after incubation of HNC homogenate with ATP in Tris buffer. The Na-K sensitive ATPase activites were calculated as the difference between total ATPase and ouabain non-sensitive ATPase. Arginine vasopressin (AVP) was measured by a radioimmunoassay.

The release of AVP from the explants was studied as follows. HNC explant of 5 days culture was used. After washing twice with MEM solution, the explants were incubated with Locke's solution twice successively for 10 min. They were then incubated with 56 mM K, Ca-free Locke's solution twice successively for 10 min, followed by two 10 min incubation periods with 56 mM K, Ca-positive Locke's solutions.

The Na-K ATPase activities of the HNC after 5 days incubation were 0.825 $\pm$ 0.276 mMPi/ mg protein/hr (mean $\pm$ S.D., $n = 7$), while the activities of fresh HNC were 1.005 $\pm$ 0.209 mMPi/mg protein/hr (mean $\pm$ S.D., $n = 6$). This difference was not significant. The uptake of [^{3}H]-thymidine into DNA in the explants was 914.5 $\pm$ 70.9 cpm/μg DNA (mean $\pm$ S.D., $n = 4$) on the 5th culture day.

Fig. 1 shows the AVP release into the culture medium from two HNC *in vitro* during the culture period. A large amount of AVP was released into the medium during the first 24 hr incubation period, and the AVP output from the explants remained fairly constant for the remaining periods.

The effect of 56 mM K Locke's solution on AVP release from HNC in organ culure is

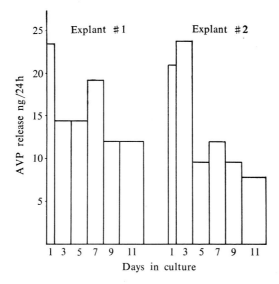

Fig. 1.　AVP release into the culture medium by HNS explants during the culture period.

summarized in Table 1. When the amounts of released AVP from HNC in 56 mM K Locke's solutions were expressed as a percentage of the amounts released during the control period, the amounts of released AVP in 56 mM K, Ca-free solutions represented 81.7% of the control, whereas those released in 56 mM K, Ca positive (2.2 mM) solutions represented 241.4% of the control.

TABLE 1.　Effects of 56 mM K and Ca ion on the release of AVP from HNC explants in organ culture

Exp. No.	AVP release pg/dish/10 min					
	control	control	56 mM K, Ca(−)	56 mM K, Ca(−)	56 mM K, Ca(+)	56 mM K, Ca(+)
1	264	150	198	192	276	284
2	81	116	96	84	109	81
3	116	280	104	114	306	370
4	10	10	11	6	70	46

These results indicate that the HNC explants cultured for 5 days *in vitro* maintained good cellular functions and also suggest that the explants were able to release AVP by depolarization. The presence of Ca ion in the incubation media was indispensable for AVP release from the explants.

REFERENCES

1. Pearson, D., Shainberg, A., Osinchak, J. and Sachs, H., The hypothalamo-neurohypophysial complex in organ culture: morphologic and biochemical characteristics, *Endocrinology*, 96 (1975) 982–993.
2. Sachs, H., Goodman, R., Osinchak, J. and McKelvy, J., Supraoptic neurosecretery neurons of the guinea pig in organ culture. Biosynthesis of vasopressin and neurophysin, *Proc. nat. Acad. Sci.* (Wash.) USA, 68 (1971) 2782–2786.
3. Sladek C.D. and Knigge, K.M., Cholinergic stimulation of vasopressin release from the rat hypothalamo-neurohypophysial system in organ culture, *Endocrinology*, 101 (1977) 411–420.

Neural inputs from the limbric structure to preoptic area and the preovulatory release of gonadotrophin in rats

MASAZUMI KAWAKAMI AND FUKUKO KIMURA

Department of Physiology, Yokohama City University School of Medicine,
Minami-ku, Yokohama 232, Japan

Cumulative evidence has shown that the preoptic-hypothalamic area constitutes an essential part in the mechanism controlling the cyclic release of gonadotrophin in female rats. We have previously demonstrated that after transection of the neural connection between the limbic structure and preoptic area on the morning of proestrus, the ovulation which was expected to occur during the next day was blocked[3]. This paper describes our recent results on the timing of the neural inputs from the limbic structure to the preoptic-hypothalamic area.

Regularly cycling female rats of Wistar strain were used. Transection of the neural connection was performed acutely under ether anesthesia at various times of the day of proestrus with either a bayonet-shaped[2] or L-shaped knife attached to a stereotaxic instrument. Blood samples were collected for determination of hormone contents either by heart puncture or through an intraatrial cannula. Ovulation was checked on the next morning. Electrochemical stimulation in combination with transection was performed under anesthesia with pentobarbital sodium (31.5 mg/kg) injected at 1345 hr.

To elucidate the neural pathways involved in the control of the ovulatory release of gonadotrophins, the effect of transection in the brain between 1200 and 1400 hr on the occurrence of ovulation was studied. Fig. 1 shows the site and size of the transection as projected on a parasagittal section. A transection placed ventrally and posteriorly to the diagonal band of Broca (DBB) blocked ovulation (Fig. 1A). This transection interrupts neural connections between the DBB, the septum (SEPT) and the bed nucleus of the stria terminalis (BST) and the preoptic area. However, ovulation was not blocked when the cut was placed more anteriorly leaving the connection between the DBB, the SEPT and BST and the preoptic area intact (Fig. 1B). A transection placed inside the medial preoptic area (MPO) (Fig. 1C) effectively blocked ovulation. A cut placed in either the upper or basal part of the DBB and a cut placed in the rostral and basal part of the preoptic area blocked ovulation. Measurements of the plasma level of pituitary hormones disclosed that a cut placed posteriorly to the DBB blocked the releases of LH, FSH and prolactin in the afternoon of the proestrous day of the surgical operation, but a cut placed in the part anterior to the DBB did not. However, additional electrochemical stimulation of the MPO in a rat bearing the former type of cut induced increases in serum LH and FSH levels as in the intact rat. These results suggest that in the intact proestrous rat, neural inputs from areas anterior and superior to the preoptic area are responsible for the activation of the MPO which in turn results in an ovulatory surge of gonadotrophin release. The limbic area concerned with the function may be the DBB, the BST and the medial part of the amygdala, since electrical and electrochemical stimulation of these areas has been shown to lead to ovulation and/or an increase in LH release in pentobarbital-blocked proestrous rats[1,4].

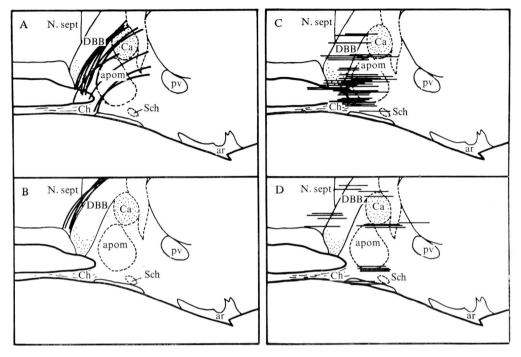

Fig. 1.   Site and size of the preoptic forebrain transection projected on a sagittal section through the rat brain. A and B represent cuts made with a bayonet-shaped knife, and C and D represent cuts with an L-shaped knife. Cuts A and C blocked ovulation, but cuts B and C did not. apom, medial preoptic area; ar, arcuate nucleus; Ca, anterior commissure; Ch, optic chiasm; DBB, diagonal band of Broca; N. sept., septal nucleus; pv, paraventricular nucleus; Sch, suprachiasmatic nucleus.

To determine until what time the limbric structure may stimulate the MPO to ensure normal pattern of preovulatory gonadotrophin release, transection of the neural connection between the limbric structure and the MPO was performed during or at the end of the "critical period" for ovulatory surge of gonadotrophins. Our animals showed peak serum levels of LH, FSH and prolactin at 1700 hr, 1700–1800 hr and 1500–1600 hr, respectively. When the cut was made anteriorly and superiorly to the MPO at 1500 hr, at which time the serum levels of LH, FSH and prolactin were in rising phases, the LH and FSH levels observed at 1500 hr were maintained for 1–2 hr thereafter and no further elevation occurred. The serum level of prolactin was more dramatically decreased to a level lower than before the critical period by 1700 hr.

Fig. 2 shows results for rats in which the neural connection between the limbric structure and the MPO was cut at 1600 hr, at which time the serum levels of the hormones were elevated considerably. The increased rate of LH release was maintained until 1700 hr and afterwards terminated quickly. The elevated FSH level was maintained for a longer period and showed a further increase to attain a maximum at 1800 hr similar to the FSH release observed in the intact rats. On the other hand prolactin release terminated promptly after the operation. These results suggest that the limbric structrue may be needed to activate the MPO during almost the whole duration of preovulatory release of LH, FSH and prolactin. In pentobarbital-blocked proestrous rats, it has been shown that bilateral retrochiasmatic transection 15 min after electrochemical stimula-

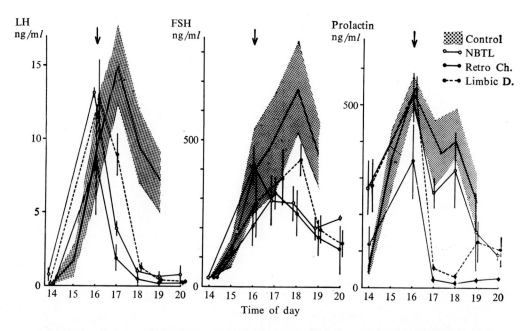

Fig. 2. Effects of limbic deafferentation (Limbic D.), retrochiasmatic cut (Retro Ch.) or pento-barbital sodium injection (NBTL, 31.5 mg/kg body wt) made at 1600 hr on the serum levels of LH (left), FSH (middle), and prolactin (right) in the afternoon of proestrus. Curves with hatched belts represent values from control animals. Arrows indicate the time of performance of the procedure. Each curve shows average values for 5 animals, with the S.E. indicated by vertical bars.

tion of the MPO did not prevent the occurrence of the normal preovulatory LH surge but such transection 5 min after the stimulation completely blocked the LH surge[5]. The reason for the discrepancy between these and our present findings remains unclear but may be attributable to a difference in the artificial and natural activations of the MPO.

The present results indicate that preovulatory FSH release may be relatively more dependent on the preoptic-hypothalamic mechanism, since the serum FSH level even tended to increase after interruption of the limbic afferents. On the other hand, preovulatory prolactin release appeared to be much more limbic-dependent than the LH release.

REFERENCES

1. Everett, J.W., Radford, H.M. and Holsinger, J., Electrolytic irritative lesions in the hypothalamus and other forebrain areas: effects on luteinizing hormone release and ovarian cycle. In Martini (Ed), *Steroid Biochemistry, Pharmacology and Therapeutics*, Academic Press, New York, 1964, pp. 251–258.
2. Halász, B. and Pupp, L., Hormone secretion of the anterior pituitary gland after physical interruption of all nervous pathways to the hypophysiotropic area, *Endocrinology*, 77 (1965) 553–562.
3. Kawakami, M. and Terasawa, E., Acute effect of neural deafferentation on timing of gonadotropin secretion, *Endocrinol. japon.*, 19 (1972) 449–459.
4. Kawakami, M., Terasawa, E. and Ibuki, T., Changes in multiple unit activity of the brain during the estrous cycle, *Neuroendocrinology*, 6 (1970) 30–48.
5. Turgeon, J. and Barraclough, C.A., Temporal patterns of LH release following graded preoptic electrical stimulation in proestrous rats, *Endocrinology*, 92 (1973) 755–761.

Indoleamine 2, 3-dioxygenase in the brain

OSAMU HAYAISHI, MOTOKAZU FUJIWARA, MASAKATSU SHIBATA,
YASUYOSHI WATANABE, TOSHIHIRO NUKIWA, FUSAO HIRATA
AND NOBORU MIZUNO

Department of Medical Chemistry, Faculty of Medicine, Kyoto University,
Sakyo-ku, Kyoto 606, Japan

Indoleamine 2, 3-dioxygenase is a hemoprotein that catalyzes oxygenative ring cleavage of the pyrrole ring of various indoleamines such as tryptophan, 5-hydroxytryptophan and serotonin. The substrate specificity of this enzyme suggests a possible role in the regulation of indoleamine metabolism in various tissues, including the brain.

TABLE 1. Distribution of indoleamine 2,3-dioxygenase activity in the rabbit brain.

	m units /mg protein	units /g tissue	Total m units in tissue
Pineal gland	84.8 ± 9.1	8.50 ± 0.70	73.2 ± 6.8
Choroid plexus	34.2 ± 6.3	4.50 ± 0.70	55.6 ± 10.1
Cerebral cortex	3.2 ± 0.6	0.08 ± 0.018	446.6 ± 97.1
Diencephalon	5.2 ± 0.6	0.12 ± 0.013	90.8 ± 9.4
Midbrain	5.8 ± 1.0	0.14 ± 0.27	94.5 ± 20.8
Cerebellum	9.8 ± 2.8	0.26 ± 0.08	323.8 ± 89.4
Pons and medulla	10.4 ± 2.0	0.23 ± 0.04	202.9 ± 35.2

One unit of enzyme is defined as the amount that forms one nmol of [^{14}C]–formic acid per hr. Results are expressed as means $\pm$ standard errors of five rabbits.

TABLE 2. Quantitative estimation of the metabolites derived from L-[methylene-^{14}C] tryptophan.

Metabolites	Exp. 1	Exp. 2
Kynurenine	14.0	12.6
5-Hydroxytryptophan	1.3	0.9
Serotonin	1.4	1.2
N-Acetylserotonin	0.2	0.2
Melatonin	1.0	0.9
5-Hydroxyindoleacetic acid	9.0	8.8
5-Methoxyindoleacetic acid	9.8	6.3
5-Hydroxytryptophol	0.6	0.5
5-Methoxytryptophol	0.8	0.8
Indoleacetic acid	0.9	1.4
Other metabolite (s)	4.3	5.2
Total metabolites	43.3	38.8
Tryptophan	36.8	45.9
Total recovered radioactivity	80.1	84.7

Total radioactivity applied to the DEAE-cellulose column was designated as 100%.

The distribution of indoleamine 2, 3-dioxygenase activity was investigated in various parts of the rabbit brain using the supernatant fraction (30,000 x g, 30 min) of homogenates. A low but significant activity was detected in all parts of the brain. The highest activity was associated with the pineal gland and choroid plexus (Table 1). Specific activities of the supernatant fractions derived from the pineal gland and choroid plexus were 84.8 and 34.2 pmol/hr/mg protein at 37°, respectively, with L-tryptophan as a substrate. When the pineal gland was cultured with L-[methylene-^{14}C]-tryptophan, L-[methylene-^{14}C] kynurenine formed by the action of indoleamine 2, 3-dioxygenase was found as one of the major products. It was isolated by DEAE-cellulose column chromatography and identified by thin layer chromatography with and without treatment with kynureninase from a pseudomonad. The amount of kynurenine thus determined accounted for approximately one-third of the total amount of tryptophan metabolites, indicating that the kynurenine pathway is one of the major metabolic pathways of tryptophan in the rabbit pineal gland (Table 2).

Morphological studies on the circadian cycle of the pineal gland of the rat

WATARU MORI, KATSUMARO KURUMADO AND AKIO HASEGAWA

Department of Pathology, Faculty of Medicine, University of Tokyo,
Bunkyo-ku, Tokyo 113, Japan

Our investigations of the pineal gland have been carried out mainly morphologically, placing emphasis on its phylogenesis and ultrastructure[1,2]. Among the results of our investigations, the demonstration of the synaptic ribbons in an infant and in an adult human pineal gland[3] is the most recent. This led us to carry out experimental studies on the rat, and we believe that these will be useful as a model for understanding the human pineal. Our attention at present is focused on the observation of circadian changes in the number of the synaptic ribbons in the pineal gland, which we believe provides a useful basis for studies on the pineal function in man and other animals.

The mean number of synaptic ribbons per unit area ($85 \times 85 \ \mu m^2 \times 5$) of the pinealocyte, irrespective of the time of day was 22.4 ± 5.9 in the proximal, 16.7 ± 5.2 in the intermediate, and 19.9 ± 3.1 in the distal part of the gland but the differences among these means were not statistically significant. The results for ribbon fields were more-or-less similar (17.2 ± 6.3, 13.1 ± 3.8, 15.2 ± 2.8), and we concluded that the interregional differences in the pineal gland of normal rats are very small.

Observations on the number of ribbon fields and synaptic ribbons over a period of 24 hr revealed that both of them changed markedly, showing a circadian rhythm; the curves for ribbon fields and synaptic ribbons were parallel. The number of ribbon fields and synaptic ribbons reached a maximum at 0200 hr and decreased to minimum level at 1400 hr. Statistical analysis of the data confirmed the increases in numbers of both ribbon fields and synaptic ribbons, from 1600 hr to 1800 hr, 2200 hr and 0200 hr, and decreases from 0200 hr to 1000 hr, 1200 hr and 1400 hr ($P < 0.05$). No significant changes were found in either ribbon fields or synaptic ribbons during the period between 1200 hr and 1600 hr.

In the next experiment using blinded rats the mean numbers of ribbon fields per unit area, irrespective of the experimental group, were 6.3 ± 2.0 in the proximal, 5.7 ± 1.5 in the intermediate, and 6.8 ± 1.4 in the distal part of the gland. The differences among these were not statistically significant, and the results with synaptic ribbons were more-or-less similar again. Therefore, we concluded that area difference was insignificant as far as this kind of experiment is concerned. When the numbers of synaptic ribbons and ribbon fields were calculated following the course after ophthalmectomy, it was apparent that the numbers of the two elements of the pinealocyte decreased remarkably after the operation. A considerable fall was noted by the 15th day, appeared to reach a minimum at around 1 month, and remained below normal even after 2 and 3 months, although it was clear that gradual recovery was occurring: the numbers returned to a normal level at around 6 months after the operation. No such change was seen in either of the control groups. Statistically, the decrease in the number of both ribbon fields and synaptic ribbons, compared with the controls of the present experiments as well as with the results of our previous study carried out under the same conditions but with normal rats, was significant 15 days and 1 month after the operation, and so was its recovery from 3 to 6 months ($P < 0.05$). On the other hand, the differences among the values for blinded rats at 6 months, the control rats, and normal rats were not statistically significant.

In the present experiments with rats we have studied the synaptic ribbons of the pineal gland according to the method of Vollrath[4], and demonstrated circadian changes quite analogous to those in guinea pigs. Thus, it is clear that there is a type of circadian change of the pineal synaptic ribbon, at least in some species of rodents. It is therefore quite possible that this phenomenon may occur in other species of mammals, including man. Furthermore, it was confirmed that the number of synaptic ribbons and ribbon fields in the pinealocyte of the rat began to show a marked decrease as early as 15 days after bilateral ophthalmectomy, and reached a minimum at around 1 month. Subsequently, a gradual increase occurred until the normal level was recovered in 6 months.

REFERENCES

1. Kurumado, K. and Mori, W., A phylogenetic study on the pineal gland, *Igaku-no-ayumi*, 94 (1975) 227–239 (in Japanese).
2. Kurumado, K. and Mori, W., A morphological study on the pineal gland of human embryo, *Acta Path. Japon.*, 27 (1977) 527–531.
3. Kurumado, K. and Mori, W., Synaptic ribbon in the human pinealocyte, *Acta Path. Japon.* 26 (1976) 381–384.
4. Vollrath, L., Synaptic ribbons of a mammalian pineal gland circadian changes, *Z. Zellforsch*, 145 (1973) 171–183.

Control of the circadian rhythm of serotonin *N*-acetyltransferase activity in the pineal gland of chicken

TAKEO DEGUCHI

Department of Medical Chemistry, Tokyo Metropolitan Institute for Neurosciences, Fuchu, Tokyo 183, Japan

The circadian rhythm of melatonin synthesis in the pineal gland is controlled by a rhythmic change of serotonin *N*-acetyltransferase activity. The neuronal pathway that regulates *N*-acetyltransferase activity in the rat has been well established[1-2,4-7]. The *N*-acetyltransferase rhythm in the rat is controlled by sympathetic nerves originating in superior cervical ganglia. In contrast, Ralph *et al.*[8] reported that the circadian rhythm of *N*-acetyltransferase activity in chicken pineal gland persists after denervation of superior cervical ganglia. The neuronal or hormonal pathway for the enzyme rhythm in the chicken has not yet been elucidated. The present study shows that in organ culture of chicken pineal gland *N*-acetyltransferase activity exhibits a circadian change.

White Leghorn chickens of both sexes were raised under diurnal lighting conditions with the light on from 0700 hr to 1900 hr for 10–12 days after hatching and were used for the study. *N*-Acetyltransferase activity was assayed by a modification of the method previously established for the rat pineal gland[3]. 5-Methyoxytryptamine (50 nmol) was used as a substrate instead of tryptamine.

N-Acetyltransferase activity in the chicken pineal gland was low during the daytime and increased 8– to 14– fold in the dark at night. The rhythm of *N*-acetyltransferase activity was not prevented by previous treatment with reserpine, α-adrenergic blockers or β-adrenergic blockers (data not shown), an observation which is in contrast to that in the rat[2]. Catecholamines or their precursor L-DOPA injected into chickens during the daytime did not elevate *N*-acetyltransferase activity. When chicken pineal gland was cultured during the daytime (from 1000 hr to 1700 hr) in the presence of catecholamines, carbachol or serotonin, *N*-acetyltransferase activity did not increase at all. Catecholamines suppressed the basal enzyme activity to one-third of the usual level in cultured chicken pineal gland. In contrast, a marked increase of *N*-acetyltransferase activity was observed in cultured pineal gland of rats in response to catecholamines[4]. Phosphodiesterase inhibitors (theophylline or IBMX) increased *N*-acetyltransferase activity 3– to 6– fold in organ culture of chicken pineal gland (data not shown).

Chickens were killed at 1200 hr and the pineal glands were cultured in the absence of such agents. *N*-Acetyltransferase activity was low during the daytime but started to increase at 2200 hr reaching a maximal level at 0200 hr (Fig. 1). The *N*-acetyltransferase activity subsequently decreased to the initial level in the next morning. The maximal level of the enzyme activity in cultured pineal gland was 40 % of the night level of the enzyme activity of *in vivo* animals. However, when chickens were killed at 1800 hr and the pineal glands were cultured, the *N*-acetyltransferase activity increased to the same level as that of *in vivo* animals (data not shown). The pattern of the increase as well as of the decrease of *N*-acetyltransferase activity in the cultured pineal was the same whenever the chickens were killed (either at 1200 hr or 1800hr). The rhythmic phase of the

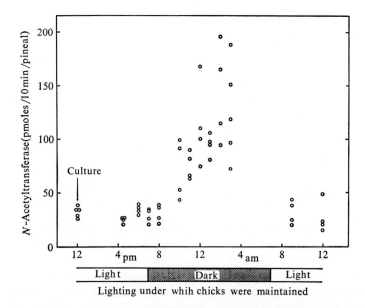

Fig. 1.   Change in serotonin *N*-acetyltransferase activity in organ culture of the chicken pineal gland.
Chickens were killed at 1200 hr and the pineal glands were cultured at 40° under 95% O_2– 5% CO_2 in darkness. Each point represents the *N*-acetyltransferase activity of an individual pineal gland.

cultured pineal gland was delayed about 3 hr compared to the *in vivo* rhythm. This autonomic rhythm of the cultured pineal gland was prevented by cycloheximide, actinomycin D or catecholamines (data not shown). The inhibitory effect of catecholamines was prevented by phentolamine, indicating that the effect of catecholamines is mediated by α-adrenergic receptors.

These observations suggest the possibility that the circadian rhythm of *N*-acetyltransferase activity in chicken pineal gland is generated by an endogenous oscillator in the gland. Zimmerman and Menaker[9] reported that pinealectomy of the sparrow abolished the free-running rhythm in constant darkness, though it was restored upon transplantation of the pineal gland. Based upon these observations, they proposed that the avian pineal gland is an endogenously rhythmic oscillator. The findings reported here are consistent with their suggestions. Thus organ culture of chicken pineal gland may offer a model for studies on the mechanism of the circadian oscillator.

References

1. Axelrod, J., The pineal gland: A neurochemical transducer, *Science*, 184 (1974) 1341–1348.
2. Deguchi, T. and Axelrod, J., Control of circadian change of serotonin N-acetyltransferase activity in the pineal organ by the β-adrenergic receptor, *Proc. natl. Acad. Sci.* (*Wash.*), 69 (1972) 2547–2550.
3. Deguchi, T. and Axelrod, J., Sensitive assay for serotonin N-acetyltransferase activity in rat pineal. *Anal. Biochem.*, 50 (1972) 174–179.
4. Deguchi, T. and Axelrod, J., Superinduction of serotonin N-acetyltransferase and supersensitivity of adenyl cyclase to catecholamines in denervated pineal gland, *Molec. Pharmacol.*, 9 (1973) 612–618.
5. Klein, D.C. and Weller, J.L., Indole metabolism in the pineal gland: A circadian rhythm in N-acetyltransferase, *Science*, 169 (1970) 1093–1095.

6. Klein, D.C., Weller, J.L. and Moore, R.Y., Melatonin metabolism: Neural regulation of pineal serotonin: acetyl coenzyme A *N*-acetyltransferase activity, *Proc. nat. Acad. Sci. (Wash.)*, 68 (1971) 3107–3110.
7. Moore, R.Y. and Klein, D.C., Visual pathway and the central neural control of a circadian rhythm in pineal serotonin *N*-acetyltransferase activity. *Brain Research*, 71 (1974) 17–33.
8. Ralph, C.L., Binkley, S., MacBride, S.E. and Kelin, D.C., Regulation of pineal rhythms in chickens: Effect of blinding, constant light, constant dark, and superior cervical ganglionectomy, *Endocrinology*, 97 (1975) 1373–1378.
9. Zimmerman, N.H. and Menaker, M., Neuronal connections of sparrow pineal: Role in circadian control of activity, *Science*, 190 (1975) 477–479.

PART VII

NEURAL MECHANISMS OF INTRINSIC BEHAVIOR:
SLEEP-WAKEFULNESS CONTROL

YUTAKA OOMURA and SHIZUO TORII*

*Department of Physiology, Faculty of Medicine, Kyushu University,
Higashi-ku, Fukuoka 812, Japan
* Department of Physiology, Faculty of Medicine, Toho University,
Ohta-ku, Tokyo 143, Japan*

Neural mechanisms of intrinsic behavior (Y. Oomura)

Ever since acceptance of the fact that the behavior of an organism is under the control of the nervous system, attempts have continued to relate specific organism functions to specific neural centers. In this respect, hunger and satiation, and related actions have been attributed to the lateral hypothalamic area (LHA) and the ventromedial hypothalamus (VMH); sex, body temperature and sleep have been related to the preoptic hypothalamic area (POA); and other similar associations have been established. Recently, sophisticated techniques such as horseradish peroxidase tracing, electron microscopy, intracellular and extracellular microelectrode recording, improved accuracy in lesioning, electrophoretic drug application with micropipettes, and computer analysis and control have contributed to further determination of control centers, and to the elucidation of the connections and interdependence between various nuclei which are involved in an organism's behavior. The aim of neurophysiological studies is an understanding of the mechanisms by which a neural system translates its inputs into efficacious behavior.

Horseradish peroxidase, intracellular staining, and retrograde degeneration have all contributed to the anatomical demonstration of interconnections between identified nuclei. The results have limitations and involve some random searching, however judicious it may be. Attempts to trace individual neurons frequently yield little more than respect for the skill, patience, discipline, and time invested by those who have already identified so many of the neurons. Computer-aided microscopy has provided savings in time and other benefits. It is now possible to map the range of neuronal processes, and to trace connections from region to region. Preliminary simple three-dimensional mapping has been carried out at a rate of about 5 neurons per day[4]. More ambitious projects may take longer, but the process is faster and more accurate than manual charting.

Hypothalamic rage, elicited by stimulation of the VMH, includes aggressive attitude and behavior, and autonomic responses. It is both emotional and well-organized, and differs from "sham rage". Lowering of the threshold of this behavior by provocation has been attenuated by amygdaloid lesion or enhanced by septal lesion. Recent studies in which the amygdala and septum were sequentially destroyed indicated that the amygdala facilitates VMH activity independent of septum, while the septum inhibits the VMH via the amygdala.[2] The amygdala may facilitate the VMH by transmission of sensory inputs.

The medial POA, in response to the presence of gonadal hormone, sends neuronal discharges down the medial forebrain bundle, which in turn elicits sexual actions such as lordosis or mounting behavior. These responses are facilitated by a section in the anterodorsal region of the anterior commisure. Hence, sexual behavior is initiated from the POA, which in turn is controlled through the anterior commisure, and inhibition is removed by section of the latter[6]. The mechanism is not yet known, but probably originates in the frontal cortex (FC). These are examples of unilateral effects in which one center is affected by, but does not affect, the other center.

Functional relations between feeding behavior and at least 4 types of neurons in three different brain regions have been demonstrated by on-line computer analysis and control of ongoing behavior experiments[3,5]. In these experiments, the LHA's function as the feeding center, and LHA (FC) cooperation in the control of effectors of overt actions were all verified. In addition, roles of the orbitofrontal cortex (OBF) in memory, the LHA in motivation, the OBFLHA relation in anticipation, and the LHA-motor cortex relation in motor behavior were all either identified or removed from the realm of doubt[5].

Electrophysiological results indicate the nature of the anatomical connections between the FC and the LHA. The electrical properties of these connections suggest functions which can be verified by behavioral experiments. The evidence indicates substantial FC influence over the LHA in its role of motivation of feeding behavior. In addition to the functional relations, an organizational pattern has also become evident in the LHA. This pattern is analogous to the organizational pattern of the motor cortex. It appears that the LHA can appraise the FC of the condition of the organism's milieu, and the FC stores the information to be used as needed by the LHA to motivate appropriate behavior.

Microelectrode recording demonstrated feeding behavior inhibition after feeding sugar to a bee. Inhibition of CNS response to sugar was produced by NaCl stimulation, demonstrating convergence. Separation of function was shown between the thoracic ganglion and the 2nd thoracic ganglion. Summation was demonstrated by an increase of CNS activity 1.5 times when sugar was applied to 2 tarsi rather than just one. These experiments demonstrate CNS mediation and control of overt behavior in response to stimulation.

The outstanding impression obtained during preparation of this commentary is that the instruments, computers, tools and techniques which are now available have improved so rapidly that there has not yet been enough time for them to achieve widespread use. When this does occur, progress in physiological research should accelerate at an even greater rate than it has in the past few years. It does not seem unreasonable to expect, in the very near future, that enough data will be available to permit detailed functional maps of midbrain regions similar to the maps which now exist for cortical areas. The hypothalamus should not be able to keep its functions and interrelations with other regions secret for very much longer. The prognosis is that within relatively few years we will have extensive, useful knowledge of many of the neural interconnections involved in the control of behavior, both normal and abnormal.

References

1. Aoki, K. and Kuwabara, M., Electrophysiological studies of gustation in honeybee (*Apis mellifica L.*). In Y. Oomura and S. Torii (Eds.) *Integrative Control Functions of the Brain*, Part VII Neural mechanisms of intrinsic behavior sleep-wakefulness control: Editor's commentary, Kodansha Scientific, Tokyo, 1978, pp. 122–123.
2. Maeda, H., Effects of septal lesions on electrically elicited hypothalamic rage response in cats, *Physiol. Behav.*, 21 (1978) in press.
3. Ono, T., Oomura, Y., Sugimori, M., Nakamura, T., Shimizu, N., Kita, H. and Ishibashi, S., Hypothalamic

unit activity related to lever pressing and eating in the chronic monkey. In D. Novin, W. Wyrwicka and G. A. Bray (Eds.) *Hunger: Basic Mechanisms and Clinical Implications*, Raven Press, New York, 1976, pp. 159–170.

4. Oomura, Y., Nakamura, M., Taniguchi, K. and Shimizu, N., Design of a semi-automatic measurement system for interconnections of neurons, *Trans. I.E.C.E.*, 60 (1977) 1117–1118.

5. Oomura, Y., Ono, T., Ohta, M., Nishino, H., Shimizu, N., Ishibashi, S., Kita, H., Sasaki, K., Nicolaïdis, S. and Van Atta, L., Neuronal activities in feeding behavior of chronic monkeys. In Y. Katsuki, M. Sato, S.F. Takagi and Y. Oomura (Eds.) *Food Intake and Chemical Senses*, Tokyo University Press, Tokyo, 1977, pp. 505–524.

6. Yamanouchi, K. and Arai, Y., Lordosis behaviour in male rats: effect of deafferentation in the preoptic area and hypothalamus, *J. Endocrinol.*, 76 (1978) in press.

Sleep-wakefulness control (S. Torii)

One approach to understanding the basic sleep mechanism is to examine the role of neurotransmitters involved in the neural pathways that regulate the sleep-waking cycle. Using the histofluorescence technique[2], it was found that serotonin-containing neurons are located in the raphe nuclei. Noradrenaline neurons are found throughout the brain stem reticular formation, with the highest concentration in the locus coeruleus[10]. Based on lesion studies on these neurons Jouvet[3] proposed a monoamine theory of sleep control. He suggested that serotonergic activity may be related to the maintenance of slow wave sleep and the priming of REM sleep. Adrenergic activity may be related to both tonic and phasic aspects of REM sleep.

In addition to the work on neurotransmitters, it should be noted that a circulating substance is responsible for regulation of sleep. Recent studies have demonstrated that this material is a nine amino acid peptide[8]. It has been also shown that a brainstem homogenate of sleep-deprived animals contains a sleep-promoting substance[5] or a sleep-promoting factor[7]. Further it was suggested that one of the constituents of their neuroactive fraction is a peptide-like substance because of its inactivation by pronase treatment[5]. Thus the possibility exists that a peptide may in fact be involved in the physiologic regulation of the sleep-waking cycle.

In this connection it is of interest to note that a number of peptide pituitary hormones are secreted in close relationship to sleep stages. Takahashi *et al.*[9] first described the close relationship between the occurrence of slow wave sleep and a rise in the secretion of growth hormone in man. Subsequent studies have suggested that growth hormone secretion may participate in the regulation of the sleep-waking cycle[1]. In order to elucidate further the underlying neuroendocrine mechanism, a number of animal species have been studied in the search for models of the human pattern. To date, the common laboratory animals have not demonstrated sleep-related growth hormone release under ordinary laboratory conditions. However Takahashi *et al.* have been successful in developing a device for automatic enforced wakefulness, by which sleep-related growth hormone secretion can be produced in dogs.

In addition to involvement in the regulation of sleep, sleep-related growth hormone may be involved in the brain protein synthesis thought to occur during sleep. A possible involvement of protein synthesis in sleep and particularly in REM sleep has been suggested by Oswald[6]. He also proposed that REM sleep is a non-specific indication of many forms of synthesis within cerebral neurons. The results of Matsumoto *et al.* support this proposal. They showed that the long-lasting complete suppression of REM sleep occurred in rats after intraventricular administration of cycloheximide, a protein synthesis inhibitor. They have suggested that cycloheximide inhibits the synthesis of receptor protein but does not decrease the neurotransmitter pool, because DOPA fails to prevent the suppression of REM sleep by heximide.

Further studies of the central effect of the peptide as well as growth hormone may reveal a basic sleep mechanism due to a non-amine sleep factor.

References

1. Drucker-Colin, R.R., Spanis, C.W., Hunyadi, J., Sassin J.F. and McGaugh, J.L., Growth hormone effects on sleep and wakefulness in the rat, *Neuroendocrinology*, 18 (1975) 1–8.
2. Falk, B., Hillarp, N. A., Thieme, G. and Torp, A., Fluorescence of catecholamines and related compounds condensed with formaldehyde, *J. Histochem. Cytochem.*, 10 (1962) 384-354
3. Jouvet, M., The role of monoamines and acetylcholine-containing neurons in the regulation of the sleep-waking cycle, *Ergeb. Physiol.*, 64 (1972) 166–307.
4. Monnier, M., Dudler, L., Gachter, R., Maier, P.F., Tobler, H.J. and Schoenenberger, G.A., The delta sleep inducing peptide (DSIP). Comparative properties of the original and synthetic nonapeptide, *Experientia*, 33 (1977) 548–552.
5. Nagasaki, H., Iriki, M., Inoue, S. and Uchizono, K., The presence of a sleep-promoting substance in the brain of sleep-deprived rats, *Proc. Japan Acad.*, 50 (1974) 241–246.
6. Oswald, I., Human brain protein, drugs and dreams, *Nature (Lond.)*, 223: (1964) 893–897.
7. Pappenheimer, J.R., Koski, G., Fence, V., Karnousky, M.L. and Krueger, J., Extraction of sleep-promoting factor S from cerebrospinal fluid and from brains of sleep-deprived animals, *J. Neurophysiol.*, 38 (1975) 1299–1311.
8. Schoenenberger, G.A., Gneni, L.B., Monnior, M. and Hatt, A.M., Humoral transmission of Sleep VII. Isolation and physical chemical characterization of the "sleep-inducing factor delta", *Pflügers Arch. ges. Physiol.*, 338 (1972) 1–17.
9. Takahashi, Y., Kipnis, D.M. and Daughaday, W.H., Growth hormone secretion during sleep, *J. clin. Invest.*, 47 (1968) 2079–2090.
10. Ungerstedt, U., Stereotaxic mapping of the monoamine pathways in the rat brain, *Acta physiol. scand. Supp.* 367 (1971) 1–48.

Neuroendocrine regulation and sexual differentiation of lordosis behavior in rats

YASUMASA ARAI, KOREHITO YAMANOUCHI AND AKIRA MATSUMOTO

Department of Anatomy, Juntendo University School of Medicine,
Bunkyo-ku, Tokyo, 113, Japan.

Summary

Lordosis is the most typical sexual behavior in female rats. This behavior is dependent on the blood levels of ovarian hormones, especially estrogen. At least two mechanisms are involved in the expression of lordosis at the hypothalamic level. The first one is facilitatory and is thought to be located in the ventromedial hypothalamic region. This region seems to be a primary site of action of estrogen to facilitate lordosis, because many estrogen-concentrating neurons have been detected there. The second one is the dorsal neural inputs coming down anterior to the anterior commissure. These dorsal afferents are considered to exert an inhibitory influence on the hypothalamic lordosis-facilitating mechanism. This inhibitory influence is disinhibited by ovarian hormones. Male rats usually do not show lordosis. This is now believed to be the result of behavioral defeminization caused by neonatal exposure to testicular hormone(s). The mechanism of behavioral defeminization is not really known, but it seems to be associated with the development of a strong inhibitory system against displaying lordosis, which is usually refractory to any priming with ovarian hormones. This may be one of the characteristic features of male rats. In addition, a possible role of sex steroids in the process of organizing adult patterns of sexual behavior is discussed based on recent electron microscopic observations.

Introduction

Sexually receptive female rats display several characteristic types of behavior in the presence of males. The most characteristic behavioral response to mounting by the male is lordosis. In order for the male to achieve penial intromission, the female arches her back so that her head and perineum are elevated, and she moves her tail to one side (Fig. 1). The occurrence of this behavior is under the control of ovarian hormones. In adult females, the display of lordosis is limited to the periovulatory period, during which estrogen and progesterone levels are much higher than in the other stages of the estrous cycle. Ovariectomy abolishes the spontaneous occurrence of lordosis behavior, while treatment with estrogen in combination with progesterone effectively restores it in ovariectomized female rats[6,22]. Several recent lines of evidence derived from direct implantation of estrogen in the brain[5,11,21] and autoradiographic studies of estrogen[40,48] indicate that the influence of ovarian hormone on sexual receptivity is the result of direct action on the neurons located in the preoptic area (POA) and hypothalamus.

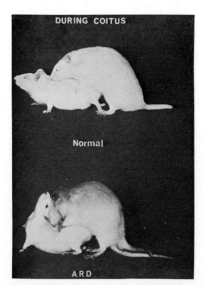
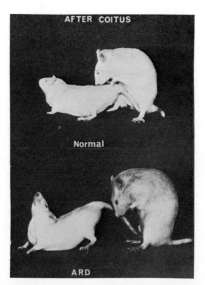

Fig. 1.   Lordosis behavior in an estrogen-progesterone-primed ovariectomized female rat (control). Note the exaggerated lordosis posture in a female which received anterior roof deafferentation (ARD, see Fig. 4) just above the level of the anterior commissure.

In the male rat, lordosis behavior is usually rare after castration in adulthood and injection with the hormone regime of estrogen and progesterone which effectively induces lordosis response in ovariectomized females[15,56]. However, removal of the testes during the first few neonatal days of life produces "feminine males" which display female levels of lordosis behavior; conversely, androgen treatment of neonatal females leads to the inability to show lordosis after sexual maturity. Thus, the inherent programing of sexual differentiation of the rat brain in both sexes is female[2,10,15]. The behavioral defeminization (loss of capacity to show feminine behavior) is dependent on the presence of endogenous or exogenous androgen during a short period after birth. This neonatal presence of androgen has been supposed to suppress the development of the female behavioral center[10,15]. This article is concerned with neuroendocrine regulation of lordosis behavior*. Particular attention is focused on the mechanism involved in behavioral defeminization in male rats. Some recent results of electron microscopic studies carried out to analyze the sexual differentiation of the neuroendocrine apparatus are also presented.

Neuroendocrine regulation of lordosis behavior

Possible sites of action of ovarian steroids and facilitation of lordosis behavior: In his pioneering study, Lisk[21] found that implants of crystalline estradiol contained in 27 and 30 gauge tubings restored lordosis behavior in ovariectomized rats when placed in the POA and anterior hypothalamus (AH). Conversely, electrolytic lesions of the POA–AH were reported to result in impairment of female sexual behavior[20,46]. Based on their earlier findings, it has been accepted

---

* For performance of lordosis, neural structures lower than the hypothalamus are also important. In particular, inputs and outputs at the spinal level contribute to expression of the lordosis reflex. In this article, however, these problems are not discussed.

that estrogen acts at the level of the POA–AH to facilitate lordosis in the female. Although these papers have been influential, there seem to be methodological problems in interpreting their results in terms of recent quantitative measures. For example, in Lisk's paper, animals were considered sexually receptive if they display one lordosis in a 10 min test. At present in many laboratories, including the authors', sexual receptivity is usually measured by a "lordosis quotient" (LQ ratio of lordosis responses to the number of mounts, times 100), which is based on at least 10 mounts. In this manner, one can distinguish between animals that occasionally lordose and those that lordose upon almost every mount.

Other than the POA–AH, the ventromedial hypothalamic region has been proposed as a possible candidate for the site of action of estrogen to facilitate lordosis by Dörner et al.[11] They implanted capillary tubes containing 1 μg of estradiol benzoate (EB) in the ventromedial hypothalamic region or the POA–AH. They found that EB implants in the former region elicited lordosis in all 10 ovariectomized rats, while implantation of EB in the latter induced lordosis in only one of 9 animals. However, in this study too, the behavioral response was evaluated as positive by the display of a single lordosis within a 5 min test.

According to recent autoradiographic studies[40,48], dense regions of estrogen–concentrating neurons are found not only in the POA, but also in the arcuate nucleus (ARC), the ventromedial nucleus (VM) and ventral premammillary nucleus. Considerable numbers of estrogen-concentrating cells are also detectable in the AH. Therefore, the distribution of the estrogen receptor sites alone is not sufficient to determine the site at which estrogen facilitates lordosis behavior. In addition, estrogen can have many functions in the brain; i.e. feedback action on the hypothalamus, food intake and running activity, etc.

Recently, however, more detailed analyses of the hypothalamic substrates for hormonal induction of lordosis in female rats have been published from two different laboratories. Barfield and Chen[5] carefully repeated similar intracerebral implantations of estrogen to verify the results reported by the earlier investigators. They implanted crystalline EB with 27 or 30 gauge hypodermic tubing in various areas of the brain in ovariectomized rats. In the group of animals receiving 27 gauge implants of EB in the hypothalamus, all were receptive. The highest LQ was recorded in the rats with EB implants in the VM region. EB implants in the POA–AH were significantly less effective. This tendency was much clearer in the rats with 30 gauge EB implants. Twenty-four of 30 animals with EB implants in the VM region exhibited lordosis, while only 8 out of 28 females with POA–AH implants showed positive responses. Implants in other areas of the brain resulted in little if any such behavior. From these results, they concluded that estrogen acted at both the VM and POA–AH in the facilitation of lordosis, but that the predominant effect of estrogen was focused on the VM region. This concept that the VM region is a primary site of estrogenic action to facilitate lordosis is consistent with the recent report of Mathews and Edwards[25]. They found that lesions placed in the VM reduced or abolished lordosis behavior in EB–progesterone–primed ovariectomized rats, while damage to the POA–AH was without apparent effect on the display of lordosis. Similar results were also reported by Malsbury et al.[24] on the hamster. These authors[24,25] stated that earlier observations of impairment of lordosis behavior after AH lesions[18,20,46] were probably related to the incidental production of damage to the anterior pole of the VM incurred in lesioning the AH. Cell bodies of the neurons located in the lateral part of the VM must be important for the mechanism of lordosis facilitation, because these neurons have been shown to concentrate estrogen[40,48].

Recently, we performed island isolation of the medial basal hypothalamus (MBH) including the VM to examine the effect of total transection of neural connections between the MBH and the rest of the brain areas by a modification of the technique of Halász and Gorski[17] (Fig. 2). As shown in Fig. 3, the MBH-island was highly effective in suppressing lordosis response in EB-progesterone-primed ovariectomized rats. This is in good agreement with the concept of VM facilitation. However, a half-dome cut placed just behind the suprachiasmatic nucleus (SC) (AD-I) was also effective in eliminating hormonally induced lordosis response. A cut placed dorsal (AD-II) or posterior (AD-III) was without any apparent suppressive effect on sexual receptivity. If these results are considered based on VM facilitation, the effect of AD-I can be ascribed to the interruption of the efferent fibers from the VM (which are related to lordosis facilitation) rather than anterior afferents to the VM. The initial course of the efferents of the VM is thought to run in an anterodorsal direction before descending to the lower brain stem[51]. However, the possibility cannot be excluded that anterior inputs from the AH or other areas are necessary for the VM facilitation of lordosis.

Although damage to the VM itself is not essential for the production of hypothalamic obesity[16], it is well known that lesions in this nucleus produce changes in growth, body weight, reactivity to different diets, diurnal feeding patterns, taste preference, behavioral sensitivity to

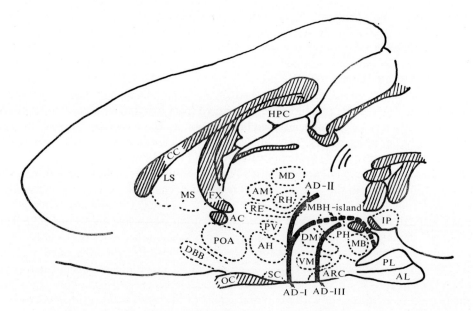

Fig. 2.   Schematic representation of the surgical cuts in the midsagittal section. A Halász knife, having a 1.4 mm lateral and 2.0 mm vertical blade was used to make 4 types of deafferentation. AD-I, anterior deafferentation type I; AD-II, anterior deafferentation type II; AD-III, anterior deafferentation type III; MBH-island, island isolation of the medial basal hypothalamus (AD-I and broken line). AC, anterior commissure; AP, anterior lobe of the pituitary; AM, anteromedial thalamic nucleus; ARC, arcuate nucleus; CC, corpus callosum; DBB, nucleus and diagonal band of Broca; DM, dorsomedial nucleus; FX, fornix. HPC, hippocampus; IP, interpeduncular nucleus; LS, lateral septal nucleus; MB, mammillary body; MD, mediodorsal thalamic nucleus; MS, medial septal nucleus; OC, optic chiasma; PH, posterior hypothalamic nucleus; PL, posterior lobe of pituitary; POA, preoptic area; PV, paraventricular nucleus; RE, nucleus reuniens, RH, nucleus rhomboideus thalami; SC, suprachiasmatic nucleus; VM, ventromedial nucleus.

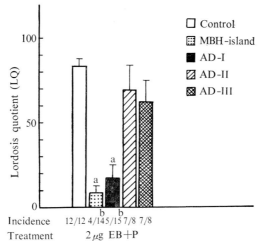

Fig. 3. Effect of hypothalamic deafferentation on the induction of lordosis and LQ in EB-pro-gesterone-primed ovariectomized rats. Behavioral tests were started 4–5 weeks after brain surgery. Each animal was treated with 2 μg of EB for 3 successive days and 0.5 mg of progesterone on the next day. a, p < 0.005 vs. control or AD-II, p < 0.01 vs AD-III (t-test). b, p < 0.005 vs. control, p < 0.05 vs AD-II or AD-III (X^2 test with Yates' correction).

hormones, and the long-term regulation of feeding behavior[35]. However, Malsbury *et al.*[24] stated that there was no correlation between degree of lordosis deficit and degree of weight gain. There-fore, it is probable that there is a dissociation of the two effects.

Inhibitory role of the dorsal inputs to the POA and hypothalamus in regulating lordosis behavior: In addition to the facilitatory mechanism described in the above section, some form of inhibition has been suggested to be involved in the control of display of lordosis behavior. Powers and Valenstein[41] postulated that the medial POA exerted an inhibitory action on the mechanism mediating estrous behavior, based on the results that medial POA lesions reduced the estrogen threshold for induction of lordosis behavior in ovariectomized rats. Recently, Nance *et al.*[36] reported that septal lesions markedly increased the behavioral responsiveness of ovariectomized rats to estrogen. Surgical decortication has been demonstrated to potentiate lordosis response in female rats[6]. These results suggest the possibility that an extrahypothalamic mechanism participat-es in regulating lordosis response.

In our own experiments[60], transection of the dorsal connections with the POA and/or hypo-thalamus was performed to examine the nature of the dorsal influence on the hypothalamic mech-anism facilitating lordosis behavior. As illustrated in Fig. 4, anterior or posterior roof deaffer-entation (ARD or PRD) was done in ovariectomized rats by lowering an L-shaped Halász knife to the level of the anterior commissure and then rotating it 180° antero– or posterohorizontally. In a number of rats, the knife was rotated 360° (RD). Fig. 5 summarizes the incidence of lordosis and LQ for various dosages of EB and progesterone in each group. RD rats showed maximal sexual receptivity in response to low doses of EB (0.5 – 1.0 μg) and 0.5 mg of progesterone, which were not sufficient to induce high levels of lordosis responses in ovariectomized or SD controls. The fact that ARD similarly potentiated lordosis while PRD had no effect indicates that the dorsal neural inputs to the POA and hypothalamus which pass only anterior to the anterior commissure exert an inhibitory influence on the lordosis facilitating mechanism, which is presumably located

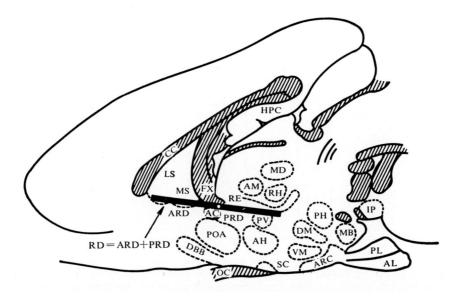

Fig. 4.   Schematic representation of the surgical cuts in midsagittal section. To make a roof cut, an L-shaped Halász knife (2.5 mm horizontal blade) was used. The horizontal black bar just above the anterior commissure indicates roof deafferentation (RD). Anterior roof deafferentation (ARD) is at the anterior part of the RD and posterior roof deafferentation (PRD) is at the posterior part of the RD[60].

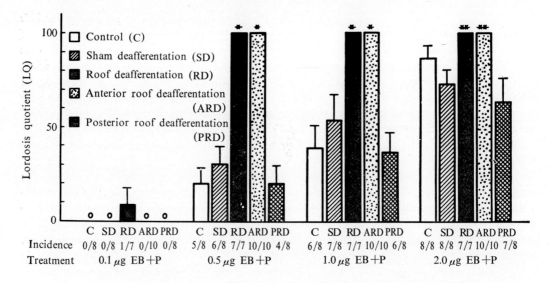

Fig. 5.   Effects of various doses of EB and 0.5 mg of progesterone (P) on the incidence of lordosis and LQ in control and experimental female rats. Each animal was treated with EB for 3 successive days and P on the next day 4–7 hr prior to testing. A series of behavioral tests was performed at 2-week intervals. * $p < 0.005$ vs. control, SD or PRD. ** $p < 0.05$ vs. control, $p < 0.005$ vs. SD or PRD[60].

in the VM region. In addition, the lordosis posture of RD and ARD rats was greatly exaggerated, as shown in Fig. 1. Soliciting behavior (ear-wiggling and hopping) that is often used as an indication of high sexual receptivity was also activated by the RD or ARD (Table 1). Since the POA does not seem to be primarily involved in inhibiting lordosis, the findings of Powers and Valestein can be interpreted as being due to interruption of the inhibitory pathway passing the medial POA.

TABLE 1. Effect of various doses of EB and 0.5 mg of progesterone (P) on the incidence of soliciting behavior (ear-wiggling and hopping) in control and experimental female rats.

Group	No. of rat	0.1 μg EB + P		0.5 μg EB + P		1.0 μg EB + P		2.0 μg EB + P	
		Incidence	(%)	Incidence	(%)	Incidence	(%)	Incidence	(%)
Control	8	0/8	0	1/8	12.5	1/8	12.5	1/8	12.5
Sham deafferentation (SD)	8	0/8	0	2/8	25.0	1/8	12.5	1/8	12.5
Roof deafferentation (RD)	7	0/7	0	7/7	100.0[†]	7/7	100.0[†]	7/7	100.0
Anterior roof deafferentation (ARD)	10	0/10	0	10/10	100.0[†]	10/10	100.0[†]	10/10	100.0
Posterior roof deafferentation (PRD)	8	0/8	0	3/8	37.5	4/8	50.0	1/8	12.5

[†] p $<$ 0.05 vs. control, SD or PRD (X^2-test).
Each animal was treated with EB for 3 successive days and 0.5 mg of P was given on the next day 4–7 hr prior to testing.
A series of behavioral tests was performed at 2-week intervals.

The origin of the inhibitory pathway is still not determined, and it is also not known whether any "relay stations" operate between the origin and the VM lordosis facilitating center. PRD interrupted the hippocampal components such as the postcommissural fornix and medial cortico-hypothalamic tract just above the level of the anterior commissure. These tracts may not participate in the inhibitory pathway, because PRD did not facilitate lordosis. Various degrees of damage were found in the septal area of rats with RD or ARD, and some with SD which exhibited facilitation of lordosis. It may be that the septum is one possible candidate for the tonic inhibitory center of lordosis behavior in female rats. Destruction of the septum has been reported to potentiate lordosis in female rats[36]; conversely, electric stimulation of the septum suppresses the display of lordosis in hamsters[62]. However, surgical decortication, as mentioned before, potentiates lordosis response in female rats[6]. Furthermore, evidence is accumulating suggesting that serotonergic or dopaminergic pathways participate in the lordosis inhibiting mechanism[12,30,63]. Most of these monoaminergic pathways have been demonstrated to ascend from the lower brain stem[13]. Recently, we found that ergocornine, a serotonergic and dopaminergic agonist, effectively suppressed lordosis, but inhibition by ergocornine failed to occur in rats with RD[4]. This suggests that the possible contact point of monoaminergic neurons with the lordosis inhibiting system may be located higher than the level of the RD, on which these ascending monoaminergic afferents may exert a tonic stimulation. Therefore, it seems premature to conclude that the septum can independently exert an inhibitory influence on the mechanism mediating lordosis.

Lordosis behavior in male rats

Table 2 shows the incidence of lordosis in Wistar male rats from 3 different sources[59]. In this series of 4 successive tests, the priming dosages of EB for castrated males were extremely high compared with that for ovariectomized females. However, the occurrence of lordosis was very infrequent in these males. Forty-three out of 51 animals never showed lordosis response throughout the series of behavioral tests. In contrast, 5 out of 8 rats which responded to mounting by the males continued to display lordosis at every test during the series of 4 tests. In the 3 other rats, the display of lordosis was limited to one or two tests (Table 3). Since the number of the animals showing different responses at each test was found to be statistically negligible (McNemar's test, p > 0.1), this consistence of individual responses may indicate the presence of individual differences in lordosis response in these males.

TABLE 2.   Incidence of males with lordosis and LQ during a series of 4 successive behavioral tests.

Group	No. of rats	1st test (50 µg EB + P†)			2nd test (100 µg EB + P)			3rd test (50 µg EB + P)			4th test (10 µg EB + P)		
		Incidence	%	LQ ± S.E.	Incidence	%	LQ ± S.E.	Incidence	%	LQ ± S.E.	Incidence	%	LQ ± S.E.
1	15	3/15[a]	20.0	12.0 ± 6.6	3/15	20.0	12.7 ± 6.8	3/15	20.0	6.0 ± 3.6	2/15	13.3	3.3 ± 2.7
2	19	3/19	15.8	5.8 ± 3.5	4/19	21.0	9.5 ± 5.0	3/19	15.8	4.7 ± 2.9	3/19	15.8	6.1 ± 3.6
3	17	0/17	0	0	0/17	0	0	0/17	0	0	0/17	0	0
Total	51	6/51[b]	11.8	6.7 ± 2.1[c]	7/15	13.7	7.3 ± 2.8	6/51	11.8	3.5 ± 1.5	5/51	9.8	3.2 ± 1.6

† 0.5 mg of progesterone
a: NS at all 4 tests, Group 1 vs. Gr. 2, Group 1 vs, Gr. 3, Group 2 vs. Gr. 3, p > 0.05 (X²-test).
b: NS in comparisons of incidence between any two of the 4 tests, p > 0.1 (X²-test).
c: NS in comparisons of LQ between any two of the 4 tests, p > 0.1 (t-test).
Castrated males were treated with EB daily for 2 days and given progesterone on the third day 4–7 hr prior to testing. Tests were performed at 2-week intervals.

TABLE 3.   Individual behavioral responses during a series of 4 tests.

Lordosis response				No. of rats	%
1st	2nd	3rd	4th		
−	−	−	−	43	84.3
−	+	−	−	1	2.0
−	+	+	−	1	2.0
+	−	−	−	1	2.0
+	+	+	+	5	9.8

+: lordosis,   −: no lordosis
NS in comparisons of response between any two of the 4 tests,
p > 0.1 (McNemar's test).

The results presented in Table 2 are consistent with the general concept that lordosis behavior is rare in adult male rats[15,56]. However, high incidence of lordosis responses has been reported in Long-Evans[9] and Danish Wistar males[47]. Although this discrepancy might be ascribed to some kind of strain difference, the fact that a small number of our Wistar males did show lordosis can be interpreted as indicating that in addition to possible strain difference, more general factors may be involved in the expression of female sexual behavior in these males. The variations in the neonatal testicular activity may be one of the critical factors. In addition, Ward[55,56] reported that male rats exposed to stressful conditions during the fetal stage of development were behaviorally feminized. The influence of changes in the maternal environment must also be considered as one of the critical factors for behavioral differentiation.

In the hamster, it has been reported that normally differentiated adult males can easily be induced to display lordosis by suitable treatment with EB-progesterone[49,52]. This was a surprise to investigators studying male rat behavior. However, it was recently found that administration of additional androgen to newborn male hamsters could suppress lordosis response in adulthood[50,39]. The bisexual behavior of the male hamster may be due to incomplete defeminization which is dependent on conditions of early steroidal deficiency or low sensitivity to testicular hormones in this species.

Behavioral defeminization following neonatal exposure to sex steroids

Importance of central aromatization of androgen: It has been reported that not only androgen but also estrogen given neonatally can induce behavioral defeminization in females[10,15]. The effect of estrogen was considered to be a pharmacological artifact by earlier investigators[15]. However, the question has recently arisen as to whether androgen is the actual organizing substance for male brain differentiation.

A non-aromatizable androgen, 5α-dihydrotestosterone, does not masculinize the brains of female or neonatally castrated male rats[1,7,23]. This steroid is regarded as the most potent androgen for stimulating the differentiation and growth of male reproductive tracts[14,45]. On the other hand, defeminization of female rats by an aromatizable androgen such as testosterone propionate can be inhibited by prior administration of antiestrogen (MER-25)[28] or by treatment with aromatizing enzyme inhibitors[29,54]. These results imply that aromatization to an estrogenic substance may be a prerequisite for androgenization[36]*. This view is supported by the demonstration of an aromatizing enzyme from testosterone or androstendione to estrogen in the neonatal brain[33,57]. However, Kato[19] recently demonstrated that receptors for dihydrotestosterone and testosterone definitely exist in the neonatal rat hypothalamus. Ohno *et al.*[38] reported that Tfm/Y mice showed no evidence of male behavior, although the level of testosterone at the neonatal stage was almost the same as that in normal males. In these mice, androgen receptors are deficient because of an X-linked Tfm mutation. These results suggest that direct action of androgen on the neonatal hypothalamus may coexist with central aromatization in the mechanism of sexual differentiation of the brain.

Mechanism involved in behavioral defeminization in rats: Regarding the mechanism of behavioral defeminization in the male, it has been proposed that the development of the female behavioral center is suppressed by aromatizable androgen or estrogen which is present in neonatal days[10,15]. This center, involved in the facilitation of lordosis, is now suggested to be located in the VM region rather than the POA–AH[5,24,25]. This is consistent with the results of Nadler[31] that the ventromedial arcuate complex is a locus of defeminizing action of androgen in the process of behavioral differentiation. He found that implants of testosterone propionate in this region of the neonatal female brain were most effective in eliminating lordosis behavior in adulthood. It is conceivable that the developmental disturbance in the VM region was caused by local exposure to a high concentration of androgen in these females.

On the other hand, we recently found that surgical transection of the dorsal afferent fibers to the POA and hypothalamus (ARD, Fig. 4) effectively potentiated the display of lordosis in EB-progesterone-primed male rats[58,61]. Again, PRD had no effect in the males (Table 4). This indicates that the dorsal neural inputs exert an inhibitory influence on the lordosis mediating

---

* Since the secretory activity of the neonatal ovary is low during the critical period of behavioral differentiation, endogenous estrogen cannot be a critical factor in defeminization.

mechanism, as demonstrated in the female rat[60]. The finding that surgical removel of these dorsal inhibitory inputs effectively facilitated lordosis indicates that the VM facilitation center for lordosis is left still intact or is only slightly affected by neonatal exposure to endogenous androgen in the male rat. This is difficult to reconcile with the view that neonatal androgen suppresses the development of the hypothalamic lordosis facilitating mechanism.

TABLE 4.   Effect of anterior or posterior roof deafferentation (ARD or PRD) on lordosis behavior in male rats treated with 2 μg of EB daily for 3 days with or without 0.5 mg of progesterone (P) on the day of test.

Group	No. of rats	2.0 μg EB + P			2.0 μg EB only		
		Incidence	(%)	LQ ± S.E.	Incidence	(%)	LQ ± S.E.
Control	8	1/8	12.5	5.0 ± 5.0	1/8	12.5	2.5 ± 2.5
ARD sham	8	2/8	25.0	20.0 ± 13.2	2/8	25.0	17.5 ± 12.1
ARD	10	10/10	100.0[a]	89.0 ± 4.8[b]	9/10	90.0[c]	68.9 ± 14.2[d]
PRD	7	0/7	0.0	0.0 ± 0.0	0/7	0.0	0.0 ± 0.0

a: $p < 0.005$ vs. control, ARD sham (X^2-test with Yates' correction).
b: $p < 0.005$ vs. control, ARD sham (t-test).
c: $p < 0.005$ vs. control, $p < 0.025$ vs. ARD sham (X^2-test with Yates' correction).
d: $p < 0.005$ vs. control, $p < 0.01$ vs. ARD sham (t-test).
The control vs. ARD sham was not significant in any case.

In normally differentiated adult male rats, behavioral defeminization seems to be associated with the development of a strong inhibitory system for lordosis, which is usually refractory to any hormonal conditioning, because the inhibition could not be released without surgical treatment. This may be one of the characteristic features of the male rat. In female rats, disinhibition of the system occurs readily following exposure to ovarian hormones. Thus, it is highly probably that the defeminizing action of aromatizable androgen or estrogen is exerted on the neural structure, presumably located higher than the level of the ARD, and stimulates the development of the lordosis inhibiting system in the male rat.

A possible organizing action of sex steroids on the neural substrates in sexual differentiation: Recently, we studied the fine structures of the arcuate nucleus (ARC), which is one of the integrative neuroendocrine stations[3,26]. As shown in Fig. 6, the neurons and the neuropil of this nucleus are morphologically undeveloped at neonatal age. The neuropil is characterized by the presence of various degrees of extracellular space and, in particular, the synapse formation of this nucleus is in an extremely immature state. A similar situation has also been reported for the neuropil of the POA[44] and the VM[32]. From these results, we might speculate that the neuropil environment of these neural substrates in neonatal rats possesses a great deal of plasticity to the organizing action of neonatal sex steroids. The neural circuit networks for operating postpubertal neuroendocrine regulation or mediating sexual behavior do not seem to be established at this period. Fig. 7 illustrates postnatal developmental changes in a number of synapses in the ARC of female rats. When EB was given neonatally, the appearance of the neuropil matrix was considerably modified[3]. Axons and dendrites were packed rather tightly in the neuropil and the extracellular space was reduced compared with the controls. Furthermore, treatment of female rats with EB during the first 30 days of life resulted in more than twice the number of axodendritic synapses compared to controls at 31 days of age (Fig. 8), and the number of axodendritic synapses of these estrogenized prepubertal rats was almost comparable to that of adult rats[3,27]. This suggests that estrogen given neonatally may stimulate afferent axonal growth, terminal arborization and/or dendritic differen-

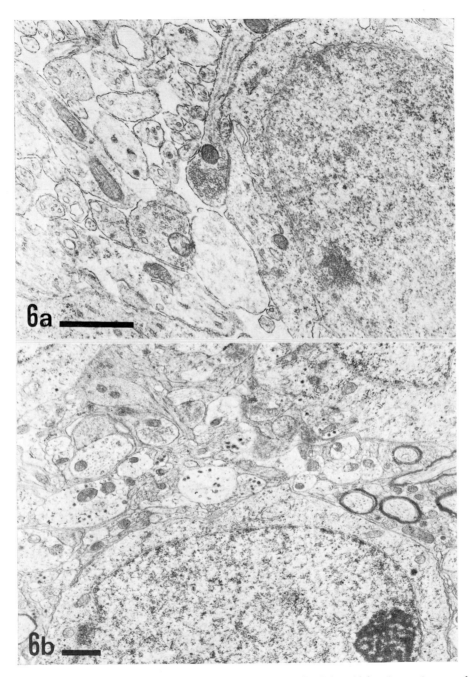

Fig. 6. (a) Cell bodies and neuropil in the arcuate nucleus of a 5-day-old female rat. Axons and dendrites are loosely packed in the neuropil. Note the larger extracellular space at this stage. x 20,000. The scale in each figure represents 1 μm. (b) Cell bodies and neuropil and the arcuate nucleus of a 150-day-old female rat. x 10,600.

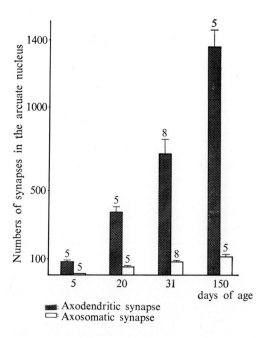

Fig. 7. Developmental changes in a number of axodendritic and axosomatic synapses of the arcuate nucleus. Numbers of synapses per field of 18,000 sq. μm in the middle level of the nucleus are presented. The vertical bars indicate S.E.M. values. Numbers at the tops of bars indicate the numbers of rats counted.

tiation, and it may have a facilitatory effect on the early postnatal organization of synaptic connections in the ARC. The fact that EB did not increase the number of axosomatic synapses in the ARC suggests that the synaptogenic effect of estrogen may be rather specific to particular afferent systems. In this connection the recent findings of Toran-Allerand[53] are of interest, i.e., that the proliferation of neuronal processes of explants from newborn mouse preoptic hypothalamic tissues was markedly accelerated by the addition of estradiol or testosterone to the culture medium. If sex steroids act on the developing hypothalamic neural substrates as a growth promoting factor, how may they participate in the process of sexual differentiation of the brain? In the presence of aromatizable androgen or estrogen, the growth rates of neurons which are going to participate in the regulatory mechanisms of sexual behavior may be influenced by whether or not they contain sufficient receptors for these steroids. It is possible that axons of sex steroid-sensitive neurons grow more rapidly and reach the target neurons earlier than those of sex steroid-insensitive neurons. Since the space for sites of synaptic contact seems to be limited, a kind of selection phenomenon of synaptic connections may be produced by the difference in responsiveness to sex steroids during the process of neural circuit formation at an early postnatal age. This may result in sex difference in the mode of termination of the afferent fibers of the endocrine hypothalamus. In this context, it is of great interest to consider the findings of Raisman and Field[42,43]. They found a sex difference in the mode of termination of the afferent fibers in the POA. This sexual dimorphism in the neuropil of the dorsomedial POA could be modified by neonatal androgen injection into female rats or by neonatal castration of male rats. In order to examine whether this sex difference could reflect a functional difference in the neuroendocrine mechanisms, they studied the effect of destruction of this sexually differentiated dorsomedial POA. Although they recognized an acute blockage of ovulation and high incidence of pseudopregnancy following lesion, lesions in this sexually dimorphic area did not result in long-term failure of ovulation[8]. Recently, Nance et al[37].

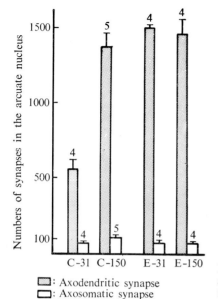

Fig. 8. Numbers of axodendritic and axosomatic synapses in the arcuate nucleus in estrogenized and control rats. E-31 and E-150 indicate estrogenized rats sacrificed at 31 and 150 days of age.

□ : Axodendritic synapse
▢ : Axosomatic synapse

demonstrated that small lesions restricted to the dorsomedial POA of female rats produced a marked increase in lordosis behavior and only marginal effects on ovarian function. This potentiation of lordosis response by dorsomedial POA lesions can be related to the removal of the dorsal inhibitory inputs[58,60,61]. It is still not clear whether damage to the neurons of this area or the fibers which pass through this area is responsible for this. It is of interest to speculate that the synaptic connections in this area play some role in the lordosis inhibiting system as a relay station to the VM facilitation center, because synaptic connections in this area have been shown to be highly plastic to neonatal androgen[42,43]. This might account for the sex difference in the degree of inhibition of the VM facilitation of lordosis. A more detailed study is required to elucidate this point.

REFERENCES

1. Arai, Y., Effect of 5α-dihydrotestosterone on differentiation of masculine pattern of the brain in the rat, *Endocrin. japon.*, 19 (1972) 389–393.
2. Arai, Y., Sexual differentiation and development of the hypothalamus and steroid-induced sterility. In K. Yagi and S. Yoshida (Eds.), *Neuroendocrine Control*, University of Tokyo Press, Tokyo, 1973, pp. 27–55.
3. Arai, Y. and Matsumoto, A., Synapse formation of the hypothalamic arcuate nucleus during postnatal development in the female rat and its modification by neonatal estrogen treatment, *Psychoneuroendocrinology*, 3 (1978) 31–45.
4. Arai, Y. Yamanouchi, K. and Suzuki, Y., Inhibition of lordosis response by ergocornine in estrogen-progesterone primed ovariectomized rats, *Proc. 5th Int. Congr. Endocrin.*, (1976) 91.
5. Barfield, R.J. and Chen, J.J., Activation of estrous behavior in ovariectomized rats by intracerebral implants of estradiol benzoate, *Endocrinology*, 101 (1977) 1716–1725.
6. Beach, F.A., Cerebral and hormonal control of reflexive mechanisms involved in copulatory behavior, *Physiol. Rev.*, 47 (1967) 289–316.
7. Brown-Grant, K., Munck, A., Naftolin, F. and Sherwood, M.R., The effect of the administration of testosterone propionate alone or with phenobarbitone and of testosterone metabolites to neonatal female rats, *Horm. Behav.*, 2 (1971) 173–182.

8. Brown-Grant, K., Murray, M.A.F., Raisman, G. and Sood, M.C., Reproductive function in male and female rats following extra- and intra-hypothalamic lesion, *Proc. Roy. Soc. Lond. B.*, 198 (1977) 267–278.

9. Davidson, J.M., Effects of estrogen on the sexual behavior of male rats, *Endocrinology*, 84 (1969) 1365–1372.

10. Dörner, G., *Hormones and brain differentiation*, Elsevier, Amsterdam, 1976.

11. Dörner, G., Döcke, F. and Moustafa, S., Differential localization of a male and female hypothalamic mating centre, *J. Reprod. Fert.*, 17 (1968) 583–586.

12. Everitt, B.J., Fuxe, K., Hökfelt, T. and Jonsson, G., Role of monoamines in the control by hormones of sexual receptivity in the female rat, *J. comp. Physiol. Psychol.*, 89 (1975) 556–572.

13. Fuxe, K., Hökfelt, T. and Ungerstedt, U., Morphological and functional aspects of central monoamine neurons, *Int. Rev. Neurobiol.*, 13 (1970) 93–126.

14. Goldman, A.S. and Baker, M.K., Androgenicity in the rat fetus of metabolites of testosterone and antagonism by cyproterone acetate, *Endocrinology*, 89 (1971) 276–280.

15. Gorski, R.A., Gonadal hormones and the perinatal development of neuroendocrine function. In L. Martini and W.F. Ganong (Eds.), *Frontiers in Neuroendocrinology, 1971*, Oxford University Press, New York, 1971, pp. 237–290.

16. Grossman, S.P., Role of the hypothalamus in the regulation of food and water intake, *Psychol. Rev.*, 82 (1975) 200–224.

17. Halász, B. and Gorski, R.A., Gonadotrophic hormone secretion in female rats after partial or total interruption of neural afferents to the medial basal hypothalamus, *Endocrinology*, 80 (1967) 608–622.

18. Herndon, J.G. and Neill, D.B., Amphetamine reversal of sexual impairment following anterior hypothalamic lesions in female rats, *Pharmacol. Biochem. Behav.*, 1 (1973) 285–288.

19. Kato, J., Cytosol and nuclear receptors for 5α-dihydrotestosterone and testosterone in the hypothalamus and hypophysis, and testosterone receptors isolated from neonatal female rat hypothalamus, *J. Steroid Biochem.*, 7 (1976) 1179–1187.

20. Law, O.T. and Meagher, W., Hypothalamic lesions and sexual behavior in the female rat, *Science*, 128 (1959) 1626–1627.

21. Lisk, R.D., Diencephalic placement of estradiol and sexual receptivity in the female rat, *Amer. J. Physiol.*, 203 (1962) 493–496.

22. Lisk, R.D., Hormonal regulation of sexual behavior in polyestrous mammals common to the laboratory. In R.O. Greep (Ed.), *Handbook of Physiology, Sect. 7, Vol. II*, Williams and Wilkins, Baltimore, 1973, pp. 223–260.

23. Luttge, W.G. and Whalen R.E., Dihydrotestosterone, androstenedione, testosterone: comparative effectiveness in masculinizing and defeminizing reproductive systems in male and female rats, *Horm. Behav.*, 1 (1970) 265–281.

24. Malsbury, C.W., Kow, L.-M. and Pfaff, D.W., Effects of medial hypothalamic lesions on the lordosis response and other behaviors in female golden hamsters, *Physiol. Behav.*, 19 (1977) 223–237.

25. Mathews, D. and Edwards, D.A., Involvement of the ventromedial and anterior hypothalamic nuclei in the hormonal induction of receptivity in the female rat, *Physiol. Behav.*, 19 (1977) 319–326.

26. Matsumoto, A. and Arai, Y., Developmental changes in synaptic formation in the hypothalamic arcuate nucleus of female rats, *Cell Tiss. Res.*, 169 (1976) 143–156.

27. Matsumoto, A. and Arai, Y., Effect of estrogen on early postnatal development of synaptic formation in the hypothalamic arcuate nucleus of female rats, *Neurosci. Lett.*, 2 (1976) 79–82.

28. McDonald, P.G. and Doughty, C., Inhibition of androgen-sterilization in the female rat by administration of an antioestrogen, *J. Endocrin.*, 55 (1972) 455–456.

29. McEwen, B.S., Lieberburg, I., Chaptal, C. and Krey, L.C., Aromatization: important for sexual differentiation of the neonatal rat brain, *Horm. Behav.*, 9 (1977) 249–263.

30. Meyerson, B.J. and Lewander, T., Serotonin synthesis inhibition and estrous behavior in female rats, *Life Sci.*, 9 (1970) 661–671.

31. Nadler, R.D., Intrahypothalamic exploration of androgen-sensitive brain loci in neonatal female rats. *Trans. N.Y. Acad. Sci., Ser. II*, 34 (1972) 572–581.

32. Naftolin, F. and Brawer, J.R., Sex hormones as growth promoting factors for the endocrine hypothalamus, *J. Steroid Biochem.*, 8 (1977) 339–343.

33. Naftolin, F., Ryan, K.J. and Petro, Z., Aromatization of androstenedione by the anterior hypothalamus of adult male and female rats, *Endocrinology*, 90 (1972) 295–298.

34. Naftolin, F., Ryan, K., Davies, I., Reddy, V., Flores, F., Petro, Z., Kuhn, M., White, R.J., Takaoka, Y. and Wolin, L., The formation of estrogens by central neuroendocrine tissues, *Recent Progr. Horm. Res.* 31 (1975) 295–319.

35. Nance, D.M., Sex differences in the hypothalamic regulation of feeding behavior in the rat. In A.H. Riesen and R.F. Thompson (Eds.), *Advances in Psychobiology, Vol. 3*, John Wiley, New York, 1976, pp. 75–123.

36. Nance, D.M., Shryne, N.J. and Gorski, R.A., Effects of septal lesion on behavioral sensitivity of female rats to gonadal hormones, *Horm. Behav.*, 6 (1975) 59–64.

37. Nance, D.M., Christensen, L.W., Shryne, J.E. and Gorski, R.A., Modifications in gonadotropin control and reproductive behavior in the female rat by hypothalamic and preoptic lesions, *Brain Res. Bull.*, 2 (1977) 307–312.
38. Ohno, S., Geller. L.N. and Young Lai, E.V., Tmf mutation and masculinization versus feminization of the mouse central nervous system, *Cell*, 3 (1974) 235–242.
39. Payne, A.P., A comparison of the effects of neonatally administered testosterone, testosterone propionate and dihydrotestosterone on aggressive and sexual behaviour in the female golden hamster, *J. Endocrin.*, 69 (1976) 23–31.
40. Pfaff, D. and Keiner, M., Atlas of estradiol-concentrating cell in the central nervous system of the female rat, *J. comp. Neurol.*, 151 (1973) 121–158.
41. Powers, B. and Valenstein, E.S., Sexual receptivity: facilitation by medial preoptic lesions in female rats, *Science*, 175 (1972) 1003–1005.
42. Raisman, G. and Field, P.M., Sexual dimorphism in the preoptic area of the rat, *Science*, 173 (1971) 731–733.
43. Raisman, G. and Field, P.M., Sexual dimorphism in the neuropil of the preoptic area of the rat and its dependence on neonatal androgen, *Brain Research*, 54 (1973) 1–29.
44. Reier, P.J., Cullen, M.J. Froelich, J.S. and Rothchild, I., The ultrastructure of the developing medial preoptic nucleus in the postnatal rat, *Brain Research*, 122 (1977) 415–436.
45. Schultz, F.M. and Wilson, J.D., Virilization of the Wolffian duct in rat fetus by various androgens, *Endocrinology*, 94 (1974) 979–986.
46. Singer, J.J., Hypothalamic control of male and female sexual behavior in female rats, *J. comp. Physiol. Psychol.*, 66 (1968) 738–742.
47. Södersten, P. and Larsson, K., Lordosis behavior and mounting behavior in male rats: effects of castration and treatment with estradiol benzoate or testosterone propionate, *Physiol. Behav.*, 14 (1975) 159–164.
48. Stumpf, W. E., Estrogen-neurons and estrogen-neuron systems in the periventricular brain, *Amer. J. Anat.*, 129 (1970) 207–217.
49. Swanson, H. H., Effects of castration at birth in hamsters of both sexes on luteinization of ovarian implants, oestrous cycles and sexual behavior, *J. Reprod. Fert.*, 21 (1970) 183–186.
50. Swanson, H. H. and Crossley, D. A., Sexual behaviour in the golden hamster and its modification by neonatal administration of testosterone propionate, In M. Hamburgh and E. J. W. Barrington (Eds.), *Hormones in Development*, Appleton-Century-Crofts, New York, 1970, pp. 677–687.
51. Szentágothai, J., Flerkó, B., Mess, B. and Halász, B., *Hypothalamic control of the anterior pituitary*, Akademiai Kiadó, Budapest, 1968.
52. Tiefer, L. and Johnson, W. A., Female sexual behaviour in male golden hamsters, *J. Endocrin.* 51 (1971) 615–620.
53. Toran-Allerand, C. D., Sex steroids and the development of the newborn mouse hypothalamus and preoptic area *in vitro*: implications for sexual differntiation, *Brain Research.*, 106 (1976) 407–412.
54. Vreeburg, J. T. M., van der Vaart, P. D. M. and van der Schoot, Prevention of central defeminization but not masculinization in male rats by inhibition neonatally of oestrogen biosynthesis, *J. Endocrin.*, 74 (1977) 375–382.
55. Ward, I. L., Prenatal stress feminizes and demasculinizes the behavior of males, *Science*, 175 (1972) 82–84.
56. Ward, I. L., Sexual behavior differentiation: prenatal hormonal and environmental control. In R. C. Friedman, R. M. Richart and L. V. Wiele (Eds.), *Sex Differences in Behavior*, Wiley, New York, 1974, pp. 3–17.
57. Weisz, J. and Gibbs, C., Conversion of testosterone and androstenedione to estrogens *in vitro* by the brain of female rats, *Endocrinology*, 94 (1974) 616–620.
58. Yamanouchi, K. and Arai, Y., Female lordosis pattern in the male rat induced by estrogen and progesterone: effect of interruption of the dorsal inputs to the preoptic area and hypothalamus, *Endocrin. japon.*, 22 (1975) 243–246.
59. Yamanouchi, K. and Arai, Y., Heterotypical sexual behavior in male rats: individual difference in lordosis response, *Endocrin. japon.*, 23 (1976) 179–182.
60. Yamanouchi, K. and Arai, Y., Possible inhibitory role of the dorsal inputs to the preoptic area and hypothalamus in regulating female sexual behavior in the female rat, *Brain Research*, 127 (1977) 296–301.
61. Yamanouchi, K. and Arai, Y., Lordosis behaviour in male rats: effect of deafferentation in the preoptic area and hypothalamus, *J. Endocrin.*, 76 (1978) 381–382.
62. Zasorin, N.L., Malsbury, C.W. and Pfaff, D.W., Suppression of lordosis in the hormone-primed female hamster by electrical stimulation of the septal area, *Physiol. Behav.*, 14 (1975) 595–599.
63. Zemlan, F.P., Ward, I.L., Crowley, W.R. and Margules, D.L., Activation of lordotic reponding in female rats by suppression of serotonergic activity, *Science*, 179 (1973) 1010–1011.

Effect of sequential destruction of amygdala and septum on hypothalamic rage in cats

HISAO MAEDA* AND HIROYUKI NAKAO

*Department of Neuropsychiatry, Faculty of Medicine, Kyushu University,
Higashi-ku, Fukuoka 812, Japan*
** Department of Neuropsychiatry, Saga Medical School,
Nabeshima, Saga 840–01, Japan*

Hypothalamic rage, which is elicited by electrical stimulation of the ventromedial hypothalamic nucleus (VMH), is a well-organized, directed emotional behavior and consists of directed attack, threat responses such as hissing, and autonomic responses such as salivation[3,7]. The thresholds for these responses are markedly lowered by the influence of a barking dog or man's threatening provocation[3,7]. Hypothalamic rage is thus not the "sham rage" proposed by Masserman[6].

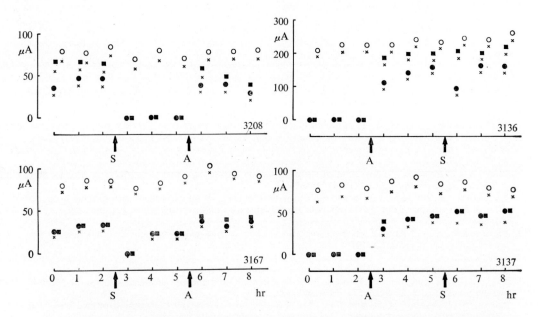

Fig. 1. Threshold changes in 4 cases. Lesions were made at the arrows. In the left two cases, the lesions were made first in the septum and then in the amygdala, and in the reverse order in the right ones. ○, Thresholds for hissing in the non-provocation situation; ● and ■, thresholds for hissing and directed attack, respectively, in the provocation situation; ×, intensities of the hypothalamic stimulation on those trials which were performed one step below each threshold. S, Septal lesion; A, amygdaloid lesion. The figures at the bottom right of each graph indicate the individual case numbers.

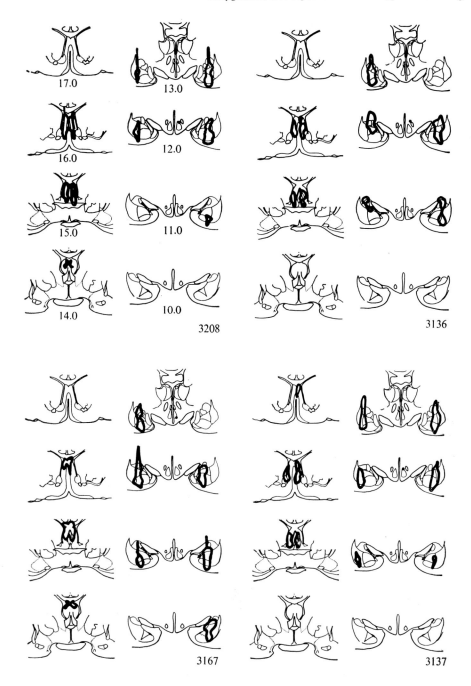

Fig. 2.   Reconstructions of the septal and amygdaloid lesions and sites of electrical stimulation for the cases in Fig. 1 (Jasper and Ajmone-Marsan[1]).

Previous studies have shown that the threshold-lowering influence of a threatening provocation was attenuated by amygdaloid lesions[4] and enhanced by septal lesions[5]. Such effects emerged most markedly immediately after such lesions and diminished gradually thereafter, ultimately returning within a 7–10 day period to the threshold level existing before such lesions.

In the present experiment, the amygdala and septum were destroyed sequentially at 3 hr intervals to clarify the relationship between the two regions. Thirty-four adult cats were used. The thresholds for hissing and directed attack were measured hourly (9 times altogether) under two situations, i.e., with threatening provocation by an experimenter and without such provocation. The amygdala and septum were destroyed electrolytically using previously implanted electrodes under unanesthetized, freely-moving conditions during the intervals between the 3rd and 4th and between the 6th and 7th threshold measurement sessions. In the 20 cats comprising group 1, the lesions were made first in the septum and then in the amygdala, and in the 14 cats comprising group 2, the lesions were made first in the amygdala and then in the septum. The detailed methods of operation, electrical stimulation, threshold measurement, formation of electrolytic lesions, and histological examination were the same as those described previously[4,5].

Typical threshold changes are shown in Fig. 1: the left two graphs are for group 1 and the right ones for group 2. In the former cases, the thresholds in the provocation situation were markedly reduced to below the control level immediately after the septal lesions and returned to the control level following the amygdaloid lesions. The thresholds in the non-provocation situation showed little change throughout the procedure. In 11 cats, the same threshold change was observed, including 5 cats in which the post-amygdaloid thresholds were elevated above the control level.

In the latter cases, the thresholds in the provocation situation were markedly elevated after the amygdaloid lesions and remained unchanged even following the septal lesions. The same threshold change was observed in 10 cats.

As shown in Fig. 2, approximately the same part of the septum, the lateral septal area, was destroyed in almost all cases.

The present findings coincide in part with the work of King and Meyer[2], and indicate that the amygdala exerts its provocation-contingent facilitatory influence on the VMH independently of septal activity, and that the septum exerts an inhibitory influence on the VMH via the amygdala. The enhancing effect after septal lesions is considered to be a result of disinhibition of amygdaloid function.

References

1. Jasper, H.H. and Ajmone-Marsan, C., *A Stereotaxic Atlas of the Diencephalon of the Cat*, National Research Council of Canada, Ottawa, 1954.
2. King, F.A. and Meyer, P.M., Effects of amygdaloid lesions upon septal hyperemotionality in the rat, *Science*, 128 (1958) 655–656.
3. Maeda, H., Behavioral construction of hypothalamic rage in cats, *Fukuoka Acta med.*, 67 (1976) 364–373 (in Japanese).
4. Maeda, H., Influence of amygdaloid lesions upon electrically elicited hypothalamic rage responses in cats, *Fukuoka Acta med.*, 67 (1976) 374–390 (in Japanese).
5. Maeda, H., Effects of septal lesions on electrically elicited hypothalamic rage response in cats, *Physiol. Behav.*, in press.
6. Masserman, J.H., Is the hypothalamus a center of emotion?, *Psychosom. Med.*, 3 (1941) 3–25.
7. Nakao, H., *Brain Stimulation and Learning. Switch-Off Behavior*, Veb Gustav Fischer Verlag Jena, Jena, 1971, pp. 19–23.

Functional relationship between the frontal cortex and lateral hypothalamus

YUTAKA OOMURA, TAKETOSHI ONO*[1], MASAHIRO OHTA*[2], NOBUAKI SHIMIZU,
HITOSHI KITA AND SHINICHIRO ISHIBASHI

*Department of Physiology, Faculty of Medicine, Kyushu University,
Higashi-ku, Fukuoka 812, Japan*
*[1] Department of Physiology, Faculty of Medicine, Toyama Medical and Pharmaceutical University,
Sugitani, Toyama 930–01, Japan*
*[2]Department of Physiology, Faculty of Dentistry, Kyushu University,
Higashi-ku, Fukuoka 812, Japan*

The frontal cortex (FC) is anatomically connected to the lateral hypothalamic area (LHA) in rats and monkeys[2]. In the rat, mutual monosynaptic connections and functional relations between these centers have been demonstrated by electronmicroscopic and neurophysiological studies[9]. FC stimulation increases the threshold of LHA stimulation and diminishes food intake[8], while lesions of the FC increase bar press activity for food[1]. These studies are in agreement with the observed inhibition of neuronal activity in the LHA when the FC is stimulated[3]. Further, procaine applied to the FC diminishes or stops self-stimulation[7]. These facts indicate that the FC exerts a considerable influence on the LHA in its motivation of feeding behavior.

In acute rat experiments, extracellularly recorded data from stimulation of FC area 10 revealed a highly ordered arrangement of neuronal types within the LHA[6]. One is a functionally oriented distinction in which those LHA neurons which respond in a specific manner to stimulation of the FC tend to group into columns with a dorsoventral direction according to their types of response. In this conformation, neurons having different functions are disposed in such a way that all neurons in one column are of the same functional type, while neurons of different type are in other columns (Fig. 1B). This type of arrangement has been confirmed to be statistically significant[6]. Intersecting these columns orthogonally is a laminar differentiation in which the neurons respond to FC stimuli, according to position in the LHA, changing from an excitation-inhibition sequence in the dorsal half to inhibition alone in the ventral half. Intracellular recordings of LHA neurons also show two response types: one is a driven spike discharge on top of the EPSP and a following IPSP with an antidromic spike occasionally appearing before the EPSP (Fig. 1A: ● Driven type), and the other is an IPSP alone (Fig. 1A :○). The latency of the former EPSP-IPSP type varied with stimulus intensity, while that of the latter IPSP type was fixed even though the stimulus intensity and/or frequency was changed. The amplitudes of both types were changed by shifting of the membrane potentials. A lesion of the rat FC revealed degenerated axon terminals on the LHA dendritic spines[9]. These indicated the monosynaptic pathway for the IPSP of inhibition type neuron. Therefore, this type is designated a Direct inhibition type neuron. The fiber conduction velocity from the FC to the LHA was calculated as approximately 3 m/sec, and 4.5 m/sec from the LHA to the FC. The FC neurons responsible for the Direct inhibition type IPSP may be located in the layer VI where relatively small sized neurons are arrayed.

In chronic monkey experiments, stimulation of the LHA evoked potentials at orbitofrontal cortex (OBF) areas 10 and 11. These were analyzed to be an antidromic spike, and a short nega-

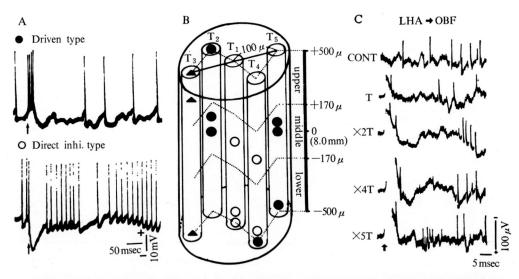

Fig. 1. Rat LHA functional organization (A, B). A, Response patierns— EPSP-IPSP (Driven type) and IPSP alone (Direct inhibition type)— of intracellular recordings from LHA neurons while stimulating FC area 10. B, Columnar organization observed by comparing the response patterns with their respective neuron positions. Responses are grouped according to response patterns. T_1, Direct inhibibition type; T_2 and T_5, driven type; T_3, no response; T_4, mixed. Note that except for T_4, all neurons in each column have the same type of response to FC area 10 stimulation. The distance between each column is 0.1 mm. C, Single spike discharges in OBF (area 11) at control, threshold intensity (T) and 2, 4, and 5 times threshold intensity stimulation (chronic monkey). Arrow: means stimulation applied. T, One antidromic spike followed by extended inhibition. ×2T, Antidromic and orthodromic spikes followed by inhibition longer than in T. In ×4T and ×5T, the first antidromic spike is probably concealed by the stimulus artifact. At ×5T, a second unit appears at 600 impulses/sec[6].

tive and positive wave sequence followed by a long negative wave. Fig. 1C shows the effect of variation of the single pulse stimulation intensity on the unit discharges. The response is an antidromic spike with a fixed and relatively short latency and one excitation spike followed by long-lasting inhibition, the duration of which is related to the stimulus intensity. The spikes which follow the inhibition may correspond to the late long negative wave. At a very high intensity of stimulation, repetitive discharges of high frequency appear during the inhibition period. This type of firing may be the activity of an interneuron responsible for the inhibition. From the latency of the anti- and orthodromic responses, the conduction velocity of the fiber from the OBF to the LHA was estimated as about 74 m/sec, and 12 m/sec from the LHA to the OBF.

These interconnections between the LHA and FC indicate that the hypothalamus can report changes in the organism's internal milieu to the FC. One third of the LHA neurons are known as chemosensitive neurons which can discriminate concentration in the blood composition[4]. Such mutual interrelations between the FC and hypothalamus could be responsible for motivation of feeding behavior[9].

References

1. Manning, F.J., Performance under temporal schedules by monkeys with partial ablations of prefrontal cortex, *Physiol. Behav.*, 11 (1973) 563–569.

2. Nauta, W.J.H., Neural associations of the frontal cortex, *Acta neurobiol. exp.*, 32 (1972) 125–140.
3. Ono, T., Oomura, Y., Sugimori, M., Nakamura, T., Shimizu, N., Kita, H. and Ishibashi, S., Hypothalamic unit activity related to lever pressing and eating in the chronic monkey. In D. Novin, W. Wyrwicka and G. Bray (Eds.), *Hunger: Basic Mechanisms and Clinical Implications*, Raven Press, New York, 1976, pp. 159–170.
4. Oomura, Y., Significance of glucose, insulin, and free fatty acid on the hypothalamic feeding and satiety neurons. In D. Novin, W. Wyrwicka and G. Bray (Eds.), *Hunger: Basic Mechanisms and Clinical Implications*, Raven Press, New York, 1976, pp. 145–157.
5. Oomura, Y., Ono, T., Ohta, M., Nishino, H., Shimizu, N., Ishibashi, S., Kita, H., Sasaki, K., Nicolaïdis, S. and Van Atta, L., Neuronal activities in feeding behavior of chronic monkeys. In Y. Katsuki, M. Sato, S.F. Takagi and Y. Oomura (Eds.), *Food Intake and Chemical Senses*, Tokyo Univ. Press, Tokyo, 1977, pp. 505–524.
6. Oomura, Y. and Takigawa, M., Input-output organization between the frontal cortex and the lateral hypothalamus. In T. Desiraju (Ed.), *Mechanisms in Transmission of Signals for Conscious Behaviour*, Elsevier, Amsterdam, 1976, pp. 163–192.
7. Rolls, E.T. and Cooper, S.J., Anesthetization and stimulation of the sulcal prefrontal cortex and brain-stimulation reward, *Physiol. Behav.*, 12 (1974) 563–671.
8. Siegel, J. and Wang, R.Y., Electroencephalographic, behavioral, and single-unit effects produced by stimulation of forebrain inhibitory structures in cats, *Exp. Neurol.*, 42 (1974) 28–50.
9. Yamamoto, T. and Shibata, Y., Fronto-hypothalamic fiber connection in the rat, *Pharmacol. Biochem. Behav.*, *Suppl. 1*, 3 (1975) 15–22.

Lateral hypothalamus—motor cortex relations in the chronic monkey

TAKETOSHI ONO, YUTAKA OOMURA*[1] HITOO NISHINO, MASAHIRO OHTA*[2],
KAZUO SASAKI, NOBUAKI SHIMIZU*[1] AND HITOSHI KITA*[1]

*Department of Physiology, Faculty of Medicine, Toyama Medical and Pharmaceutical University,
Sugitani, Toyama 930-01, Japan.*
*[1]Department of Physiology, Faculty of Medicine, Kyushu University,
Higashi-ku, Fukuoka 812, Japan*
*[2]Department of Physiology, Faculty of Dentistry, Kyushu University,
Higashi-ku, Fukuoka 812, Japan*

This report gives electrophysiological evidence for direct mutual connections between the feeding center, the lateral hypothalamus (LHA), and the motor cortex (MC). It may also help to explain the temporal course of activity and neural emission observed in certain behavioral circumstances[2,3].

Six 3–5 kg macaque monkeys (*Macaca mulata*) were used. All experiments were performed on unanesthetized animals just prior to bar-press feeding experiments[2,3]. Stimulating electrodes were implanted bilaterally in the pyramidal tracts (PT) of all 6 animals, in the left LHA in 3, and over the hand area of the MC in the other 3. Unit discharges were recorded from the left LHA or MC while stimulating the PT of either side and the ipsilateral MC or LHA.

Of 26 LHA neurons tested for response to MC stimulation, 8 responded with the following sequence (Fig. 1A): antidromic excitation with a latency of 2.9 msec, about 140 msec of extended inhibition, and subsequent multiple excitation. Five others responded in a similar manner, but without the antidromic excitation. A poststimulus time histogram of summed responses and its cumulative frequency distribution are shown in Figs. 1B and C, respectively. The dashed line in C represents an extension of the prestimulation discharge rate. The data plotted in B and C indicate average latency of 2.7 msec for the initial antidromic excitation and 116 msec for the final excitation. The conduction velocity of the projecting fibers from LHA to MC averaged 14 m/sec over the estimated 40 mm distance.

LHA stimulation produced three different types of response in 20 PT neurons tested in the MC: 4 responded with an antidromic spike at 0.5 msec, 4 with the antidromic spike followed by 25 msec of inhibition, and 6 with the antidromic spike followed by orthodromic activity having a further latency of about 3.6 msec. Six neurons showed no significant response. The three types of response are illustrated in Figs. E, F, and G, respectively. A typical PT neuron in the MC responded to PT stimulation as shown in D, and to LHA stimulation as shown in E. No non-PT neuron exhibited a consistent, significant response with a relatively short latency, to LHA stimulation.

These results, i.e., the consistent antidromic responses and the less frequent but distinctly evident orthodromic action, establish the existence of direct neuronal connections in both directions between the LHA and MC. Late excitation after intense inhibition might be due to either rebound or polysynaptic paths. The existence of direct connections from the LHA to the MC has been demonstrated in the monkey using the horseradish peroxidase method[1]. Our recent studies

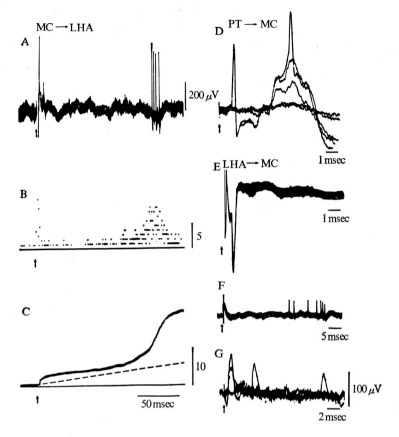

Fig. 1. Typical stimulation responses. A, Single antidromic LHA spike followed by inhibition and late excitation after MC stimulation. B, Poststimulus time histogram of summed responses for 50 stimuli at 1 Hz; total discharges per 0.5 msec over a 200 msec period for 50 stimuli; vert. bar, 5 discharges. C, Cumulative frequency distribution of responses in B; dashed line, extension of the prestimulus cumulative slope; vert. bar, average of 10 counts per single response. Stimuli were applied at the arrows. D, PT neuron responses in MC to stimulation of PT. The initial antidromic spike, absent in the case of non-PT neurons, shows this to be a PT neuron. E. F, G, MC responses to LHA stimulation. E, The same neuron as in D but LHA stimulation produces antidromic spike (upward) with after-potential (downward). F, Antidromic spike followed by inhibition and excitation. G, The same as E, but plus orthodromic spike.

with horseradish peroxidase have also revealed direct anatomical connections in the opposite direction, at least in some MC areas.

The above results indicate that LHA neurons which may initiate feeding motivation intercommunicate with MC neurons which innervate feeding behavior effectors.

REFERENCES

1. Kievit, J. and Kuypers, H.G.J.M., Subcortical afferents to the frontal lobe in the rhesus monkey studied by mean of retrograde horseradish peroxidase transport, *Brain Research*, 85 (1975) 261–266.
2. Ono, T., Oomura, Y., Sugimori, M., Nakamura, T., Shimizu, N., Kita, H. and Ishibashi, S., Hypothalamic unit

activity related to lever pressing and eating in the chronic monkey, In D. Novin, W. Wyrwicka and G.A. Bray (Eds.), *Hunger: Basic Mechanisms and Clinical Implications,* Raven Press, New York, 1976, pp. 159–170.

3. Oomura, Y., Ono, T., Ohta, M., Nishino, H., Shimizu, N., Ishibashi, S., Kita, H., Sasaki, K., Nicolaidis, S. and Van Atta. L., Neuronal activities in feeding behavior of chronic monkeys, In Y. Katsuki, M. Sato, S.F. Takagi and Y. Oomura (Eds.). *Food Intake and Chemical Senses*, Tokyo Univ. Press, Tokyo, 1977, pp. 505–524.

Semi-automatic measurements of neuronal processes by a computer controlled optical microscope

MASAO NAKAMURA, KEIJI TANIGUCHI[*1], KOOZO TSUCHIDA[*1], YUTAKA OOMURA[*2], AND NOBUAKI SHIMIZU[*2]

Department of Information Science, Faculty of Engineering, Fukui University, Bunkyo, Fukui 910, Japan
*[*1]Department of Electronics, Faculty of Engineering, Fukui University, Bunkyo, Fukui 910, Japan*
*[*2]Department of Physiology, School of Medicine, Kyushu University, Higashi-ku, Fukuoka 812, Japan*

A computer controlled optical microscope has been developed[1] for measuring the three dimensional coordinates of sampling points along neuronal processes in Golgi-stained preparations. It differs from similar systems[2,3] in that no separate coordinate digitizer is required other than a monitor TV and stepping motors.

A block diagram of the whole system is given in Fig. 1. The microscope image can be viewed either directly with the eye or through a TV camera. The display control permits the display of characters designated by either the computer or the keyboard on the TV receiver in one line up to 32 characters. It also controls the display of a cross cursor (consisting of a horizontal and vertical line) on the TV receiver in response to key maneuvering on the control desk by an operator.

The cursor is used to pinpoint a sampling point on the picture frame. When an operator presses a request key, the computer responds to it by first reading the cursor position and then commanding the interface circuitry to send pulses to stepping motors attached to the microscope stage to bring the sampling point precisely to the frame center on the TV receiver. When this latter step is completed, the operator keys in a code to identify the sampling point and requests the computer to read the code and stage position data. In this way, data acquisition proceeds interactively between the operator and computer.

Automatic focusing of the microscope has not been dealt with in the references[2,3] cited. To implement it, the gray level information for 16×16 points around the frame center is produced through an A–D converter. This information is then fed into the computer, and the gray level gradient across a dendrite or axon is computed and used as a parameter for optimizing the vertical position of the microscope stage.

The system has been used for preliminary tracking of neuronal processes in the lateral hypothalamic area of a young cat. The number of cells so far examined is about 50. Approximately 10 days of routine work are required for handling this number of cells. However, it is not always possible to trace all processes of each cell due to detrimental situations such as imperfection in the preparation or intermingling of processes from other cells. For closer scrutiny, however, a portion in question can be repeatedly brought into view by computer control.

The way in which various neuronal processes branch out from a cell could be readily grasped by making perspective projections of the stereoscopic neuronal structure. This has not in fact been done yet, but with a simple program, it has been possible to display plane projections in arbitrary directions on a TEKTRONIX 4010 display. Fig. 2 shows examples obtained from two cells. In the figure, (a) and (c) show normal projections, i.e., those corresponding to the microscope image, while (b) and (d) show vertical projections of the same two cells, respectively.

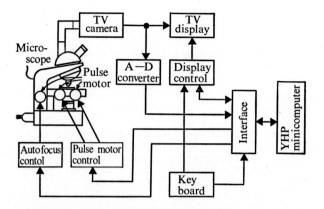

Fig. 1.   Block diagram of the cell process tracking system.

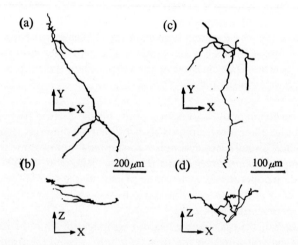

Fig. 2.   Plane projections of neuronal processes of two cells sampled from the lateral hypothalamic area of a young cat.

Data are at present being analyzed to ascertain differences in branching features of processes according to cell type. It is hoped that neuronal connections will eventually be found by extending this work.

REFERENCES

1. Oomura, Y., Nakamura, M., Taniguchi, K. and Shimizu, N., Design of a semi-automatic measurement system for interconnections of neurons, *J. Inst. Electro. Commun. Eng. Japan,* 60-D (1977)1117–1118 (in Japanese).
2. Llinas, R. and Hillman, D.E., A multipurpose tridimensional reconstruction computer system for neuroanatomy. In M. Santini (Ed.), *Golgi Centennial Symposium Proceedings,* Raven Press, New York, 1975, pp. 519–528.
3. Lindsay, R.D. (Ed.), *Computer Analysis of Neuronal Structures,* Plenum Press, New York, 1977.

Electrophysiological studies on the depolarization shift of hippocampal pyramidal cells *in vitro*

NOBUAKI HORI AND NOBUO KATSUDA

Department of Pharmacology, Faculty of Dentistry, Kyushu University,
Higashi-ku, Fukuoka 812, Japan

Many investigators have described the "depolarization shift" (DS) associated with interictal epileptic spikes[1,2,4]. The present study concerns the generation mechanism of DS in guinea pig hippocampal pyramidal cells *in vitro*. The procedures for preparation, incubation and recording described by Yamamoto and McIlwain[5] were used with minor modifications. Slices were perfused with Krebs-Ringer solution, which was replaced by a medium of modified ionic concentrations or containing the convulsant, pentetrazol (PTZ). Evoked responses to single mossy fiber stimuli were recorded intracellularly from pyramidal cells of the CA_3 area or extracellularly from various layers with glass microelectrodes filled with 0.5 M potassium citrate. Pyramidal cells were identified physiologically from the presence of antidromically evoked spike potentials or anatomically by Procion yellow injection into the cell. Moreover, they were usually identifiable by visual observation of the portion of the slice under the microscope during the experiment. The resting membrane potential of the pyramidal cells was around -50 mV in normal Ringer solution.

Mossy fiber stimulations induced IPSPs (5–10 mV, 100–200 msec), presumably mediated by basket cells, during which spontaneous firings were suppressed (Fig. 1A). If PTZ was added to the perfusate at a concentration of 10^{-3} M, 5 min later a DS (20–25 mV, 100–200 msec) was produced by mossy fiber stimulations (0.2–0.5 Hz) on which several abortive spikes were superimposed. Repetitive stimulations at 1 Hz, however, produced short latency (5 msec) spike(s) followed by an almost normal IPSP, or produced an IPSP followed by a delayed DS (Fig. 1B).

The membrane conductance measured by the application of short current pulses (10^{-7}–10^{-8}A) showed no change during the DS except for a slight increase at the initial phase, which coincided in time with the initial phase of the IPSP. Thus, the IPSP was intact but only concealed by a large DS. Also, stimuli during various grades of depolarizing or hyperpolarizing current injections provoked DS of almost unchanged amplitude, i.e., the DS amplitude was independent of the level of the membrane potential. In laminar analysis on the field potentials, the largest and steepest slow negative potential, the time course of which coincided with that of the intracellularly recorded DS, could be obtained at the apical dendritic layer 200–300 μm apart from the pyramidal cell layer. The slow negative potential was clearly different from the primary mossy fiber responses obtained within 100 μm from the pyramidal cell layer in normal Ringer solution. These recordings, therefore, clearly indicated that the DS did not arise at the pyramidal cell soma but resulted from electrotonic spread of the potentials produced at the dendrites into the pyramidal cell body. Thus, it is considered that the DS was not spikes of the apical dendrites; rather, it is likely that the DS results from the summated EPSPs.

To detect the presumed excitatory interneurons responsible for the DS, various layers of the CA_3 area were examined from extracellular recordings. As shown in Fig. 1C and D, specific neurons responding with repetitive firings at 400–500 impulses/sec which were strikingly synchroniz-

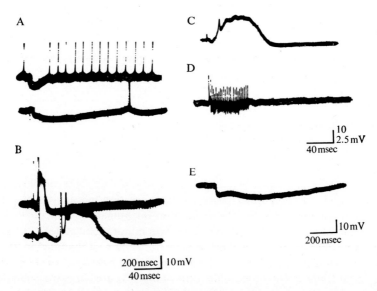

Fig. 1.   Intracellular activities of pyramidal cells in hippocampal slices. A and B: Intracellular responses of a pyramidal cell to mossy fiber stimulation before (A) and after administration of pentetrazol (10 mM) (B). The upper and lower traces show the same responses, the upper being 1/5 the sweep speed of the lower. The stimulus frequency was 0.5 Hz in A and 1 Hz in B. Note the dissociation of the DS comlex, i.e., short latency spike, IPSP and DS envelope (lower record in B) and long-lasting hyperpolarization after the DS envelope (upper record in B). C and D: DS recorded in a pyramidal cell (C) and repetitive firings (about 400 impulses/sec) of a presumed interneuron in the stratum oriens (D). This represents the same preparation under pentetrazol. E: Hyperpolarizations of a pyramidal cell induced by mossy fiber stimulation in normal Ringer solution. Note the step-wise development of the IPSP and long lasting hyperpolarization.

ed with the DS in the same preparation, could be obtained by single mossy fiber stimulations in the stratum oriens. Constancy of discharge rate and amplitude of trains of spikes was noted. This is not observed in the discharge patterns of pyramidal or basket cells. For morphological labeling of these repetitively firing neurons, a new method was introduced using horseradish peroxidase (HRP). The tip of a glass pipette (30–50 μm pore size) was filled with crystalline HRP powder, inserted into the apical dendritic layer approximately 200 μm apart from the pyramidal cell layer, and positioned quietly there. After mossy fiber stimulations at 1 Hz for 7 hr, enzyme uptake by neurons was clearly demonstrated. A few small neurons and 3–5 pyramidal cells could be found histochemically in the stratum oriens. Several fine axons originating from one of the former cells interlaced with the apical dendritic shafts of the latter cells. These small cells, probably interneurons, correspond to those previously reported by Lorente de Nó[3] in silver stained preparations.

It was concluded on the basis of the above data that the DS induced by PTZ in the hippocampal pyramids was generated by powerful activation of the interneurons or at least of neuronal pathways containing these neurons. Recurrent excitatory loops may well be composed of recurrent collaterals of pyramidal cells, excitatory interneurons in the stratum oriens, and their axons which made synapses on the apical dendritic shaft. This positive feedback system could be activated by PTZ.

Another component of the DS complexes was a long lasting hyperpolarization (1–2 sec) after DS envelopes (Fig. 1B, upper record). In some cells, a usual IPSP was followed by a delayed long lasting hyperpolarization in normal Ringer solution (Fig. 1E). Long lasting hyperpolarizations were temperature-dependent and decreased by cooling of the perfusate. They completely disappeared on addition of 2,4–dinitrophenol (10^{-5} M) or ouabain (10^{-6} M). This suggests the presence of certain metabolic mechanisms in their genesis apart from the involvement of synaptic events described by others[1]. The presence of the delayed long lasting hyperpolarization could represent one of the potent inhibitory factors for DS generation.

REFERENCES

1. Ayala, G.F., Dichter, M., Gumit, R.J., Matsumoto, H. and Spencer, W.A., Genesis of epileptic interictal spikes. New knowledge of cortical feedback systems suggests a neurophysiological explanation of brief paroxysms, *Brain Research,* 52 (1973) 1–17.
2. Dichter, M. and Spencer, W.A., Penicillin-induced interictal discharges from the cat hippocampus. II. Mechanisms underlying origin and restriction, *J. Neurophysiol.*, 32 (1969) 663–687.
3. Lorente de Nó. R., Studies on the structure of the cerebral cortex. II. Continuation of the study of the ammonic system, *J. Psychol. Neuroe. (Leipzig),* 46 (1934) 113–177.
4. Prince, D.A., The depolarization shift in "epileptic" neurons, *Exp. Neurol.*, 21 (1968) 467–485.
5. Yamamoto, C. and McIlwain, H., Electrical activities in thin sections from the mammalian brain maintained in chemically-defined media *in vitro, J. Neurochem.*, 13 (1966) 1333-1343.

The laminated organization of the cytoarchitecture of the dog brain in relation to domestication

HIDEO MASAI*[1], KOICHI TAKATSUJI*[1] AND YASUKO SATO*[2]

*[1]Department of Anatomy, Osaka University Medical School,
Kita-ku, Osaka 530, Japan
*[2]Department of Anatomy, Yokohama City University School of Medicine,
Minami-ku, Yokohama 232, Japan

Brain morphology from the viewpoint of domestication has been one of the most important problems in the field of animal husbandry and evolutionary biology. Klatt[7] investigated the external features and weight of dog brains, and Herre[5] and his co-workers carried out a series of important studies on variations of brain patterns in connection with domestication. These studies were concerned with the external shape of the whole brain and the allometry of each brain division, such as the telencephalon, diencephalon, and so on, and areas of the cerebral cortex, but rarely dealt with internal structures, including cytoarchitecture. An attempt was therefore made to discover whether there were variations of laminated structures in the prefrontal cortex and the dorsal lateral geniculate nucleus among dog breeds, since the prefrontal cortex is considered to have an inhibitory function in performance[2] and to be the associative cortex, and the dorsal lateral geniculate nucleus is one of the typical laminated structures of the subcortical nuclei, as well as being a relay station in the pathway of visual information, which may participate in releasing animal behavior.

The breeds used in this study were three adults each of German shepherds and collies as working breeds, beagles as a hound breed, and two Japanese spaniels as a "toy" breed. Each breed shows diversification in both body form and habits. After the animals had been sacrificed by an intravenous overdose of pentobarbital, the gyrus proreus and gyrus orbitalis in the prefrontal cortex and the lateral geniculate body were removed and embedded in celloidin. The prefrontal cortex was sectioned at 25 μm perpendicularly to the cortical surface and the gyri, and the lateral geniculate body was serially sectioned at 25 μm through the frontal, sagittal, and horizontal planes of the diencephalon. The sections were stained by the Nissl method. Those of the lateral geniculate body were alternatively stained by the Heidenhain-Woelcke method. The thickness in the crown part of the gyri of the prefrontal cortex was calculated from photographs taken of the relevant sections.

The prefrontal cortex on the lateral surface of the hemisphere is delimited by the anterior rhinal fissure, the presylvian fissure, and on the medial surface of the hemisphere, by the genual fissure posteriorly (Fig. 1 a,b,c,d). In the shepherd and collie, the two fissures, i.e., the fissura prorea and fissura infraorbitalis, are distinct and the presylvian fissure is greatly deepened. In general, the surface of the prefrontal cortex is greatly expanded in the shepherd and collie, which have long snouts. The Japanese spaniel with its short snout rarely shows any fissures within the prefrontal cortex, and thus the whole surface of the prefrontal cortex is reduced. In the beagle the features of this cortex are intermediate between those of the shepherd-collie breed and the Japanese spaniel. As for cytoarchitecture, layer IV is delimited indistinctly except in the Japanese spaniel. In the crown part of the gyrus proreus and gyrus orbitalis, the ratio of the thickness of the supragranular layers, including the granular layer (layers II–IV), to that of the infragranular layers (layers V–VI) is increased in the shepherd, collie, and beagle, while this ratio is reduced in the Japanese spaniel, as shown in Table 1 and Fig. 1 e,f,g.

Regarding the dorsal lateral geniculate nucleus, grossly the posterolateral region of the thalamus containing this nucleus is swollen and extended posteriorly beyond the level of the habenular commissure in the shepherd, collie, and beagle. In contrast, the nucleus in the Japanese

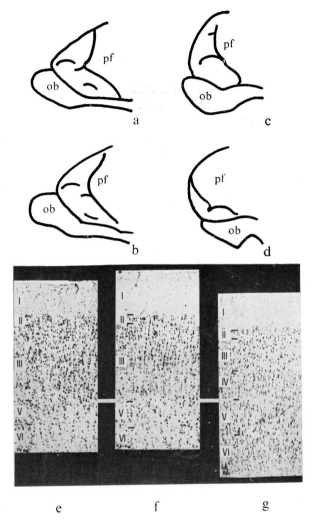

Fig. 1. Upper: Lateral view of the prefrontal cortex. ob, Olfactory bulb; pf, presylvian fissure; a, German shepherd; b, collie; c, beagle; d, Japanese spaniel. In the shepherd and the collie, the fissura prorea (upper) and the fissura infraorbitalis (lower) can be seen. Lower: Cytoarchitecture of the gyrus proreus. Nissl staining. The Roman numerals show cortical layers; for comparison the boundary between layer III/IV and layer V is placed at the same level. e, German shepherd; f,collie; g, Japanese spaniel. Partly from H. Masai, *Kagaku,* 45:427–433 (1975); *Brain and Nerve,* 28:867–882 (1976); *Metabolism and Disease,* 14(supp.):441–451 (1977); *J. Clin. Sci.,* 13:1422–1430 (1977).

Table 1.   The ratio of the thickness of the supragranular layers, including the granular layer (layers II–IV), to that of the infragranular layers (layers V–VI).

	Shepherd	Collie	Beagle	Japanese spaniel
Gyrus proreus	1.6	1.4	1.4	
	1.5	1.9	1.3	1.0
	1.6	1.7	1.2	0.6
Gyrus orbitalis	1.5	1.4	1.6	
	1.8	1.8	1.4	1.1
	1.7	2.3	1.2	0.6

spaniel remains at the level of the habenular commissure (Fig. 2 a,b). In each breed the nucleus consists of four main layers, and the laminar pattern is found to be differentiated most clearly in sagittal section. In all breeds each lamina is curved forward, and no confusion of the laminae is observed. The representation site of the optic disk lacks nerve cells, but it contains a high density of myelinated fibers. In the shepherd, collie, and beagle the optic disk disruption is located at the level of one third to one-half below the dorsal edge of lamina A, and in the middle in a medio-lateral direction. On the other hand, the optic disk discontinuity in the Japanese spaniel is further towards the dorsal edge of the lamina than in other breeds. In all breeds the lamina A and AI are prominently developed and distinguished (Fig. 2 g,h). In the beagle and Japanese spaniel which are highly evolved, the lateral segment of lamina A shows distinct folding, in comparison with that of the shepherd and collie, which probably approaches that of certain wild types (Fig. 2 c,d,e,f).

In the prefrontal cortex, an increase in the thickness of the supragranular layers in proportion to that of the infragranular layers was also recognized in the other cortical sensory areas, that is, the somatic sensory, auditory, and visual cortices[8]. An increase in the thickness of the supra-granular layers, which receive afferent fibers, was observed in the wild boar, in contrast to the domestic pig[9]. The areal expansion of the prefrontal cortex and the increase in the thickness of the supragranular layers in working breeds, such as the shepherd and collie, may be related to the representation of ancestral pack social structure, based on its inhibitory function in animal behavior.

An evoked potential mapping study in the cat[1] and the cell discontinuity of the optic disk can help in determining the representation of the visual field on the dorsal lateral geniculate nucleus. In particular, the central biocular visual field is projected onto the medial matched pair segments of both lamina A and AI, and the peripheral monocular field is represented on the lateral unpaired segment of lamina A. The upper and lower parts of the visual field correspond with the dorsal and ventral subdivisions of the nucleus, respectively. The folding of the lateral segment of lamina A suggests some disturbance of orderly representation of the outside world, probably accompanied by a certain abnormality of the retino-geniculate projection, as the fusion and disruption of laminae had already suggested[3,4]. In a highly evolved breed[5] such as the Japanese spaniel or beagle, as compared with the shepherd and collie, the folding of the lateral segment extends conspicuously in a direction from the dorsal to the ventral subdivision, including the tapetum, of the nucleus, which corresponds to the upper to lower peripheral visual field. In association with the variations in ophthalmoscopic fundus appearance in domestic dogs[6], the occurrence of folding in lamina A may result from a phenotypic representation of genetic abnormality caused by domestication.

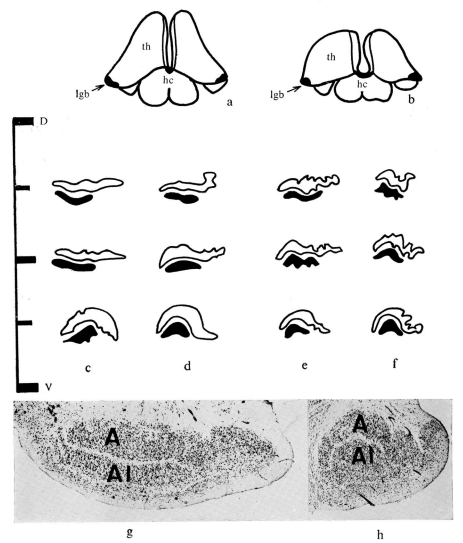

Fig. 2. Upper: Dorsal view of the thalamus. th, Thalamus; hc, habenular commissure; lgb, lateral geniculate body; a, German shepherd; b, Japanese spaniel.
Middle: Schematic drawing of horizontal sections of the dorsal lateral geniculate nucleus. The scale shows the levels between the dorsal pole (D) and ventral pole (V) of the nucleus.
Open, lamina A; solid, lamina Al; a, German shepherd; b, collie; c, beagle; d, Japanese spaniel.
Lower: Horizontal sections of laminae A and Al of the dorsal lateral geniculate nucleus at its middle level. Nissl staining. g, German shepherd; h, Japanese spaniel. Partly from H. Masai, *Brain and Nerve,* 28:867–882 (1976); *Metabolism and Disease,* 14(supp.):441–451 (1977); *J. Clin. Sci.,* 28: 1422–1430 (1977).

ACKNOWLEDGEMENT: We express our sincere appreciation to the staff of publishing companies for their generous permission to reproduce and partly redraw the materials, which were already published by Hideo Masai in the review articles in Kagaku (Iwanami Shoten), Brain and Nerve

(Igaku Shoin), Metabolism and Disease (Nakayama Shoten) and Journal of Clinical Science (Sekai Hoken Tsushinsha).

REFERENCES

1. Bishop, P. O., Kozak, W., Levick, W. R. and Vakkur, G.J., The determination of the projection of the visual field on to the lateral geniculate nucleus in the cat, *J. Physiol. (Lond)*, 163 (1962) 503–539.
2. Brutkowski, S., Prefrontal cortex and drive inhibition. In J. M. Warren and K. Akert (Ed.) *The Frontal Granular Cortex and Behavior*, McGraw-Hill, New York, 1964, pp. 242–270.
3. Guillery, R. W., Visual pathways in albinos, *Scient. Amer.*, 230 (1974) 44–54.
4. Guillery, R.W., Okoro, A. N. and Witkop, Jr. C. J., Abnormal visual pathways in the brain of a human albino, *Brain Research*, 96 (1975) 373–377.
5. Herre, W., Fragen und Ergebnisse der Domestikationsforschung nach Studien am Hirn. In *Verhandl. Deutsch. Zool. Gesell.Erlangen,* Akad. Verlag, Leibzig, 1955, pp. 144–214.
6. Johnson, G. L., Ophthalmoscopic studies on the eyes of mammals, *Phil. Trans. B*, 254 (1968) 207–220.
7. Klatt, B., Studien zum Domestikationsproblem, Untersuchungen am Hirn. In E. Bauer (Ed.) *Bibliotheca Genetica*, Gebrüder Borntraeger, Leipzig, 1921, pp. 1–179.
8. Masai, H. and Sato, Y., The variation of brain patterns under domestication in the dog, *Acta Anat. Nippon*. 48 (1973) 58 (in Japanese).
9. Stephan, H., Vergleichende Untersuchungen über den Feinbau des Hirnes von Wild- und Haustieren (nach Studien am Schwein und Schaf), *Zool. Jb. Abt. Anat.*, 71 (1951) 487–586 (cited from W. Herre, Fragen und Ergebnisse der Domestikationsforschung nach Studien am Hirn. In *Verhandl. Deutsch. Zool. Gesell. Erlangen*, Akad. Verlag, Leipzig, 1955).

Sleep-related growth hormone secretion in dogs after 8–hr forced wakefulness

YASURO TAKAHASHI, SHIGEMITSU EBIHARA, YOSHIKO NAKAMURA AND
KIYOHISA TAKAHASHI

*Departments of Psychology and Medical Chemistry, Tokyo Metropolitan Institute for Neurosciences,
Fuchu, Tokyo 183, Japan*

It has been established that growth hormone (GH) is secreted during slow wave sleep shortly after the onset of sleep in man[1]. Further experiments are required to elucidate the neuroendocrine mechanisms underlying this phenomenon. Dogs were chosen as experimental animals due to their adequate blood volume for serial sampling, good adaptability to an experimental environment and human handling, similarity to man in GH response to various stimuli, and the availability in our laboratory of a sensitive radioimmunoassay for canine growth hormone (CGH).

Our preliminary studies[2,3] indicated that there was no close temporal relation between spontaneous CGH peaks and sleep when the dog was left without interference, and that CGH secretion occurred during high voltage slow wave sleep shortly after the onset of recovery sleep following 6–9 hr of sustained forced wakefulness (FW). These findings suggest that the length of sustained waking prior to sleep onset is an important factor in connection with the relation between sleep and GH secretion in dogs as well as in man.

Recent improvement in techniques has enabled us to repeat 24–hr blood samplings concomitant with polygraphic monitoring in the same dog: this involves (1) blood transfusion, (2) long-term indwelling of a venous catheter without obstruction, and (3) a device for automatic forced wakefulness. With this device, sleep is automatically detected every 5 sec when 5-sec integrated values of the δ band of cortical and hippocampal EEG exceed a preset level and those of neck EMG and body movements are simultaneously below a preset level. When sleep is detected, a sound stimulus is given as a conditioned stimulus to the dog. If the animal remains unawakened by this sound, an electroshock is applied to the neck to cause waking. When such avoidance conditioning has been established, the device easily keeps the dog awake for as long as 12 hr without electroshocks.

The purpose of the present study was to compare the effect of this automatic FW on sleep-related CGH secretion with that of manual FW, and to examine the effect of time of 8-hr automatic FW and the reproducibility of sleep-related CGH secretion produced by this method. Seven adult male mongrel dogs and 2 beagles aged 18–20 months were used. Sleep was polygraphically monitored and the records were scored in 1-min epochs into 4 stages: waking (W), light sleep (L), high voltage δ wave sleep (D) and REM sleep (REM). One ml of blood was drawn without disturbing the dog's sleep through long tubing connected to the venous catheter from the outside of an animal chamber. The sampling intervals were 15 min during 2 hr after 8-hr FW and 30 min for the remainder of the experimental period. Blood samples were analyzed for their plasma CGH and cortisol concentrations.

The spontaneous secretion patterns of CGH and cortisol concomitant with sleep stages were studied during a 24-hr period in all 9 dogs. They showed polyphasic sleep patterns: sleep was frequently disrupted by periods of awakening of less than 1 hr in duration during the 24-hr period. CGH peaks occurred 1 to 6 times over the 24-hr period in each dog. It was difficult, however, to correlate these CGH peaks with sleep onset or any specific stages of sleep.

Eight dogs were subjected to 8-hr FW on 3 consecutive days: manually from 09:00 to 17:00 (Day-M), automatically from 09:00 to 17:00 (Day-A), and automatically from 21:00 to 05:00 (Day-rA). When a CGH peak occurred within 60 min after the onset of recovery sleep and its level was higher than 3 ng/ml above the baseline level, it was defined as a sleep-related CGH peak.

The incidences (and mean levels $\pm$ SE) of sleep-related CGH peaks were 5/8 (10.1 $\pm$ 2.1 ng/ml) on Day-M, 6/8 (9.7 $\pm$ 2.2 ng/ml) on Day-A and 7/8 (9.4 $\pm$ 2.1 ng/ml) on Day-rA, respectively. There were no significant differences in incidence and peak level of sleep-related CGH secretion among these 3 days. Three of the 8 dogs had a sleep-related CGH peak on each of the 3 days. An example is given in Fig. 1.

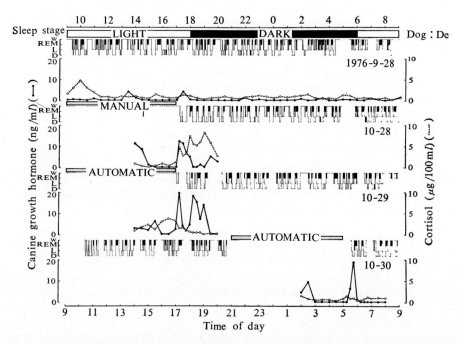

Fig. 1. Twenty-four hr sleep stages and concomitant plasma CGH and cortisol levels in a dog. The data show, from top to bottom, a 24-hr control study and 3 consecutive days of manual 8-hr FW, automatic 8-hr FW, and reversal of automatic 8-hr FW.

The sleep-related CGH peaks were associated with stage D. High voltage δ activity almost always preceded the initial rise in CGH level. Stages L and REM of 1–2 min duration sometimes occurred during the 8-hr FW periods. During short sleep periods without high voltage δ activity, there was no CGH secretion. These findings suggest that neural mechanisms responsible for high voltage δ activity at sleep onset trigger GH release in dogs as well as in man.

Sleep-related CGH secretion was effectively produced by the automatic 8-hr FW even if the time of FW was shifted by 12 hr. This means that GH secretion at sleep onset is sleep-dependent not only in man but also in the present animal model.

Four dogs were subjected to automatic 8-hr FW (09:00–17:00) on 5 consecutive days. Blood was sampled on the last 3 days. Three of the 4 dogs had a sleep-related CGH peak on each of the 3 days. Another dog failed to have one on the first day, but did have one on the 2 subsequent days. The mean CGH peak level $\pm$ SE in this series was 7.0 ± 0.8 ng/ml. This result indicates that the effect of the automatic 8-hr FW on sleep-related CGH secretion is highly reproducible ($11/12 = 0.92$).

It is concluded that the present sleep-related CGH secretion of high incidence and reproducibility in dogs can be utilized as an animal model to study the mechanisms of human sleep-related GH secretion.

REFERENCES

1. Takahashi, Y., Kipnis, D.M. and Daughaday, W.H., Growth hormone secretion during sleep, *J. clin. Invest.*, 47 (1968) 2079–2090.
2. Takahashi, Y., Takahashi, K., Kitahama, K. and Honda, Y., A model of human sleep-related release of growth hormone in dogs, *Sleep Res.* 3 (1974) 147.
3. Takahashi, Y., Takahashi, K., Higuchi, T., Inoue, K. and Honda, Y., A model of human sleep-related release of growth hormone in dogs: twenty-four-hour secretory patterns of canine growth hormone (CGH) and effects of 3, 6 and 9 hours of sleep deprivation, *Sleep Res.* 4 (1975) 288.

Sleep-promoting fractions obtained from the brain-stem of sleep-deprived rats

KOJI UCHIZONO*1, AKIFUMI HIGASHI*1, MASAMI IRIKI*2, HIROAKI NAGASAKI*2, MASAYUKI ISHIKAWA*3, YASUO KOMODA*3, SHOJIRO INOUE*3 AND KAZUKI HONDA*3

*1National Institute for Physiological Sciences,
  Okazaki, Aichi 444, Japan
*2Department of Physiology, Tokyo Metropolitan Institute of Gerontology,
  Itabashi-ku, Tokyo 173, Japan
*3Institute for Medical and Dental Engineering, Tokyo Medical and Dental University,
  Bunkyo-ku, Tokyo 113, Japan

Partially purified active fractions showing inhibitory effects on crayfish stretch receptors were obtained from brain-stem extract of 24 hr sleep-deprived rats[5]. The active fractions contained at least two components: a peptide-like substance which immediately blocked impulse discharges, and a slow-acting substance which blocked the impulse discharge for 10 min. The activity of the latter was not lost on pronase treatment (Fig. 1). It was also confirmed by bioassay in crayfish stretch receptors that the substances differed from previously reported compounds such as γ-

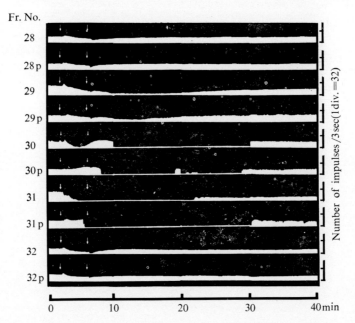

Fig. 1. Effects of serial fractions on the discharge of crayfish stretch receptor. Solution containing fractionated materials was perfused between the two arrows. In all experiments, the concentration of the material was 1 unit/ml Van Harreveld's solution. A small p after the fraction No. (left ordinate) indicates perfusion of solution containing the respective pronase-treated fractions. Note that an "immediate effect" was observed in fraction Nos. 30 to 32 which was diminished by pronase treatment, while a "delayed effect" was observed in fraction Nos. 29 to 31 which was unaffected by the treatment.

aminobutylic acid, γ-amino-β-oxybutyric acid, guanidoacetic acid, β-guanidopropionic acid, β-guanidobutyric acid, γ-hydroxybutyric acid, γ-guanidobutyric acid[1,7], 2,4-diaminobutyric acid[9,11] and γ-butyrolactone[2]. It was proposed that they might represent new substances in the brain[5]. Although purification of the active fractions was not yet refined, infusion of active fraction into mouse and rat brain ventricle induced a striking decrease in locomotor activity and prolongation of sleeping time. Fig. 2 shows results for infusion of active fraction (Fr. No. 30, Fig. 1) into mouse lateral ventricle. In EEG at mouse occipital cortex, components of 2–4 Hz were extracted and integrated at every 10 sec. According to the power of the delta component, a level voltage was set, and with the comparator, the EEG stages were conventionally classified as "1" and "0". On the other hand, after amplifying signals from the body movement transducer (BM transducer), a slicer voltage was set somewhat above the vibration pulse peak voltage caused by respiration of the mouse. Body movement stages (BM stages) were conventionally classified as "1" and "0" according to whether signals from the BM transducer exceeded the set voltage more than once in 10 sec. The classified digital signals were combined and converted into 3 steps such as active, sleeping, and other stages. The "active stage" meant that the BM stage was "1"; the "sleeping stage" meant that the EEG and BM stages were "1" and "0" respectively; and the "other stage" meant that the EEG and BM stages were both "0". In the graphic display, the ratios of the 3 stages calculated in 1 hr were plotted against time.

The mode of sleep of mice is of the multiphasic type, repeating sleep and waking several hundred times a day. It was therefore extremely difficult to assess the real effects of the treatment.

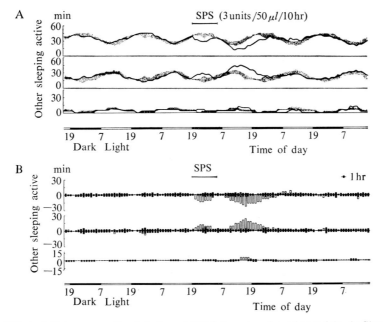

Fig. 2. Effect of 10–hr consecutive infusion of SPS into mouse lateral ventricle. A: Sleep-waking rhythm before and after administration, smoothed by the method of moving averages (order 7). Dotted bands show the maximum variability over several days before administration. B: Variation after balancing the averaged control curve against the above-mentioned sleep-waking rhythm every hr. White parts are interpreted as significant. Light on at 07:00, and off at 19:00. Ordinate: occupied time in min per hr.

It was necessary to determine whether the sleep-waking rhythm before treatment was proceeding naturally. Standardization of the natural pattern of the mouse was thus essential. For this purpose, a smoothing operation by the method of moving averages was adopted[3]. The sleep-waking rhythm was smoothed for several days before infusion of the fractions, and the average control curve of the rhythm per day and its variability were obtained. The size of the area by which the sleep-waking rhythm overflowed beyond the limit of maximum variability of the control after the application of active fraction was taken to show the effect of the fraction. A chronic pharmacological experimental system related to EEG and locomotor activity of free moving mice is to be described elsewhere[4].

The sleep-promoting substance (SPS) in Fig. 2 represents the effect of 3 units of active fraction dissolved in 50 μl saline which was infused continuously into the lateral ventricle for 10 hr: 1 unit was approximately equivalent to the active material extracted from one sleep-deprived rat. Before and after infusion of the active fraction, saline was continuously infused at 5 μl/hr. In this example, for about 7 hr after starting treatment, the locomotion of the mice became remarkably reduced and the sleeping time lengthened dramatically in comparison with the normal condition. No change was observed in the behavior of recipient mice for another 7 hr, but at about 13 hr after commencing treatment, a dramatic decrease in locomotion and remarkable extension of sleeping time occurred which continued for over 13 hr before returning to the control state. Even at a smaller dose (0.5 unit/50 μl/10 hr), a tendency towards increased sleeping time was maintained for more than 24 hr.

Fig. 3 shows the night-time locomotor activity of mice with continuous infusion of the same fraction (5 units/200 μl/10 hr) into the third ventricle for 10 hr. The active fraction induced about 50% reduction of the night-time locomotor activity.

In 1913, Lengendre and Piéron[6] reported that injection of cerebrospinal fluid (CSF) from sleep-deprived dogs into recipients caused behavioral sleep. Humoral sleep-inducing factors from various sources have subsequently been studied. In 1975, Pappenheimer et al.[10] reported the extraction and partial purification of sleep promoting factor (Factor S) from CSF, cortex and brain-stem of sleep-deprived goats and sheep. In 1975, Uchizono et al.[12] reported the extraction of sleep-promoting substances (SPS) from 24-hr sleep-deprived rat brain-stems. Recently, Monnier et al.[8] purified delta sleep-inducing peptide (DSIP) from hemodialysate of rabbit kept asleep by electrical stimulation of the thalamic center. They gave the sequence of this nonapeptide as Trp–Ala–Gly–Gly–Asp–Ala–Ser–Gly–Glu. It induced a drastic increase in both delta and spindle activity with organized biorhythms (5–6 cycles/hr) by ventricle infusion, and they insisted that DSIP passes the blood brain barrier. The effect of DSIP appears about 10 min after application and persists for about 50 min after ventricle infusion in rabbits. However, it appears that the chemical and physiological properties of DSIP definitely differ from those of Factor S and SPS, since the short-lived (50 min) effect of DSIP strikingly contrasts with the long-lasting (7 hr–1 day) increase in slow wave sleep induced by Factor S and SPS. Based on the results of the above series of experiments, it appears that the fractions blocking impulse generation in crayfish stretch receptors may contain the SPS or Factor S investigated independently by the Uchizono and Pappenheimer groups, respectively.

Acknowledgement: The authors are grateful for assistance in the biochemical technique by Dr. M. Hoshino and computer technique by Dr. Y. Tani, without whose help the experiments could not have been conducted successfully.

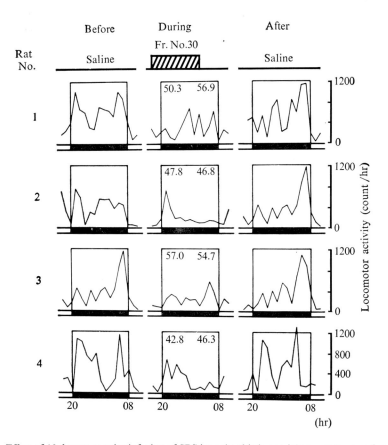

Fig. 3. Effect of 10-hr consecutive infusion of SPS into the third ventricle on rat locomotion. Values of relative percentage for night-time locomotor activity are shown on both sides of the upper part of the central frames, taking the value of the night-time locomotor activities before and after sample infusion as 100%

REFERENCES

1. Edwards, C. and Kuffler, S.W., The blocking effect of γ-aminobutyric acid (GABA) and the action of related compounds on single nerve cells, *J. Neurochem.,* 4 (1959) 19–20.
2. Giarman, N.K. and Roth, R.H., Differential estimation of gamma-butyrolactone and gamma-hydroxybutyric acid in rat blood and brain, *Science,* 145 (1964) 583–584.
3. Hannan, E.J., *Time Series Analysis*, Methuen, London, 1960.
4. Higashi, A., Uchizono, K., Hoshino, M., Tani, Y., Yano, T. and Yazawa, K., A new technique for EEG recording in the free-moving mouse, *Med. biol. Engineering and Computing,* (1978) in press.
5. Higashi, A., Uchizono, K., Iriki, M., Nagasaki, H., Ishikawa, M., Inoue, S., Komoda, Y. and Honda, K., in preparation.
6. Legendre, R. and Piéron, H., Recherches sur le besoin de sommeil consécutif à une veille prolongée, *Z. a llg. Physiol.,* 14 (1913) 235–262.
7. McLennan, H., The identification of one active component from brain extracts containing factor I, *J. Physiol.,* 146 (1959) 358–368.
8. Monnier, M., Dudler, L., Gächter, R., Maier, P.F., Tobler, H.J. and Schoenenberger, G.A., The delta sleep inducing peptide (DSIP): comparative properties of the original and synthetic nona-peptide, *Experientia,* 33 (1977) 548–552.

9. Nakajima, T., Wolfgra, F. and Clard, W.G., Identification of 1,4–methylhistamine, 1,3–diaminopropane and 2, 4-diaminobutyric acid in bovine brain, *J. Neurochem.*, 14 (1967) 1113–1118.

10. Pappenheimer, J.R., Koski, G., Fencl, V., Karnovsky, M.L. and Krueger, J., Extraction of sleep promoting factor S from cerebro-spinal fluid and from brains of sleep deprived animals, *J. Neurophysiol.*, 38 (1975) 1299–1311.

11. Riggs, T.R., Coyne, B.A. and Christensen, H.N., Amino acid concentration by a free cell neoplasm: structural influences, *J. biol. Chem.*, 209 (1954) 395–411.

12. Uchizono, K., Inoué, S., Iriki, M., Ishikawa, M., Komoda, Y. and Nagasaki, H., Purification of the sleep-promoting substances from sleep-deprived rat brain. In R. Walter and J. Meienhofer (Eds.), *Peptides: chemistry, structure and biology,* Ann Arbor Science, Ann Arbor, 1975, pp.667–671.

The circadian rhythm of tryptophan hydroxylase in rat pineal gland

MICHIO TORU, SHUZO WATANABE, HARUO SHIBUYA AND YASUO SHIMAZONO[*1]

Department of Psychobiology, National Musashi Research Institute for Mental and Nervous Diseases, Kodaira, Tokyo 187, Japan
[*1] *Department of Neuropsychiatry, School of Medicine, Tokyo Medical and Dental University, Bunkyo-ku, Tokyo 113, Japan*

The purpose of this study is to describe the presence of the circadian changes of tryptophan hydroxylase activity in rat pineal gland, together with the physiological and pharmacological properties of the circadian rhythm.

Adult male Wistar rats (200–300g) were housed in a light-tight room under diurnal lighting conditions (lights on from 0700 hr to 1900 hr) for about 3 weeks before experiments. The room was illuminated with overhead cool-white fluorescent lamps providing 100–120 lux as measured at the bottom of the cage. Oriental MF rat chow, containing 24.6% protein and 0.22% tryptophan, and tap water were available *ad libitum*. Rats were killed by decapitation every 4 hr from 1000 hr. During the dark period they were handled under a dim red light. The pineals were rapidly removed in a cold box which was kept at around 0°C and homogenized in 0.1 ml of ice-cold 0.01M Tris acetate buffer, pH 7.4, containing 1% Lubrol-WX using a glass-Teflon homogenizer. Tryptophan hydroxylase activity was assayed according to the method of Ichiyama *et al*.[4,11]

More than 1.5-fold increase in the activity of pineal tryptophan hydroxylase occurred during the first 3 hr of the dark period and persisted until the lights went on. The differences between the high values during the dark period and the low values during the light period were found to be significant ($p < 0.0005$).

When the rats were left in light-on conditions for 3 hr from 0700 hr following a 12-hr light period, there was no increase in the enzyme activity. The daily rhythmic fluctuation in pineal tryptophan hydroxylase activity persisted in rats placed under total darkness for 9 days. 1–Propranolol injection blocked the dark period increase in the activity at 2200 hr while decreased activity was obtained at 1000 hr after the drug injection. Cycloheximide administered 3 hr before greatly decreased the activity measured at 1000 hr and 2200 hr. The time course of the activity following cycloheximide injection was studied between 1900 hr and 2200 hr. It gradually decreased with a half-life between 60 min and 120 min. 1-Isoproterenol injected at 1000 hr increased the activity 3 hr after the administration. The nocturnal increase of activity was completely prevented in rats in which the superior cervical ganglions had been removed.

Using a double-reciprocal plot of tryptophan hydroxylase activity as a function of 1-tryptophan concentration, the enzyme preparations obtained from the rats at 1000 hr and 2200 hr were kinetically compared. The Km values of the hydroxylase for 1-tryptophan were calculated to be identical (25 μM) whereas the Vmax of the enzyme from rats at 2200 hr was 1.8 times higher than that from rats at 1000 hr. The finding of a clear 24-h rhythm in the pineal body is of special interest, because of the suggestion that the pineal tryptophan hydroxylase in rat may have a different nature from that in the brain[2].

In the pineal body, 5-hydroxytryptamine shows a rhythm[9] with the opposite phase of the marked circadian rhythms of N-acetyltransferase[6], N-acetylserotonin[7] and melatonin[10]. The inverse rhythm of 5-hydroxytryptamine has been explained by an insufficient production to keep pace with the increased rate of its N-acetylation[6]. The activity of the pineal tryptophan hydroxylase has been considered to be low[8], and the presence of a circadian rhythm in this enzyme has been denied[2].

The higher activity obtained in our experiments by employment of preincubation and optimal assay conditions separating the steps of decarboxylation and hydroxylation has allowed us to identify the rhythm. The use of a detergent in the homogenizing buffer and of tetrahydrobiopterine as a cofactor was also useful to increase the activity.

1-Propranolol, a β-adrenergic blocking agent, or cycloheximide, a protein synthesis inhibitor, injected immediately before the onset of darkness, blocked the increase of pineal tryptophan hydroxylase activity in animals placed in darkness for 3 hr after injection. Also significant is the finding that the increase of the enzyme activity was prevented when the rats were exposed to continuous lighting for 3 hr from 1900 hr to 2200 hr. The daily cycle in the enzyme activity is endogenously generated because it persists in rats placed in continuous darkness for 9 days.

In contrast, the effect of *1*-isoprotelenol, a β-adrenergic stimulator, of increasing the activity to the nocturnal level during the light period is interesting.

The effects of drugs, β-agonist, -antagonist or cycloheximide, and lighting conditions on the enzyme activity are similar to those on pineal N-acetyltransferase as reported by Deguchi and Axelrod[1].

The activity of N-acetyltransferase is thought to be under the control of noradrenaline released from sympathetic nerve endings innervating the pineal body. Klein *et al.*[5] postulated, from their experiments using cultured rat pineal, that cyclic AMP stimulated by noradrenaline increases the formation of N-acetyltransferase.

Whether the effect of noradrenaline on the tryptophan hydroxylase activity is direct or indirect, the fact that ganglionectomization abolishes the rhythm of pineal tryptophan hydroxylase clearly demonstrates noradrenergic control.

The main functions of the pineal body in rodents are the production and secretion of melatonin. N-acetyltransferase is considered to be the rate-limiting enzyme in melatonin synthesis[6]. Our experimental results using 1-propranolol seem consistent with the evidence that bilateral superior cervical ganglion ectomization abolishes the circadian changes of 5-hydroxytryptamine in the pineal body[3]. As 5-hydroxytryptamine does not have any effect on N-acetyltransferase[6], the blocking effect of 1-propranolol on pineal tryptophan hydroxylase might be via an effect on N-acetyltransferase. These findings suggest that tryptophan hydroxylase in the pineal body mainly functions as one of the melatonin synthesizing enzymes. This view is also supported by the suggestion that this enzyme in the pineal body of rats is different from that in the brain.

From the results of the kinetic study we conclude that increases and decreases in enzyme protein level regulate the rhythmicity of pineal tryptophan hydroxylase.

References

1. Deguchi, T. and Axelrod, J., Control of circadian change of serotonin N-acetyltransferase activity in the pineal organ by the β-adrenergic receptor, *Proc. Nat. Acad. Sci.* (*Wash.*), 69 (1972) 2547–2550.
2. Deguchi, T. and Barchas, J., Comparative studies on the effect of parachlorophenylalanine on hydroxylation

of tryptophan in pineal and brain of rat. In J. Barchas and E. Usdin (Eds.), *Serotonin and Behavior*, Academic Press, New York, 1973, pp. 33–47.

3. Fiske, V.M., Serotonin rhythm in the pineal organ: control by the sympathetic nervous system, *Science*, 146 (1964) 253–254.
4. Ichiyama, A., Hasegawa, H., Tohyama, C., Dohmoto, C. and Kataoka, T., Some properties of bovine pineal tryptophan hydroxylase. In *Iron and Copper Proteins*, Plenum, New York, 1976, p. 103.
5. Klein, D.C., Berg, G.R. and Weller, J., Melatonin synthesis: adenosine 3′, 5′-monophosphate and norepinephrine stimulate N-acetyltransferase, *Science*, 168 (1970) 979–980.
6. Klein, D.C. and Weller, J.L., Indole metabolism in the pineal gland: a circadian rhythm in N-acetyltransferase, *Science*, 169 (1970) 1093–1095.
7. Klein, D.C. and Weller, J.L., The role of N-acetylserotonin in the regulation of melatonin production, *Excerpta Med. Int. Congr. Ser.*, 256 (1972) 52.
8. Lovenberg, W., Jequier, E. and Sjoerdsma, A., Tryptophan hydroxylation: measurement in pineal gland, brain stem, and carcinoid tumor, *Science*, 155 (1967) 217–219.
9. Quay, W.B., Circadian rhythm in rat pineal serotonin and its modifications by estrous cycle and photoperiod, *Gen. comp. Endocrinol.*, 3 (1963) 473–479.
10. Ralph, C.L., Mull, D., Lycnh, H.J. and Hedlund, L., A melatonin rhythm persists in rat pineals in darkness, *Endocrinology*, 89 (1971) 1361–1366.
11. Shibuya, H., Toru, M. and Watanabe, S., A circadian rhythm of tryptophan hydroxylase in rat pineals, *Brain Research*, 138 (1977) 364–368.

Nervous and humoral factors in sleep mechanisms

JUNJI MATSUMOTO, YUSUKE MORITA, ATSUKO SANO, NOBUHIDE ISHIKAWA, HIROMASA SENO AND EIKO UEZU

Department of Physiology, School of Medicine, Tokushima University, Kuramoto, Tokushima 770, Japan

Our previous study[3] demonstrated the synchronized occurrence of slow wave sleep (ss) and paradoxical sleep (PS) between parabiotic rats. It was suggested that SS is regulated predominantly by nervous factors, while humoral factors play the major role in PS.

Nervous factors: Our study[4] on temperature changes in the skin surface of the hand both in infants and adults suggested that attenuation of the sympathetic tonus may induce SS. The ventromedial nucleus of the hypothalamus (VMH, a sympathetic center of the autonomic nervous system) was electrically stimulated (1.0 V, 0.5 msec, 14–1 Hz, 2–5 min) in 6 cats. An apparatus for applying the electrical stimulation was newly devised in our laboratory in collaboration with the Homer-Ion Institute. Sleep could be induced a few sec after the stimulus onset and it continued after its cessation. A slow wave appeared in the EEG, heart rate decreased drastically, and respiration became slower and regular. The heart rate during 20–sec periods before and after the stimulation was significantly different ($P < 0.001$).

It should be noted that this stimulus effect was observable only during the moderate vigilante state. It was not induced if the animal was feeding or grooming at a state of higher vigilance. If the stimuli were applied through the cranial bone, sleep was similarly induced. Stimulation of the lateral nucleus of the hypothalamus (parasympathetic center) did not induce sleep.

During the electrical stimulation (14 Hz, 1 min.) of the VMH, EEG of the frontal region was analyzed by the power spectrum method. Before the stimulation fast components of the EEG frequency were predominant, but during the stimulation peak value was observed at 13.7 Hz in the first 20 sec. spectrum, and the peak moved to slower components thereafter, notwithstanding continuance of the stimulation of 14 Hz. These results indicated that the sleep was induced by an increase of parasympathetic tonus due to a suppression of the sympathetic center activity by hypothalamic stimulation. Thus, induction of SS may be attributable to the electrical synchrony of the cerebral cortex by the 14 Hz stimulation, corresponding to the frequency of the spindle wave. The effectiveness of the electrical stimulation through the cranial bone may be interpreted according to the above-mentioned considerations. We applied this method in man. Stimuli (1.0–3.0 V, 0.5 msec) were given via electrodes placed on the frontal and occipital regions for 3 min. In 6 insomniacs, during and after the stimulation, a high voltage slow wave appeared in the EEG, and heart rate decreased gradually. Further experiments are now in progress to confirm the effectiveness of our method of "electrosleep".

Humoral factors: The relationships between protein and ribonucleic acid synthesis and the two phases of sleep were studied. Cycloheximide, puromycin and actinomycin D were administered to male Wistar rats, weighing 200–300 g. A cannula was chronically implanted in the right lateral ventricle, and screw electrodes were placed on the frontal and occipital cortices for EEG recording and stainless wires for eye movement. The rats were kept in an observation chamber with a 12–hr light-dark cycle (06:00–18:00 light, 18:00–06:00 dark).

After 1 week, the rats were continuously subjected to polygraphic recording for 48 hr. The first 24-hr records were taken as untreated control records. One of the inhibitors or saline was tested in 5 rats, respectively, by administration at 06:00 on the second day. After cycloheximide administration (2.5 mg/kg) into the ventricle, PS was completely suppressed for 8–12 hr. The SS period was also decreased, but a rebound in SS was observed during 24 hr. Intraperitoneally injected cycloheximide produced identical results. Puromycin (2.5 mg/kg) also suppressed PS for 6–10 hr, but exerted no effect on SS. When injected intraperitoneally, it had no effect on either SS or PS. Intraperitoneal injection of DOPA (50 or 100 mg/kg) did not eliminate the suppresssion of PS by cycloheximide. Actinomycin D (0.1 mg/kg) caused disappearance of EEG for 10–20 min (brain death), although ECG and respiration were maintained. A smaller dose (0.05 mg/kg) showed no effect on EEG, or on sleep patterns.

According to the monoamine theory of sleep[1,2], the neurotransmitter participating in the induction of PS is thought to be noradrenergic. On the basis of the above results, it is suggested that cycloheximide inhibits the synthesis of receptor protein and does not decrease the neurotransmitter pool, since DOPA did not eliminate the suppression of PS induced by cycloheximide administration.

REFERENCES

1. Jouvet, M., Biogenic amines and the state of sleep, *Science*, 163 (1967) 32–41.
2. Matsumoto, J. et Jouvet, M., Effets de réserpine, DOPA et 5HTP sur les deux états de sommeil, *C. r. Soc. Biol.*, 158 (1964) 2137–2140.
3. Matsumoto, J., Sogabe, K. and Hori-Santiago, Y., Sleep in parabiosis, *Experientia*, 28 (1972) 1043–1044.
4. Matsumoto, J., Kiuchi, T. and Morita, Y., Relation between the skin temperature and sleep in human subjects, *Sleep Res.*, 3 (1974) 76–77.

PART VIII

BRAIN MECHANISMS FOR LEARNING AND MEMORY

MASAO ITO

*Department of Physiology, Faculty of Medicine, University of Tokyo,
Bunkyo-ku, Tokyo 113, Japan.*

The importance of investigating mechanisms of *memory* in elucidating higher brain functions has long been emphasized. Any brain function without support by memory could be nothing more than a stereotyped reflex, just as a computer equipped with no memory can manage only a relatively simple task. *Learning* is a modification of behavior based upon a memorized preceding experience. Its simplest form is *adaptation* in which an experience leads to modification of succeeding behavior in the course of the same trial. Learning in the usual sense involves an improvement of behavior by referring to experiences in preceding trials. Adaptation and learning enable an animal to survive under continuously altering environmental conditions. Ultimately, learning is essential in the development of the elaborate human mental capability.

The progress of investigation of memory and learning, however, has been rather slow. One of the difficulties involved arises from the fact that the focus sites of the memory process have not been well localized in the central nervous system. Vagueness of the cortical localization of learning in the monkey led Lashley[3] to assume that the memory is distributed over the extent of the cerebral cortex. If the memory is indeed stored in such a distributed manner, it is impossible in principle to find a specific localization for memory. However, this possibility could have been overemphasized if a functional deficiency arising from ablation of a small area of the CNS can be compensated for by the learning capability of remaining intact tissues in the surroundings. An example of such compensation has long been known to occur in the cerebellar cortex. Another factor which might also have led to an overemphasis of vague localization is that memory and learning are borne by a large-scale system including a number of separate areas of the CNS. Lesions located in, or electric stimuli applied to, various parts of the CNS would therefore influence memory and learning diffusely. Hence, the possibility still remains that memory and learning are represented in a rather specific and concentrated, rather than distributed, manner.

What is apparently needed at the present stage of investigation is identification of structures of memory and learning systems and localization of their components. Efforts have been made to specify the system for conditioned reflexes taking advantage of the simplest conditioned reflex, i.e., the glabella tap reflex[4]. In the study of cerebellar motor learning, the center for adaptation of the vestibuloocular reflex has been located in the cerebellar flocculus (cf. Ito[1]). Habituation in *Aplysia* has been taken as a simplified model of the memory and learning system[2]. As will be introduced in Part VIII, delayed response seemingly executed by the cerebral frontal lobe provides an interesting system for short memory holding (Kubota). Reverberation of nerve impulses provides another model for learning and memory (Tsukahara *et al.*). It is important to expand our knowledge of structure and mode of operation to many other memory and learning systems, including human intelligence (Ueki and Konno). Chemical destruction techniques now offer a new tool for specific elimination of a certain component of the CNS (Murakami; Tsukada and Kohsaka). Once a focal site is localized specifically, electrophysiological, biochemical and theoretical (Amari) investigations can be brought to bear in order to uncover the neuronal mechanisms of memory and learning.

References

1. Ito, M., Learning control mechanisms by the cerebellum investigated in the flocculo-vestibulo-Ocular system. In D.B. Tower (Ed.), *The Basic Neurosciences*, Vol. 1, Raven Press, New York, 1975, pp. 245–252.
2. Kandel, E., Neuronal plasticity and the modification of behavior. In J.M. Brookhart and V.B. Mountcastle (Ed.), *The Nervous System*, Handbook of Physiol, Vol. 1, Am. Physiol. Soc., Bethesda, pp. 1137–1182.
3. Lashley, K.S., *Brain Mechanisms and Intelligence: A Quantitative Study of Injuries to the Brain*, Chicago University Press, Chicago, 1929.
4. Woody, C.D. and Engel, J., Jr., Changes in unit activity and thresholds to electrical microstimulation at coronal-pericruciate cortex of cat with classical conditioning of different facial movements. *J. Neurophysiol.*, 35 (1972) 230–241.

Neuron activity in the dorsolateral prefrontal cortex of the monkey and initiation of behavior

KISOU KUBOTA

Department of Neurophysiology, Primate Research Institute, Kyoto University, Inuyama, Aichi 484, Japan

A technique to record single neuron activity in brain areas of the unanesthetized, unrestrained monkey[7] offers a new approach to an understanding of highly integrated functions of the nervous system, particularly of the so-called association cortex. This technique was applied to the frontal eye field of the monkey in 1968 by Bizzi,[4] and subsequently to the mid-principalis area by Kubota and Niki[27]. Since then, our knowledge of how prefrontal neurons are involved in the integration of complex sensory stimuli and in the control of behavior has been extended considerably. This short review deals with the activity related to the intiation of movement or behavior in which the prefrontal cortex is involved, and on the basis of previous reports aims to suggest areas which will repay study in the near future.

Cytoarchitecturally speaking, the dorsolateral prefrontal cortex may be divided into various areas[1]. Walker's classification (areas 8a, 8b, 45 and 46)[51] is adopted in this paper, because of its simplicity. Discussions on the orbital gyrus (Walker's area 9) are not included in this review.

Function of the prefrontal cortex from the viewpoint of anatomical input-output relations

Nauta summarized efferent connections of the prefrontal cortex in the Pennsylvania Symposium in 1962[35] and later in the Jablonna Symposium held near Warsaw in 1971[36] he added further efferent connections to the scheme. No new connections have so far been found though new staining methods such as the retrograde HRP labeling technique[28] or Fink-Heimer's method[9] have been introduced.

Detailed discussions on efferent connections will not be attempted in this review, which is limited to anatomically described connections. Fig. 1 illustrates schematically efferent connections from the prefrontal cortex, (1) cortico-cortically to the anterior temporal cortex, inferior parietal lobule and limbic cortex, (2) cortico-striatally to the caudate nucleus and putamen, (3) cortico-thalamically to the dorsomedial, intralaminar, and reticularis nuclei, (4) cortico-hypothalamically to the preoptic area, ventromedial nuclei, mammilary body, etc., (5) cortico-subthalamically to the subthalamus, (6) cortico-tegmentally to the midbrain tegmentum, including the rostral part of the central grey matter of the midbrain and (7) cortico-pontinely to the pontine nuclei. Panadya and Kuypers[41] added a connection from areas 45 and 8a (arcuate area) to the postarcuate-premotor area, which in turn sends axons to the motor area. Further, it was shown that the prearcuate cortex gains access to the premotor cortex via projections to the post-arcuate region[6,17,42,43]. It is expected that integrated motor tasks from the prefrontal cortex may be executed via this route.

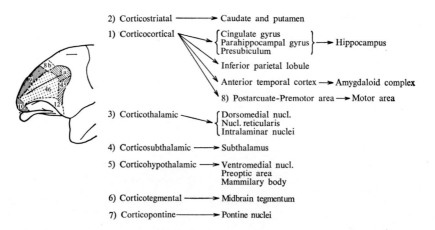

2) Corticostriatal ——————→ Caudate and putamen

1) Corticocortical ⟨Cingulate gyrus
Parahippocampal gyrus⟩——→ Hippocampus
Presubiculum

Inferior parietal lobule

Anterior temporal cortex ——→ Amygdaloid complex

8) Postarcuate-Premotor area ——→ Motor area

3) Corticothalamic ⟨Dorsomedial nucl.
Nucl. reticularis
Intralaminar nuclei

4) Corticosubthalamic ——————→ Subthalamus

5) Corticohypothalamic ——→ Ventromedial nucl.
Preoptic area
Mammilary body

6) Corticotegmental ——————→ Midbrain tegmentum

7) Corticopontine——————→ Pontine nuclei

Fig. 1.   Schematic illustrations of various efferent connections from the prefrontal cortex. The diagram shows the cytoarchitectural areas of the macaque prefrontal cortex as defined by Walker[51].

Although various efferent connections are known, in none of the above efferent pathways has the physiological function been identified.

According to Nauta,[36] the unique feature of the neural circuitry of the prefrontal cortex is that it places the frontal cortex in a reciprocal relationship with two great functional realms, namely: i) parietal and temporal regions involved in the processing of visual, auditory and somatic sensory information, and ii) the telencephalic limbic system and its cortical correspondence, in particular, the hypothalamus and meso- and diencephalic structures associated with the hypothalamus. The reciprocal nature of these entails a need to view the frontal lobe at once as a "sensory" and as an "effector" mechanism. Thus, the frontal cortex is interpreted as a higher-order processing mechanism for visual, auditory and somesthetic information for integrated behavior, rather than for simple reflex-like behavior. It could also be capable of modulating earlier stages in the processing of such information. Because of its reciprocal connections with the limbico-hypothalamic axis the frontal cortex could be viewed as a modulator of hypothalamic mechanisms. Recently Mesulam et al,[30] after studying the connections of the inferior parietal lobule area, emphasized that the periarcuate cortex may subserve a role of efferent integration for the initiation or inhibition of attentive behavior. On the other hand, a stage of afferent integration may occur at the inferior parietal lobule where a 'supramodal' representation of the sensory space is formed and the cingulate cortex may constitute a locus for limbic integration at which the motivational relevance of ongoing events is assessed. The efferent interaction among these three stages of integration may be indispensable for the effective execution of attention. Thus, they emphasized the role of the pariarcuate area as indispensable for attentive integration.

Corollary discharge hypothesis vs. command hypothesis

If the prefrontal neuron activity is involved in the control of voluntary movement or behavior, two possible influences may be considered on the neuron activity prior to the onset of movement. The first possibility was proposed by Teuber,[49,50] who suggested on the basis of his experience with human traumatic patients that the prefrontal cortex sends a discharge from motor to sensory structures for an anticipated change (corollary discharge hypothesis). The second possibility may be called the "command hypothesis", that neuronal discharges related to the task performance will lead to the activation of the mortor system. This hypothesis has been proposed in the parietal association cortex by Mountcastle *et al.*[34] However, this hypothesis is challenged by Robinson *et al.*[44] because area 7 neurons are activated by visual stimuli and this, they believe, makes it difficult to suggest "command" functions. As will be shown later, presently available evidence does not exclude either of these views.

In order to assess timing relations of movement-related neurons, movement-related discharges of prefrontal neurons were compared with those of the motor system, usually with those of the pyramidal tract neurons (PTNs) obtained in motor control studies. These comparisons have not been made in the same animal, that is, PTNs were not recorded from the same animal from which prefrontal neurons were recorded. Even in the same movement, such as hold key release, the temporal sequence of muscle activations may be different. Further, it has been shown that before movement onset there is an anticipatory or preparatory activity in the PTNs without any measurable movement[15,48]. Therefore it seems likely that PTNs are activated as soon as movement-related prefrontal neurons are activated. It may be misleading to compare discharge timings of motor cortex neurons and prefrontal neurons obtained in different task situations. In order to determine precise timing relations, it is necessary to record activities of PTNs and prefrontal neurons in the same task, preferably in the same monkey.

Single neuron activity related to the task

Since the introduction of the extracellular unit recording technique for the dorsolateral prefrontal cortex, more than 20 papers (short or final) have appeared. Table 1 lists these papers chronologically, together with the areas searched, tasks employed, electrodes used, etc. Except for two papers on the frontal eye field neurons, all neuron activities were recorded while the monkeys were performing operantly conditioned tasks, such as delayed response (DR), delayed alternation (DA), conditional position reponse (CP), cue-guided choice reaction task (cue-choice) and visual fixation task (VFT). It is noteworthy that except in one paper visual stimuli were used as stimulus cues and response cues. Lever depression by hand movement or eye movement was reinforced. In one paper, sound was used as the "go" signal. No kinesthetic cues were used.

In these papers suggestions were made on possible functions on attention, anticipation, short-term memory and initiation of the goal-directed movements. The right-hand column of Table 1 indicates the major interest of the paper, i.e., whether it is related to attentive mechanism (A), short-term memory mechanisms (ST) or goal-directed movement or behavior (M). This short review deals only with the relations between the prefrontal neuron activity and goal-directed movement.

The studies listed in Table 1 simply sought correlations of the neuron activity with some aspect of behavior, particularly operantly reinforced behavior, such as pressing of a specified lever or an eye movement to a specific position. Therefore it is not easy to infer causal relations, e.g. that a given neuron activity represents efferent activity from the prefrontal cortex, even though there is a correlation between discharge rates and task movements. As the eye movement-related activity always occurred after eye movement was initiated[4], it appears that the prefrontal cortex does not initiate the eye movement. In contrast, the inferior parietal lobule is more concerned with the eye movement initiation, since neuron activity preceding operantly conditioned saccadic eye movement has been found (saccade neurons)[29].

When we compare the results obtained in different laboratories, even in the same task situa-

TABLE 1.   List of papers on neuron activity of the prefrontal cortex in the unanesthetized, chronic state.
Papers are listed in chronological order with authors (year of publication), task employed, cortical areas in which neurons were recorded (areas 8a, 8b, 45, 46 and premotor area), kind of electrode (Pt, platinum; W, tungsten or Fe, stainless steel), and the major interests of papers: attention mechanism (A), motor aspects (M) or the short-term memory process (ST). Tasks: DR, delayed response; DA, delayed alternation; CP, conditional positional response; VCR, visual cue choice reaction; DMS, delayed matching to sample task and VFT, visual fixation task.

No. of authors	(Year)	DR	DA	CP	VCR	DMS	VFT	Areas searched	Electrodes	Subject
1 Bizzi[4]	(68)							8a	Pt	M
2 Bizzi and Schiler[5]	(70)							8a	Pt	M
3 Kubota and Niki[27]	(71)	○						46	W	M
4 Fuster[10]	(73)	○						8a, 8b, 45, 46	W	A
5 Mohler, Goldberg, and Wurtz[33]	(73)						○	8a	Pt	A
6 Kojima and Kubota[18]	(74)	○						45, 46	W	A
7 Kubota[21]	(74)	○	○					45, 46	W	ST, M
8 Kubota, Iwamoto and Suzuki[27]	(74)		○					8a, 45, 46	W	ST
9 Niki[37]	(74a)	○						46	Pt	ST
10 Niki[38]	(74b)	○	○					46	Pt	ST
11 Niki[39]	(74c)			○				46	Pt	M
12 Sakai[45]	(74)	○						46	W	A
13 Kojima and Tobias[19]	(75)				○		○	45, 46	Pt, W	A
14 Kubota[22]	(75)	○						8a, 8b, 45, 46, premotor	W	M
15 Fuster and Bauer[12]	(76)	○				○		—	?	ST
16 Kubota[23]	(76)	○	○		○			8a, 45, 46	W	M, ST
17 Niki and Watanabe[40]	(76)		○	○				46	Pt	M
18 Wurtz and Mohler[52]	(76)			○				8a	Pt	A
19 Kubota[24]	(77)	○						8a, 45, 46	Pt, W	M, ST, A
20 Suzuki and Azuma[47]	(77)						○	45, 46	W	A
21 Kubota and Mikami[25]	(78)					○		8a, 45, 46	Pt, W	M
22 Mikami, Ito and Kubota[31]	(78)					○	○	45, 46	Pt	M
23 Azuma and Suzuki[2]	(78)						○	45, 46	Fe	A

tion, care is required regarding sampling problems of neurons inherent in the selection of the micro-electrode (Pt, tungsten or stainless steel). As pointed out by Humphrey and Corrie[16] in the monk-key motor cortex, a glass-coated Pt electrode tends to pick up activities of larger-sized neurons and a tungsten electrode medium- or small-sized neurons, in addition to larger-sized ones. Since it appears that this holds true in the prefrontal cortex, we should be cautious in interpreting results obtained with different kinds of electrodes, though large pyramidal neurons are not found in the prefrontal cortex.

Neuron activity prior to lever pressing in the prefrontal cortex was described for the first time by Kubota and Niki[27] in a delayed alternation (DA) task. Tungsten electrodes were used. As soon as the screen was raised, indicating the end of the delay period, the monkey in the primate chair pressed one of two levers alternately. Onset latency of the discharge was about 300 msec and the monkey depressed the lever with about 1000 msec latency. Discharge onset was about 200 msec earlier than the arm stretching, as seen in the EMG of the triceps muscle. They have designated such neurons as E-type neurons. This onset timing was compared with that of PTNs[8] and it was inferred that the E neuron activity preceded the PTN activity of the motor cortex by more than 150 msec.

This observation was further extended by Niki.[37] He tested DA with visual cues. There was a panel with two choice keys and a central 'hold' key at the bottom. The trial started by depress-ing the hold key and then the two choice keys were lighted. The monkey pressed the choice keys alternately to obtain reward juice. He classified task-related units into 3 types (I, II and III). In one-third of task-related units there was a neuron discharge immediately before the choice key press (type I unit). Half of these (26 units) showed the same pattern of discharge irrespective of the position of the correct response (non-directionally selective type I unit) and the other half (29 units) showed a differential firing pattern depending on the correct side for that trial (directional-ly selective type I unit). If these neuron activities were tested in a visual cue-guided task (illumina-tion of one key lamp, instead of two lamps, as a response cue in DA), the change in activity was the same as that in DA. The earliest change of the EMG appeared in the supraspinate muscle (in-dicating relatively large bodily movements were necessary for key pressing in this task situation) and this was 120 msec before the release of the hold key. Since the response cue was the same in both right and left presses, the difference in the activity before the pressing movement is inter-preted as indicating that the activation is coupled to some aspect of lever pressing. The non-direc-tional type I unit was said to be related to the initiation and execution of operant key-pressing and the directional one to be involved in the initiation and execution of a response to a given position. Though the type I unit is claimed to respond to other visual stimuli, it was not determined how much of the non-directional activation by the cue was due to the visual stimuli, that is, sensory effect. Niki further tested whether the directional selectivity of the discharge is related to the ab-solute or relative position of the choice keys[38]. Monkeys performed a DA task in which 2 arbitrari-ly chosen choice keys out of 4 aligned horizontally were used. He found 182 directional units in the task. How many differential type I units are included in these 182 directional units is not clear. A unit in Fig. 3 of ref. 39 is a type I unit according to his criteria[37]. Pressing key 3, when it was right-most, was said to show slightly greater activity than pressing the same key when it was left-most. He did not make any suggestions regarding relative vs. absolute positions and related type I unit activities. It appears that these two factors may contribute to the discharges of type I units.

The prefrontal neurons in the delayed response (DR) with visual cues were tested by 3 dif-ferent groups. Firstly, Fuster[10] analyzed neurons of the prefrontal cortex by a classical direct method with tungsten electrodes in which the monkey faced a window giving a view of the test objects (two identical white wooden blocks covering shallow food wells, on the right and left of the animal's field of vision. Two openings covered by spring-loaded doors gave the monkey manual access to the bait. During the delay period the screen was down and the two doors remained locked. At the end of the delay, the screen was raised and the doors were unlocked. After the object had been chosen, the animal retrieved the food from under it. Because of this direct method situation it was difficult to determine exactly neuron activity related to the bait picking movement. He classified related prefrontal units into 6 types (A, B, C, D, I, O units); the type B and C units increased their rate during this retrieval period. However, it is difficult to correlate this increase to some aspect of the retrieval movement because the onset timings, movement distances, etc., are not well described. Secondly, Kubota et al.[25] analyzed DR with visual cues in an indirect method. Results consistent with Fuster's were found on discharges related to the movement. A left or right lamp signal was presented as a visual cue and both lamps as a response cue. They used tungsten electrodes. As soon as the response cue was presented, the monkey released the hold key and depressed one of levers located just below the lamp. Neurons activated with about 100 msec latency after the response cue were also activated by the visual cue. However, the increase of discharge rate was greater in the former than the latter case. They designated such neurons as visuokinetic neurons because these neurons were not only activated by the visual cue but also prior to lever pressing, and were considered to be essential in executing the DR. Some of them were activated during lever pressing on either side and some others during lever pressing on only one side (non-differential and differential). Activations before lever pressing were always associated with the response cue stimulus, so it was impossible to determine how many of the discharges are due to visual activation or related to motor activation. Thirdly, Niki[39] tested DR in a similar manner to Kubota et al.[25], but with platinum electrodes. One hundred and forty-two units showed changes for both cue and choice (response) periods and 114 for the choice period only. Some of the former units showed higher or lower rates in a delay period than in intertrial intervals. He found 95 units with differential response for right and left trials during stimulus-response events. Of these, 16 showed differential response during both cue and choice periods and 60 at the choice response. It is clearly important to determine how these neurons differ from those of Fuster[10] and Kubota et al.[25] In particular, it is desirable to determine whether and how these activations are related to the response movement. A unit illustrated in Fig. 1 of ref. 39 appears to be responding to visual stimulus, being unrelated to the lever pressing. Neurons responding only to visual stimulus were not described by Kubota et al.[25] This discrepancy may be partially due to sampling differences of the electrodes and should be examined further. Niki[39] showed a differential activity at the choice phase, which may be a reflection of the intention to select a given position; this is consistent with the data of Kubota et al.[25] Later, Niki and Watanabe[40] analyzed neuron activities during 3 kinds of spatial tasks (right-left DR, up-down DR and conditional position discrimination with delays). Among neurons activated during the delay period (32 neurons) there were neurons with a clear dependence on the direction of the response (up, down, left or right lever; 7 neurons). A unit in Fig. 4 of this paper showed a differential increase during the delay period of left side pressing in DR and CP. It is not clear whether there is a specific increase before right choice key pressing. This neuron does not seem to be a visuokinetic neuron, though there is a differential activity during cue and delay periods.

Kubota[22] tested the same prefrontal neurons in both DR and DA tasks. In DA visuokinetic neurons behaved as predicted from data in DR. In DA they showed an increase for no-go two-lamp signals given during the delay period and also for go signals. The E neuron in DA appears to be a visuokinetic neuron with little spontaneous activity in the delay and weak activation by visual cues. This group constituted a fraction of the visuokinetic group. Niki's type I seems to belong to the visuokinetic category. Visuokinetic patterns of neurons were recorded not only from the periprincipal area, but also from the post-arcuate area[22]. This suggests the possibility that the efferents of the prefrontal cortex may be conveyed to the motor cortex via the post-arcuate-pre-motor area.

Finally, neuron activity was tested in a DR without go signals by Kojima *et al.*[18,23] After a delay period of 1 sec the monkey had to release the hold key and depress one of levers. There were neurons active during periods before the lever pressing. In this task the delay period cannot be separated clearly from the response period, so it was called the delay-preresponse period. During this period some neurons were activated differentially and others non-differentially. Such activations were considered to represent activity related to the lever pressing. Figs. 2 and 3 show 3 examples of neurons activites in DR without a go signal. In both left (L) and right (R) trials an activity was induced during cue periods of Fig. 2A and during delay-preresponse periods of Fig. 2B.

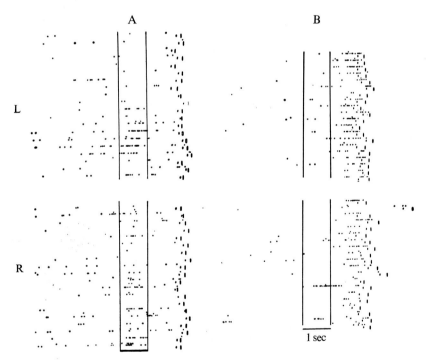

Fig. 2.   Dot displays of 2 prefrontal neurons (A and B) in a delayed response with visual cues and without go signal. After a 3 sec intertrial interval started by hold key depression, left (L) or right (R) lamp cue was presented for 1 sec and then the monkey was allowed to release the hold key 1 sec after cue stimulus offset. Dots below dot trains indicate timings of hold key release and vertical bars indicate the timings of lever pressing. In A and B 20 left and right trials are shown, respectively. Periods between vertical lines indicate cue presentation. One bin represents 20 msec. If more than two spikes appeared in a single bin, this is shown by a dot above the base line dots. Neuron "A" was activated non-differentially mostly during the cue period and neuron "B" was activated non-differentially mostly during delay-preresponse periods.

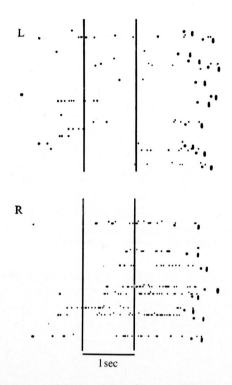

Fig. 3.   Dot display of a prefrontal neuron with differential activation before lever pressing in a delayed response without go signal. Similar to Fig. 2.

Hence these neurons are non-differentially activated. Fig. 3 shows an example of differential activation. A right cue induced increased activity, while a left cue had no effect. In the right trials there was higher activity from the cue period through the delay-preresponse period until hold key release, although discharges during right side delay were variable the discharge peak was several hundred msec earlier than the moment of hold key release. This indicates that the activity before the lever pressing movement is not like that of PTNs. Kubota and Mikami[26,24,32] tested neuron activities in a Konorski task[20] (one of the short-term memory tasks) in which red or right color sample stimulus was presented for a short period and then there was a delay period followed by a matching red or green stimulus. After these stimuli, a go signal (sound of 1 KHz) was presented, then the monkey released the hold key and pressed the levers (one side if the sample and matching colors are the same, the other side if the colors are different). A group of visually activated neurons were also activated during the sound go signal; this increase was not due to a sensory response to the sound but has been related to the lever pressing. Therefore this neuron was correctly designated as visuokinetic. Thus, activity prior to the reinforced movement was again demonstrated. Similarly, some neurons were activated during pressing on one side and others during pressing on both sides.

The presence of prefrontal activity prior to movement has been demonstrated in several task[3] such as DR, DA, CP, Konorski. Some of these neurons showed relatively higher discharge rates prior to the movement to be reinforced than to movements to other directions. Precise correlations of the neuron activity in the motor system remain to be examined. It is presumed that these neurons are efferents from the prefrontal cortex and send their axons to an unknown locus of the motor or sensory system.

Side dependence to lever position as seen in incorrect response

The presence of location-dependent activity prior to lever pressing was observed in incorrect trials of DA[22] or DR[39]. If the monkey pressed incorrectly, an increase of the discharge persisted during the delay and go periods. This indicates that the increase is related to the lever location rather than the correctness of the performance.

Summary and final comments

Extracellular neuron studies at the prefrontal cortex have shown that there is neuron activity prior to hand-arm movement to a specified location during task performance. Two kinds of activity were differentiated; one is related differentially to a specified location and the other non-differentially to 'any' location of the movement goal. Some of these neurons were activated by visual cue. It remains to be determined where these terminate. The timing relations of movement-related prefrontal neurons with neurons of the motor system such as PTNs in the same task also require examination. It is desirable to stain neurons and their axons which show activity prior to movement. Azuma and Suzuki's effort[2,46] seems promising. They stained the electrode site by Fe ion infusion in chronic monkeys.

It is known that cooling of the prefrontal cortex itself does not disturb the control of voluntary movements, such as visual tracking, motor coordination, and strength of muscles in the hand and arm; only the correct choice of the lever to be pressed[3,11] was disturbed. Lesion studies of the cortico-frontal connections disrupted fine finger movements[13,14]. Therefore, it is likely that the pathway from an efferent prefrontal neuron to the motor system is not included in the main pathway of movement control from receptors to the motor neurons, but inputs and outputs of the prefrontal cortex may constitute a parallel pathway attached to the main pathway of motor control from receptors to the motor neurons. Either of the hypotheses, corollary discharges or command, can account for the findings.

References

1. Akert, K., Comparative anatomy of frontal cortex and thalamofrontal connections. In J.M. Warren and K. Akert (Eds.) *The Frontal Granular Cortex and Behavior*, McGraw-Hill, New York, 1964, pp. 372–396.
2. Azuma, M. and Suzuki, H., Laminar distributions of gaze neurons in the prefrontal cortex, *J. physiol. Soc. Japan* (1978) (in press).
3. Bauer, R.H. and Fuster, J.M., Delayed-matching and delayed-response deficit from cooling dorsolateral prefrontal cortex in monkeys, *J. comp. Physiol. Psychol.*, 90 (1976) 293–302.
4. Bizzi, E., Discharge of frontal eye field neurons during saccadic and following eye movements in unanesthetized monkeys, *Exp. Brain Res.*, 6 (1968) 69–80.
5. Bizzi, E. and Schiller P. H., Single unit activity in the frontal eye fields of unanesthetized monkeys during eye and head movement, *Exp. Brain Res.*, 10 (1970) 151–158.
6. Chavis, D.A. and Pandya, D.N., Further observations on corticofrontal connections in the rhesus monkey, *Brain Res.*, 117 (1976) 369–386.
7. Evarts, E.V., Methods for recording activity of individual neurons in moving animals. In R.F. Rushmer (Ed.) *Methods in Medical Research*, vol. 2, Year Book, Chicago, 1966, pp. 241–250.

8. Evarts, E.V., Pyramidal tract activity associated with a conditioned hand movement in the monkey, *J. Neurophysiol.*, 29 (1966) 1011–1027.
9. Fink, R. P. and Heimer, L., Two methods for selectives silver impregnation of degenerating axons and their synaptic endings in the central nervous system, *Brain Research*, 4 (1967) 369–374.
10. Fuster, J.M., Unit activity in prefrontal cortex during delayed-response performance: Neuronal correlates of transient memory, *J. Neurophysiol.*, 36 (1973) 67–78.
11. Fuster, J.M., Cryogenic and microelectrode studies of the prefrontal cortex. In S. Kondo., M. Kawai., A. Ehara and S. Kawamura (Eds.) *Proceedings from the Symposia of the Fifth Congress of the International Primatological Society*, Japan Science Press, Tokyo, 1975, pp. 445–458.
12. Fuster, J.M. and Bauer, R.H., Prefrontal unit activity during retention of spatial and nonspatial information, *Neurosci. Abstr.*, vol. 2 (1976) 429.
13. Haaxma, R. and Kuypers, H., Role of occipito-frontal, cortico-cortical connections in visual guidance of relatively independent hand and finger movements in rhesus monkeys, *Brain Research*, 71 (1974) 361–366.
14. Haaxma, R. and Kuypers, H.G.J.M., Intrahemispheric cortical connections and visual guidance of hand and finger movement in the rhesus monkey, *Brain*, 96 (1975) 239–260.
15. Hamada, I. and Kubota, K., Preparatory activity of monkey pyramidal tract neurons during visual tracking performance of single step, *J. physiol. Soc. Japan*, 39 (1977) 347.
16. Humphrey, D.R. and Corrie, W.S., Properties of pyramidal tract neuron system within a functionally defined subregion of primate motor cortex, *J. Neurophysiol.*, 41 (1978) 216–243.
17. Jacobson, S. and Trojanowski, J. Q., Prefrontal granular cortex of the rhesus moneky. I. Intrahemispheric cortical afferents, *Brain Research*, 132 (1977) 209–233.
18. Kojima, S. and Kubota, K., Prefrontal neuron activity and delayed response without go signal, *Abstract of 38th Annual Meeting of Japan Psychol. Soc.*, (1974) 368–369 (Japanese).
19. Kojima, S. and Tobias, T., Reward related visual stimuli: Single unit recording in monkey prefrontal cortex (PFC), *Exp. Brain Res.*, 23 (1975) p. 111.
20. Konorski, J., A new method of physiological investigation of recent memory in animals, *Bull. Acad. pol. Sci.*, 7 (1959) 115.
21. Kubota, K., A neurophysiological approach to study the functions of the prefrontal cortex, *Seitai no Kagaku*, 25 (1974) 196–208 (Japanese).
22. Kubota, K., Prefrontal unit activity during delayed-response and delayed-alternation performances, *Jap. J. Physiol.*, 25 (1975) 481–493.
23. Kubota, K., Prefrontal programming of lever pressing reactions in the monkey. In T. Desiraju (Ed.) *Mechanisms in Transmission of Signals for Conscious Behaviour*. Elsevier, Amsterdam, 1976, pp. 61–80.
24. Kubota, K., Visual discrimination tasks with short-term memory and neuronal activities of prefrontal and inferotemporal cortex of rhesus monkeys, *Electroenceph. clin. Neurophysiol.*, 43 (1977) 893.
25. Kubota, K., Iwamoto, T. and Suzuki, H., Visuokinetic activities of primate prefrontal neurons during delayed-response performance, *J. Neurophysiol.*, 36 (1974) 1197–1212.
26. Kubota, K. and Mikami, A., Prefrontal cortex and behavioral execution: Integrative controls of brain, *Progress report of "Special Project of the Ministry of Education"*, vol. 1 (1978) 133–134 (Japanese).
27. Kubota, K. and Niki, H., Prefrontal cortical unit activity and delayed alternation performance in monkeys, *J. Neurophysiol.*, 34 (1971) 337–347.
28. La Vail, J.H. and La Vail, M.M., The retrograde intraaxonal transport of horseradish peroxidase in the chick visual system: a light and electron microscopic study, *J. comp. Neurol.*, 157 (1974) 303–357.
29. Lynch, J.C., Mountcastle, V.B., Talbot, W.H. and Yin, T.C., Parietal lobe mechanisms for directed visual attention, *J. Neurophysiol.*, 40 (1977) 362–389.
30. Mesulam, M-M, Hoesen, G.W.V., Pandya, D.N. and Geschwind, W., Limbic and sensory connections of the inferior parietal lobule (area PG) in the rhesus monkey: A study with a new method for horseradish peroxidase histochemistry, *Brain Research*, 136 (1977) 393–414.
31. Mikami, A., Ito, S. and Kubota, K., Responses of prefrontal neurons to extrafoveal slit stimuli in visual fixation task of monkeys, *J. physiol. Soc. Japan*, (1978) (in press).
32. Mikami, A., Kubota, K. and Tonoike, M., Inferotemporal unit activity and a color memory task, *J. physiol. Soc. Japan*, 38 (1976) 115–116.
33. Mohler, C.W., Goldberg, M.E. and Wurtz, R.H., Visual receptive fields of frontal eye field neurons, *Brain Research*, 61 (1973) 385–389.
34. Mountcastle, V.B., Lynch, J.C., Georgopoulos, A., Sakata, H., and Acuna, C., Posterior parietal association cortex of the monkey: Command functions for operations within extrapersonal space, *J. Neurophysiol.*, 38 (1975) 871–908.
35. Nauta, W.J.H., Some efferent connections of the prefrontal cortex in the monkey. In J.M. Warren and K. Akert (Eds.) *The Frontal Granular Cortex and Behavior*, McGraw-Hill, New York, 1964, pp. 397–409.
36. Nauta, W.J.H., Neural associations of the frontal cortex, *Acta neurobiol. exp.*, 32 (1972) 125–140.

37. Niki, H., Prefrontal unit activity during delayed alternation in the monkey. I. Relation to direction of response, *Brain Research*, 68 (1974) 185–196.
38. Niki, H., Prefrontal unit activity during delayed alternation in the monkey. II. Relation to absolute versus relative direction of response, *Brain Research*, 68 (1974) 197–204.
39. Niki, H., Differential activity of prefrontal unit during right and left delayed response trials, *Brain Research*, 70 (1974) 346–349.
40. Niki, H. and Watanabe, M., Prefrontal unit activity and delayed response: Relation to cue location versus direction of response, *Brain Research*, 105 (1976) 79–88.
41. Pandya, D.N. and Kuypers, H.G.J.M., Cortico-cortical connections in the rhesus monkey, *Brain Research*, 13 (1969) 13–36.
42. Pandya, D.N. and Vignolo. L.A., Intra- and interhemispheric projections of the precentral, premotor and arcuate areas in the rhesus monkey, *Brain Research*, 26 (1971) 217–233.
43. Pandya, D.N., Dye, P. and Butters, N., Efferent cortico-cortical projections of the prefrontal cortex in the rhesus monkey, *Brain Research*, 31 (1971) 35–46.
44. Robinson, D.L., Goldberg, M.E. and Stanton, G.B., Parietal association cortex in the primate: Sensory mechanisms and behavioral modulations, *J. Neurophysiol.*, 41 (1978) (in press).
45. Sakai, M., Prefrontal unit activity during visually guided lever pressing reaction in the monkey, *Brain Research*, 81 (1974) 297–309.
46. Suzuki, H. and Azuma, M., A glass-insulated "elgiloy" microelectrode for recording unit activity in chronic monkey experiments, *Electroenceph. clin. Neurophysiol.*, 41 (1976) 93–95.
47. Suzuki, H. and Azuma, M., Prefrontal neuronal activity during gazing at a light spot in the monkey, *Brain Research*, (1977) 497–508.
48. Tanji, J. and Evarts, E.V., Anticipatory activity of motor cortex neurons in relation to direction of an intended movement, *J. Neurophysiol.*, 39 (1976) 1062–1068.
49. Teuber, H.-L., The riddle of frontal lobe function in man. In J.M. Warren., and K. Akert (Eds.) *The Frontal Granular Cortex and Behavior*, McGraw-Hill, New York, 1964, pp. 410–444.
50. Teuber, H. L., Unity and diversity of frontal lobe functions, *Acta neurobiol. exp.*, 32 (1972) 615–656.
51. Walker, A.E., *The Primate Thalamus*, The University of Chicago Press, Chicago, 1938, 319 pp.
52. Wurtz, R.H. and Mohler, C.W., Enhancement of visual responses in monkey striate cortex and frontal eye fields, *J. Neurophysiol.*, 39 (1976) 766–793.

The visual learning area in the inferotemporal cortex of monkeys

EIICHI IWAI

Tokyo Metropolitan Institute for Neurosciences,
Fuchu, Tokyo 183, Japan

The inferotemporal cortex (IT) in monkeys is a crucial area for visual discrimination learning (visual learning area or focus). Even a small and partial lesion made within the IT produces a marked impairment of visual learning[29,30]. The exact locus and extent of the IT visual area and its functional nature are not clear, however. This paper presents studies concerning the localization of the visual learning area in the temporal lobe of the monkey. In the absence of well-defined boundaries, IT lesions made for the purpose of analyzing the nature of the resulting visual impairment have varied widely within and between studies.

The discovery of the visual area in the temporal lobe in the monkey stemmed from two studies by Brown and Schäfer[2] and by Klüver and Bucy[33], which reported some drastic changes in the behavior of monkeys following bilateral temporal lobectomy, known as Klüver-Bucy syndrome. Perhaps the most striking and interesting effect was the symptom of "psychic blindness" or "visual agnosia", connoting an inability of their monkeys to recognize objects by vision. Klüver[32] considered the visual disturbance to be but one manifestation of a more profound disturbance in behavior.

The "Klüver-Bucy syndrome" was subsequently studied by Lashley's associates, e.g., Blum[1], Chow[6,7], Pribram, etc. They showed that the component symptoms could be produced independently by smaller and different lesions. Impairment of visual discrimination learning unaccompanied by other symptoms, followed lesions of the neocortex of the posterior association cortex, including the temporal cortex, whereas the remaining aspects of the syndrome resulted from destruction of rhinencephalic structures of the temporal lobe, particularly of the amygdala.

Mishkin[37] and Mishkin and Pribram[41] demonstrated that the cortex crucial for normal visual discrimination learning is the IT, comprising the middle and inferior gyri of the temporal lobe. By contrast, a number of studies up to the present have indicated that lesions of regions of the association cortex other than IT have no effect on visual discrimination. Even frontal or parietal lesion had no or a negligible effect on visual discrimination, when the animals were tested on a pair of objects or on the usual pattern discriminations presented simultaneously.

On the other hand, the IT lesion has no effect on the discrimination learning in other sensory or on spatial tasks. The evidence indicates that the IT is involved in vision only, that is, that it has a modality-specific function. As for the cortical mechanisms of the sensory modalities other than vision, it has been generally considered that the superior temporal cortex is involved in auditory discrimination learning, the parietal association cortex in tactile, the insular cortex in gustatory, and the temporal pole and the lateral orbital cortex in olfactory discrimination learning. Moreover, the frontal cortex is concerned with spatial function. These findings indicate that several regions within the association cortex have a modality-specific function (see reviews[13,18,22–27,38,51]).

The studies in which the visual area in the temporal lobe was first described[6,37,41] identified

419

the area only in broad terms of the IT region, and there has been no systematic attempt since then to delineate it more precisely. For a standard or reproducible lesion, however, the view gradually evolved that the IT visual area coincided with the cytoarchitectural area TE in terms of von Bonin and Bailey[48] or, equivalently, Brodmann's areas 20 and 21.

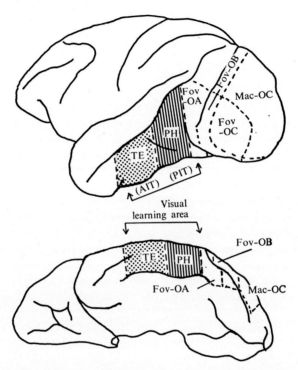

Fig. 1. Two visual learning foci in the temporal association cortex of monkeys, and diagrammatical representations of various cortical visual areas.
    The visual learning area consists of two anatomically and functionally distinguishable sub-areas. The anterior inferotemporal subarea (AIT) or Area TE (dotted area) is concerned with visual memory or associative learning, and the posterior inferotemporal subarea (PIT) or Area PH (or TEO) (hatched area) is involved in pattern perception or selective attention in visual discrimination learning[30,39]. The foveal prestriate cortex (Fov-Prest) is shown here outside the visual learning area, and consists of Fov-OA and Fov-OB as indicated in the figure.

The nature of the underlying visual impairment resulting from IT lesions (IT impairment) has been interpreted in many very different ways. Some investigators[4,5,8,9,15,16,40,45] have proposed that the underlying disorder is a perceptual or an attentional disturbance; others[3,10,14,20,34, 36,50,53] have suggested that the basic deficit is in memory or in stimulus-reward association; and still others[42,47] have proposed that it is a subtle sensory loss.

Delineation of the visual learning area

As mentioned above, the IT visual area was first defined in a broad sense, and many work-ers have considered that it occupies approximately the middle third of the temporal lobe; the an-terior half of the IT or Area TE.

Some results were obtained, however, which did not conform to this view and suggested rather that the posterior portion of the IT, outside Area TE, was also crucial for visual learning. For example, Mishkin and I found a relatively close correlation between backward extension of lesions beyond the posterior TE boundary and degree of visual deficit in pattern discrimination. On the other hand, there was no significant correlation between anterior extension of the lesions beyond the anterior TE boundary and degrees of visual impairment. Fig. 2a shows two examples of monkey with IT lesions (Iwai and Mishkin, unpublished). Both the bilateral lesions of the monkey on the left apparently invaded the portion posterior to the TE boundary, whereas neither of the bilateral lesions on the right extended into the posterior. The monkey with the former lesion required nearly 5 times as many trials to relearn as the monkey with the latter lesion. The degree of deficit in terms of relearning scores may be influenced by various factors. The large difference among relearning scores in the above cases might be due to the presence of invasion into the portion posterior to the TE area. Fig. 2b shows two examples of monkeys with crossed lesions. The monkey on the left failed to relearn even after 2000 retraining trials, while the monkey on the right retained the preoperatively learned habit perfectly. Again, the difference in the results might be attributable to the presence vs. absense of bilateral lesions of the portion between the inferior occipital sulcus and the posterior boundary of Area TE.

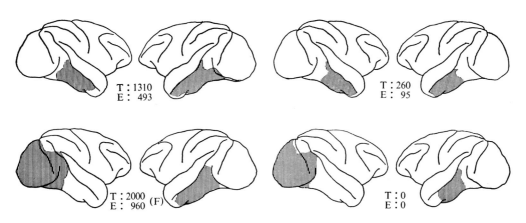

Fig. 2. Examples of analyses for localization of the inferotemporal visual area (Iwai and Mishkin).
a: Inferotemporal lesions and relearning scores on pattern discrimination. b: Crossed lesions of the unilateral prestriate and striate cortices and of the contralateral inferotemporal cortex, and relearning scores on pattern discrimination.
Note that the relearning scores of the two monkeys in each experiment were quite different. T, Relearning trials; E, errors. Hatching, lesioned area. (F), failure of relearning.

Mishkin and I undertook, therefore, to examine this possibility and, simultaneously, to investigate the other presumed boundaries of the visual learning area. For this purpose, we tested the effects of very small lesions distributed along the entire length of the IT upon pattern discrimination relearning[29]. The lesions made in this experiment are shown schematically in Fig. 3b and the postoperative relearning results are indicated in Fig. 3a.

As a result, the visual learning area could be fairly closely defined. Beginning at the ascending limb of the inferior occipital sulcus (specifically, at the downward vertical extension from the limb toward the occipitotemporal sulcus), the visual learning area extends forward along the combined middle and inferior temporal gyri for about 2 cm, or approximately to the posterior portion

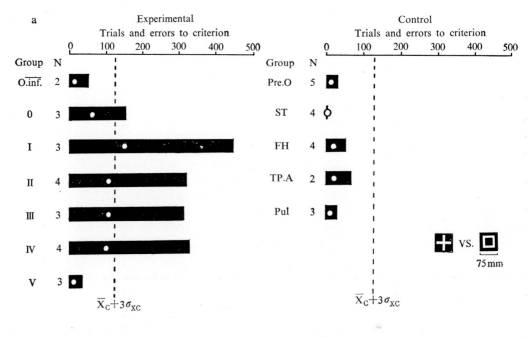

a

Experimental
Trials and errors to criterion

Control
Trials and errors to criterion

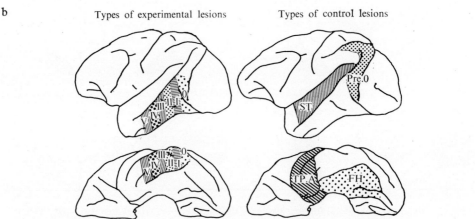

b   Types of experimental lesions   Types of control lesions

Fig. 3.   Results of a small strip lesion study (Iwai and Mishkin).
     a: Group mean scores for pattern discrimination relearning after various lesions.   b: Diagram-
matic representation of various lesions made within the inferotemporal cortex (IT) and lateral prestriate cortex (lateral Prest) (experimental lesions, left) and made outside the above experimental lesioned areas (control lesions, right).
     Each experimental group received one of seven different types of bilateral small strip lesions
(O-V and O. $\overline{\text{inf}}$), which were sequentially arranged along the IT and Prest. Each of the I-V lesions
was made rostrocaudally 5 mm wide, and extended dorsoventrally from the bottom of the superior
temporal sulcus to the bottom of the occipitotemporal sulcus. Lesion type O was an ablation of the
lateral part of the Prest, extending from posterior to Type 1 into the lunate sulcus and including both
banks of the inferior occipital sulcus and the anterior bank of the lunate sulcus. Lesion type O. inf was
the same as Type O lesion, but leaving intact both banks of the inferior occipital sulcus. Control lesions
were much larger ones. For Pre. O lesion, ablation of the preoccipital gyrus and the dorsolateral portion of the inferior parietal lobule. For ST lesion, ablation of the superior temporal gyrus. For lesion
Type FH, ablation of the fusiform, parahippocampal gyri and anterior half of the lingual gyrus. For
lesion TP.A, ablation of the temporal pole and amygdala. For lesion Pul (not presented in Fig. 2b),
damage to the pulvinar nuclei. Each type of lesion was made bilaterally and symmetrically, including
banks adjacent to the intended lesioned part in the gyrus. The insert in Fig. 2a shows the task employed; + - pattern was positive, i.e. baited with a piece of peanut (30 trials, daily sessions). Ninety
correct responses out of 100 trials was used as the learning criterion.

of the anterior middle temporal sulcus. Although we did not attempt to delineate the dorsal and ventral limits more clearly in this study, it may be concluded that these limits are the bottom of the superior temporal sulcus, and the bottom of the occipitotemporal sulcus, respectively (Fig. 1), since lesions of Types ST and FH were without effect on visual discrimination performance.

This redefinition is important on several counts. (1) The visual learning area clearly extends quite far backwards, contrary to earlier views, including the posterior half as well as the anterior half of the IT. (2) Correlation with data from neuroanatomical studies suggests that this behaviorally defined visual area may be composed of two neurally distinguishable subareas, the anterior and posterior portions of the visual learning area (AIT and PIT, respectively). In correlation with the cytoarchitectural charts, these subareas AIT and PIT correspond to Areas TE and PH (or TEO)[29,43,49], respectively. (3) Subsequent studies[30,39] have indicated that these subareas play functionally distinguishable roles in visual discrimination learning: the anterior subarea or Area TE contributes predominantly to memory or associative learning, whereas the posterior subarea or Area PH (TEO) primarily serves perception or selective attention in visual learning. (4) On this basis, dual mechanisms for the visual learning in IT can be proposed, contrary to the earlier view of a unitary mechanism[23,27,30].

Reinvestigation of the localization of the posterior visual learning subarea

Our findings in the above localization study have been confirmed by many subsequent studies. On reviewing these subsequent studies, however, some important differences can be seen among them as to their definition of the locus and extent of the visual learning area, and their nomenclature for the subareas. Representative studies are listed in Table 1, showing their approximate correlations.

TABLE 1.   Loci and extents of visual learning subareas and their nomenclature according to various investigators

Cytoarchitectural areas[29,48,49] / Investigators	Area TE	Area PH	Area OA (Foveal representation only†)	Area OB
Iwai et al.[22,29]	Anterior Inferotemporal (or Area TE)	Posterior Inferotemporal (or Area PH, or TEO)	Foveal OA	Foveal OB
			Foveal Prestriate	
Iversen[21]	Anterior Inferotemporal	Posterior Inferotemporal (including a part of ventral OA)	——	
Gross et al.[18]	Inferotemporal	Foveal Prestriate	——	
Pribram[12]	Inferotemporal (corresponding to classical Inferotemporal)	Foveal Prestriate (sometimes including Macular Prestriate†)		
Keating[31]	Inferotemporal (corresponding ·to classical Inferotemporal)	Prestriate (corresponding to subtotal OA and OB areas in color map by von Bonin and Bailey)		

†Refer to Fig. 1.

The delineation of the rostral, dorsal and ventral limits of the visual area are all in fairly good accord, but the posterior boundary is still not generally agreed upon; some workers (e.g., Iwai *et al.*[22],[29], Iversen *et al.*[21]) have drawn it at the ascending limb of the inferior occipital sulcus; others (e.g., Gross[11],[18]) have placed it at the lunate sulcus; and still others (e.g., Pribram *et al.*[12], Keating[31]) have put it at the OB-OC boundary.

No localization study on the visual learning area has been reported since our small strip lesion study, to my knowledge. Thus, the above discrepancy as to the posterior extent seems to be caused by our results on Type O lesion, which produced a significant but small deficit, as well as the other types of small strip lesions (Fig. 3). Although we pointed out that the small deficit following the Type O lesion was probably due to damage to the anterior portion within the Type O area, this might not be taken as the case. I decided therefore to reexamine the localization of the visual learning area, particularly as regards its posterior extent.

In order to delineate the posterior extent of the visual learning area more precisely and, simultaneously, to check the functional nature of the cytoarchitecturally classified areas, Kikuchi, Ichinose and I investigated the effects of bilateral lesions of the Foveal OA (Fov-OA), Foveal OB (Fov-OB), Macular OC (Mac-OC), and partial PH upon pattern discrimination learning (preparing for publication). The locus and extent of each lesion made in this study are diagrammed in Fig. 1. The task, procedure and apparatus employed in this study were essentially the same as were used in the previous experiments.

The results are shown in Fig. 4. Only the PH group showed a marked deficit. It may therefore be concluded from the present and foregoing results that the posterior boundary is located at the ascending limb of the inferior occipital sulcus, and that only Area PH (or TEO) is involved in the posterior visual learning area; Areas OA and OB are not.

The anatomical identification, including the cytoarchitectural features, of the posterior subarea of the visual learning area as defined by us in the monkey are not necessarily definitive. von Bonin and Bailey depicted this area as a part of Area OA in their original charts[48], but they later adopted a suggestion by Petr *et al.*[43] who labeled this area PH, and they relabeled this transitional portion between Areas OA and TE proper as Area TEO(PH)[49], although they did not establish this classification on cytoarchitectural grounds.

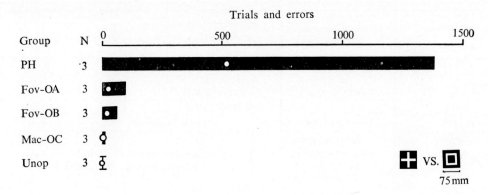

Fig. 4.   Group mean scores of relearning on pattern discrimination following ablations of areas of the PH, Fov-OA, Fov-OB and Mac-OC (Kikuchi, Ichinose and Iwai).

Insert, discrimination task; + - pattern, positively baited with a raisin (30 trials, daily sessions). Ninety correct responses out of 100 trials was used as the learning criterion. Refer to Fig. 1 for details of lesions.

In attempt to obtain anatomical evidence supporting our behavioral distinctions for the visual cortical areas as presented in Fig. 1, Kido, Umitsu, Yukie and I have investigated the distribution patterns of the labeled cells following injection of horseradish peroxidase (HRP) into various cortical areas (preparing for publication). Here, only the results that appear to support our view that the posterior subarea (PIT) is distinguishable from the prestriate, Areas OA and OB, are presented. The main findings pertained to the lateral geniculate nucleus (LGN). No labeled cell was found in the LGN following injection into the PIT. Contrary to previous reports based on anterograde degeneration studies, however, retrogradely labeled cells were found in the LGN following injection of HRP into the Prest (OA and/or OB), showing a clear topographical relation between them. The result was not artifactual, due to diffusion of HRP into the adjacent striate cortex and optic radiation, since the labeled cells in the LGN of the monkey following injections of HRP into striate and prestriate cortices were different in shape and location. I once assumed that this transitional area of the PIT in the monkey might be a possible OA subdivision, not a TE subdivision, mainly after von Bonin and Bailey's original charts and partly based on the finding of a topographical relation between the pulvinar nuclei and cortical areas. The above finding strongly suggests, however, that the posterior subarea is anatomically distinguishable from Areas OA and OB.

Our conclusion that the visual learning area is distinct from Areas OA and OB appears to be supported by another recent finding[28] in our laboratory. We found that complete ablation of the foveal prestriate (Fov-Prest), i.e., combined ablations of Fov-OA and Fov-OB, produced a marked impairment of visual discrimination learning, whereas ablations of Fov-OA, Fov-OB, Exra-Fov-Prest or Mac-OC alone did not result in visual deficit. Thus, both the total removal of the IT visual area and of Fov-Prest showed a similar severe visual deficit. On the other hand, the findings following small or partial lesions were different: partial lesions made within the IT visual area affected visual learning significantly, whereas partial lesions made within Fov-Prest did not. These findings indicate that Fov-Prest plays a different role in visual discrimination performance from that of the IT visual area. Presumably, the Fov-Prest sends visual efferents into the IT visual learning area. As is well-established[35], the striate cortex sends its fibers into both Areas OA and OB (the prestriate), and in turn these areas project their fibers to the IT. Thus, even after partial ablation of Fov-Prest, there is still a reliable interaction between the striate and IT through the portion within the Fov-Prest which remains intact, resulting in no deficit in visual discrimination. On the other hand, the complete removal of the Fov-Prest makes it impossible for the IT visual area to receive visual input or information, resulting in a marked impairment similar to the severe deficit following removal of the IT visual area (so-called disconnexion symptom[17]). Our finding thus throws a new light upon the long-standing question of prestriate functions from a neurobehavioral viewpoint.

Finally, we will consider the nomenclature for these subareas of the visual learning area (see Table 1). The above findings indicate that neither the OA nor OB area is a part of the visual learning area. Generally speaking, the prestriate cortex consists of two anatomically distinguishable areas of the OA or peristriate and the OB or parastriate cortices. The visual learning area here defined is located within the IT. On this basis, I believe, the term foveal prestriate for the posterior subarea of the IT visual learning area seems to be at least inadequate. The term inferotemporal for the anterior subarea may also be unsuitable, since the anterior subarea occupies a rostral part of the IT and does not represent the whole IT. We therefore tentatively propose calling these two subareas of the visual learning area the anterior and posterior inferotemporal subareas (AIT and PIT), respectively, and using the term (total) inferotemporal visual learning area (TIT) for the combination of these subareas. Also, we propose using the term foveal prestriate (Fov-Prest; Fov-OA and Fov-OB) for that cortex caudal to the TIT within the prestriate cortex (Areas OA and OB) and anteriorly and ventrally adjacent to the foveal striate (Fov-OC)[19,46,52], as shown diagrammatically in Fig. 1.

Acknowledgment: I thank my co-workers, Prof. M. Mishkin (NIH), Drs. R. Kikuchi and T. Ichinose, Messrs. Y. Osawa, K. Umitsu and M. Yukie and Miss S. Kido for their advice, discussions and co-operation.

References

1. Blum, J.S., Chow, K.L. and Pribram, K.H., A behavioral analysis of the organization of parieto-temporo-preoccipital cortex, *J. comp. Neurol.*, 93 (1950) 53–100.
2. Brown, S. and Schäfer, E.A., An investigation into the functions of the occipital and temporal lobes of the monkey's brain, *Phil. Trans.*, 179 (1888) 303–327.
3. Buffery, A.W.H., Attention and retention following frontal and temporal lesions in the baboon, *Proc. Amer. psychol. Ass.*, 73 (1965) 103–104.
4. Butter, C.M. and Gekoski, W.L., Alterations in pattern equivalence following inferotemporal and lateral striate lesions in rhesus monkeys, *J. comp. physiol. Psychol.*, 61 (1966) 309–312.
5. Butter, C.M., Mishkin, M. and Rosvold, H.E., Stimulus generalization in monkeys with inferotemporal and lateral occipital lesions. In D.J. Mostofsky (Ed.) *Stimulus Generalization*, Stanford University Press, California, 1965, pp. 119–133.
6. Chow, K.L., Effects of partial extirpation of posterior association cortex on visually mediated behavior in monkeys, *Comp. psychol. Monog.*, 20 (1951) 187–217.
7. Chow, K.L., Further studies on selective ablation of associative cortex in relation to visually mediated behavior, *J. comp. physiol. Psychol.*, 45 (1952) 109–118.
8. Chow, K.L., Effects of temporal neocortical ablation on visual discrimination learning sets in monkeys, *J. comp. physiol. Psychol.*, 47 (1954) 194–198.
9. Chow, K.L. and Orbach, J., Performance of visual discriminations presented tachistoscopically in monkeys with temporal neocortical ablations, *J. comp. physiol. Psychol.*, 50 (1957) 636–640.
10. Cordeau, J.P. and Mahut, H., Some long-term effects of temporal lobe resections on auditory and visual discrimination in monkeys, *Brain*, 87 (1964) 177–190.
11. Cowey, A. and Gross, C.G., Effects of foveal prestriate and inferotemporal lesions on visual discrimination by rhesus monkeys, *Exp. Brain Res.*, 11 (1970) 128–144.
12. Christensen, C.A. and Pribram, K.H., The visual discrimination performance of monkeys with foveal prestriate and inferotemporal lesions, *Physiol. Behav.*, 18 (1977) 403–407.
13. Dean, P., Effects of inferotemporal lesions on the behavior of monkeys, *Psychol. Bull.*,183 (1976) 41–71.
14. Dean, P. and Cowey, A., Inferotemporal lesions and memory for pattern discrimination after visual interference, *Neuropsychologica*, 15 (1977) 93–98.
15. Ettlinger, G., Visual discrimination with a single manipulandum following temporal ablations in the monkey, *Quart. J. exp. Psychol.*, 11 (1959) 164–174.
16. Ettlinger, G., Relationship between test difficulty and the visual impairment in monkeys with ablations of temporal cortex, *Nature (Lond.)*, 196 (1962) 911–912.
17. Geschwind, N., Disconnexion syndromes in animals and man: Parts (1) and (11), *Brain*, 88 (1965) 237–294 and 585–644.
18. Gross, C.G., Visual functions of inferotemporal cortex. In R. Jung (Ed.) *Handbook of Sensory Physiology, Vol. VII, Pt. 3, Central Processing of Visual Information B*, Springer-Verlag, Berlin, 1973, pp. 451–482.
19. Hubel, D.H. and Freeman, D.C., Projection into the visual field of ocular dominance columns in macaque monkey, *Brain Research*, 122 (1977) 336–343.
20. Iversen, S.D., Interference and inferotemporal memory deficits, *Brain Research*, 19 (1970) 277–289.
21. Iversen, S.D., Brain lesions and memory in animals. In A.J. Deutsch (Ed.) *The Physiological Basis of Memory*, Academic Press, New York, 1973, pp. 305–364.
22. Iwai, E., Experimental visual agnosia, *Advanc. neurol. Sci.*, 15 (1971) 71–86 (in Japanese).
23. Iwai, E., Review of neurobehavioral studies on visual mechanisms in the temporal lobe: (I) and (II), *Igaku-no-Ayumi (Progr. Med. Japan)*, 83 (1972) 514–518 and 565–571 (in Japanese).

24. Iwai, E., Central mechanisms of visual learning and its plasticity. In J. Nagumo and H. Mannen (Eds.) *The Contemporary Neurosciences, Vol. II*, 1976, pp. 175–203 (in Japanese).

25. Iwai, E., Experimental studies on agnosia, apraxia, and aphasia in the monkey and ape, *Advanc. neurol. Sci.*, 21 (1977) 1029–1039 (in Japanese).

26. Iwai, E., Function of the posterior association cortex, *Advanc. neurol. Sci.*, 21 (1977) 1116–1130 (in Japanese).

27. Iwai, E., The association cortex. In T. Tokizane, K. Iwama and H. Shimazu (Eds.) *Physiology of the Brain*, Asakura-shoten, Tokyo (in press) (in Japanese).

28. Iwai, E. and Ichinose, T., Visual impairment following ablation of prestriate association cortex in monkeys, *Japan Acad.*, 53 (1977) 83–86.

29. Iwai, E. and Mishkin, M., Further evidence on the locus of the visual area in the temporal lobe of the monkey, *Exp. Neurol.*, 25 (1969) 585–594.

30. Iwai, E. and Mishkin, M., Extrastriate visual focus in monkeys: Two visual foci in the temporal lobe of monkeys. In N. Yoshii and N.A. Buchwald (Eds.) *Neurophysiological Basis of Learning and Behavior*, Osaka University Press, 1968, pp. 23–33.

31. Keating, E.G., Effects of prestriate and striate lesions on the monkey's ability to locate and discriminate visual forms, *Exp. Neurol.*, 47 (1975) 16–25.

32. Klüver, H., Brain mechanisms and behavior with special reference to the rhinencephalon, *Lancet*, 12 (1952) 567–577.

33. Klüver, H. and Bucy, P.C., Psychic blindness and other symptoms following bilateral temporal lobectomy in rhesus monkeys, *Amer. J. Physiol.*, 119 (1937) 352–353.

34. Kovner, R. and Stamm, J.S., Disruption of short-term visual memory by electrical stimulation of inferotemporal cortex in the monkey, *J. comp. physiol. Psychol.*, 81 (1972) 163–172.

35. Kuypers, H.G.J.M., Szwarcbart, M.K., Mishkin, M. and Rosvold, H.E., Occipitotemporal corticocortical connections in the rhesus monkey, *Exp. Neurol.*, 11 (1965) 245–262.

36. Lashley, K.S., Functional interpretation of anatomic patterns, *Res. Publ. Ass. Ner. Ment. Dis.*, 30 (1950) 529–547.

37. Mishkin, M., Visual discrimination performance following partial ablations of the temporal lobe: II. Ventral surface vs. hippocampus, *J. comp. physiol. Psychol.*, 47 (1954) 187–193.

38. Mishkin, M., Visual mechanisms beyond the striate cortex. In R. Russell (Ed.) *Frontiers in Physiological Psychology*, Academic Press, New York, 1966, pp. 93–119.

39. Mishkin, M., Cortical visual area and their interactions. In A.G. Karczmar and J.C. Eccles (Eds.) *Brain and Human Behavior*, Springer-Verlag, New York, 1972, pp. 187–208.

40. Mishkin, M. and Hall, M., Discrimination along a size continuum following ablation of the inferior temporal convexity in monkeys, *J. comp. physiol. Psychol.*, 48 (1955) 97–101.

41. Mishkin, M. and Pribram, K.H., Visual discrimination performance following partial ablations of the temporal lobe: I. Ventral vs. lateral, *J. comp. physiol. Psychol.*, 47 (1954) 14–20.

42. Pasik, T., Pasik, P., Battersby, W.S. and Bender, M.B., Factors influencing visual behavior of monkeys with bilateral temporal lobe lesions, *J. Comp. Neurol.*, 115 (1960) 89–102.

43. Petr, R., Holden, L.B. and Jirout, J., The efferent intercortical connections of the superficial cortex of the temporal lobe (*Macaca mulatta*), *J. Neuropathol. exp. Neurol.*, 8 (1949) 100–103.

44. Pribram, H.B. and Barry, J., Further behavioral analysis of parieto-temporo-preoccipital cortex, *J. Neurophysiol.*, 19 (1956) 99–106.

45. Stepien, L.S., Cordeau, J.P. and Rasmussen, T., The effect of temporal lobe and hippocampal lesions on auditory and visual recent memory in monkeys, *Brain*, 83 (1960) 470–489.

46. Talbot, S.A. and Marshall, W.H., Neural mechanisms of visual localization, *Amer. J. Ophthal.*, 24 (1914) 1255–1263.

47. Valciukas, J.A. and Pasik, P., Influence of illumination on pattern discrimination thresholds in monkeys with temporal lesions, *Fed. Proc.*, 24 (1965) 274.

48. von Bonin, G. and Bailey, P., *The Neocortex of Macaca mulatta*, University of Illinois Press, Urbana, Ill., 1947.

49. von Bonin, G. and Bailey, P., *The Isocortex of the Chimpanzee*, University of Illinois Press, Urbana, Ill., 1950.

50. Weiskrantz, L., Impairment of learning and retention following experimental temporal lobe lesions. In M.A.B. Brazier (Ed.) *Brain Function, Vol. II, RNA and Brain Function, Memory and Learning*, University of California Press, California, 1964, pp. 203–231.

51. Weiskrantz, L., The interaction between occipital and temporal cortex in vision: An overview. In O. Schmitt and F.G. Worden (Eds.) *The Neurosciences, The Third Study Program*, MIT Press, Cambridge, Mass., 1974. pp. 189–203.

52. Whitteridge, D., Projection of optic pathways to the visual cortex. In R. Jung (Ed.) *Handbook of Sensory Physiology, Vol. VII, Pt. 3, Central Visual Information B*, Springer-Verlag, Berlin, 1973, pp. 247–268.

53. Wilson, M., Further analysis of intersensory facilitation of learning sets in monkeys, *Percep. Mot. Skills*, 18 (1964) 917–920.

Effect of destruction of microtubules upon the memory function of mice

TETUHIDE H. MURAKAMI

Department of Physiology, Okayama University Medical School,
Shikata-cho, Okayama 700, Japan

Recently, microtubules have been found to be related to a number of functions, in addition to their roles in mitosis, such as the formation of cytoskeleton, cilia and flagella, granule movement, secretion and neuronal activities. Antimitotic agents, e.g. colchicine and vinblastine, which are known to disrupt microtubules, impede these functions. Our work has been concerned with the effect of vinblastine on learning behavior in mice[4], as it produces extensive paracrystal formation in myelinated axons of the hippocampal cortex[3].

In order to test learning, we used a training apparatus called a jump-box[2]. It was made of opaque plastic board, 30 × 30 × 30 cm in size with an electric grid floor. An escape net was attached 10 cm above the floor. The conditioning stimulus (CS) was either a light and buzzer presented for 3 sec. Termination of the CS was followed by the onset of an electric shock, as an unconditioning stimulus (UCS) of 40 V (AC) for 20 sec through the grid floor. The average interval from the start of one trial to that of the succeeding one was approximately 30 sec. When the animal jumped onto the escape shelf before the onset of the UCS, we judged that an avoidance response had occurred. One session of training consisted of 30 or 60 successive trials.

ddN strain mice with high training scores were selected for genetic improvement through avoidance training[1]. When the mice jumped up after a conditioned stimulus (CS) in more than 20 times out of the first 60 trials, they were allowed to mate. In the 7th and later generations of brother and sister matings, the mice showed the response more than 15 times out of the first 30 trials. The standard deviation of the scores in the 10th generation (ddN-F10) was significantly different, as compared with the earlier generations of inbred mice. There was no appreciable difference between the male and female as to learning ability.

Memory formation was compared using avoidance training between ddN-F10 strain and the following inbred strains; C3H, DBA, C57-BL, RF, AKR, C58, D103, C6 and CBA. The results are shown in Fig. 1.

Vinblastine sulfate (Lilly Co.) was dissolved in physiological saline solution. Under light anesthesia by either inhalation, 0.5 μg of vinblastine was injected into each of the right and left frontal lobes at a depth of 3 mm below the cortical surface, or 50 μg of vinblastine was given intraperitoneally. Control mice received the same volume of physiological saline solution.

The mice injected with vinblastine did not show any appreciable change in their open field activity, but there were some changes in their learning capability. When vinblastine was injected intraperitoneally one week before the first training session, learning was blocked. When it was injected immediately after the first training, memory acquisition was slightly retarded. After consolidation of the memory, intraperitoneal administration of vinblastine was no longer effective.

Intracerebral administration one week before the first training session affected learning significantly, the effect being apparent even in the second session (Fig. 2-A). Upon injection immediate-

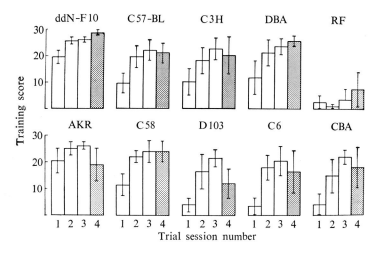

Fig. 1. Comparison of memory formation in avoidance training with an average of 24 mice for each
group in various mouse strains. Ordinates show training scores in 30 trials. Hollow columns are for
three sessions performed with one-week intervals and the doted one indicates that 4 weeks after the
3rd session. Bers attached to columns show standard deviations.

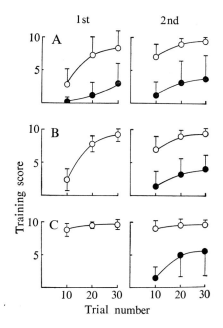

Fig. 2. Learning curves in mice intracerebrally injected with saline (0) and vinblastine. A, Injected
one week before the first training session; B, injected immediately after the first session; C, injected
after consolidation. Ordinates show mean training scores in 10 trials.

ly after the first session, memory of the training was obliterated (Fig. 2-B). Even the consolidated memory was profoundly impaired by intra-cerebral injection (Fig. 2-C).

An electronmicroscopic study of the hippocampus showed extensive paracrystal formation in myelinated axons 5 hr to 7 days after vinblastine administration.

REFERENCES

1. Hara, T., Genetic improvement of mouse through the avoidance learning, *Okayama Igakkai Zasshi*, 89 (1977) 1549–1560 (in Japanese).
2. Hayakawa, M., The effect of cycloheximide on mouse learning, *Acta Med. Okayama*, 31 (1977) 161–175.
3. Hirano, A., The pathology of the central myelinated axon. **In**: The structure and function of nervous tissue, ed. by Bourne, G.H. Academic Press, New York and London, Vol. 5, (1972) pp. 73–162.
4. Murakami, T.H., Microtubules and memory, *Igakuno Ayumi*, 93 (1975) 306–307, (in Japanese).

Neurochemical correlates of learning disability in experimental phenylketonuric rats and postnatal undernourished rats

YASUZO TSUKADA AND SHIN-ICHI KOHSAKA

Department of Physiology, Keio University School of Medicine,
Shinjuku-ku, Tokyo 160, Japan

This study aimed to clarify certain mechanisms involved in higher nervous activities such as learning and memory. It is well known that phenylketonuria accompanies severe mental retardation, and that growth restriction due to undernutrition at certain ages results in many children in irreversible deficit of mental function[3]. Experimental phenylketonuric rats (PKU rats) and postnatal undernourished rats (C-D rats) were therefore produced, and neurochemical changes in these animals which could be a correlate of learning disability were investigated.

PKU rats were produced by feeding with a diet containing 7% L-phenylalanine for several months starting from the 22nd day after birth. Some PKU rats were rehabilitated by feeding with a normal diet from 3 months after birth (rehabilitated PKU rats). In order to produce postnatal undernourished rats, dams were fed on a low protein diet (12% casein) just after delivery for 21 days, and after weaning, pups were fed on the same diet throughout the experiment.

The DNA content in the cerebrum was measured by the method of Burton[1] following the fractionation procedures of Schmidt-Thannhauser[7] and Schneider[8]. The content of 5-hydroxy-tryptamine (5-HT) and 5-hydroxyindol acetic acid (5-HIAA) in the cerebrum was estimated by the method of Fischer *et al.*[4] 2′, 3′-Cyclic nucleotide 3′-phosphohydrolase (CNPase) activities were measured in several parts of the brain by the method of Kurihara and Tsukada[5]. The tryptophan content in the cerebrum was determined by the method of Denckla and Dewey[2]. Protein content was determined by the method of Lowry *et al.*[6]. The operant brightness discrimination learning test (variable interval schedule; VI-15″) was performed using the procedure of Tsukada *et al.*[9].

Gains in body weight and cerebral weight were suppressed in PKU rats and in C-D rats, but the total DNA content in the cerebrum did not differ from that of control rats (Table 1). The cell number in the cerebrum thus appeared to be maintained in the experimental rats.

The 5-HT and 5-HIAA content in the cerebrum of PKU rats decreased remarkably at 50 days of age. The tryptophan content in the cerebrum also decreased significantly. On the other hand, the contents of 5-HT, 5-HIAA and tryptophan in the cerebrum of rehabilitated PKU rats showed normal values at the age of 4 months. On the basis of these results, it was suggested that the transient decrease in 5-HT and 5-HIAA contents was due to depletion of tryptophan in the cerebrum caused by inhibition of tryptophan uptake into the cerebrum as a result of elevation of phenylalanine in the plasma. The contents of 5-HT and 5-HIAA in the cerebrum of C-D rats did not differ from those of the controls. It was proposed therefore that synaptogenesis of mono-aminergic neurons occurred normally in PKU rats, rehabilitated PKU rats and C-D rats.

To investigate the grade of myelination in the cerebrum of these experimental rats, the activity of CNPase which was considered to represent a good marker enzyme of the myelin sheath

TABLE 1.   Neurochemical changes in the brain of phenylketonuric (PKU) and undernourished (C-D) rats[†1]

	DNA (mg/cerebrum)	5-HT (μg/g.w.w.)	CNPase (U/mg protein)	Learning ability
Control	1.08 ± 0.03 (4)[†2]	0.79 ± 0.01 (5)[†2]	3.16 ± 0.04 (3)[†3]	
PKU rats	1.03 ± 0.01 (4)[†2]	*0.33 ± 0.05 (5)[†2]	*2.76 ± 0.06 (3)[†3]	disturbed
Rehabilitated PKU rats		0.90 ± 0.05 (3)[†3]	*2.57 ± 0.09 (4)[†4]	disturbed
Control	1.19 ± 0.04 (5)[†5]	0.63 ± 0.04 (3)[†3]	3.74 ± 0.12 (5)[†5]	
C-D rats	1.11 ± 0.07 (5)[†5]	0.59 ± 0.04 (3)[†3]	*2.91 ± 0.08 (5)[†5]	disturbed

[†1] All values are means ± S.E. Numbers in parentheses show no. of rats used in each case. Asterisks indicate $P < 0.01$.

[†2] 50–day-old rats.

[†3] 4–month-old rats.

[†4] 7–month-old rats.

[†5] 8–month-old rats.

in the central nervous system[5], was determined. The CNPase activity in the cerebrum decreased significantly in PKU rats and C-D rats at the age of 4 months or 8 months. These results suggested that myelination was disturbed by the accumulation of phenylalanine in the cerebrum or under-nourishment at early postnatal stages of cerebral development. In rehabilitated PKU rats, the CNPase activity in the cerebrum also showed a lower level at the age of 7 months. It was con-cluded that the dysmyelination which occurred in the early postnatal period could not be reha-bilitated by feeding with a normal diet after the age of 3 months.

The operant brightness discrimination learning ability of the experimental rats was ex-amined. In control rats, the correct response ratio (no. of correct responses/(no. of correct responses + no. of errors)) increased gradually by training, and attained the criterion of discrimination learning within 35 sessions. In the case of PKU rats, rehabilitated PKU rats and C-D rats, the correct response ratio also increased gradually by training, but the animals were unable to attain the criterion of discrimination learning within 40 sessions. It was concluded that the discrimina-tion learning ability of these experimental rats was poor compared to the control rats.

The above results strongly suggested that the disability of discrimination learning in PKU rats, rehabilitated PKU rats and C-D rats was closely related to dysmyelination of the cerebrum rather than other neural factors such as cerebral weight, DNA content or monoamine content. It is proposed that myelination in the cerebrum in the early postnatal stage represents an impor-tant event in the establishment of the ability of operant discrimination learning.

REFERENCES

1. Burton, K., A study of the conditions and mechanism of the diphenylamine reaction for the colorimetric estima-tion of deoxyribonucleic acid, *Biochem. J.,* (1956) 315–322.
2. Denckla, W.D. and Dewey, H.K., The determination of tryptophan in plasma, liver and urine, *J. lab. clin. Med.,* 69 (1967) 160–169.
3. Dobbing, J., Undernutrition and the developing brain: The use of animal models to elucidate the human problem. In *Normal and Abnormal Development of Brain and Behavior*, Leiden University Press, 1971, pp. 20–30.
4. Fischer, C.A., Kariya, T. and Aprison, M.H., A comparison of the distribution of 5–HIAA and 5–HT in four specific brain areas of the rat and pigeon, *Comp. gen. Pharmacol.,* 1 (1970) 61–68.
5. Kurihara, T. and Tsukada, Y., The regional and subcellular distribution of 2′, 3′-cyclic nucleotide 3′–phospho-hydrolase in the central nervous system, *J. Neurochem.,* 14 (1967) 1167–1174.

6. Lowry, O.H., Roberts, N.R., Leiner, K., Wu, M. and Farr, L., The quantitative histochemistry of brain, *J. biol. Chem.*, 207 (1954) 1–17.
7. Schmidt, G. and Thannhauser, S.J., A method for the determination of deoxyribonucleic acid, ribonucleic acid and phosphoproteins in animal tissues, *J. biol. Chem.*, 161 (1945) 83–89.
8. Schneider W.C., Phosphorus compounds in animal tissues, *J. biol. Chem.*, 161 (1945) 293–303.
9. Tsukada, Y., Nomura, M., Nagai, K., Kohsaka, S., Kawahata, H., Ito, M. and Matsutani, T., Neurochemical correlates of learning ability. In *Behavioral Neurochemistry*, Spectrum Pub. Inc., New York, 1977, pp. 63–84.

A neurochemical analysis of hemispherectomized rats

YUICHI KOMAI, YUKIO KOBAYASHI, YASUHO NAGANO, SHIGEKO ARAKI, MASAHIDE OKUDA AND MEI SATAKE

Department of Neruochemistry, Brain Research Institute, Nigata University,
Asahi-machi, Niigata 951, Japan

Rats hemispherectomized in the early postnatal stage exhibit rather normal behavior. We attempted to find some neurochemical change specific to these rats which might have relevance to the molecular mechanisms of neural plasticity.

Wistar rats were operated on within 24 hr after birth. After craniotomy performed using a razor blade, the cerebral hemisphere on one side was removed by suction through a glass capillary. The operated rats were reared with their litter mates. Within a month their behavior became apparently indistinguishable from that of their control litter mates. After six months the animals were decapitated under light ether anaesthesia and their central nervous tissues were dissected in a cold room at 0–4° C.

Macroscopically, there was an enlargement of the olfactory bulb contralateral to the side of hemispherectomy, a decrease in the diameter of the contralateral optic nerve, and disappearance of the white line running longitudinally in the ventromedial portion of the medulla oblongata. The intact cerebral hemisphere, both cerebellar hemispheres, the brain stem and the spinal cord were separated by one worker (K.K.) and subjected to the following chemical analyses. The water content was determined from the difference of weight of the tissue before and after drying at 105° C for 4 hr; protein by the method of Lowry et al.[1]; the colchicine-binding activity of the homogenate according to the filter assay of Weisenberg et al.[2] with a minor modification; cerebroside plus sulfatide by the method of Scott and Melvin[3]; ganglioside by the method of Aminoff[4];

TABLE 1. Changes in constituents of the CNS of rats after hemispherectomy

Constituents	Changes (% of the control)	Regions
Tissue weight	100–113	cerebrum, cerebellum
Water content	100	
Total protein per tissue weight	100	
Water-soluble protein per tissue weight	92–100	brain stem
Colchicine binding activity per total protein	100–130	cerebellum, brain stem, spinal cord
DNA per tissue weight	100	
RNA per tissue weight	100–122	cerebrum, cerebellum, brain stem
	84–100	spinal cord
Ganglioside per tissue weight	86–100	cerebrum, brain stem
Phospholipid per tissue weight	90–100	cerebellum, spinal cord
Cholesterol per tissue weight	100–117	brain stem
Cerebroside + sulfatide per tissue weight	100–112	brain stem
Oxygen consumption	100	

phospholipid by the method of Keenan[5]; cholesterol by the method of Searcy and Bergquist[6]; DNA by the method of Burton[7] with some modifications; RNA by the method of Fleck and Munro[8] as modified by Satake and Abe[9]; oxygen consumption of slices of the cerebral cortex with Warburg's apparatus using 10 mM D-glucose as a substrate.

Biochemical data thus obtained are summarized in Table 1. Only those values of statistical significance are shown as percentages of the control ones, together with the regions where the differences were observed. Values of statistical insignificance are expressed as 100% without describing the regions.

This study shows that the constituents of the rat central nervous system remain fairly constant in spite of a large lesion in the cerebrum. The DNA content, an index of the number of cells, was not changed in any region of the CNS. Of the constituents whose variations were small but statistically significant, the increase in cholesterol, cerebroside plus sulfatide, and colchicine-binding protein, which constitute the nerve cell processes in the lower regions of the CNS may be relevant to the recovery of behavioral activities by the hemispherectomized rats.

REFERENCES

1. Lowry, O.H., Rosebrough, N.J., Farr, A.L. and Randall, R.J., Protein measurement with the Folin phenol reagent, *J. biol. Chem.*, 193 (1951) 265–274.
2. Weisenberg, R.C., Borisy, G.G. and Taylor, E.W., The colchicine-binding protein of mammalian brain and its relation to microtubules, *Biochemistry*, 7 (1968) 4466–4479.
3. Scott, T.A. and Melvin, E.H., Determination of dextran with anthrone, *Anal. Chem.*, 25 (1953) 1656–1661.
4. Aminoff, D., Methods for the quantitative estimation of N-acetylneuraminic acid and their application to hydrolysates of sialomucoids, *Biochem. J.*, 81 (1961) 384–392.
5. Keenan, R.W., Schmidt, G. and Tanaka, T., Quantitative determination of phosphatidylethanolamine and other phosphatides in various tissues of the rat, *Anal. Biochem.*, 23 (1958) 555–566.
6. Searcy, R.L. and Bergquist, L.M., A new color reaction for the quantitation of serum cholesterol, *Clin. chem. Acta*, 5 (1960) 192–199.
7. Burton, K., A Study of the conditions and mechanism of the diphenylamine reaction for the colorimetric estimation of deoxyribonucleic acid, *Biochem. J.*, 62 (1956) 315–323.
8. Fleck, A. and Munro, H.N., The precision of ultraviolet absorption measurements in the Schmidt-Thannhauser procedure for nucleic acid estimation, *Biophem. biocphys. Acta*, 55 (1962) 571–583.
9. Satake, M. and Abe, S., Preparation and characterization of nerve cell perikaryon from rat cerebral cortex, *J. Biochem.*, 59 (1966) 72–75.

Reorganization of the cerebello-cerebral response following hemicerebellectomy or cerebral cortical ablation in kittens

SABURO KAWAGUCHI, TETSURO YAMAMOTO AND AKIO SAMEJIMA

Department of Physiology, Institute for Brain Research, Faculty of Medicine, Kyoto University, Sakyo-ku, Kyoto 606, Japan

It has been reported that stimulation of the cerebellar nucleus in cats induces two distinct types of responses contralaterally in the two separate domains of the cerebral cortex, i.e., the frontal motor and parietal association cortex[5]. In the frontal cortex, it is a positive followed by negative wave in the superficial cortical layer which reverses polarity at a certain depth of the cortex and becomes a negative followed by positive wave in the deeper layer. In the parietal cortex, it is a surface negative-deep positive wave.

Studies on the postnatal development of the cerebello-cerebral response in kittens have revealed that basically the same type of response as in adult cats can be strongly evoked in the frontal cortex already at birth and in the parietal cortex at 2 days after birth (Kawaguchi, Yamamoto and Samejima, in preparation).

Changes in the cerebello-cerebral response after hemicerebellectomy or cerebral cortical ablation were studied in kittens by laminar field potential analysis in the cerebral cortex.

Kittens ranging in age from newborn to adolescent were hemicerebellectomized or had their cerebral cortices unilaterally or bilaterally ablated, i.e., in those areas which receive the cerebellar projection via the VA-VL complex of the thalamus[1,3]. Electrophysiological experiments were carried out at various stages of postoperative survival in 25 hemicerebellectomized and 23 decorticated kittens. Morphological studies were performed by the retrograde and anterograde horseadish peroxidase (HRP) tract-tracing methods in 7 kittens hemicerebellectomized before the 10th postnatal day and permitted to survive for 30–35 days.

In all 11 kittens hemicerebellectomized before 11 days of age and permitted to survive for more than 16 days after surgery, marked cerebello-cerebral responses with a clear-cut potential reversal at a certain depth of the cortex were evoked not only contralaterally as in normal animals but also ipsilaterally. The latter situation was quite different from that in normal animals in which the evoked potential in the ipsilateral cerebral cortex was, if at all, small and ambiguous, and usually devoid of appreciable potential reversal on the depth profile.

Neuronal connections for this ipsilateral response were investigated by extracellular recording from the cerebellar nuclear neurons activated antidromically on stimulation of the thalamus, and by destruction of the VL nucleus of the thalamus. In the former study, a remarkable increase in the number of bilateral cerebellothalamic projection neurons was found in the operated animals. The latter study confirmed that such neurons are responsible for the ipsilateral cerebellocerebral response. Morphological studies by the retrograde HRP tract-tracing method revealed that in the lateral nucleus of the cerebellum ipsilateral to the thalamus injected with HRP, HRP-labeled neurons were far more numerous in the operated animals than in the controls. The anterograde HRP tract-tracing studies revealed that presumed terminals of ipsilateral cerebellothalamic fibers were distributed more densely and extensively in the VA-VL complex of the operated animals.

It was concluded therefore that after neonatal hemicerebellectomy in kittens, nuclear neurons in the remaining cerebellum sprout axon collaterals growing into the thalamus ipsilateral to the spared nucleus.

In all 4 kittens hemicerebellectomized at 17–196 days of age, no ipsilateral cerebello-cerebral response could be evoked. However, a significant change was observed in the contralateral cerebello-cerebral response, i.e., there was appearance of the motor cortical response in the parietal cortex.

Unilateral or bilateral ablation of the cerebral cortical areas which receive the cerebellar projection led to an extensive reorganization of the contralateral cerebello-cerebral response while no appreciable ipsilateral response was observed. Unusual responses were found to appear in usually responsive areas and usual responses were recorded not only in the usual responsive areas but also in usually unresponsive areas. In kittens whose frontal cortex was previously ablated, the response in the parietal association cortex tended to resemble the response in the frontal cortex of normal animals. In the postcruciate sensory cortex or in the rostral portion of the ectosylvian gyrus, which is usually an unresponsive area, responses appeared which resembled those usually observed in the precruciate cortex. Responses similar to those in the parietal cortex of normal animals were frequently found to appear in the most caudal portion of the middle suprasylvian gyrus and in the caudal portion of the ectosylvian gyrus, which are usually unresponsive areas.

Despite the quite early ontogenesis and established synaptic connections at birth, cerebello-cerebral projections are predisposed towards an extensive reorganization after lesioning of their related structures. The appearance of an ipsilateral cerebello-cerebral response after neonatal hemicerebellectomy is evidently due to collateral sprouting of cerebellothalamic neurons. There is clearly a susceptible period for such collateral sprouting.

Tsukahara *et al.*[7]. have reported electrophysiological findings which indicate the formation of new terminals in corticorubral pathways even in adult cats after destruction of the interpositus nucleus. In the septal nucleus[4] and hippocampus[2,6], detailed research has confirmed collateral sprouting from neighboring axons in response to deafferentation in adult rats. Evidently, the susceptible period varies widely in different structures. It should be emphasized that lesioning of certain structures, as in the case of hemicerebellectomy, may bring about qualitatively different outcomes depending on the age of the animals at the time of surgery.

The functional significance of the extensive reorganization of the cerebello-thalamo-cerebral projection system following hemicerebellectomy or cerebral cortical ablation is open to question. It would correspond to a very strong capacity for functional recovery after traumatic or operative injury of the cerebellum, particularly in children.

ACKNOWLEDGEMENT: We wish to express our gratitude to Prof. K. Sasaki for his constant encouragement and helpful advice.

REFERENCES

1. Itoh, K. and Mizuno, N., Topographical arrangement of thalamocortical neurons in the centrolateral (CL) nucleus of the cat, with special reference to a spino-thalamo-motor cortical path through the CL, *Exp. Brain Res.*, 30 (1977) 471–480.

2. Lynch, G., Gall, C., Rose, G. and Cotman, C., Changes in the distribution of the dentate gyrus associational system following unilateral or bilateral entorhinal lesion in the adult rat, *Brain Research*, 110 (1976) 57–71.
3. Mizuno, N., Konishi, A., Sato, M., Kawaguchi, S., Yamamoto, T., Kawamura, S. and Yamawaki, M., Thalamic afferents to the rostral portions of the middle suprasylvian gyrus in the cat, *Exp. Neurol.*, 48 (1975) 79–87.
4. Raisman, G. and Field, P., A quantitative investigation of the development of collateral regeneration after partial deafferentation of the septal nuclei, *Brain Research*, 50 (1973) 241–264.
5. Sasaki, K., Kawaguchi, S., Matsuda, Y. and Mizuno, N., Electrophysiological studies on cerebello-cerebral projections in the cat, *Exp. Brain Res.*, 16 (1972) 75–88.
6. Steward, O., Cotman, C.W. and Lynch, G.S., Growth of a new fiber projection in the brain of adult rats: reinnervation of the dentate gyrus by contralateral entorhinal cortex following ipsilateral entorhinal lesions, *Exp. Brain Res.*, 20 (1974) 45–66.
7. Tsukahara, N., Hultborn, H., Murakami, F and Fujito, Y., Electrophysiological study of formation of new synapses and collateral sprouting in red nucleus neurons after partial denervation, *J. Neurophysiol.*, 38 (1975) 1359–1372

Control of the cerebellar reverberatory activities by local cooling of the cerebellar peduncles

NAKAAKIRA TSUKAHARA, TAKEHIKO BANDO, FUJIO MURAKAMI AND
NORIYASU OZAWA

*Department of Biophysical Engineering, Faculty of Engineering Science, Osaka University,
Machikaneyama, Toyonaka 560, Japan*

The dynamic (reverberating circuit) hypothesis of the short-term memory in the nervous system is of long standing, but the presence of a reverberating circuit in the central nervous system has never been established. Evidence suggesting such a circuit between the cerebellar nuclei and some of the precerebellar nuclei (PCN) has been reported previously[1,2]. These studies were based on the postulate that the long-lasting depolarization and repetitive impulse discharges produced in the neurons of the red nucleus (RN) which could be observed after picrotoxin injection represent reverberatory activities due to circulation of impulses along the interposito-precerebellar loop.

This article reports that a similar long-lasting depolarization can be produced in RN cells in a preparation in which the cerebellar intermediate cortex has been ablated. It will also be shown that this long-lasting excitation of RN neurons is abolished reversibly by cooling the inferior and middle cerebellar peduncles in accordance with the view that long-lasting excitation of RN cells is due to impulse reverberation between the nucleus interpositus (IP) and the PCN.

The experiments were performed on adult cats. The procedures and techniques were the same as those employed previously[2]. Cooling of the cerebellar peduncles was performed by inserting a cooling probe into the cerebellum between the inferior and middle cerebellar peduncles stereotaxically. The cooling probe was made of two concentric stainless-steel tubes (Fig. 1A), forming a closed circulating system. The outer tube had a diameter of about 1.3 mm. The inner tube had an orifice at the tip from which liquid Freon was ejected into the outer tube by means of a compressor. The liquid Freon evaporated rapidly, thus producing local cooling around the tip of the probe. In order to control the temperature of the tissue around the probe, the compressor was switched on and off by an electric circuit controlled by the local temperature which was monitored continuously with a thermometer (the diameter of the tip of the probe was about 1 mm).

Fig. 1B illustrates a prolonged depolarization produced in an RN cell by a single shock to the IP in a cat in which the intermediate part of the cerebellar cortex had been ablated chronically. Fig. 1 C–G show other examples of the prolonged depolarization of another RN cell by a single shock to the nucleus reticularis tegmenti pontis (NRTP). With an increase of the stimulus intensities from Fig. 1C to G, the depolarization appeared in an all-or-none manner, as shown in the superimposed traces in Fig. 1C. The depolarization returned to the resting state after several tens of milliseconds. As far as its regenerative nature is concerned, the depolarization illustrated here is essentially the same as that reported previously under picrotoxin injection[1,2].

If the prolonged depolarization is due to reverberation of impulses along the IP-PCN loop, blockage of impulse conduction by local cooling of the inferior and middle cerebellar peduncles would abolish the prolonged depolarization and repetitive impulse discharges of RN cells. If the prolonged depolarization is due to pacemaker properties of IP neurons, the prolonged depolarization would persist after cooling the inferior and middle cerebellar peduncles.

439

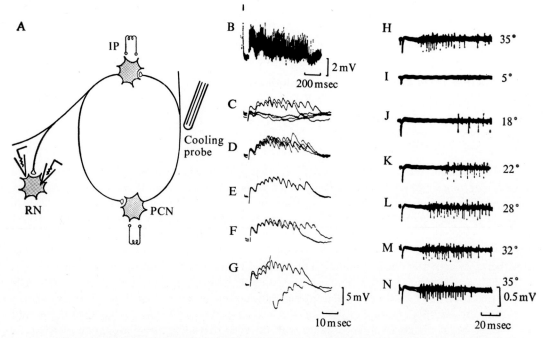

Fig. 1.   A, Diagram of the experimental arrangement for study of the reverberating circuit between the nucleus interpositus (IP) and the precerebellar nuclei (PCN). Intracellular and extracellular recordings were made from red nucleus (RN) neurons. Stimulation was applied to the IP and the PCN. The cooling probe was inserted between the inferior and middle cerebellar peduncles. B, Intracellular recording from an RN cell. A prolonged depolarization induced by a single shock to IP. C–G, Intracellular recording from another RN cell. A prolonged depolarization induced by a single shock to one of the PCN, nucleus reticularis tegmenti pontis, of increasing stimulus intensities from C to G. H–N, Extracellular recording from an RN cell. Repetitive discharges induced by a single shock to IP before (H), during (I) and after (J–N) cooling at the temperature of peduncles given to the right-hand side of each trace. Voltage and time calibration in G and N also apply to C–F and H–M, respectively.

Fig. 1 H–N exemplify the records obtained from an RN cell by stimulating IP before (H), during (I) and after (J–N) cooling the inferior and middle cerebellar peduncles. The repetitive discharges of the RN unit disappeared at 5°C except for the initial brief excitation and recovered gradually on rewarming the probe. Similar results were obtained from all nineteen RN cells tested.

Based on these results, it was concluded that reversible interruption of conduction of the IP-PCN loop abolished the prolonged excitation of RN cells. This is taken to indicate that the prolonged excitation of RN cells is not due to pacemaker activities of IP neurons but to reverberation of impulses along the IP-PCN loop.

References

1. Tsukahara, N., Bando, T., Kitai, S.T. and Kiyohara, T., Cerebello-pontine reverberating circuit, *Brain Research*, 33 (1971) 233–237.
2. Tsukahara, N., Bando, T. and Kiyohara, T., The properties of the reverberating circuit in the brain. In K. Yagi and S. Yoshida (Ed.), *Neuroendocrine Control*, Tokyo University Press, Tokyo, 1973, pp. 3–26.

Neuronal correlates of timing behavior in the monkey

HIROAKI NIKI AND MASATAKA WATANABE

*Department of Psychology, Faculty of Letters, University of Tokyo,
Bunkyo-ku, Tokyo 113, Japan.*

While various characteristics of performance under temporal schedules such as fixed interval (FI), variable interval (VI) and differential reinforcement of low rate (DRL) have been extensively studied, little information is yet available on the neuronal correlates of timing behavior. The results of ablation studies of the prefrontal cortex for such behavior in the monkey are not consistent[2-4,7]. In recent work on prefrontal unit activity in delayed alternation (DA)[5] and delayed response (DR)[6], many prefrontal units showed an anticipatory change in discharge rate toward the time of responding in the later part of the delay period.

The central question in the present study was whether such an anticipatory change in unit firing could be found in association with timing behavior. Using approximation procedures, monkeys (N = 3) were trained in the performance of a modified differential reinforcement of long latencies (DRLL) task. The testing-panel contained a "hit-button" and a "hold-lever". The monkey first had to depress the "hold-lever" for several sec (which changed randomly from 3 to 5 sec) in order to illuminate the "hit-button". If he continued depressing the lever for at least 2 sec (the delay period) after the onset of illumination and hit the "button," a drop of fruit juice was delivered and the illumination was turned off. Thus, in this task situation, the animal had to estimate the lapse of time after the onset of illumination since there was no external stimulus indicating the end of the delay period. On completion of training for this task. the animal was surgically prepared for chronic unit recording using the standard technique developed by Evarts[1].

Many units which were found in the dorsolateral prefrontal cortex (N = 252) and in the anterior cingulate cortex (N = 218) showed changes in firing (either an increase or decrease) in association with one or more of the events in the DRLL task.

Concerning the main question of the present study, 106 prefrontal units and 87 cingulate units showed an anticipatory change in firing rate toward the time of responding. The results indicated that there were two types of timing units. The first type (Fig. 1A) showed a sustained increase in discharge rate immediately after the onset of illumination and an abrupt cessation of firing at the time of initiation of the response (release of the hold-lever). The duration of the sustained elevation of this type of neurons was dependent on the animal's behavioral response latency: if the latency was short (long), the duration was also short (long). The duration of sustained changes in firing may be considered to reflect the monkey's subjective delay interval. Consequently, this type of neurons may participate in the time estimation process. However, another interpretation is possible. This type of neurons may be involved in the process of withholding the behavioral response during the delay period. The second type (Fig. 1B) exhibited a gradual increase in firing rate toward the time of responding, and reached maximum at the time of response. The start of the gradual change in firing was dependent on the latency of the animal's response: when

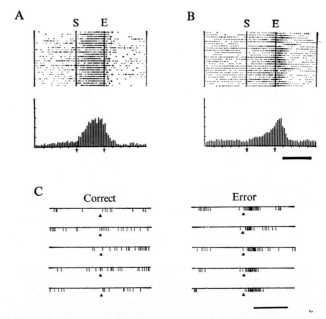

Fig. 1.   A and B, Raster and histogram displays of two types of timing units. The heavier dot in each trial indicates the time of response initiation (release of the hold lever). Below each raster is a histogram which sums raster activity in 120 msec bins. The ordinate scale in each histogram is 36 spikes/division. The time bar indicates 2 sec. S, Stimulus onset; E, end of delay. C, Example of an error-recognition unit. The triangles indicate the time of button pressing. The time bar indicates 2 sec.

the latency was short (long), the firing change occurred earlier (later). The firing change of the second type of neurons may reflect the preparatory set for responding.

Of special interest is the unexpected discovery of units showing a differential change in incorrect trials. Twenty units (prefrontal cortex, N = 3; cingulate cortex, N = 17) showed a marked increase in firing only when the animal made errors (i.e., the animal responded within 2 sec after illumination onset and received no juice). These units exhibited little or no change in correct trials. An example of these possible error-recognition units is shown in Fig. 1C. Such units were also responsive to omission of reinforcement (juice) for correct response.

REFERENCES

1. Evarts, E.V., A technique for recording activity of subcortical neurons in moving animals, *Electroenceph. clin. Neurophysiol.*, 24 (1968) 83–86.
2. Glickstein, M., Quigley, W.A. and Stebbins, W.C., Effect of frontal and parietal lesions on timing behavior in monkeys, *Psychol. Sci.*, 1 (1964) 265–266.
3. Manning, F.J., Performance under temporal schedules by monkeys with partial ablations of prefrontal cortex, *Physiol. Behav.*, 11 (1973) 563–569.
4. Pribram, K.H., A further experimental analysis of the behavioral deficit that follows injury to the primate frontal cortex, *Exp. Neurol.*, 3 (1961) 432–466.
5. Niki, H., Prefrontal unit activity during delayed alternation in the monkey: I. Relation to direction of response, *Brain Research*, 68 (1974) 185–196.
6. Niki, H., Differential activity of prefrontal units during right and left delayed response trials, *Brain Research*, 70 (1974) 346–349.
7. Stamm, J.S., Function of prefrontal cortex in timing behavior of monkeys, *Exp. Neurol.*, 7 (1963) 87–97.

Changes in visual responsiveness of prefrontal cortical neurons related to gazing behavior

HISAO SUZUKI AND MASAO AZUMA

Department of Physiology, Hirosaki University Faculty of Medicine,
Zaifu-cho, Hirosaki 036, Japan

In the inferior dorsolateral area of the prefrontal cortex, many neurons showed increased discharge rates when the monkey was continuously gazing at a small light spot that had a reward significance[1]. Though this increase in discharge rate was rather independent of stimulus parameters, such as location in the visual field, and the size and intensity of the light spot, it was considerably dependent on the behavioral state of the animal. Therefore, there may be two factors that take part in producing activation of the neurons: stimulus (light target) and behavioral (gazing) factors. In this report, we have tried to separate these factors and to test the extent to which each factor contributes to the neuronal reaction.

For this purpose, we trained the animal under the following multiple schedules. In the first schedule (SI), the monkey must press a key after an intertrial interval as soon as a light spot appears on the screen. The light spot remained for 1–4 sec and then increased slightly in brightness. On this brightness change, rapid key-release resulted in reinforcement with orange-flavored juice. Under SI, we obtained continuous gazing at the small light spot for several seconds (gaze-at-target situation). In the second schedule (SII), the spot appeared after the intertrial interval. When the monkey pressed the key, the spot was turned off for 1–4 sec and reappeared at the same location on the screen as before. Upon spot appearance, rapid key-release was rewarded. During the light turn-off period of SII, the animal continued to gaze at the place where the light spot was to appear again. Thus, we obtained a kind of gazing behavior in the absence of the target light (target-free gaze situation). We compared the neuronal behavior under the "gaze-at-target" situation in SI with that of the "target-free gaze" situation in SII. It was expected that if neuronal activation occurs only under light stimulus presentation, the activation will cease under the latter situation. In contrast, it will continue firing in the absence of the target light if the behavioral state of the animal is an important factor for the activation.

Under these multiple schedules, we found two extreme types of neurons from the prefrontal cortex that showed contrasting neuronal behavior under the "target-free gaze" situation. Fig. 1 illustrates the activities of the neurons. In this figure, A and B refer to one extreme type of neuron. "A" represents the discharge pattern of the neuron during SI performance. The light spot was turned on at the triangle marks, and the monkey pressed the key at the vertical broken line. The spot was brightened at the vertical solid line and key-release occurred at the arrow. The lower two traces refer to horizontal and vertical electroculograms for monitoring eye movements of the animal. We obtained constant base lines indicating that the monkey's eyes were fixed on the light target. As shown in the uppermost trace, this unit fired continuously during the fixation period. Under SII, the discharge pattern of the unit was changed as shown in B. We observed firing only in the presence of the target light. This indicates that for this unit the light target or stimulus as well as gazing behavior was necessary for activation.

443

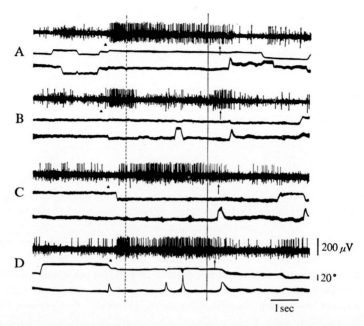

Fig. 1. Two types of prefrontal neurons. A and B show the activity of the first type of neurons during SI and SII performance, respectively. C and D show the activity of the second type of neurons. Triangles represent the times at which the light spot was turned on. A vertical broken line shows the onset of lever pressing, and a vertical solid line, the onset of brightening of the light target (A, C) or reappearance of the light spot (B, D). Arrows indicate the onset of lever release. Notice that first-type neurons stopped firing during the light interruption period in SII (B), while second-type neurons continued firing (D).

The activity of the other extreme-type neuron is illustrated in C and D. As shwon in C, the neuron also maintained firing in SI, but this unit showed quite different neuronal behavior from that of the first type of neuron in SII. As shown in D, the activation was maintained in SII despite the off period of the light target.

Between the two neuron types showing extreme reactions, there were many neurons with continuously graded properties, i.e., those maintaining discharge to some degree during the "target-free gaze" situation but with a reduced discharge rate as compared with that in the "gaze-at-target" situation.

Such a gradation of neuronal reaction during the "target-free gaze" situation may indicate that there are two processes in the prefrontal cortex: one requires the light target for neuronal activation ("visual" process). The other does not require the light target, but is probably related to an intentional process. Association of these processes in various degrees produces a gradation in the neuronal population of the prefrontal cortex. It is also possible that such association may produce a higher nervous function such as attention.

REFERENCE

1. Suzuki, H. and Azuma, M., Prefrontal neuronal activity during gazing at a light spot in the monkey, *Brain Research*, 126 (1977) 497–508.

A hemispheric asymmetry of performance of a visual conditional discrimination task in split-brain monkeys

KIYOKO MUROFUSHI

Department of Psychology, Primate Research Institute ,Kyoto University,
Inuyama, Aichi 484, Japan

Although hemispheric specialization of cognitive functions is well documented in humans, in the monkey no consistent data are yet available. As for discrimination learning, no differential abilities have been found between the two hemispheres of split-brain monkeys[3], or between dominant and nondominant hemispheres subjected to unilateral cortical ablations[6,7]. However, interhemispheric asymmetries are observed in complex auditory-dependent activities after cortical ablation[1], or in reaction times in split-brain monkeys[4], and cortical macropotentials are seen during delayed-response performance[5], suggesting that the two hemispheres in monkeys are not equipotent for perceptual processing or for memory storage.

The following experiment was designed to detect possible functional a symmetries between the cerebral hemispheres in split-brain monkeys with a dichotic viewing paradigm. It seems possible under binocular viewing conditions that the split-brain monkeys use both cerebral hemispheres relatively independently in a visual discrimination task. It is expected that if one of the hemispheres is superior in the visual processing task it should arrive at a solution more rapidly than the other hemisphere and thus control the ensuing motor response.

Three adolescent monkeys (*Macaca mulatta*) received a midline section of the optic chiasm, the anterior commissure, and the corpus callosum about three years ago. The subjects were restrained in primate chairs and trained in a successive conditional discrimination task under monocular viewing. Pressing of the start lever by the monkey turned vertically arranged conditional stimulus lights on (red or green). Three seconds later, left and right response keys were lit with white light to inform the animals that the response was available. When both stimulus lights were red (or green), left (or right) key press was correct and pressing was reinforced by orange juice. A total of 100 trials was run a day. After reaching a criterion of 90% correct responses for two days, training was transferred to the other eye. A pair of polaroid filters were adjusted using the experimenter's eyes at the beginning of each session to a position such that the stimulus light reached the brain only through one eye. When the monkey had completed learning with each eye independently, 100 test trials were given for two days under dichotic viewing conditions in which one eye was exposed to red light and the other to green light. All responses were reinforced in test trials. Hands were free throughout the experiment so that the monkey could use its preferred hand.

In the monkeys (Nos. 353, 385 and 382) the numbers of trials required to reach the criterion in training with the first eye were 2000, 1600 and 1800, respectively, while those with the second eye were 1800, 2000, and 600, respectively. In the first two monkeys the test was started with the right eye, and in the third one it was with the left eye. The second monkey failed to reach the criterion for the second eye. Training was interrupted at the 85% correct level, at which performance was maintained for 7 days after reaching 90% correct in one day. Response distributions on test days are shown in Table 1. On the first day, No. 353 used stimulus colors presented to the right eye significantly more than those presented to the left eye for correct choices of responses ($X^2 = 43.58$, $p < .005$). The other two monkeys did not show any significant difference between response numbers dependent on each eye. On the second day, the response dependency on the right hemisphere of No. 353 was still significant ($X^2 = 6.76$, $p < .01$). No. 385 became controlled by left eye stimulus significantly more than by right eye stimulus ($X^2 = 19.36$, $p < .005$). Since No. 353 used its left hand and No. 385 used its right hand, an established functional dominance seems to be contralaterally related to the hand involved in task acquisition. No. 385's result is somewhat ambiguous because its response bias to the right key appeared on the second day. No. 382 reacted slowly as test trials increased, so the experiment was discontinued early on the second day.

TABLE 1.   Response distributions in tests for 3 monkeys. The hand used by individual animals and eye exposed to stimulus light are indicated by R for right, L for left. Results of X^2 tests are shown by †2 for $p < .005$, and by †1 for $p < .01$

Monkey No.	Hand used			Test					
				Day 1				Day 2		
		Eye	Red Left	Green Right	Total	Eye	Red Left	Green Right	Total
353	L	R	42	41	83	R	34	29	63
		L	9	8	17†2	L	21	16	37†1
385	R	R	20	28	48	R	5	23	28
		L	22	30	52	L	27	45	72†2
382	L	R	20	38	58	R			
		L	10	32	42	L			

To examine the degree of independent use of both cerebral hemispheres by split-brain monkeys, the variance of reaction times (RTs) and response evocation characteristics (REC), as defined by Grice[2], by the dominant hemisphere in test trials were compared with those by the same hemisphere in the criterion trials for monocular training. Homogeneity of variance to training RTs was statistically confirmed for No. 353's first test day and No. 385's second test day. REC is a plot of probability of response for green-right against probability of response for red-left,

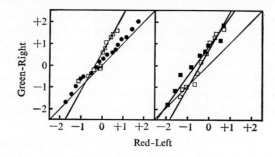

Fig. 1.   REC plots of reaction times for monkey No. 353 (cf. 2). Training data are shown on the left and test data on the right. Filled circles represent left-eye data in training, open squares represent right-eye data in training and test Day 1, and filled squares represent right eye data in test Day 2. The abscissa and ordinate are scaled in standard deviation units.

as shown in Fig. 1. The RECs in No. 353 show that features of the RTs in monocular viewing remain in dichotic viewing for the relatively dominant right hemisphere. If the mean and standard deviations of RTs in green-right responses are very similar to those in red-left responses, REC is obtained along the diagonal line as indicated by the left eye training data in Fig. 1. However, the mean and standard deviations of RTs with the right eye in training were much smaller for green-right than for red-left response, and this response bias was still observed during test days. These investigations of RT distributions suggest that split-brain monkeys utilize the relatively dominant hemisphere independently for information processing required by a visual discrimination task. Thus, it is concluded from these observations that the hemisphere contralateral to the hand involved in task acquisition plays a disproportionate role in the determination of choice behavior by monkeys in dichotic viewing.

REFERENCES

1. Dewson, J.H., III, Preliminary evidence of hemispheric asymmetry of auditory function in monkeys. In S. Harnad *et al.* (Eds.) *Lateralization in the Nervous System*, Academic Press, New York, 1977, pp. 63–71.
2. Grice, G.R., Application of a variable criterion model to auditory reaction time as a function of the type of catch trial, *Percept. Psychophysics*, 12 (1972) 103–107.
3. Hamilton, C.R., Investigations of perceptual and mnemonic lateralization in monkeys. In S. Harnad *et al.* (Eds.) *Lateralization in the Nervous System*, Academic Press, New York, 1977, pp.45–62.
4. Murofushi, K., Variable criterion analysis of simple reaction time distributions in normal, chiasm-sectioned and chiasm-callosum-sectioned monkeys (*Macaca mulatta*), *Ann. Anim. Psychol.*, 25 (1975) 1–17.
5. Stamm, J.S., Rosen, S.C. and Gadotti, A., Lateralization of functions in the monkey's frontal cortex. In S. Harnad *et al.* (Eds.) *Lateralization in the Nervous System*, Academic Press, New York, 1977, pp. 385–402.
6. Warren, J.M., Handedness and cerebral dominance in monkeys, In S. Harnad *et al.* (Eds.), *Lateralization in the Nervous System,* Academic Press, New York, 1977, pp. 151–172.
7. Warren, J.M. and Nonneman, A.J., The search for cerebral dominance in monkeys, *Ann. N. Y. Acad. Sci.*, 280 (1976) 732–744.

Analysis of memory disturbance using speech tests in human cerebral disorders

KOMEI UEKI AND KIMIKAZU KONNO

Department of Neurosurgery, Brain Research Institute, Niigata University,
Asahi-machi, Niigata 951, Japan

As is well known, memory comprises three functions: registration, retention and recall. It is impossible, however, to test these three functions separately. For example, even with a relative simple registration test such as Benton's test[1], registration ability can be examined only through the procedure of recall. The amnesia known as a disorder of recall is also, at the same time, a disorder of retention. The three functions do not exist independently but are in closely associated relation. Furthermore, since various underlying factors such as age, intelligence, biography, educational history, consciousness, emotion, attentiveness, interest, etc. exert a complicated influence on memory, analysis of memory disorders must be performed with great caution taking all these factors into consideration.

In our department, a "standard language test for aphasia (SLTA)"[2] has been employed since December 1974, on patients more or less suspected of mental dysfunctions or aphasia. The SLTA enables the speech behavior of individuals to be expressed in relatively objective "numerals". We have analyzed such SLTA data from the viewpoint of the three functions of memory and thereby attempted to evaluate disorders of memory in patients with organic brain diseases.

Since memory disturbance cannot be evaluated by the SLTA in cases of severe aphasia, our analysis was limited to patients who scored 70 or higher in a verbal IQ test (an IQ of 70–79 is regarded as borderline). Those patients who obtained fully normal scores in the SLTA test or who displayed no detectable organic lesion were excluded. The following observations were made on 67 patients (51 male, 16 female). The diseases involved were as follows: cerebral infraction, 21; intracerebral hematoma, 10; arterio-venous malformation, 8; malignant brain tumor, 16; benign brain tumor, 4; normo-pressure hydrocephalus, 3; and abnormal vascular network at the base of the brain (Moyamoya disease), 1. The 51 men ranged in age from 17 to 73 yr (mean 49.9 yr), and the 16 women from 13 to 62 yr (mean 39.6 yr).

The SLTA test covers hearing, speaking, reading, writing and calculation, and consists of 26 items. Of these, the following were specifically selected: (1) Item No. 10, as principally related to recall; (2) Item Nos. 4, 11, 12, 15 and 16, for retention; and (3) Item Nos. 6 and 9, for registration. The forward and backward recitations of WAIS and Benton's test were also adopted as registration tests.

In Item No. 10 of the SLTA, each subject is instructed to mention as many names of animals as possible within 1 min. We consider that recall is predominantly involved. The average score for the 67 subjects was 9.5 ± 3.2, which was, compared to an average of 12.6 ± 4.5 for a control group of 150 normal subjects[2], significantly low ($P < 0.01$). However, there was no clear dependence of the low scores on the localization of the cerebral changes (frontal lobe, parietal lobe, temporal lobe, occipital lobe or basal ganglia of each side) or on the type of disease.

The SLTA test items related to the written language, i.e., Item No. 4 (to listen to and choose a single *kana* (Japanese phonetic) letter), Item No. 11 (to read aloud a word written in Chinese characters), Item No. 12 (to read aloud a word written in kana letter), Item No. 15 (to read a word written in Chinese characters and point to the corresponding picture), and Item No. 16 (to read a word written in *kana* letters and point to the corresponding picture), were selected on the basis of the assumption that, although the procedure of recall is necessarily involved, they are relevant to old memory primarily obtained by learning. However, no significant decreases in scores were observed, and there were no significant differences according to type of disease or damaged region in the present subjects.

SLTA Items No. 6 (recitation of words) and No. 9 (recitation of short sentences) are tests relevant to auditory registration. The average scores in the 67 subjects were 9.9 ± 0.5 for Item No. 6 and 4.1 ± 1.0 for Item No. 9, compared to an average for 150 normal humans[2] of 10.0 ± 0.1 in Item No. 6 and 4.5 ± 0.8 in Item No. 9. There was thus no significant difference between the groups at the 5% level of significance. Data analysis with regard to the damaged regions failed to show any region with particularly low values.

The average of the forward recitation scores for the 67 patients in WAIS was 4.6 ± 1.06, while the average of the backward recitation scores was 3.13 ± 0.8 (number of places). These values are significantly low ($P < 0.01$) compared to the average scores for 30 normal humans (i.e., 5.7 ± 1.2 for forward recitation, and 4.0 ± 0.9 for backward recitation).

Benton's[1] visual registration test was performed on 29 of the 67 subjects. The average score of 5.38 ± 2.48 represented a moderate decrease from the normal score of not less than 8. Eight cases scoring 4 or less were selected for scrutiny of their SLTA data. This analysis revealed that, even when their data for Item Nos. 6 and 9 for auditory registration and Item Nos. 4, 11, 12, 15 and 16 for retention were substantially normal, the patients scored remarkably low in Item No. 10 pertinent to recall.

Both the SLTA and WAIS tests were repeated more than twice in 20 of the 67 subjects. Concerning verbal IQ, 10 cases showed improvement, 3 decrease, 3 remission, and 4 no appreciable change. The scores for SLTA Item Nos. 4, 11, 12, 15 and 16 (mainly related to retention) remained almost the same, while the scores for Item No. 10 (related to recall) changed according to the scores for verbal IQ.

The above results for patients with very minor mental dysfunction or very slight aphasia due to organic lesions suggest that, in the functions of memory, "recall" is first impaired, while "retention" may remain relatively unaffected.

REFERENCES

1. Benton, A.L., *The Revised Visual Retention Test: Clinical and Experimental Applications*, The Psychological Corporation, New York, 1955.
2. Hasegawa, T., *Standard Language Test of Aphasia Manual of Directions* (Japanese), Homeido Shoten, Tokyo, 1977.

Mathematical theory of self-organizing nerve cells

SHUN-ICHI AMARI

Department of Mathematical Engineering and Instrumentation Physics, Faculty of Engineering, University of Tokyo, Bunkyo-ku, Tokyo 113, Japan

The brain has a self-organizing ability which is thought to be based on plastic changes in the synaptic weights of nerve cells. Many models of memory and learning have been proposed from the engineering viewpoint, most of which involve nerve cells with modifiable synapses. The present paper proposes a unified theory for the synaptic modfication of nerve cells.[2,3] This theory not only gives a mathematical basis to various learning systems but also elucidates the automatic formation mechanism of feature detecting cells (especially abnormal formation in an abnormal environment).

General law of synaptic modification: Consider a nerve cell which receives n inputs x_1, x_2, ..., x_n and emits an output z. The signals x_i and z take in general analog values representing the respective pulse rates. Let w_i be the so-called synaptic weight of x_i, which represents the efficiency of the input x_i. We assume the following simple model where the output z is determined as a function of inputs x_i by

$$z = f(\sum_{i=1}^{n} w_i x_i - h),\tag{1}$$

where h is a constant and f is a non-linear function satisfying

$$f(u) = 0 \quad \text{for } u \leq 0.$$

The cell self-organizes by changing its synaptic weight w_i according to the inputs and output (and also to a teacher signal y when the cell receives it). We propose the following law of synaptic modification. In the learning phase, the synaptic weight w_i increases in proportion to rx_i and decays with a time constant τ, where r is a quantity called the learning signal of the cell. The learning signal is a function of the weighted sum of inputs (and teacher signal y, when it exists),

$$r = r(\sum w_i x_i, y).\tag{2}$$

Different types of cells would use different learning signals, so that the nervous system could realize a rich self-organizing ability. The learning equation is written as

$$\tau \dot{w}_i = -w_i + cx_i r,\tag{3}$$

where $\dot{w}_i$ denotes the time derivative dw_i/dt and c is a constant.

We use vector notation and write a set of inputs by a vector $x = (x_1, \ldots, x_n)$, calling it a pattern signal. We also denote a set of weights w_i by $w = (w_1, \ldots, w_n)$. Let $x(t)$ be a pattern signal at time t. A cell receives *a* time sequence of signals $x(t)$ (and $y(t)$) from the environment to which it adapts by learning the signals. We assume that the environment is an ergodic information source, which includes a set of pattern signals and emits one of them randomly after every fixed time interval. A cell can thus adapt to the environment by learning a time sequence $x(t)$, of which the time average is equal to the ensemble average over the environment.

Let us put

$$R(w, x, y) = \frac{1}{2}|w|^2 - c\int_0^{w\cdot x} r(u, y)du .$$ (4)

We can then rewrite the learning equation as

$$\tau\dot{w}_i = -\partial R/\partial w_i .$$ (5)

Let us define a function $L(w)$ by taking the ensemble average $< >$ over x, y of $R(w, x, y)$,

$$L(w) = <R(w, x, y)> .$$ (6)

By replacing R in Eq. (5) by its average L, we obtain the average learning equation

$$\tau\dot{w}_i = -\partial L(w)/\partial w_i .$$ (7)

Eq. (7) means that $w(t)$ converges to a minimum of $L(w)$ on the average. We can show that, for a large τ, the fluctuation of a real $w(t)$ from the average is sufficiently small. Hence, the synaptic weight w of a cell converges to a value which minimizes $L(w)$. When $L(w)$ has a unique minimum, the average learning equation is monostable, converging to the unique minimum. When $L(w)$ has many minima, the equation is multi-stable, and the weight w converges to one of the minima. Most of the learning rules which make use of a teacher signal are monostable, while rules without teacher signals are multi-stable, representing diversity of the environment.

Various types of learning signals: Most of the synaptic modification rules so far proposed can be studied in a unified manner by the average learning equation with appropriate learning signals, as follows.

(1) Perceptron learning. The perceptron is a model of learning decision systems, where the environment has two subsets S_1 and S_0 of patterns. A nerve cell self-organizes to be excited by any pattern belonging to S_1 but by none of S_0. The teacher signals $y = 1$ and $y = 0$ accompany patterns of S_1 and S_0, respectively, in the learning phase. The rule of perceptron learning is given by

$$r(w \cdot x, y) = y - 1(w \cdot x - h) ,$$ (8)

where $1(u)$ is the unit step function ($1(u) = 1$ for $u > 0$ and 0 otherwise).

(2) Correlation learning and orthogonal learning[1]. When the learning signal r is put equal to the teacher signal, i.e., $r = y$, the rule of correlation learning is obtained. The synaptic weight converges, in this case, to

$$w = c < yx > .$$ (9)

When a cell uses the following learning signal,

$$r = y - w \cdot x ,$$ (10)

the weight converges approximately to

$$w = < yx^* > ,$$ (11)

where x^* is the orthogonal dual vector of x with respect to the patterns in the environment. By these learning rules, a cell becomes to output, for any pattern x, the accompanying signal y which the teacher has taught it to output.

(3) Formation of pattern detectors[4]. When a cell self-organizes under an environment without teacher signals, it can use

$$r = 1(w \cdot x - h) \tag{12}$$

as the learning signal. We can prove that, by the above learning rule, the detectors of each pattern can automatically be formed. When some patterns form a cluster, the detector of the cluster can also be formed.

REFERENCES

1. Amari, S., Neural theory of association and concept formation, *Biol. Cybernetics*, 27 (1977), 77–87.
2 Amari, S., Mathematical approach to neural systems. In J. Metzler (Ed.), *Systems Neuroscience*, Academic Press, New York, 1977, pp. 67–117.
3. Amari, S., *Mathematical Theory of Nerve Nets* (Japanese), Sangyo Tosho, Tokyo, 1978, 323 pp.
4. Amari, S. and Takeuchi, A., Mathematical theory on formation of category detecting nerve cells, *Biol. Cybernetics*, 29 (1978), 127–136.

Subject Index

A

abortive spike, 124
acetylcholine (ACh), 36, 39, 292
—— sensitivity, 40, 41
——-— neuron, 302
——-synthesis, 36
acid secretion, 290
action potentials, 312, 314
adaptation, 405
adenohypophysis, 330
β-adrenergic agent, 398
afferent fiber, 333
air gap method, 124
—— puff stimulation, 205
γ-aminobutyric acid (GABA), **45**
—— receptor, 43
alimentary canals, 268
alpha-motoneuron, 172
amygdala, 370
amylase output, 292
anatomy, 157
ankle movements, 168
anophthalmia, 100
anterior pituitary, 311, 327
—— gland, 325
antidromic responses, 196
aphasia, 448
arcuate nucleus, 333
area 2 neuron, 74
aromatization of androgen, 363
association cortex, 184
ATP, 32
ATPase, 336
automatic focusing, 379
autoradiography, 102
avoidance training, 428
axonal polypeptide migration, **53**
—— transport, 44
axon of crayfish, 45

B

basal ganglia, 136, 199
baroreceptor, 232
behavioral defeminization, 355
—— mutation, 58
bicuculline, 43
bifurcating axons, 53
bipolar cell, 82, 83
blastoderm fate map, 58
blink reflex, 205
blood pressure, 242, 247
bradykinesia, 200
bradykinin-induced activation, **114**
brain, 100, 265
—— slice, 382
bulbar locomotor region (BLR), 209

β-bungarotoxin (β-BT), 48

C

calcium ion, 44–7
canine duodenum, 296
cardiac sympathetic afferents, **239**
cardio-inhibitory reflex, 244
cardiovascular center, 247
carotid sinus nerve (CSN), 244
—— stimulation, 239
carp, 83
cat, 106, 130, 145, 164, 180, 189
cation, 33
CCK-PZ, 294
cells of origin, 201
central integration, 260
—— noradrenaline, 290
—— patterning, 136
centrolateral nucleus (CL), 106
cerebellar cortex, 49, 194, 212
cerebellum, 102, 439
cerebello-cerebral projection, 436
cerebral cortex, 174
cerebral decortication, 436
—— disorder, 448
cerebro-cerebellar communication, **135**
——-— interactions, 187
chemoreceptor, 231
chick embryo, 48
chicken, 346
chloralose-anesthetized cat, 87
chlorotetracycline (CTC), 44–7
cholinergic agents, 38, 51
chorea, 202
choroid plexus, 342
chronic monkey, 409
cingulate cortex, 441
circadian rhythm, 343, 345, 397
circulatory regulation, 222
climbing fiber (CF) response, 184
cochlear nerve, 130
—— nucleus, (CN), 112
colon, 269, 274
conditional discrimination, 445
cone, 82
constant illumination, 331
cooling, 212, 213
correlation analysis, 254
—— learning, 452
—— time, 172
coordinate digitizer, 379
cord pithing, 247
—— section, 247
coronary constriction, 239
cortical function, 135
corticospinal (CS) neuron, 137
—— tract (CST), 180
cranial nerve, 256

crayfish, 30, 126
cross-correlation, 65
— -correlogram, 172
cuneiform nucleus, 210
2′,3′-cyclic nucleolide 3′-phosphohydrolase (CNPase), 431
cycloheximide, 397

D

decerebrate cat, 212
defecation, 283
delayed response (DR), 411
delta sleep-inducing peptide (DSIP), 394
2-deoxy-d-glucose (2-DG), 298
depolarization shift (DS), 383
diameter, 164
differential reinforcement, 443
digestive, 265
discriminator, 182
disinhibition, 257
dog, 296, 389
— breeds, 384
— brain, 384
domestication, 384
dopamine release, 32
dorsal lateral geniculate nucleus, 384
— motor nucleus of vagus (DMNV), 244
double O₂ test, 260
Drosophila, 58

E

EEG, 130, 393
EMG, 205
electron microscopy, 106
electrophysiology, 187
electrosleep, 400
embryonic chick atrium, 40, 41
endogenous oscillator, 346
β-endorphin, 51
entric plexus, 265
enterogastrone, 294
EPSP, 373
equilibrium potential, 42
error-recognition, 442
estrogen, 355
evoked brain-stem response, 130
excitatory post-synaptic potential, 172
exocrine pancreas, 292

F

fast and slow fiber, 180
Fast green FCF, 207
feedback control, 307
feeding behavior, 352, 376
fiber
  A-δ—, 242
  C—, 242
field potential, 131
flickering-pattern, 96
flocculus, 93
fluorescent probe, 44

forced wakefulness (FW), 389
fractography, 55
frog, 124
frontal cortex (FC), 373
functional surface, 78

G

gastric acid secretion, 294
— inhibitory polypeptide (GIP), 294
— motility, 285
— mucosal blood flow, 290
gastrin, 288
gastrointestinal hormone, 265, 288, 294
— motor activity, 288
gaze control, 91
gazing behavior, 443
genetic mosaics, 58
glucose, 298
glycogen synthetase, 301
Golgi preparation, 26, 29
group Ia fiber, 164
growth hormone (GH), 389

H

habemula, 51
hair cell-afferent fiber synapse, 104
heart rate, 242
hemiballism, 202
hemicerebellectomy, 436
hemisection, 170
hemispherectow, 434
hemispheric asymmetry, 445
hepatic nerve, 298
hippocamps, 381
homeostasis, 235
honeybee, 122
hormone secretion, 311
horseradish peroxidase (HRP), 93, 102, 106, 164, 190, 207, 333, 382, 436
H-reflex, 168
human stereotaxy, 157
humoral sleep-promoting substances, 394
HVEM (high voltage electron microscope), 26, 29
6-hydroxydopamine, (6-OHDA), 252
hypertension, 247, 249, 252
hypothalamic behavior, 351
— nucleus, 128
— rage, 370
hypothalamico hypophysial-adrenal axis, 303
— -vagal neural pathway, 303
hypothalamo-neurohypophysial complex (HNC), 336
hypothalamus, 379
hypoxia, 233, 260

I

image processing, 379
indoleamine, 341
inferotemporal cortex (IT), 419
infundibuls-preoptic projection, 331
inhibitor
  of protein synthesis, 400

of RNA synthesis, 400
inhibitory postsynaptic current (IPSC), 30
inner ear, 48
intention tremor, 202
intraaxonal staining, 164
intracellular recording, 373
interdigestive gut motility, 288
interneuronal connectivity, 67
interneuron, 126
internodal length, 164
interpeduncular nuleus, 51
intestinal reflex, 269
IPSP, 373

J, K, L

Japanese quail, 329

kinetics, 397

labyrinth, 90
laminated organization, 384
lateral geniculate nucleus (LGN), 85
— hypothalamic area (LHA), 351, 373, 376
— hypothalamus (LH), 301, 329
— tegmentum, 209 (→ BLR)
learning, 405, 450
— ability, 431
— equation, 450
lethal mutation, 58
leucine-enkephalin (Leu-enk), 114
lidocaine, 296
lingual afferents, 120
locomotor activity, 393
locomotion, 212
locus coeruleus (LC), 112, 252, 290
lordosis, 355
luteinizing hormone releasing hormone (LH-RH)
   receptor, 327

M

man, 168
masseteric motoneurons, 281
mastication, 281
matrix cell, 55
maximal saccadic velocity (MSV), 200
median eminence, 329, 331
medulla oblongata, 245
melatonin, 345
memory, 405, 448
mesencephalic locomotor region (MLR), 209
methionine-enkephalin (Met-enk), 114
α-methyldopa (α-MD), 253
α-methylnoradrenaline (α-MeNA), 253
micro-fluorospectrometer, 44
microphthalmia, 100
nicrostimulation, 140
mitral cell, 117
modulating control, 307
monkey, 106, 146, 170, 177, 187, 419, 441
morphine, 114
mossy fiber, 93

motilin, 288
motility, 268
motor cortex (MC), 139, 196, 376
— effort, 203
— instruction, 174
— unit spike, 172
mouse, 428
multicompartment model, 105
muscular afferents, 242
muscle spindle, 124
mutant mouse, 194
mutant strain, 100
myelination, 431
myenteric plexus, 283

N

nerve VIII, 131
neural connections, 376
neural mechanism, 63
neural plasticity, 434
neural regulation, 267
neural transmitter, 265
neuroblast, 55
neurochemistry, 434
neuroendocrine control, 307
— reflex, 307
neurogenesis, 58
neuromuscular junction, 31
neuron processes, 379
noradrenaline (NA), 112, 252
non-homogenous distribution of sympathetic nerve,
   217
non-invasive method, 217
nucleus ambiguus (NA), 244
nucleus centralis lateralis, 87
— reticularis tegmenti pontis (Bechterew), 93
nucleus of solitary tract (NTS), 244

O

ocular movement, 199
olfactory bulb, 117
olive, 102
optical microscope, 379
optic inputs, 102
optic nerve, 93, 100
—— afferent, 85
orbital gyrus, 207
orbitofrontal cortex (OBF), 373
organ culture, 43, 336
orthogonal learning, 451
ovaluation, 332
oxygenase, 341

P

pacemaker activity, 217
pain, 242
pallidum, 196
pancratic juice flow, 292
pancreozymin-producing endocrine cells, 296
paracrine, 265
paradoxical sleep (PS), 400

paraneurons, 265
Parkinson's disease, 199
parvocellular red nucleus (RN), 184
peptide, 354
peptide-like substance, 392
peripheral chemoreceptor, 261
peroxidase, 329
phenylketonuric (PKU) rat, 431
photic driving (PD), 96
phrenic nerve, 256
physiology, 159
picrotoxin, 257
pineal body, 397
— gland, 342, 343, 346
plain synaptic vesicles, 32
polymodal nociceptor, 242
pons, 103
pontine locomotor region (PLR), 209
pontine nucleus (PN), 93
——cell, 180
pontobular locomotor region, 209
position compensation, 177
postsynaptic potentials, 281
postural tremor, 202
— spectra analysis, 256
precerebellar nuclei (PCN), 439
prefrontal cortex, 384, 441, 443
— neuron, 407
preoptic area (POA), 333, 355
preoptic hypothalamic area, 351
primary afferent neuron, 42
primate, 152
proboscis extension reflex, 122
proprioceptive afferent, 156
psychological effort, 202
Purkinje cell, 182
— shift, 83
pyramidal tract, 180
——neurons (PTNs), 177

Q, R

quadriceps motoneuron, 170

rabbit, 117, 257
rage reaction, 351
rat, 85, 100, 120, 285, 329, 331, 343
— central nervous system, 435
reaction time (RT), 200
recall, 448; see also memory
receptive field, 74
—-— property, 85
recovery of motor function, 170
rectal motility, 284
red-flicker (RF), 96
red nucleus (RN), 439
reflex, 285
regional sympathetic activity, 222
relay cell, 85
REM sleep, 354
reorganization, 436
respiration, 257
respiratory center, 254
— discharge, 256

— neuron, 255
reticular formation, 209
— neuron, 207
retina, 83, 91
reverberating circuit, 439
rhythmicity, 259
rhythmic jaw movements, 281
rod, 82, 83
rolling mouse Nagoya (RMN), 194

S

secretin, 288, 294
self-organization, 450
sensation, 63
sensory adaptation, 104
septum, 372
sequential destruction, 370
serotonin N-acetyltransferase, 346
sexual behavior, 352
sex steroid hormone, 327
simple and complex spike, 182
single-unit recording, 174
sleep, 389
—-promoting factor (Factor S), 394
—-related growth hormone secretion, 354
—-wakefulness cycle, 354
slow wave sleep (ss), 400
small intestine, 273
solitary tract nucleus neurons, 120
somatosensory cortex, (SI), 73
somatostatin, 294
somatotopic organization, 109
speech test, 448
split-brain monkey, 446
spinal axon branching, 139
spinal cord, 164, 170
spinal dorsal lamina V neuron, 114
spinal mechanism, 135
spinal trigeminal complex, 249
spinal trigeminal nucleus (STN), 112
spinocerebellar tract, 190
spinothalamic fiber, 106
spontaneously hypertensive rat (SHR), 247, 252
starvation, 122
statocyst, 126
stellate cell, 325
stereotyped response in autonomic functions, 218
stimulus feature extraction, 81
stomach, 269
stretch receptor, 392
——cell, 36, 37
— reflex, 172
subesophageal ganglion, 122
substance P, 51
substantia nigra, 39
superior cervical ganglion, 397
— colliculus, 91
supplementary motor area (SMA), 174
sympathetic nerve, 285
—tonus, 400
—vasoconstrictor fiber, 249
synaptic connection, 65
—junction, 32

— membrane, 32
— modification, 450
— plasticity to sex steroids, 363
— ribbon, 343
— transmission, 38
synaptogenesis, 48

T

tactile form discrimination, 75
—— representation, 109
—— sensation, 75
tanycytes, 329
tarsus, 122
temperature regulation, 222, 351
terminal hyperpolarization, 124
thalamus, 154, 196
thoracic ganglion, 122
time-to-peak, 172
timing behavior, 441
tonic synpathetic discharge, 250
transmitter depletion, 104
tremor at rest, 202
trigeminal depressor response, 249
— motoneuron, 207
— subnucleus caudalis, 109
tryptophan hydroxylase, 397
tubero-infundibular (TI) neuron, 331
tyrosine aminotransferase, 302

U

ultrastructure, 325
undernourished rat, 431
unit activity, 443
unit discharge, 119, 374, 376
unitary EPSP (excitatory postsynaptic potential), 170
— visual response, 87
uropod, 126

V, W

vagal inhibition, 257
vagal nuclei, 290
vagus, 292
vagus nerve, 244, 292
vasopressin, 336
ventialis intermedius (Vim) nucleus, 152
ventromedial hypothalamus, 355
vestibular nucleus (VN), 112
— nerve, 130
vinblastine, 428
visual cortex, 65
— learning, 419
— message, 443
— tracking, 177

withdrawal test, 260